CANCER   4

A COMPREHENSIVE TREATISE

BIOLOGY OF TUMORS: Surfaces, Immunology, and
Comparative Pathology

Therapies will be covered in subsequent volumes.

CANCER 4

A COMPREHENSIVE TREATISE

BIOLOGY OF TUMORS: Surfaces, Immunology, and Comparative Pathology

Frederick F. Becker, EDITOR

New York University School of Medicine

PLENUM PRESS • NEW YORK AND LONDON

Library of Congress Cataloging in Publication Data

Becker, Frederick F
  Biology of tumors.

  (*His* Cancer, a comprehensive treatise; v. 4)
  Includes bibliographies and index.
  1. Cancer cells. 2. Cancer—Immunological aspects. 3. Oncology,
Experimental. 4. Tumors, Plant. I. Title. [DNLM: 1. Neoplasms.
QZ200 C2143]
RC261.B42 vol. 4 [RC262]   616.9'94'008s   75-28176
ISBN 0-306-35204-4 (v. 4)   [616.9'94'07]

© 1975 Plenum Press, New York
A Division of Plenum Publishing Corporation
227 West 17th Street, New York, N.Y. 10011

United Kingdom edition published by Plenum Press, London
A Division of Plenum Publishing Company, Ltd.
Davis House (4th Floor), 8 Scrubs Lane, Harlesden, London, NW10 6SE, England

Printed in the United States of America

Contributors

to Volume 4

A. C. Allison, Clinical Research Centre, Harrow, Middlesex, England

Tadao Aoki, Viral Oncology Area, Division of Cancer Cause and Prevention, National Cancer Institute, National Institutes of Health, Bethesda, Maryland

Ettore Appella, Laboratory of Cell Biology, National Cancer Institute, Bethesda, Maryland

Robert W. Baldwin, Cancer Research Campaign Laboratories, University of Nottingham, Nottingham, England

Armin C., Braun, The Rockefeller University, New York, New York

Isaiah J. Fidler, University of Pennsylvania, Philadelphia, Pennsylvania

Sidney H. Golub, Division of Oncology, Department of Surgery, and Department of Microbiology and Immunology, University of California School of Medicine, Los Angeles, California

Lloyd W. Law, Laboratory of Cell Biology, National Cancer Institute, Bethesda, Maryland. Present address: Frederich Cancer Research, Frederich, Maryland

Garth L. Nicolson, Department of Cancer Biology, The Salk Institute for Biological Studies, San Diego, California, and Department of Developmental and Cell Biology, University of California, Irvine, California

Jan Pontén, The Wallenberg Laboratory, University of Uppsala, Uppsala, Sweden

Michael R. Price, Cancer Research Campaign Laboratories, University of Nottingham, Nottingham, England

James C. Robbins, Department of Cancer Biology, The Salk Institute for Biological Studies, San Diego, California

Dante G. Scarpelli, The University of Kansas Medical Center, College of Health Sciences and Hospital, Kansas City, Kansas

Louis R. Sibal, Viral Oncology Area, Division of Cancer Cause and Prevention, National Cancer Institute, National Institutes of Health, Bethesda, Maryland

HAROLD L. STEWART, Registry of Experimental Cancers, National Cancer Institute, National Institutes of Health, Bethesda, Maryland

MARY J. TEVETHIA, Department of Pathology and Cancer Research Center, Tufts University School of Medicine, Boston, Massachusetts

SATVIR S. TEVETHIA, Department of Pathology and Cancer Research Center, Tufts University School of Medicine, Boston, Massachusetts

Preface

As was shown in the first two volumes of this series, great strides have been made in identifying many of the agents or classes of substances responsible for carcinogenesis and in delineating their interactions with the cell. Clearly, the aim of such studies is that, once identified, these agents can be eliminated from the environment. Yet, despite these advances and the elimination of some important carcinogenic agents, one major problem exists. It is a constant monitor of all oncologic study and diminishes the importance of every experiment and of every clinical observation. *As we noted earlier, that problem is our inability to define the malignant cell.* It is through studies of the fundamental biology of tumors that we seek this definition.

A vast amount of information has been gathered which describes *what* this cell does and—to a lesser extent—*how* it does it. But the *why* evades us. We have been unable to define the malignant cell, save in broad terms by comparing it to its normal counterpart. The major problem appears to be that the malignant cell does so much. It is a chimera, mystifyingly composed of normal activities and structures, of phenotypic schizophrenia with embryonic, fetal, and adult characteristics and, occasionally, a hint of an unclassifiable capacity unique to malignant cells.

The clues as to the *why* of cancer function must be derived directly or by induction from the *what* and *how*. Malignant cells replicate when replication is not required. Whether by escaping the normal inhibitory controls of the host, or by suprasensitivity to stimulation, or by some defect other than these, the tumor grows. The growth is noncompensatory and nonfunctional. The malignant cell also lives beyond its normal span. Together, growth and increased life span result in disruptive cellular accumulation. And what is more, malignant cells compete rather than participate with their normal neighbors and then competitively invade and destroy. The malignant cell itself evades destruction by humoral, immunological, and cellular defense mechanisms. It is therefore characterized by autonomous behavior, living off the host rather than with it. Are these abnormal activities the result of a single alteration or many? One integrated pattern or many? And what genetic or epigenetic or genetic–epigenetic alteration is responsible for this successful, this deadly capacity? An examination of the biology of tumors presented in Volumes 3 and 4 serves many purposes. It may enable us to better understand normal cell biology. It may suggest crucial cellular alterations induced by carcinogenic agents. And, by understanding its aberrations of control and the advantages thus gained by the malignant cell, we may be better able to find a means of reversing them and halting their destructive processes.

New York   Frederick F. Becker

Contents

Spread of Tumors

Surfaces of Normal and Transformed Cells 1

JAMES C. ROBBINS AND GARTH L. NICOLSON

Contact Inhibition 2

JAN PONTÉN

Mechanisms of Cancer Invasion and Metastasis   3

Isaiah J. Fidler

Immunology

Studies of Soluble Transplantation and Tumor Antigens   4

LLOYD W. LAW AND ETTORE APPELLA

RNA Oncogenic Virus-Associated Antigens (and Host Immune Response to Them)   5

TADAO AOKI AND LOUIS R. SIBAL

DNA Virus (SV40) Induced Antigens   6

SATVIR S. TEVETHIA AND MARY J. TEVETHIA

Immunobiology of Chemically Induced Tumors   7

MICHAEL R. PRICE AND ROBERT W. BALDWIN

Immunological Surveillance Against Tumor Cells   8

A. C. ALLISON

Host Immune Response to Human Tumor Antigens   9

SIDNEY H. GOLUB

Comparative Pathology

Comparative Aspects of Certain Cancers   10

HAROLD L. STEWART

Neoplasia in Poikilotherms 11

DANTE G. SCARPELLI

Plant Tumors   12

Armin C. Braun

Spread of Tumors

Surfaces of Normal and Transformed Cells

James C. Robbins and Garth L. Nicolson

1. Introduction

Considerable data implicate events at the cell surface as having a primary role in the growth, development, and communication of normal animal cells and in the multiplication of cancer cells. For example, surface changes are of particular relevance in determining whether neoplastic cells provoke a host immune response and whether they survive or succumb to that response. Surface characteristics are also at least partially involved in the ability of cancer cells both to establish a primary growth site and to metastasize to secondary sites. A variety of additional factors are involved in each case, but progress in distinguishing neoplastic from normal cell surfaces will surely help to understand and to combat the development and growth of neoplastic cells.

Little detailed biochemical knowledge of animal cell surface structure and behavior has been available until recently. In the last few years, several new techniques and approaches—for example, freeze-fracture electron microscopy, lectin biochemistry, convalent labeling of cell surface molecules, and electron spin resonance spectroscopy—have produced vast quantities of data on normal and neoplastic cell surfaces. The data are still somewhat fragmentary, and in some areas contradictory, but a coherent picture of the cell surface is gradually emerging.

Actual tumors arise from unknown precursor cells, so most basic studies have relied on model systems such as tumor virus transformation of "normal" cells

James C. Robbins and Garth L. Nicolson • Department of Cancer Biology, The Salk Institute for Biological Studies, San Diego, California, and Department of Developmental and Cell Biology, University of California, Irvine, California.

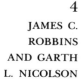

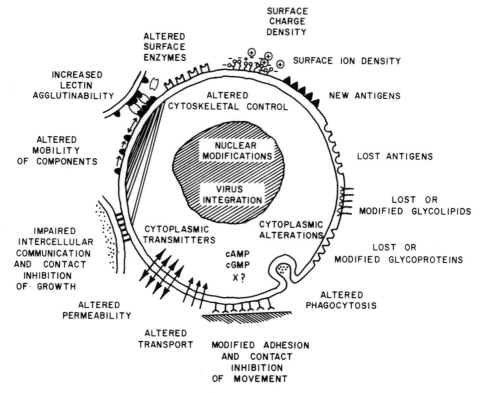

FIGURE 1. Some changes after neoplastic transformation.

cultured *in vitro* to permit comparison of normal and malignant cells. Several differences between normal and malignant cell surfaces have been found (Fig. 1), but it is not yet clear which changes are relevant to tumors in general and which are more relevant to peculiarities of the model system or the cancer studied. In particular, host influences on the cancer cell surface, such as serum enzymes, hormones, and humoral and cellular immune reactions, are lacking or greatly altered with cells cultured *in vitro*. None of the biochemical differences between normal and malignant cells has yet been shown to be the primary determinant of the neoplastic state, from which the other differences would normally arise. Different kinds of cancer may arise in different ways from different cells, so that multiple alterations should not be discouraging.

We describe in this chapter the normal animal cell surface, as presently conceived, and some of the surface changes which seem to be associated with cancer *in vivo* and transformation *in vitro*. We hope that this review of present knowledge will aid further progress in expanding and integrating that knowledge. It is, of course, not possible to cover thoroughly all relevant areas in one chapter, and the reader is urged to consult other recent reviews. Tooze (1973) discusses the normal cell surface very comprehensively and also covers tumor virus transformation. The book edited by Clarkson and Baserga (1974) includes several chapters on the cell surface role in the control of cell division in normal and malignant cells. Herschman (1972) and Wallach (1969) discuss membrane changes in cancer. Two areas which will not be covered in this chapter, electrical and structural junctions between normal and tumor cells, have been adequately described elsewhere (McNutt and Weinstein, 1973; Weinstein and McNutt, 1972; Loewenstein, 1969; Martinez-Palomo, 1970; Staehelin, 1974).

2. Organization of Cell Surfaces

2.1. Basic Principles of Membrane Structure

The cell surface is loosely defined as the structure which forms the cell's outer semipermeable barrier, the plasma membrane, but it also contains extracellular, cell-associated components that are bound to the plasma membrane. In addition, it is necessary to define arbitrarily as part of the cell surface structure some intracellular components such as the membrane-bound cell cytoskeletal components, even though these components may only transiently interact with the plasma membrane. The plasma membrane has been the subject of a number of reviews (Nicolson, 1974a; Singer, 1971, 1974; Steck, 1974; Green et al., 1973; Guidotti, 1972; Capaldi and Green, 1972; Singer and Nicolson, 1972), thus it will be dealt with only briefly here. The plasma membrane is composed of lipids, glycolipids, proteins, and glycoproteins dynamically organized into structural configurations of minimum free energy. Lipids and glycolipids appear to form the matrix of most plasma membranes (Singer and Nicolson, 1972). To assume their lowest free energy configuration, membrane phospholipids and glycolipids present the hydrophilic head portions of their structure to the bulk aqueous phase and sequester the hydrophobic tail portions inside the hydrophobic portions of the membrane away from the aqueous environment. The phospholipids and glycolipids are therefore arranged in a bilayer configuration as originally proposed by Danielli and Davson (1935), except that the bilayer is not continuous but is interrupted in certain regions. Neutral lipids such as cholesterol appear to be intercalated into the lipid bilayer, with the more hydrophilic parts of their structures facing the aqueous environment. The evidence supporting a bilayer configuration for the bulk membrane lipid is overwhelming: X-ray diffraction (Blaurock, 1971; Wilkins et al., 1971; Engelman, 1970; Blasie and Worthington, 1969), differential scanning calorimetry (Papahadjopoulos et al., 1973; Steim et al., 1969), electron spin resonance (Jost et al., 1973; Scandella et al., 1972; Kornberg and McConnell, 1971a,b; Keith et al., 1970; Tourtellotte et al., 1970; Hubbell and McConnell, 1968), and nuclear magnetic resonance (Lee et al., 1972; Glaser et al., 1970). In some plasma membranes, the lipids appear to be asymmetrically distributed across the two halves of the phospholipid bilayer (Bretscher, 1973). By using chemical labeling techniques, Bretscher (1972) demonstrated that amino-containing lipids (phosphatidylethanolamine and phosphatidylserine) are overwhelmingly on the inner membrane surface of the human erythrocyte. More convincing enzymatic data from Zwaal et al. (1973) indicate that in intact

6

JAMES C.
ROBBINS
AND GARTH
L. NICOLSON

erythrocytes 70% of the membrane phosphatidylcholine is susceptible to cleavage by phospholipase A_2, while sphingomyelin, phosphatidylserine, and phosphatidylethanolamine are resistant to enzymatic cleavage. When intact erythrocytes are lysed, all of the above phospholipids are accessible to enzymatic digestion. This indicates that phosphatidylcholine is predominantly in the outer half of the lipid bilayer. In addition, more than 80% of the sphingomyelin in intact cells is degraded by sphingomyelinase, indicating that its predominant location is also in the outer half of the lipid bilayer (Zwaal *et al.*, 1973). From these experiments and from the chemical labeling studies of Bretscher (1972), it appears that phosphatidylethanolamine and phosphatidylserine are predominantly in the inner half of the bilayer. The importance of lipid asymmetry in the organization and function of plasma membranes is unknown, but specific partitioning, orientation, association, and structure of membrane proteins and glycoproteins may depend on associations with an asymmetrical lipid bilayer.

Membrane proteins and oligosaccharides also appear to be asymmetrically distributed on the inner and the outer side of the bilayer. This has been extensively studied in the human erythrocyte membrane, where the oligosaccharides are known to be expressed only on the exterior surface of the membrane (Steck, 1972*a*; Nicolson and Singer, 1971; Eylar *et al.*, 1962) while most membrane proteins are expressed on the inner surface (Phillips and Morrison, 1971; Nicolson *et al.*, 1971). These observations have been extended to more complex cells (Nicolson and Singer, 1974).

2.1.1. Integral Membrane Proteins

Plasma membrane proteins and glycoproteins fall loosely into two major classes depending on whether or not they have strong hydrophobic interactions with membrane lipids. One class of membrane proteins and glycoproteins, called integral (Singer, 1974; Singer and Nicolson, 1972) or intrinsic (Green *et al.*, 1973; Vanderkooi, 1972) components, tend to seek hydrophobic environments (interacting with lipid acyl groups) where they are thermodynamically most stable. The integral proteins which have been isolated and characterized have amphipathic structures. That is, they are asymmetrical or bimodal with regard to their hydrophilic and hydrophobic structural portions and have the following general properties: they are usually unstable in low ionic strength neutral pH buffers; strong chaotropic agents (organic solvents, detergents, etc.) are required to solubilize and then stabilize them in aqueous solutions (Steck and Yu, 1973); and when isolated they quite often have some strongly bound lipid. The integral membrane proteins and glycoproteins that have been isolated and purified have distinct hydrophilic and hydrophobic regions which can be enzymatically separated (Segrest *et al.*, 1973; Gahmberg *et al.*, 1972; Winzler, 1970; Ito and Sato, 1968; Morawiecki, 1964). Although integral membrane proteins have been reported to contain a large percentage of globular character due to the amount of α-helical peptide structure (Glaser and Singer, 1971; Wallach and Zahler, 1966), their interaction in two phases, aqueous and hydrocarbon, requires that their three-dimensional structures be asymmetrical.

Such integral glycoproteins as glycophorin, the major sialoglycoprotein of the human erythrocyte membrane, have been proposed to penetrate the membrane. Evidence for glycophorin's transmembrane disposition comes from controlled proteolysis experiments and chemical labeling data (Morrison *et al.*, 1974; Segrest *et al.*, 1973; Bretscher, 1971*a*; Winzler *et al.*, 1967). The hydrophilic portions of its peptide structure probably radiate into the aqueous environment on both sides of the membrane matrix formed by the phospholipid bilayer. Glycophorin is approximately 60% carbohydrate by weight, and is composed of a single peptide with multiple oligosaccharide chains attached to hydrophilic amino acid residues near the *N*-terminal region (Segrest *et al.*, 1973; Winzler, 1970). Another region of predominantly hydrophilic amino acid residues exists at the *C*-terminal end of the molecule separated by an internal region of hydrophobic residues from the *N*-terminal hydrophilic region. Glycophorin bears a number of cell receptors in its *N*-terminal domain: Ss, ABO, and MN antigens, lectin receptors for wheat germ agglutinin and phytohemagglutinin, and influenza and other virus receptors. In the human erythrocyte membrane, another major integral membrane glycoprotein exists called component *a* (Bretscher, 1971*b*) or band III component (Steck, 1972*a*). It contains less carbohydrate (5–8%) than glycophorin and is slightly larger (mol wt ∼100,000 by SDS-polyacrylamide gel electrophoresis). Similar to glycophorin, it is exposed at the cell surface (Hubbard and Cohn, 1972; Bretscher, 1971*b,c*; Phillips and Morrison, 1971) and can be labeled from either side of the membrane, indicating that it also traverses the membrane bilayer (Bretscher, 1971*b,c*). This component (or more properly a component of this molecular weight) has been implicated as being involved in membrane anion transport (Guidotti, 1973) and can be phosphorylated in association with membrane Mg^{2+}-dependent, Na^+, K^+-stimulated ATPase (Avruch and Fairbanks, 1972). It is reported to contain one receptor per molecule for the lectin concanavalin A (Con A) (Findlay, 1974). Electron microscopy utilizing freeze-etch replica techniques has been used to localize the receptors borne by glycophorin and component *a*. During fracture of the membrane, particles (membrane intercalated particles) are revealed that penetrate deeply into the lipid bilayer. In the human erythrocyte, these particles are approximately 85 Å in diameter and are known from localization experiments to contain at least one copy of glycophorin per particle, although the number of glycophorin molecules per cell, and its size, precludes it from being the sole component of the freeze-etch membrane intercalated particle. Guidotti (1972) has suggested that glycophorin and band III component(s) form an intramembrane oligomeric complex which traverses the membrane bilayer and is revealed as a particle during freeze-cleavage experiments. Evidence in favor of this proposal is that the Con A binding sites on human erythrocytes, which are borne by component III or *a*, are exclusively associated with the membrane-intercalated particles (Pinto da Silva and Nicolson, 1974), and that glycophorin and other glycoproteins can be selectively crosslinked in the membrane using short-chain bifunctional imidates (Ji, 1973, 1974). The association of transport functions with components in this transmembrane structure (Carter *et al.*, 1973; Cabantchik and Rothstein, 1972) led to the term "permeaphore" for this class of membrane structure (Pinto da Silva and Nicolson, 1974) (Fig. 2). Functions such

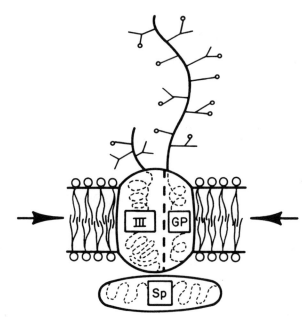

FIGURE 2. "Permeaphore" integral glycoprotein complex of the human erythrocyte membrane. See text for details. GP, Glycophorin; Sp, spectrin; III, band III component or component *a*; arrows indicate fracture plane during freeze-etch experiments. From Pinto da Silva and Nicolson (1974), by permission.

as transport and ion passage which are dependent on transmembrane events may require specific structures that provide continuity between the inner and outer membrane surfaces.

2.1.2. Peripheral Membrane Proteins

The other major class of membrane proteins, peripheral or extrinsic proteins, is characterized by properties that are quite different from those of the integral proteins and glycoproteins. Peripheral membrane proteins are more loosely associated with the membrane and are not stabilized by extensive hydrophobic bonding with membrane lipids. Mild treatments usually remove peripheral proteins from membranes without disruption of integral membrane structures, and, once removed, peripheral proteins are usually stable in neutral aqueous buffers. A classic example of a peripheral membrane protein is human erythrocyte membrane spectrin. Spectrin constitutes approximately 20–25% of human erythrocyte membrane protein by weight (Marchesi and Steers, 1968) and can be easily removed from the membrane without its denaturation by low ionic strength buffers containing chelating agents (Marchesi *et al.*, 1969; Marchesi and Steers, 1968; Mazia and Ruby, 1968). It is composed of two ~210,000–240,000 mol wt peptides (Clarke, 1971; Fairbanks *et al.*, 1971; Marchesi *et al.*, 1969), and it is quite stable in aqueous solutions. Spectrin has been localized exclusively at the inner erythrocyte membrane surface by labeling with ferritin-antibody (Nicolson *et al.*, 1971) and by controlled proteolysis experiments (Steck, 1972*b*).

In the human erythrocyte membrane, oligomeric complexes appear to be the rule rather than the exception. The major glycoproteins (glycophorin and component *a*) seem to be in the permeaphore complex, and further evidence has implicated several additional proteins in this complex: a protein kinase (Ji and Nicolson, 1974), enzymes such as glyceraldehyde-3-phosphate dehydrogenase (Kant and Steck, 1973), and at least some spectrin (Ji and Nicolson, 1974; Nicolson and Painter, 1973). Spectrin is associated with actin-like molecules at the inner surface, and Steck (1974) has proposed that the actin–spectrin system forms a dense network at the inner membrane surface, a sort of "two-ply" membrane structure, that is responsible for defining cell shape and deformability. The linkage of this spectrin-containing complex to the permeaphore (Ji and Nicolson, 1974; Nicolson and Painter, 1973) ties the integral and peripheral membrane components together and may account for the low mobility of the permeaphore complex in intact cells (Fig. 2). Elgsaeter and Branton (1974) found that partial disruption of the spectrin-containing network at the inner surface was necessary in order to induce membrane intercalated particle movement. The "two-ply" linked system probably provides the tough and inextensible support for the deformable lipid bilayer so that the erythrocyte can withstand the rigors of shearing forces encountered in the circulatory system.

In other plasma membranes, a system analogous to the spectrin–actin complex is usually made up of microfilaments, microtubules, and perhaps other energy-dependent contractile systems. The plasma membrane associated micro-filament–microtubule systems of some cell types are extensive (Perdue, 1973; McNutt *et al.*, 1971), and these systems have been implicated in a variety of cellular processes requiring membrane and cell movement and shape changes, such as endocytosis and secretion.

2.2. Fluid Nature of Membranes

There is good evidence for the mobility of membrane components in the plane of the membrane. Estimates of phospholipid planar diffusion from nuclear magnetic resonance and electron paramagnetic resonance spin-label studies indicate rapid motion of these components ($D \cong 10^{-8}$ cm s^{-1}) (Jost *et al.*, 1973; Lee *et al.*, 1972; Scandella *et al.*, 1972; Kornberg and McConnell, 1971*a*), but little or no "flip-flop" or rotation from one side of the membrane to the other (Kornberg and McConnell, 1971*b*). Certain protein components also appear to diffuse rapidly in the membrane plane, although less rapidly than the membrane lipids. After Sendai virus induced fusion of two unlike cells to form a heterokaryon, it takes about 30–40 min at 37°C to intermix completely specific surface antigens such as H-2 histocompatibility antigens (Edidin and Weiss, 1972; Frye and Edidin, 1970). Cell surface Ig (de Petris and Raff, 1972, 1973; Taylor *et al.*, 1971) and H-2 antigens (Davis, 1972; Edidin and Weiss, 1972; Kourilsky *et al.*, 1972) aggregate into a cap on lymphoid cells in even less time. Results with antibody-induced aggregation of surface antigens have led to a general proposal that essentially all cell surface components are capable of rapid redistribution (Sundqvist, 1972). Using fluorescent antibody techniques, Edidin and Fambrough (1973) estimated the diffusion constant for certain antigens on muscle fibers to be $D \cong 10^{-9}$ cm s^{-1}. Since glycoproteins are much larger than membrane lipids, the finding that certain glycoproteins could diffuse laterally at approximately one-tenth the rate of the phospholipids is reasonable. Saccharides attached to membrane glycoproteins can also be quickly aggregated with lectins on certain cells, but not on others (Huet and Bernhard, 1974; Garrido et al., 1974; Comoglio and Filogamo, 1973; Inbar and Sachs, 1973; Inbar et al., 1973; Rosenblith et al., 1973; Comoglio and Guglielmone, 1972; Bretton et al., 1972; Nicolson, 1972, 1973b, 1974b). The point should be made that different membrane protein components may move laterally at quite different rates (Comoglio and Filogamo, 1973; Pinto da Silva, 1972; Edidin and Weiss, 1972, 1974; Frye and Edidin, 1970), from very fast to very slow or almost not at all, depending on the types of restraints that have been applied on these moieties from outside and/or inside the cell.

In the fluid mosaic membrane model (Fig. 3), lipids are postulated to be rapidly diffusing laterally and intermixing in the membrane. Proteins and glycoproteins are postulated to move laterally at a range of rates, from somewhat less rapidly than lipids for free proteins to very slowly for molecules relatively "frozen" by various restraints. Although the membrane is basically fluid, several types of restraints have been proposed to restrict or control the mobility of some membrane proteins—for example, intercellular junctions (reviewed by McNutt and Weinstein, 1973, and Loewenstein, 1969), subsurface contractile networks, complexing into large assemblies by external peripheral proteins, and frozen lipid domains. Cell membrane associated energy-driven contractile structures such as the microtubule–microfilament systems may under certain conditions be involved in an energy-dependent lateral movement of surface components. Such a system may control antibody- and lectin-induced capping of aggregated or patched receptors on lymphocytes (Edelman et al., 1973; Karnovsky et al., 1972; Loor et al., 1972; de Petris and Raff, 1972, 1973; Yahara and Edelman, 1972, 1973a,b; Taylor et al., 1971), cell motility (de Petris and Raff, 1972; Taylor et al., 1971), and endocytosis (Berlin, 1972; de Petris and Raff, 1972; Karnovsky et al., 1972). But under resting conditions in the absence of contraction of the membrane-associated contractile systems, the lateral mobilities of certain (linked) proteins and glycoproteins may be impeded (Edelman et al., 1973). The linkage between outer membrane surface components and inner surface peripheral and membrane-associated contractile components has not been directly demonstrated, but it will probably turn out to be of the noncovalent type, probably mediated through proteins involved in hydrophilic or hydrophobic interactions with integral membrane components. Alternatively, the existence of a network of membrane-associated contractile components tightly opposed to the inner membrane surface may increase the rigidity and reduce the deformability of the cell surface; thus membrane-associated components may indirectly affect cell adhesion, agglutina-

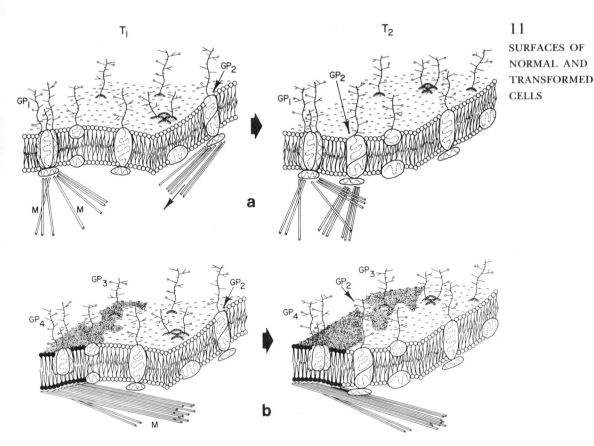

FIGURE 3. Modified version of the fluid mosaic model of membrane structure. T_1 and T_2 represent different points in time. (a) Impedence of membrane receptor mobility by cell cytoskeletal attachment. Certain hypothetical integral membrane glycoprotein components are free to diffuse laterally in the membrane plane formed by the fluid lipid bilayer, while others such as the integral glycoprotein complex GP_1 may be impeded by a microfilament–microtubule complex (M). Under certain conditions, some integral membrane complexes (GP_2) can be displaced by membrane-associated contractile components in an energy-dependent process. From Nicolson (1974a). (b) Impedence of membrane receptor mobility by sequestration into less mobile lipid domains. Certain integral glycoprotein complexes are free to move in the fluid lipid bilayer regions, but others such as the complexes GP_3 and GP_4 are sequestered into a "less fluid" lipid domain (shaded area with solid lipid headgroups). In the "less fluid" region, the viscosity is such that lateral mobilities are relatively much lower than the fluid lipid regions. In addition, cell cytoskeletal components may interact with the "less fluid" domains.

tion, etc. (Fig. 3). These interactions of exterior and integral membrane proteins with internal structures may be very important in the communication of cells with their environment.

Another possible restriction of mobility is that glycoproteins at the outer surface may interact with a variety of proteoglycans or complex polysaccharide-containing components that form a peripheral matrix at the outer cell surface. Hynes (1973) has suggested this possibility as a mechanism for the retardation of mobility of plasma membrane components on normal cells. If "islands" or domains of integral membrane components linked by extracellular peripheral glycoproteins exist, then these domains would naturally be expected to diffuse at a much lower rate than their constituent components. Cell surface glycoproteins that may fit this scheme have recently been isolated and partially purified (see Section 3.1.3).

The mobility and topography of certain receptors could also be controlled by sequestering them into "frozen" (solid-phase) lipid domains (Fig. 3b). That some lipid may exist in a solid state and the remainder in a fluid state at physiological temperatures has not been experimentally demonstrated in mammalian cells.[1] However, using bacterial fatty acid auxotrophs, Kleemann and McConnell (1974) have shown by changing the fatty acid composition of membrane lipids that discrete fluid–solid lipid phase separations occur when the bacteria are cooled below their membrane lipid fluidius phase transition temperature. At temperatures above the fluidius phase transition, membrane lipid is in a completely fluid state as monitored by electron spin resonance probes, and the plasma membrane intercalated particles revealed by freeze-fracture electron microscopy are distributed in a dispersed netlike arrangement. Below the transition temperature, when both solid and fluid domains can be found by spin resonance, the membrane particles are pushed together into continuous areas, leaving other large areas of the membrane free of particles. Fixation prevents the movement of particles into the large, tightly packed particle domains. In this case, it appears that the solid lipid phase excludes the membrane intercalated particles, but the converse might also be possible. In summary, membrane lipids seem generally to move freely within the membrane plane. Proteins and glycoproteins may be seen to move with more or less freedom, depending on the particular molecules studied and the conditions of observation. Of course, the mobility of some lipids is probably reduced by association with proteins (Jost et al., 1973), and such association may result in the sequestration of lipoprotein complexes in relatively immobile membrane domains that could exist as islands in fluid "seas" of lipid. Possible changes in membrane fluidity related to neoplasia are discussed in Section 3.4.2.

3. Differences Between Normal and Transformed Cell Surfaces

3.1. Composition

3.1.1. Carbohydrate

Most animal cell surface carbohydrates are components of glycoproteins (Section 3.1.3), glycosaminoglycans (Nigam and Cantero, 1972), or glycolipids (Section 3.1.2). Glycoproteins are principally proteins with relatively small attached oligosaccharide chains consisting largely of neutral and amino sugars including sialic acid (Winzler, 1970). Glycosaminoglycans (mucopeptide, mucopolysaccharide), on the other hand, are a mixture of oligosaccharides containing substantial amounts of hexuronic acids and hexosamines, sometimes covalently attached to small proteins. They include hyaluronic acid and chondroitin sulfate,

[1] See Fox (1975) for an extensive discussion of lipid phase changes and their relationship to lateral separation, transport, and receptor mobility.

and largely make up the "glycocalix" or "fuzz" outside the integral zone of the
plasma membrane.

Early observations on the differential histochemical staining of normal and
cancerous tissue (Defendi and Gasic, 1963) led to investigation of cell surface
carbohydrates, but the molecules involved are diverse, and useful generalizations
are limited. There are several reports that animal cell line cultures *in vitro* contain
less total or membrane-associated sialic acid (Grimes, 1973; Perdue *et al.*, 1972;
Ohta *et al.*, 1968) and other sugars (Grimes, 1974; Wu *et al.*, 1969) after viral
transformation, although Hartmann *et al.* (1972) did not find these differences.
Rous sarcoma virus transformed chick embryo fibroblasts were reported to
contain more sialic acid accessible to enzymatic removal than nontransformed
fibroblasts, but total content was not measured (Bosmann *et al.*, 1974*a*). Mitotic
normal cells are somewhat more similar to transformed cells than are nongrowing
normal cells, in lectin agglutinability and external glycopeptide size (Section
3.1.3), and nontransformed BHK cells contain less sialic acid (though more
fucose) during mitosis (Glick and Buck, 1973).

Increases in sialic acid content, however, have been reported for human tumors
of the colon, stomach, breast (Barker *et al.*, 1959), pancreas, liver, skin, and lymph
node (Mabry and Carubelli, 1972). Sialic acid and several other sugars are
increased in human lung tumors (Bryant *et al.*, 1974), and in the plasma
membrane of a rat hepatoma (Benedetti and Emmelot, 1967) compared to
normal tissue levels. The amount of sialic acid in human leukemic lymphocytes is
the same as (Lichtman and Weed, 1970) or less than (McClelland and Bridges,
1973) that in normal lymphocytes, so a general increase in sialic acid may be more
characteristic of solid tumors (Bryant *et al.*, 1974). Weiss (1973) has reviewed the
literature on cellular sialic acid content and neuraminidase effects on cell
interactions such as tumor rejection and found few useful generalizations relating
to malignancy. Virus-transformed cell lines are frequently used as *in vitro* models
for malignant tumor cells, but the growth conditions and selective pressures *in
vitro* and *in vivo* may be expected to affect cells differently. The changes in
carbohydrate content reported for several transformed animal cell lines do not
correlate well with the changes seen in several human tumor tissues, implying that
care is necessary in application of the model. In any case, gross changes in
carbohydrate content may be less important than changes in particular molecules
with key roles in growth control. If these controlling molecules were not very
numerous, their changes would not be detectable in measurements of total cell
composition.

Glycosaminoglycans seem to be important in cell recognition and adhesion
(Section 3.4.3), but their precise functions are unknown. The molecules involved
are heterogenous and have not yet been completely defined structurally. Several
reports indicate that transformation changes cellular glycosaminoglycan
composition—for example, cultured green monkey kidney cells contain more
glycosaminoglycan after transformation (Makita and Shimojo, 1973).
Glucosamine-containing surface material of rat liver cells is a relatively
homogeneous material as judged by gel filtration and electrophoresis, but

comparable material from several ascites hepatoma cells is a mixture of several components (Yamamoto and Terayama, 1973). Hyaluronic acid content rises with transformation of hamster embryo fibroblasts (Satoh *et al.*, 1973) and chick embryo fibroblasts (Ishimoto *et al.*, 1966), with increased release by added hyaluronidase in the latter case (Bosmann *et al.*, 1974*a*). Several cultured cell lines show by histological methods an increase in glycosaminoglycan with transformation (Martinez-Palomo *et al.*, 1969; Defendi and Gasic, 1963).

Cells growing in culture attached to glass or plastic leave a glycosaminoglycan layer on the substrate when the cells are removed with EDTA. The material deposited by mouse 3T3 cells seems to be largely hyaluronic acid covalently linked to small proteins, and SV40-transformed cells (SV3T3) deposit less of this material than do 3T3 cells (Terry and Culp, 1974). On the other hand, the thickness of the film deposited on glass by a cell monolayer is greater in the case of several transformed cell lines, including mouse fibroblasts (although SV3T3 was not included in this study) (Poste *et al.*, 1973). EDTA removes equal amounts of a sulfated glycosaminoglycan—probably heparan sulfate—from normal and transformed BHK cells. Subsequent treatment with trypsin then releases more of this material from the normal cells than from transformed cells, but the relative amount released by each treatment is not clear (Chiarugi *et al.*, 1974). The growing body of glycosaminoglycan literature is presently difficult to fit into a unifying hypothesis. It seems likely that better structural definition of glycosaminoglycan species would facilitate studies on the functions of this material and possible changes with cancer. Changes in only a few of the diverse species might be relevant.

3.1.2. Lipids and Glycolipids

Lipids and glycolipids form the bulk structure of cell membranes (Section 2), and so are quite important in establishing cell surface properties. At least some malignant human tumors contain more phospholipid and cholesterol than benign tumors and the corresponding normal tissue (Christensen Lou *et al.*, 1956; Haven and Bloor, 1956). Substantial differences were not found in nonglycosylated lipids between normal chicken cells and tumor or virus-transformed cells (Quigley *et al.*, 1971; Figard and Levine, 1966), although the fatty acid composition of the phospholipids does tend to shift with transformation toward more oleate and less arachidonate (Yau and Weber, 1972, 1974). Mouse and rat leukemic lymphocytes have a somewhat lower ratio of cholesterol to total phospholipid than normal lymphocytes (Vlodavsky and Sachs, 1974; Inbar and Shinitzky, 1974). The more striking lipid differences presently associated with malignancy or transformation, though, are in membrane glycolipids.

Most cellular glycolipids are found in membranes, particularly the plasma membrane, and several glycolipids change markedly after transformation. The most common glycolipids of animal cell membranes are derivatives of ceramide (sphingosine fatty acyl amide, Fig. 4). Sugar residues are transferred sequentially by glycosyltransferases from sugar nucleotides to the primary hydroxyl of

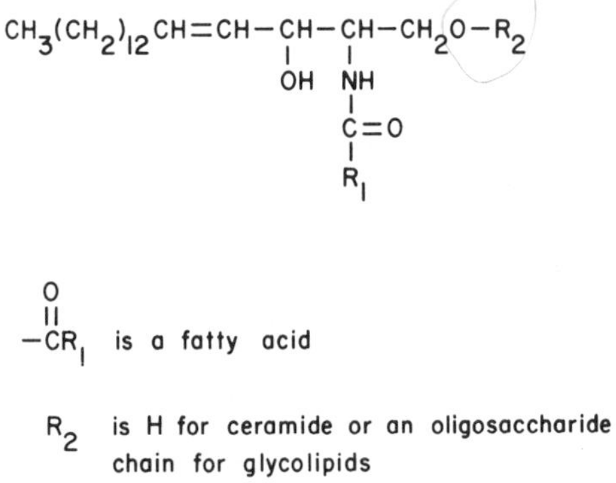

$$CH_3(CH_2)_{12}CH=CH-CH-CH-CH_2O-R_2$$

$$\underset{OH}{|}\quad\underset{\underset{\underset{R_1}{|}}{\underset{C=O}{|}}{NH}}{|}$$

$^{1°CH}$

glycolipid

$$\overset{O}{\overset{||}{-CR_1}}\quad \text{is a fatty acid}$$

R_2 is H for ceramide or an oligosaccharide
chain for glycolipids

FIGURE 4. The structure of ceramide.

ceramide to form several glycosylceramides. The assortment of these glycolipids present in any cell varies with species and cell line, and may even vary between clones of a cell line (clonal variation of glycolipids was reported by Sakiyama *et al.*, 1972, but not by Critchley and Macpherson, 1973).

Partially because of this variability and because of difficulties in determining glycolipid structure, a certain confusion exists in the literature on glycolipid changes and malignant transformation. To illustrate the present knowledge and its limitations, we will first present the findings on a well-studied system, the hamster NIL cell line, and then discuss the applicability of these findings to other systems. Recent reviews should be consulted for more extensive discussion of neutral glycolipids (Hakomori, 1973, 1975a,b; Hakomori *et al.*, 1972) and gangliosides—those glycolipids containing sialic acid (Brady and Fishman, 1974).

Three main changes occur in NIL glycolipids upon viral transformation: (1) decreased concentrations of complex glycolipids, (2) failure of glycolipid synthesis to respond to contact between cells growing in culture, and (3) increased accessibility of the glycolipids to macromolecules such as antibodies, enzymes, and lectins. Increased concentrations of simpler precursor glycolipids sometimes accompany disappearance of the more complex species.

Hakomori *et al.* (1972) reported that hamster NIL cells contain six glycolipids (Fig. 5): ceramide mono- through pentahexoside, and hematoside. There is a question as to whether some NIL clones may contain less than this full complement (Critchley and Macpherson, 1973; Sakiyama *et al.*, 1972). The "higher" glycolipids—ceramide tri-, tetra-, and pentahexoside—and sometimes hematoside, are present in greater concentration in confluent than in sparse cells. These glycolipids showing a dependence on cell density in normal NIL cells are all decreased substantially or missing entirely in NIL cells transformed by polyoma or hamster sarcoma virus. Remaining glycolipids in transformed cells do not vary with cell density (Critchley and Macpherson, 1973; Hakomori *et al.*, 1972; Sakiyama *et al.*, 1972).

These changes in glycolipid composition with cell density and transformation can be explained by alterations in a synthetic enzyme. Kijimoto and Hakomori (1971) measured the activity of the α-galactosyltransferase, which catalyzes synthesis of the first higher glycolipid, ceramide trihexoside, from the dihexoside.

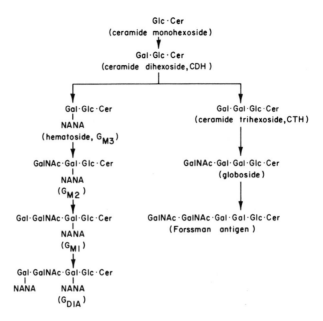

FIGURE 5. Some glycolipid structures. Symbols: Cer, as in Fig. 3, with R_2 the sugar chains shown here; Glc, glucose (all sugars are D); Gal, galactose; GalNAc, N-acetylgalactosamine; NANA, sialic acid. From Sakiyama *et al.* (1972), Hakomori (1973), and Brady *et al.* (1973).

The activity of this enzyme is two- to threefold higher in confluent NIL than in sparse cells, and only 10–50% as high in polyoma-transformed NIL (sparse or confluent) as in sparse NIL. The β-galactosyltransferase involved in synthesis of ceramide dihexoside neither rose with confluence nor fell with transformation. In addition to changes in synthetic enzymes, transformed cells may have higher glycosidase activities for degradation of glycolipids (Section 3.2.3).

While the population of glycolipids varies with species and cell line, a simplification of a glycolipid structure is frequently seen to accompany transformation by tumor viruses. Reductions in at least some higher glycolipids related to transformation or tumorigenesis have been reported with cells of hamster (Gahmberg and Hakomori, 1974; Critchley and Macpherson, 1973; Den *et al.*, 1971; Sakiyama *et al.*, 1972), mouse (Brady and Fishman, 1974), human (Steiner and Melnick, 1974; Hakomori, 1970; Hakomori *et al.*, 1967), chicken (Hakomori *et al.*, 1971), rat, and baboon (Steiner *et al.*, 1973a), although there are some dissenting reports (Diringer *et al.*, 1972; Warren *et al.*, 1972a; Yogeeswaran *et al.*, 1972). Chemical transformation also leads to a more simplified glycolipid population in hamster cells (Den *et al.*, 1974). Increased synthesis of higher glycolipids as cells grow and contact each other has been seen with hamster cells (Critchley and Macpherson, 1973; Sakiyama *et al.*, 1972; Kijimoto and Hakomori, 1971; Hakomori, 1970), and smaller increases with human (Hakomori, 1970) and chicken (Hakomori *et al.*, 1971) cells, but was not seen with mouse cells (Brady and Fishman, 1974; Critchley and Macpherson, 1973). The glycolipid differences between sparse and confluent

cells do not seem to be due simply to presence or absence of growth since sparse
cells made quiescent by serum deprivation did not resemble confluent cells in
glycolipid pattern (Critchley and Macpherson, 1973).

Glycosyltransferase activities (Section 3.2.1) involved in the synthesis of higher
glycolipids have been reported to decrease with viral transformation of hamster
(Yogeeswaran *et al.*, 1974; Den *et al.*, 1971, 1974; Kijimoto and Hakomori, 1971)
and mouse (Brady and Fishman, 1974; Patt and Grimes, 1974; Fishman *et al.*,
1974; Mora *et al.*, 1973) cells. A given transforming virus may lead to reductions in
different transferase activities in different cell lines, and even more than one
activity in a particular line. Glycosyltransferase activity increases have been
reported for confluent hamster cells compared to sparse (Kijimoto and
Hakomori, 1971), but these changes were not found with mouse cells (Brady and
Fishman, 1974). In sum, part but not all of the conclusions reached from the study
of NIL cell glycolipids seem applicable to other systems (discussed below).

A potential problem with DNA tumor virus transformed cells is that viruses
such as polyoma and SV40 transform only a small percentage of cells exposed to
them, so it can be argued that transformation merely selects a few cells with
preexisting glycolipid abnormalities. Certain RNA tumor viruses, such as sarcoma
viruses, however, transform essentially all cells in culture, so sarcoma virus
transformed cells have been used to test this possibility. Sarcoma virus transformation of mouse cells reduces the amount of higher ganglioside and the activity of
an appropriate glycosyltransferase (Fishman *et al.*, 1974; Mora *et al.*, 1973).
Sarcoma virus transformation of chick embryo fibroblasts in culture has been
reported to cause similar changes and also a loss of contact extension of glycolipids
(Hakomori *et al.*, 1971), but another group failed to find these differences
(Warren *et al.*, 1972*a*).

The increased synthesis of complex glycolipids as normal cells grow into contact
with each other, termed "contact extension" by Hakomori (1973), could be
involved in the growth control which stops growth of nontransformed cells in
culture at approximately a monolayer–density-dependent inhibition of growth. If
complex glycolipids or their synthetic enzymes are involved in growth control, the
control mechanism must be complex, because studies of phenotypic revertants of
transformed cells, a temperature-sensitive viral transformant, and spontaneous
transformants do not completely support a simple relationship between contact
inhibition of growth and contact extension of glycolipids. Revertant cell lines can
be obtained from transformed cells by selection for restoration of contact
inhibition of growth, inability to grow in soft agar, or resistance to killing by some
drugs or lectins. Although they are not "normal" cells, revertants do have growth
control and morphology resembling those of nontransformed cells, and they
generally show low tumorigenicity when injected into animals. Morphological
revertants of transformed hamster and mouse cells only partially regain glycolipid
patterns characteristic of normal cells (Brady and Fishman, 1974; Den *et al.*, 1974;
Critchley and Macpherson, 1973).

Temperature-sensitive cell lines can be obtained which have transformed
morphology and growth control at one temperature but normal characteristics at

another temperature. These lines result from infecting cells with temperature-sensitive virus mutants or from subjecting transformed cell lines to selection for normal growth characteristics at one temperature and retention of transformed characteristics at another. Virus production is generally maintained at both temperatures. Temperature-sensitive transformation permits comparison of normal and transformed characteristics in the same cell line and genetic background, reducing the complications involved in comparing separate normal and transformed cell lines. It also permits more detailed kinetic studies on the process of transformation than do other systems. BHK fibroblasts infected with a temperature-sensitive polyoma virus grow as transformed cells at 31°C and revert to normal growth control at 39°C; yet their synthesis of ceramide trihexoside is greatly depressed at both temperatures (Hammarström and Bjursell, 1973). This finding shows that the synthesis of ceramide trihexoside is not required for normal growth control in BHK cells.

Useful cancer theories must apply not only to cancer induced by added tumor viruses but also to spontaneously arising malignancy. Spontaneously transformed mouse cell lines, however, do not undergo the ganglioside simplifications characteristic of viral transformation, although some simplification does occur over many generations in culture (Brady and Fishman, 1974). One of eleven spontaneous tumors arising from injection of hamsters with nontransformed NIL cells retained the NIL glycolipid composition, although the other ten tumors did have reductions in higher glycolipid (Critchley and Macpherson, 1973). These experiments with reversion, temperature-sensitive transformation, and spontaneous transformation demonstrate that higher glycolipids and density-dependent growth control, while frequently lost together upon viral transformation, may be gained and lost independently in other cases. The simplifying hypothesis that higher glycolipids are synthesized by contact extension, and that altered glycolipid compositions of transformed cells can be explained by a lack of this contact extension, currently seems well established only for the hamster NIL cell line. The picture is further complicated by work of Gahmberg and Hakomori (1975a) showing that hamster NIL cells have a total of seven neutral glycolipids (hematoside and other gangliosides were not measured). In agreement with previous work, polyoma-transformed NIL cells have reduced higher glycolipid and lack contact extension, but the transformed cells also contain a small amount of a different ceramide tetrasaccharide not present in normal cells, and therefore not attributable to incomplete synthesis. More work is necessary to clarify completely the role of contact extension in NIL cells, and particularly to elucidate the control of glycolipid synthesis in those cell lines where contact extension has not been demonstrated.

While virus-transformed cells generally contain less complex glycolipid than do untransformed cells, the remaining molecules of higher glycolipid have been found to be more reactive with macromolecular reagents, such as antibodies and enzymes. Although BHK and 3T3 cell lines contain less hematoside after transformation by any of several viruses, the transformed cells are more sensitive to lysis by antihematoside antibody plus complement (Hakomori et al., 1968).

However, trypsinization of the normal cells made them as sensitive as the transformed cells (which were not affected by trypsin). Similar findings were reported for Forssman antigen on normal and transformed BHK cells (Burger, 1971) and their plasma membranes (Makita and Seyama, 1971).

Chemical labeling of glycolipids has also been used to detect changes in glycolipid accessibility. Gahmberg and Hakomori (1973b) have adapted a method for tritium-labeling glycolipids and glycoproteins to cell surface studies. Cells are treated with galactose oxidase, which oxidizes carbon atom 6 of nonreducing terminal galactose and galactosamine residues to the aldehyde, and the resulting aldehydes are then reduced back to [^{3}H]galactose and [^{3}H]galactosamine by tritiated sodium borohydride. Inability of the galactose oxidase to penetrate easily into healthy cells limits incorporation of tritium to glycolipids and glycoproteins exposed on the cell surface. Using this technique, Gahmberg and Hakomori (1975a) have found that, while polyoma-transformed NIL contains much less higher neutral glycolipid than NIL, the remaining glycolipid molecules are more accessible to (or reactive with) added galactose oxidase. That is, the transformed cells incorporate more tritium into each milligram of complex ceramide. The amount of complex ceramide in NIL changes little over the cell cycle (Gahmberg and Hakomori, 1974), but it is more efficiently surface-labeled during G_1 and less during S. The complex ceramide of transformed cells, although reduced in quantity, is labeled well throughout the cell cycle.

The glycolipids of NIL cells, but not of polyoma-transformed NIL, were made more accessible to galactose oxidase–[^{3}H]sodium borohydride labeling by addition of a low concentration of *Ricinus communis* lectin, which binds galactoselike residues (Nicolson *et al.*, 1974). Gahmberg and Hakomori (1975b) suggest that a large glycoprotein of NIL cells, missing from transformed cells (Section 3.1.3), hinders interaction of the galactose oxidase with glycolipid until the glycoprotein is clumped into patches by the lectin.

3.1.3. Proteins and Glycoproteins

In addition to differences in cell surface enzymatic activities (Section 3.2), cancer-associated changes in cell surface proteins have been studied directly. For example, a particular glycoprotein which seems to protect a murine mammary adenocarcinoma from immune killing by allogeneic recipient animals has been shown to be a surface component (Cooper *et al.*, 1974). Most work, however, has been done with tumor virus transformation of cells in culture. Transformed cells are frequently smaller than nontransformed cells of the same strain and so tend to have less protein per cell. Results are generally reported per milligram of cellular protein, or—ignoring possible size differences—per cell. Polyacrylamide gel electrophoresis (PAGE) in the presence of the powerful detergent sodium dodecylsulfate (SDS) resolves complex mixtures of proteins into distinct components, largely according to molecular weight (SDS-PAGE techniques are well reviewed by Maizel, 1971). One may study surface proteins by using isolated membranes or may label the surface proteins of intact cells, disrupt the cells, and study the labeled material.

The most popular surface labeling technique is currently iodination with lactoperoxidase (Phillips and Morrison, 1971). This enzyme uses iodide and hydrogen peroxide to generate a reactive iodine species, which then forms mono- and di-iodo derivatives of "exposed" protein tyrosine residues. Radioactive iodide makes the iodinated proteins easily distinguishable by autoradiography or scintillation counting. Lactoperoxidase (mol wt $\sim$78,000) does not easily penetrate intact cell membranes and so does not label interior proteins of intact cells significantly. It is to be expected, however, that some proteins which are partially exposed on the cell surface will not be labeled, because of steric hindrance to the approach of lactoperoxidase or because the exposed protein segment contains no accessible tyrosine. Also, if a protein cannot be iodinated in isolated or solubilized membranes, no positional inferences may be drawn from failure to iodinate it in whole cells (Stone *et al.*, 1974). Reported molecular weights based on SDS-PAGE may be expected to vary somewhat, especially for glycoproteins (Segrest and Jackson, 1972), and the evidence that particular proteins are glycoproteins—such as coincidence of carbohydrate- and protein-stained bands in PAGE gels—is frequently suggestive rather than definitive.

Gahmberg and Hakomori (1973*b*) have applied galactose oxidase treatment followed by tritiated sodium borohydride (NaB^3H_4) reduction to label galactose and galactosamine residues at the nonreducing termini of cell surface glycoproteins and glycolipids (Section 3.1.2). Other chemical labeling techniques have been developed (Bretscher, 1971*a*; Bender *et al.*, 1971) but with less certainty that the reagents exclusively label surface components. Vidal *et al.* (1974) have reported a procedure for attaching trinitrobenzene to cell surface amino groups. The derivatized proteins can then be isolated by affinity chromatography with insolubilized antibody against the trinitrophenyl moiety. Stein and Berestecky (1975) have developed an arginine-specific label.

Viral transformation of cultured fibroblasts particularly decreases the amount of high molecular weight membrane glycoprotein(s). Transformation of hamster NIL cells substantially reduces the labeling of a glycoprotein of molecular weight about 250,000 daltons ("250 K") with lactoperoxidase (Hynes, 1973) or galactose oxidase–B^3H_4 (Critchley, 1974; Gahmberg and Hakomori, 1973*a*). This glycoprotein or a fragment of it is easily removed from normal cells by trypsinization of intact cells, leading to the designation "large external trypsin-sensitive (LETS) protein." It is more available to surface labeling during the G_1 phase of the cell cycle than in other phases and is better labeled in confluent than in sparse cultures (Hynes, 1974; Hynes and Bye, 1974; Gahmberg and Hakomori, 1974; Pearlstein and Waterfield, 1974). After growth of cells in media containing [^{14}C]fucose or [^{14}C]glucosamine, the 250 K glycoprotein is visible upon autoradiography after SDS-PAGE of extracts of normal but not transformed cells. It therefore seems to be missing from the transformed cells, not simply hidden from lactoperoxidase (Hynes and Humphreys, 1974). Its absence may be caused by surface proteolysis or by decreased synthesis in transformed cells. Transformed BHK cells do release into the medium more of several glycoprotein species, particularly components of high molecular weight, than do untransformed cells, although with unknown degrees of degradation (Voyles and Moskowitz, 1974). Normal 3T3 cells, however, release a 150 K glycoprotein into the medium while transformed cells do not (Sakiyama and Burge, 1972). The 250 K glycoprotein of NIL cells also seems to bear the primary receptors for the lectins Con A and RCA$_1$ (Gahmberg and Hakomori, 1975b). A similar glycoprotein has been reported to be unavailable for surface labeling after transformation of the hamster BHK cell line (Gahmberg et al., 1974[2]; Hynes, 1973). SV40 virus transformation of hamster embryo fibroblasts also decreases the amount of a high molecular weight glycoprotein (Steiner et al., 1973b), as detected by autoradiography after SDS-PAGE of cells grown with [^{14}C]sugars. While a surface location was not demonstrated for this component, most cellular glycoproteins are surface components.

Hogg (1974) found a trypsin-sensitive, 250 K glycoprotein to be lactoperoxidase-iodinated in normal but not transformed mouse 3T3 cells. SDS-PAGE of isolated membrane proteins, followed by a protein stain, gave one wide protein-staining band in normal cells corresponding to the ^{125}I-labeled 250 K glycoprotein. Transformed cells gave three discrete, smaller protein-stained bands in the 250 K region without significant radioactivity. These smaller bands could be related to the 250 K glycoprotein of normal cells, or could simply be lesser components made visible by the absence of the major band. These were the main protein changes found by Hogg (1974), although an earlier study (Sheinin and Onodera, 1972) found more extensive differences between normal and transformed surface proteins. Some differences were seen in the galactose oxidase–B^{3}H$_4$ labeling of normal and transformed mouse cells if the cells were treated with neuraminidase before labeling, but the magnitude of the changes was small (Gahmberg and Hakomori, 1973a). Lactoperoxidase labeling of other tumorigenic mouse lines and of a human HeLa cell line has been reported, but without normal cells for comparison (Huang et al., 1974; Shin and Carraway, 1973; Marchelonis et al., 1971). Decreased amounts of a 210 K protein were found in Rous sarcoma virus transformed rat kidney cells compared to the nontransformed cells (Stone et al., 1974).

A very useful system for studying cellular changes accompanying transformation is the chick embryo fibroblast cell line, with transformation by regular and temperature-sensitive strains of Rous sarcoma virus. Chick embryo fibroblast surface proteins have been studied by several groups, before and after transformation by RSV or by shifting cells infected with temperature-sensitive RSV to the permissive temperature. Transformation-dependent reduction or loss of a large glycoprotein (200–250 K) upon SDS-PAGE has been seen using lactoperoxidase iodination of whole cells (Hynes, 1974; Wickus et al., 1974; Stone et al., 1974), radioactive amino acid incorporation (Stone et al., 1974; Wickus et al., 1974; Wickus and Robbins, 1973), and protein staining (Vaheri and Ruoslahti, 1974; Bussell and Robinson, 1973). A glycoprotein quite similar to that detected by labeling studies has been partially purified (Yamada and Weston, 1974). It is

---

[2] One report that lactoperoxidase labeling does not detect protein changes with transformation (Poduslo et al., 1974) is complicated by the use of trypsinized cells and the presence of relatively high background labeling in the absence of lactoperoxidase. This laboratory did find transformation-dependent reductions in several hamster membrane proteins, as measured by staining of SDS-PAGE gels (Greenberg and Glick, 1972).

probable but not certain that the large glycoprotein detected by each approach is the same—differences in cell lines and in handling techniques may affect the results, particularly with peripheral proteins associated only loosely with the plasma membrane, as the LETS protein may be (Graham et al., 1975).

Beyond the transformation-dependent decrease in labeling and amount of 200–250 K glycoprotein in several cultured cell lines, there is less agreement on protein changes after transformation. Differences in experimental procedure may be more critical with less numerous molecules. An 85 K glycoprotein on hamster NIL cells was better labeled by the galactose oxidase–B^{3}H$_4$ method after transformation (Gahmberg and Hakomori, 1973a), but this difference was seen only with labeling after neuraminidase treatment. Transformation of chick embryo fibroblasts has been reported to increase the amounts of two 70–95 K proteins (Stone et al., 1974). Vaheri and Ruoslahti (1974) also found increases in two similar or identical proteins, as well as decreases in the amount of 145 and 210 K proteins. The latter proteins are the molecular counterparts of a fibroblast surface antigen (also found in serum) which is decreased in amount upon transformation. The larger of these components strongly resembles the high molecular weight glycoprotein revealed by surface labeling (Critchley, 1974; Hynes and Bye, 1974). A similar antigenic protein is found on human fibroblast surfaces (Vaheri and Ruoslahti, 1974).

Before surface-labeling reagents were widely available, Warren and others began studying the glycoprotein fragments released by mild (nonlytic) trypsinization of cultured cells. This work has been reviewed by Warren et al. (1973). Roughly 25% of the cellular sialic acid is released by this treatment without loss of cell viability. After removal of cells, thorough digestion of the trypsinate with pronase leaves glycopeptides (primarily carbohydrate) of around 4000 daltons. Normal cell glycopeptides elute from gel filtration columns in a wide peak, but glycopeptides from several different lines of transformed cells elute as a peak slightly shifted toward higher molecular weight, or with a higher molecular weight shoulder on the main peak, compared to the corresponding normal cell. This shift in the size of protease-released glycopeptides has been found with BHK (Buck et al., 1970), hamster embryo cells (Glick et al., 1974), 3T3 (Meezan et al., 1969), and chick embryo fibroblasts (Lai and Duesberg, 1972; Warren et al., 1972a). A wide-ranging study also found the shift in viral, chemical, and spontaneous transformants of several lymphoblast, fibroblast, and epithelial cell lines (van Beek et al., 1973). Mitotic BHK cells also seem to have more of the larger glycopeptides than nonmitotic cells, although still less than transformed cells (Glick and Buck, 1973). Sakiyama and Burge (1972) have reported that confluent 3T3 cells have less of the larger glycopeptides than do SV40-transformed 3T3 cells but that exponentially growing 3T3 have as much as do the transformed cells.

Treatment of transformed-cell glycopeptides with neuraminidase produces a gel filtration elution pattern quite similar to that of normal-cell glycopeptides (van Beek et al., 1973; Warren et al., 1973). Transformed BHK and chick embryo fibroblasts have a higher sialyltransferase activity specific for the cell surface glycopeptides, compared to untransformed cells, to add the additional sialic acid. Sialyltransferase activity toward added glycoproteins changes little with transformation (Warren *et al.*, 1973). Nongrowing transformed cells have less of the

specific activity, similar to that of growing normal cells, but nongrowing normal cells exhibit still lower activity. The presence of elevated neuraminidase activity in nontransformed, confluent cells has not been precluded, however, and would also explain these results. For example, while transformed 3T3 cells have a higher sialyltransferase activity toward surface glycoproteins, they still have less-sialylated glycoproteins than normal cells, possibly due to higher hydrolytic activities (Bosmann, 1972c, and see Sections 3.2.2 and 3.2.3).

The extra sialylation of transformed cell surface glycopeptides supports the idea that sialic acid changes are involved in transformation, but the importance of the glycopeptide changes is unclear. The number of different glycopeptide species, by size or by carbohydrate composition, in either the main group or the higher molecular weight portion is unknown. The disappearance of the heavier population after neuraminidase treatment does not show increased sialylation to be the only distinctive feature of transformed glycopeptides. For example, the glycoprotein of vesicular stomatitis virus grown in BHK cells gives glycopeptides of the same size distribution as those of virus grown in polyoma-transformed BHK, but the sugar composition and sensitivity to a mixture of glycosidases are different (Moyer and Summers, 1974). Differences have been found in the mixture of carbohydrate–peptide linkage regions of glycopeptides isolated from growing vs. confluent nontransformed human diploid cells (Muramatsu *et al.*, 1973). In addition, decreases in large glycopeptides with transformation can be found in some of the published data (Sakiyama and Burge, 1972; Meezan *et al.*, 1969), and there is a report that while glycoproteins spontaneously released by transformed BHK cells are more glycosylated than those released by normal cells the remaining membrane proteins are less glycosylated in the transformed cells (Chiarugi and Urbano, 1972).

Glick *et al.* (1973) studied the correlation of these glycopeptides with both *in vitro* and *in vivo* criteria of malignancy. They analyzed the glycopeptides of hamster embryo cells, a chemically transformed derivative, a nontransformed second derivative, a retransformed third derivative, and tumors from all these lines. Presence of the heavier glycopeptide fraction correlated well with *in vivo* tumorigenicity, but not with transformed behavior *in vitro* (e.g., growth to high density or growth in soft agar). In addition to dissociating the appearance of the fraction of large glycopeptides from lack of normal growth control *in vitro*, this report also emphasizes the limitations of applying *in vitro* tissue culture studies to the *in vivo* spread of cancer. Further understanding of the significance of the glycopeptide changes may well depend on progress in resolving the present mixture of glycopeptides into distinguishable components, and in relating them to the glycoproteins from which they were cleaved.

3.2. Enzymes

3.2.1. Glycosyltransferases

Glycosyltransferases are the enzymes which catalyze transfer of a sugar residue from a donor, generally a sugar nucleotide such as UDP-D-galactose, to an acceptor, such as the nonreducing terminal sugar of a glycolipid or glycoprotein. Most cellular glycosyltransferase activity is associated with the golgi apparatus, where most glycoproteins receive their oligosaccharide portions. Cell surfaces, however, also seem to contain glycosyltransferases. Roseman (1970) has suggested that intercellular adhesion and communication may involve binding of cell surface enzymes to their substrates on the surfaces of other cells, with or without reaction actually taking place (depending perhaps on availability of cofactors). There is evidence that some surface glycosyltransferases are involved in such communication (Section 3.4.3; Roth, 1973).

Transformation-dependent changes in glycosyltransferase activities have been found in several experimental systems, although the significance of these changes is very difficult to assess. One difficulty is that the enzymes have most often been studied in cell homogenates in the presence of detergent. Assay conditions are therefore very different from *in vivo* reaction conditions, and enzyme activity varies with such parameters as detergent concentration (Mårtensson *et al.*, 1974). The number of different enzymes in any preparation capable of transfering the added sugar donor to the acceptor or acceptors being studied is unknown, as is their normal location on or inside the cell. Whether cell surface acceptors normally glycosylated by the enzymes are similar to those endogenous or exogenous acceptors glycosylated by the homogenate is also unknown. In addition, there is recent evidence that polyisoprenoid lipids may participate in glycosyltransferase reactions as intermediate sugar donors (Dorsey and Roth, 1974; Hsu *et al.*, 1974; Yogeeswaran *et al.*, 1974). Experiments using unbroken cells avoid some of these difficulties—detergents are not required and the measured transferase activities are assumed to reside on the cell surface. It must be remembered, however, that glycosylation of endogenous acceptors by cells (whole or broken) is affected by amount of active enzyme, amount of suitable donor, amount of suitable acceptor, and the mutual accessibility of all three. Deppert *et al.* (1974) conclude that several cell types do *not* have surface-located galactosyltransferase activity, and that reports of such activity have failed to allow for external hydrolysis of UDP-galactose followed by uptake and internal metabolism of the galactose. This conclusion is strongly contradicted by galactosylation by whole cells of glycolipid covalently linked to glass beads (Yogeeswaran *et al.*, 1974; see below). A resolution of the conflict will require further research.

Some glycosyltransferases which use glycolipids as acceptors show marked reductions upon viral transformation. The gangliosides of mouse cell lines have been studied by Brady and Fishman (see their 1974 review for details and primary references) as well as others. Correlating with changes in glycolipid composition accompanying transformation (Section 3.1.2), homogenates of several mouse cell lines transformed by SV40, polyoma, or the Moloney isolate of murine sarcoma virus have substantially decreased N-acetylgalactosaminyltransferase activity, responsible for synthesis of ganglioside G_{M2} from G_{M3} (Fig. 5). There is some viral specificity, as transformation by the Kirsten isolate of murine sarcoma virus causes a reduction in a different enzyme—the galactosyltransferase for the synthesis of G_{M1} from G_{M2}. Morphological revertants regain partially or fully the non-transformed activities. The relevance of ganglioside changes to tumor growth is in question, however, since spontaneously-transformed cell lines do not show these changes. A decrease in the ganglioside N-acetylgalactosaminyltransferase was also seen upon transformation of hamster embryo cells, but morphological reversion did not restore activity (Den *et al.*, 1974). Decreases were reported for several transferase activities in polyoma-transformed BHK cells, with sialyltransferase (CDH → G_{M3}) particularly reduced (Den *et al.*, 1971).

Hakomori and coworkers have studied the neutral glycolipids of hamster cell lines. Correlating with changes in complex ceramides, the α-galactosyltransferase for synthesis of CTH from CDH rose with confluence in normal cells and fell sharply upon transformation (Kijimoto and Hakomori, 1971), while the β-galactosyltransferase (CMH → CDH) did not change with cell density or transformation.

The activities of some cell surface transferases which use lipid acceptors have been measured with unbroken cells and found lower on transformed than normal cells. Viral transformation of 3T3 reduces the transfer of added sialic acid, galactose, and N-acetylgalactosamine from sugar nucleotides to endogenous lipid, while increasing the transfer of mannose (Patt and Grimes, 1974). Polyoma-transformed NIL and BHK whole cells transfer less sialic acid and galactose than do nontransformed cells from added sugar nucleotides or endogenous sugar donors to ceramide dihexoside covalently attached to glass beads or plates (Yogeeswaran *et al.*, 1974). This demonstration argues strongly for cell surface glycosyltransferase activities.

The situation is confused with glycosyltransferases, which use glycoproteins as acceptors—transformation causes both substantial increases and decreases in these activities. Bosmann and Hall (1974) found that homogenates of human breast and colon tumor tissue (not cultured cell lines) have higher sialyltransferase activity toward endogenous or added glycoprotein than do homogenates of the nearest nonmalignant tissue. On the other hand, homogenates of cultured mouse and hamster cell lines transformed spontaneously or by several tumor viruses show reduced sialyltransferase activity toward added glycoprotein (Grimes, 1973). One exception was polyoma-transformed 3T3, while polyoma-transformed BHK and NIL did show the decrease. In each case (including polyoma-transformed 3T3), this activity correlated with the total cellular sialic acid content. Galactose and fucose transferase activities sometimes rose with transformation and sometimes fell.

Using as acceptors the glycoproteins released by mild trypsinization of cells (Section 3.1.3), or the glycopeptides remaining after pronase digestion of these glycoproteins, Warren *et al.* (1972*b*) found that homogenates of growing virally transformed BHK and chick embryo fibroblasts have a higher sialyltransferase activity than do the nontransformed cells. The activity is reduced in all non-growing cells, but transformation still gives higher values. Bosmann (1972*c*) obtained similar results with 3T3, and further found that the glycoproteins released by mild trypsinization of transformed cells are better sialic acid acceptors than those from nontransformed cells, apparently because of a larger proportion of "incomplete" glycoprotein. These results emphasize the specificity of enzyme reactions. If the substrate added to assay an enzyme is not very similar to the natural endogenous substrate, or if the reaction conditions are not similar, any conclusions based on the assay are likely not to represent fully the *in vivo* situation. This danger is particularly apparent when the normal endogenous substrate is not known, and a substitute is chosen on the basis of convenience.

Transformation is reported to increase the glycosylation of endogenous surface glycoproteins by unbroken cells of 3T3 (Patt and Grimes, 1974; Den *et al.*, 1971) and chick embryo fibroblasts (Bosmann *et al.*, 1974*a*). Bosmann (1972*b*) reported the activities to be similar in growing normal and transformed 3T3, but to decrease upon confluence of the normal cells. Roth and White (1972) have suggested that transferases and acceptors on the same cell surface are not accessible to each other, so that glycosylation on normal cell surfaces occurs only when two cells make contact. Transformed cells were suggested to have surface differences such that transferase and acceptor on the same cell surface are accessible to each other, possibly due to increased lateral mobility of the enzyme and/or substrate (Section 3.4.2). Patt and Grimes (1974) were unable to verify these conclusions, but they used a different strain of 3T3 cells and different experimental conditions. It seems certain that some cell surface glycosyltransferase activities do change upon viral transformation of cultured cells, but it is not yet clear how much these changes relate to changes in amount and distribution of enzymes and how much to availability of the appropriate acceptors. Availability of sugar nucleotide donors might also be limiting under at least some conditions *in vivo*.

3.2.2. Proteases

Mild proteolytic treatment—without cell lysis—of confluent nontransformed cells in culture transiently gives the cells several properties attributed to transformed cells. Glucose transport (Section 3.3) and agglutinability with lectins (Section 3.4.2) are increased. Some antigens become more reactive with antibodies (Section 3.1.1) and surface glycoproteins are removed from fibroblasts (Section 3.1.3). The confluent cells may also go through another cell cycle, doubling in number (Burger, 1970; Sefton and Rubin, 1970). These findings have led to hypotheses that proteolysis at the cell surface may be important in normal growth control (discussed by Hynes, 1974, and Talmadge *et al.*, 1974). Increased release of lysosomal and other hydrolytic enzymes at certain stages in the cell cycle of normal cells, and continuously in malignant cells, could cause surface alterations ("sublethal autolysis") necessary for growth or other cell functions (Bosmann *et al.*, 1974*b*; see also Poste, 1972).

Transformed and tumor cell homogenates have elevations in some protease activities compared to normal cells. Using hemoglobin as a substrate, Bosmann and coworkers have found elevations in cathepsin-like (pH 3.4) protease activity in human breast and colon tumor tissue (Bosmann and Hall, 1974) as well as in virally transformed mouse cells (Bosmann, 1972*a*) and chick cells (Bosmann *et al.*, 1974*b*). Neutral (pH 7.4) protease activity was increased with transformation of the mouse cells, but not significantly in the other cases. Using a mixture of exogenous proteins as substrate, Schnebli (1972) found proteolysis by whole cells lower with 3T3 than with transformed 3T3, but equal if the nontransformed cells were first given a mild hypotonic treatment. His results are consistent with surface-associated proteases being more accessible after transformation, rather than being increased in amount. In contrast, nontransformed cells in culture apparently have greater breakdown and replacement of at least some surface proteins when confluent than when growing (Borek et al., 1973; Baker and Humphreys, 1972; but see also Pearlstein and Waterfield, 1974). Minced fragments of some human tumor tissues exhibited higher collagenase activity than healthy tissue, but several other tumors did not (Dresden et al., 1972). The elevated enzymes resembled those isolated from normal human skin.

Transformed cells in culture release a serine protease which has been characterized by Christman and Acs (1974) and Unkeless et al. (1974b). This protease is measured by its conversion of serum plasminogen to the protease plasmin, which in turn hydrolyzes fibrin.[3] This two-step fibrinolysis has been reported to be higher with transformed than with normal cell lines of chick (Weber et al., 1975; Goldberg, 1974), hamster, mouse, and rat fibroblasts (Ossowski et al., 1973a), and also high with three human tumor cell lines (Rifkin et al., 1974). The importance of this activity in cancerous growth is uncertain, since an active fibrinolytic system is necessary but not sufficient for expression of some morphological changes associated with transformation (Ossowski et al., 1974). Also, reduction of fibrinolytic activity, by growth of transformed cells with serum containing endogenous protease inhibitors (Quigley et al., 1974), with plasminogen-depleted serum (Ossowski et al., 1973b), or with a synthetic inhibitor of fibrinolysis (Chou et al., 1974b) still permits growth of transformed cells to a higher density than normal cells. Furthermore, a similar plasminogen activator is released by some nonmalignant mouse cells (Unkeless et al., 1974a). Chou et al. (1974b), using somewhat different assay conditions, have found that nontransformed 3T3 cells cause as much fibrinolysis as do SV40-transformed cells while actively growing, but production by the nontransformed cells decreases at confluence. For those morphological traits which do seem to require activation of plasminogen, the substrate on which plasmin acts is not known. Transformation-dependent fibrinolysis not dependent on serum plasmin has also been found (Chen and Buchanan, 1975).

Reports that protease inhibitors selectively retard the growth of transformed cells (Talmadge et al., 1974; Schnebli, 1974; Schnebli and Burger, 1972; Goetz et al., 1972) gave emphasis to hypotheses that proteases are involved in growth control. More recent work, though, has shown that at least some protease inhibitors affect growth primarily by inhibiting protein *synthesis*, and inhibit growth of normal as well as transformed cells (Chou et al., 1974a,b,c). Schnebli (1974) reported that several protease inhibitors selectively stop the growth of transformed but not normal 3T3 cells, but not at the G_1 stage of the cell cycle. This inhibition is therefore not an imposition of normal growth control, but is more

[3] Some human cancer patients do have abnormal blood clotting (Peck and Reiquam, 1973).

likely a toxicity effect. In addition, protease-induced increases in lectin agglutinability of confluent normal cells can occur without stimulation of cell division (Glynn *et al.*, 1973), and protease stimulation of sugar transport does not reach levels characteristic of transformed cells (Weber *et al.*, 1975).

Lipkin and Knecht (1974) reported that a hamster cell line subject to density-dependent inhibition produces a protein factor which imposes density-dependent inhibition of growth on a related malignant line. The surface of the malignant cells contains an abundance of the protease cathepsin B_1, as measured by binding of fluorescent antibody. The related nonmalignant cell surfaces do not bind this antibody, due to a reduction in either amount or exposure of the surface protein. The protein factor from nonmalignant cells prevents binding of the anticathepsin antibody to the malignant, non-density-inhibited cells (Lipkin, 1974; Lipkin and Knecht, 1974). These results support the hypothesis that surface proteases play a role in the control of cell division.

3.2.3. Glycosidases

Glycosidases are the hydrolytic enzymes which cleave the hemiacetal linkages between sugar residues. If their activities differ between normal and malignant cells, then differences in carbohydrate-containing molecules could result, regardless of whether synthetic rates were similar or different. As with other enzymes, it is difficult to demonstrate that substrates added for activity measurements are representative of normal endogenous substrates. Nitrophenyl sugars are most often used to measure glycosidase activities, for convenience, but it must be recognized that other glycosidic specificities might be seen if other substrates and assay conditions are used. One may draw conclusions based only on the activities actually measured, and should beware of extrapolating to apparently related activities. Measurements are generally made in cell or tissue homogenates, so that no conclusions may be drawn about cellular location of the enzymes, although even soluble enzymes may act on cell surfaces after release into the medium.

Bosmann and Hall (1974) compared glycosidase and protease activities of malignant human tissue with those of the nearest nonmalignant tissue removed from the same patients. Malignant breast and colon tissue homogenates have substantially greater β-galactosidase, α-mannosidase (assayed with nitrophenyl substrates), neuraminidase (sialoglycoprotein substrate), and acid protease (hemoglobin substrate) activities, with lesser increases in other hydrolases. Apparent premalignant lesions give intermediate activities. Histological examination did not show unusual numbers of leukocytes in the malignant tissue, but they are a possible source of the enzymatic activity. Elevated human serum glycosidase levels have been reported with cancer and some other diseases (Woollen and Turner, 1965).

Transformation of cultured cells also increases some cellular glycosidase activities. With glycolipids as substrates, transformation raises α-galactosidase (ceramide trihexoside substrate, Kijimoto and Hakomori, 1971) and neuraminidase (ganglioside substrates, Schengrund *et al.*, 1973) activities in hamster cells, but neuraminidase activity (ganglioside substrates) of a mouse cell line is not increased by transformation (Cumar *et al.*, 1970). With nitrophenyl sugars as substrates, transformation substantially increases several glycosidic activities of mouse (Bosmann, 1972a) and chicken (Bossmann *et al.*, 1974b) cell lines. The elevated enzymes are those commonly associated with lysozomes and could be involved in sublethal autolysis (Section 3.2.2; Bosmann *et al.*, 1974b; Poste, 1972).

3.3. Transport

Cells, both prokaryotic and eukaryotic, have specific mechanisms for transporting polar small molecules through the apolar plasma membrane. Without these transport systems, polar nutrients would enter the cell quite slowly, and polar waste products would tend to accumulate (see Oxender, 1972, for a general transport review).

Viral transformation of cultured animal cells increases some but not all transport activities in every case examined to date. Increased sugar transport is particularly striking and has been well reviewed by Hatanaka (1974). That work is only summarized here, and the reader is referred to Hatanaka's review for details and primary references. Transport of glucose and the glucose analogues 2–deoxyglucose and 3-O-methylglucose are increased about 3–4 times concurrently with morphological appearances of transformation. 2-Deoxyglucose has been used extensively in transport studies because of a belief that it is not metabolized beyond phosphorylation. While Steiner *et al.* (1973b) have now shown 2-deoxyglucose to be incorporated into cellular glycoproteins and glycolipids, transport studies involving less than 30-min incubations are not complicated by significant 2–deoxyglucose metabolism beyond phosphorylation. These incubations may be too long on other grounds, though—Kletzien and Perdue (1974a) have recently reemphasized the necessity of demonstrating actual passage of substrate through the membrane to be rate limiting in transport studies. Transport of mannose, galactose, and glucosamine also rises with transformation, while that of fructose, ribose, deoxyribose, fucose, sucrose, glucose-1-phosphate, and glucose-6-phosphate does not (Hatanaka, 1974).

Despite a report to the contrary (Romano and Colby, 1973), measurements of increased sugar entry with transformation are due to increased transport, not simply to increased phosphorylation (Hatanaka, 1974; Kletzien and Perdue, 1974a). The increases result from increased maximum velocity, with some disagreement remaining over changes in Michaelis constant.

Transformed animal cells also have higher transport activity for some amino acids. Increases were reported for glutamine (Foster and Pardee, 1969), arginine, and glutamic acid (Isselbacher, 1972), with both reports finding higher transport of the amino acid analogues α-aminoisobutyric acid and cycloleucine. Phosphate transport, too, is increased with transformation (Cunningham and Pardee, 1969), insulin (Rozengurt and Jiménez de Asúa, 1973), trypsin (Sefton and Rubin, 1971), or neuraminidase (Vaheri *et al.*, 1972). Stimulation by serum has been studied particularly for the association of transport changes with the release of the growth restriction of quiescent cells, and the possible involvement of cAMP. Addition of serum—which is, of course, a diverse mixture of components—to quiescent chick embryo fibroblasts causes a two-stage increase in 2-deoxyglucose transport capacity (Kletzien and Perdue, 1974b). A doubling of maximum velocity occurs within 10 min, independent of protein and RNA synthesis, and an additional doubling, dependent on protein but not RNA synthesis, is seen in about an hour. Sefton and Rubin (1971) reported a similar increase caused by serum or trypsin, to be completely dependent on protein synthesis, but Fig. 4 of their paper does show a rapid doubling in 2-deoxyglucose transport in the presence of cycloheximide (Rubin and Fodge, 1974; Kletzien and Perdue, 1974b). Serum addition to quiescent 3T3 cells also increases the transport of phosphate and uridine (Rozengurt and Jiménez de Asúa, 1973; Cunningham and Pardee, 1969).

Addition of serum to quiescent cells sharply reduces the intracellular level of cAMP, and there is evidence for involvement of cyclic nucleotide changes in growth control. The evidence for association of decreases in cAMP levels with stimulation of mammalian cell growth has been reviewed by Abell and Monahan (1973; see also Bannai and Sheppard, 1974, and Pardee et al., 1974). Recent work also suggests that increases in cGMP may stimulate growth (Seifert and Rudland, 1974; Rudland et al., 1974), although Hovi et al. (1974) have concluded that neither cyclic purine nucleotide has a specific role in the growth control of chick embryo fibroblasts.

The increase in uridine transport after serum addition to quiescent cells does seem to be dependent on an intervening fall in cAMP, but the increase in phosphate transport seems not to depend on this fall (Jiménez de Asúa et al., 1974; Rozengurt and Jiménez de Asúa, 1973). The rapid increase in sugar transport with serum addition or with transformation also seems not to depend on cAMP changes (Hatanaka, 1974; Kletzien and Perdue, 1974a,b). Dibutyryl cAMP does reduce the 2-deoxyglucose transport of polyoma-transformed 3T3 cells to the 3T3 level and stop the growth of the transformed cells, but the growth restriction is not a restoration of the nontransformed-type density-dependent inhibition (Grimes and Schroeder, 1973). Paul (1973) suggests that dibutyryl cAMP retards the growth of transformed 3T3 cells by inhibiting leucine transport.

Some thought has been given to the possibility that the transport changes which do not depend on the fall in cAMP levels could actually be responsible for that fall (Jiménez de Asúa et al., 1974). Kasărov and Friedman (1974) have found that the sodium–potassium dependent adenosine triphosphatase activity (Na^+-K^+-ATPase) of mouse and rat fibroblasts is four- to five-fold higher after transformation. While transport measurements were not made, this enzymatic activity is normally closely associated with the coupled transport of sodium out of and potassium into cells. Transport measurements by Kimelberg and Mayhew (1975) support these observations. Kasărov and Friedman suggest that the reduction in cAMP in transformed cells is due to competition of adenyl cyclase (which synthesizes cAMP) with greatly increased Na^+-K^+-ATPase for limited amounts of the precursor, ATP. They further suggest that the sodium fluoride stimulation of adenyl cyclase in crude preparations and the stimulation of animal cell cAMP levels by some bacterial toxins result from inhibition of Na^+-K^+-ATPase. These interesting ideas will no doubt encourage further progress.

Small quantitative transport changes might affect cells' ability to grow when nutrient concentrations are marginal. Pardee (Pardee et al., 1974; Pardee, 1964) and Holley (1972, 1974) have suggested that transport changes are very important in the escape of malignant cells from normal growth control. Holley suggested that a primary change in conversion to malignancy is an increase in cellular ability to transport from the medium various molecules which stimulate growth. Pardee et al. (1974) suggest that transformation causes a permanent cell surface change inhibiting adenyl cyclase. The resulting drop in cAMP would increase the uptake of various components of the medium—stimulating transport either directly or by membrane changes—so that nutrients would be less likely to fall below the critical minimum concentrations which would cause a regulatory mechanism (Pardee, 1974) to stop cell growth at the restriction point during G_1 of the cell cycle. However, in contact-inhibited nontransformed cells (stopped at the presumed restriction point: Pardee et al., 1974) stimulated with serum, some transport changes do not depend on cAMP changes (Kletzien and Perdue, 1974a; Jiménez de Asuá et al., 1974; Rozengurt and Jiménez de Asúa, 1973). The hypothesis of Pardee et al. (1974) should probably be adapted, therefore, to include other controls of cAMP level or other effectors between a primary membrane change and transport activity. While it is not possible at present to demonstrate a primary cellular change among the many changes found with malignancy, the hypotheses of Holley (1972) and of Pardee et al. (1974) have helped greatly in focusing attention on cell surface changes in cancer. Transport measurements require particularly close attention to comparing cells grown and treated as similarly as possible, making studies with actual human cancer cells, as opposed to cultured cell lines, quite difficult. Nevertheless, progress in understanding the importance of transport activities in growth control calls for these studies.

3.4. Other Surface Properties

3.4.1. Electrokinetic Properties of Tumor Cells

The charge characteristics of normal and tumor cells have been measured by examining their electrophoretic mobilities, which reflect the ζ-potential of a cell at its hydrodynamic slip plane (border between the bulk fluid and the fluid moving with the cell: see Mehrishi, 1972, or Weiss, 1967). Early literature indicated higher surface charge densities on tumor cells than on similar normal cells. Ambrose et al. (1956) and Lowick et al. (1961) found higher electrophoretic mobilities for malignant cells from solid tumors than for their normal analogues. Forrester (1963) found that the mean electrophoretic mobilities of "normal" and polyoma-transformed hamster kidney fibroblasts were approximately equivalent, but that the spread of mobilities was much greater with the transformed cells. Neuraminidase treatment lowered the mobility of the normal and transformed cells to the same level, indicating that the difference in electrophoretic mobility was due to more sialic acid residues on the tumor cell surfaces. Fuhrmann (1963) obtained similar results with normal and malignant rat liver cells—only the malignant cell mobilities were reduced with neuraminidase.

Other investigators have reported higher cell surface charge densities on tumor cells (Simon-Reuss *et al.*, 1964; Doljanski and Eisenberg, 1963), but several have failed to find a correlation between malignancy and increased electrophoretic mobility. Mehrishi and Thomson (1968) and Thomson and Mehrishi (1969) failed to find differences between the electrophoretic mobilities of normal human lymphocytes and a variety of leukemia cells, and several other studies have confirmed these results (Schubert *et al.*, 1973; Lichtman and Weed, 1970; Patinkin *et al.*, 1970). Vassar (1963) examined several different types of human solid tumors (including cells from malignant epithelium and mesenchyma) and their normal cell counterparts. The cells were dispersed by mechanical means and their electrophoretic mobilities were determined, with no significant differences found between tumor cells and normal cells from the tissue of origin of the tumor.

A serious complication in the determination of cell surface charge density and surface biochemistry as well is the variation in surface properties with the stage of the cell cycle. Mayhew (1966) found that normal and tumor cell electrophoretic mobility varies with the cell cycle and is highest at mitosis. He also found that neuraminidase treatment of cells at any phase of the cycle results in a reduction of mobility to a common level. Also, cell electrophoretic mobility varies with temperature.

In conclusion, although some tumor cells have higher surface charge densities than their normal cell counterparts, enhanced electrophoretic mobility does not seem to be a general characteristic of malignant cells.

3.4.2. Antigens and Lectin Receptors

Cells transformed *in vitro* or *in vivo* have been characterized by the appearance of new tumor-specific transplantation antigens (TSTA) on their surfaces. Presumably, TSTA serve a function in establishing or maintaining the tumor cell in the transformed state. TSTA are capable of eliciting humoral or cellular tumor-specific immune responses in autochthonous or syngeneic hosts. Although TSTA may play an important role in the immune destruction of tumor cells bearing them, these antigens are not well characterized (Meltzer *et al.*, 1972). Other surface antigens appear after transformation and these may represent derepressed host antigens (in some cases embryonic antigens) or virus-coded surface antigens that are not part of the tumor virus's antigenic structure (Black, 1968). This latter property has been demonstrated immunologically by the lack of effect of antiviral antibodies on tumor growth or direct complement-mediated cytotoxicity. Also, some tumor cells appear to be free of infectious virus and viral antigens (Butel *et al.*, 1972; Khera *et al.*, 1963). Certain tumor cells may express normal surface antigens in abnormally high or low amounts (Lengerová, 1972), or they can express virus-specific antigens, particularly if viruses are being released from the cell. Since the antigens of tumor cells form the topic of other chapters, they will

not be discussed in detail here. Detailed information can also be found in reviews by Boyse (1973), Klein (1973), Old and Boyse (1973), Butel *et al.*, (1972), and Coggin and Anderson (1974).

Another property of cells after transformation is an increase in agglutinability by plant lectins, proteins and glycoproteins that bind specific saccharide determinants (for review, see Nicolson, 1974a; Burger, 1973; Lis and Sharon, 1973). Aub *et al.* (1963, 1965a,b) found that a wheat germ (*Triticum vulgaris*) preparation agglutinated certain transformed cells but not their normal counterparts. Burger and Goldberg (1967) purified the agglutinating activity and characterized the responsible molecule as a lectin, wheat germ agglutinin (WGA), that binds to cell surface N–acetyl-D-glucosamine-like residues. To explain the difference in lectin-mediated agglutination between normal and transformed cells, Burger (1969) advanced the theory that the agglutinability of transformed cells was due to an exposure of "cryptic" lectin binding sites during transformation. The sites were reasoned to be cryptic or masked on normal cells because brief proteolysis rendered normal cells as agglutinable as transformed cells but did not enhance the agglutinability of transformed cells (Burger, 1969).

A variety of alternate theories have been proposed to explain differential agglutinability by lectins and to account for the subsequent finding that normal, protease-treated, and transformed cells have equivalent numbers of lectin receptors per cell (Phillips *et al.*, 1974; Nicolson, 1973a, 1975; Barbarese *et al.*, 1973; Inbar *et al.*, 1972; Arndt-Jovin and Berg, 1971; Cline and Livingston, 1971; Ozanne and Sambrook, 1971) with transformed cells having even fewer receptors in one case (Nicolson *et al.*, 1975). Inbar *et al.* (1972) proposed that cell agglutination is due to special metabolically linked lectin agglutination sites (distinct from lectin binding sites) which are altered on the transformed cell surface. Simultaneously, it was proposed that the difference in agglutinability might be due to a clustering in the topographic distribution of lectin binding sites that allows multiple lectin cross-bridging between adjacent cells (Nicolson, 1971).

Fluorescent, ferritin, peroxidase, and hemocyanin labeling techniques have been used to determine the distribution and mobility of lectin binding sites on normal and transformed cells. Although several investigators did not report differences in the distribution of Con A binding sites using fluorescent Con A (Shoham and Sachs, 1972; Mallucci, 1971; Cline and Livingston, 1971; Ozanne and Sambrook, 1971) or hemocyanin–Con A (Smith and Revel, 1972), Nicolson (1971) reported that ferritin–Con A binds to mounted SV40-transformed 3T3 cell membranes at 20°C in more clustered distribution than to 3T3 cell membranes, and proposed that the more clustered Con A receptor state is responsible for the differential agglutination of transformed cells. Using Con A–peroxidase techniques, Martinez-Palomo *et al.* (1972) and Bretton *et al.* (1972) found that normal, polyoma-, and SV40-transformed hamster cell lines bind Con A–peroxidase, but the peroxidase product is generally more patchy on the transformed cells labeled at room temperature than at 0°C. Also, two adenovirus-12 hamster tumor lines of differing malignancy were discontinuously labeled with Con A–peroxidase compared to the normal parental line (Huet and Bernhard,

1974; Rowlatt *et al.*, 1973). Francois *et al.* (1972) used peroxidase-coupled Con A and WGA to study the surface distribution of lectin binding sites on normal and transformed human fibroblasts and found patchy distribution on some cells but uniform distribution on others. Similar observations were made by Huet and Bernhard (1974) using WGA–peroxidase labeling. The fact that uniform rather than clustered Con A or WGA distributions have been found on some transformed cell lines, although they are more agglutinable, suggests that other surface properties must also be important in determining lectin agglutinability. In particular, transformed rat embryonic fibroblasts labeled with Con A–peroxidase at room temperature do not show dramatic clustering of their Con A binding sites (Garrido *et al.*, 1974; Roth *et al.*, 1973; Bretton *et al.*, 1972).

Protease treatment of normal cells renders them as agglutinable by lectins as transformed cells, but does not increase the number of lectin binding sites (Cuatrecasas, 1973; Nicolson, 1973*a*; Ozanne and Sambrook, 1971; Inbar *et al.*, 1971). Nicolson (1972) examined briefly trypsinized 3T3 cells and found clustering of ferritin–Con A sites. The clustered Con A sites were reasoned to be directly involved in cell agglutination, because trypsinized cells specifically agglutinated with ferritin–Con A into small cell aggregates, which when carefully removed, fixed, and embedded in plastic had high concentrations of ferritin between adjacent agglutinated cells as seen by electron microscopy of thin sections. The agglutination was reversible by α-methyl-D-mannoside, and the ferritin reagent was not nonspecifically trapped between agglutinated cells. This latter control was performed using another lectin to agglutinate trypsinized cells in ferritin–Con A solutions containing α-methyl-D-mannoside, and the ferritin reagent was not trapped between agglutinated cells. These results were also found with SV3T3 cells (Nicolson, 1974*b*).

Mobile lectin sites are directly involved in the agglutination of cells at room temperature, but the clusters seem to arise from a uniform distribution by lectin-induced effects on the cell surface. Inbar and Sachs (1973) and Nicolson (1973*b*) used fluorescent Con A to show that transformed cells have inherently dispersed distributions of their Con A binding sites at low temperature (or on aldehyde-fixed cells), and these dispersed sites can rearrange into clusters at or above room temperature in the presence of Con A. Normal cells seem to have dispersed distributions of Con A binding sites which do not dramatically cluster with lectin, even in several minutes at 37°C. Similar results were obtained by Rosenblith *et al.* (1973) and Garrido *et al.* (1974) using Con A–hemocyanin techniques on 3T3 and SV3T3 cells labeled *in situ*. They found, on transformed cells labeled at low temperature and subsequently warmed, that rearrangement of cell surface-bound Con A occurred, ranging from uniform, random distributions to clustered distributions. These results seem to indicate a difference in the relative mobility of Con A binding sites on transformed cells at and above room temperature.

The relative mobilities of antigens on normal and transformed cells have been studied with the aid of fusion heterokaryons. Edidin and Weiss (1974) used techniques developed earlier by Frye and Edidin (1970) to study the mobility and

restriction of mobility of antigens on mouse and human normal and transformed cells and their normal–transformed fusion heterokaryons. The normal cells they examined failed to form caps after incubation with antisera and anti-immunoglobulin, but several transformed cells capped readily under identical conditions in suspension or on substrate. When intermixing of antigens on mouse–human heterokaryons was followed, normal–normal heterokaryons failed to intermix within the time of the experiment, transformed–transformed heterokaryons mixed rapidly, and normal–transformed heterokaryons showed intermediate rates.

Differences in the relative mobility of antigens and lectin binding sites on certain transformed cells could be due to a variety of possible membrane changes after transformation: (1) the intrinsic fluidity of the lipid bilayer could be increased after transformation; (2) the antigen or the lectin binding determinant could be structurally modified by transformation to a component which is more readily crosslinked or diffuses more rapidly in the membrane; or (3) there could be alterations in peripheral structures attached at the inner or outer membrane surface which influence the mobility of lectin binding or antigenic membrane components. Proposals (1) and (2) seem less likely than (3).

Extraction and analysis of phospholipids from normal and Rous sarcoma virus transformed chick embryo cells have revealed little change in lipid composition (Quigley *et al.*, 1974) (see Section 3.1.2), although Yau and Weber (1974) have demonstrated some changes in acyl group composition correlating with transformation and density-dependent inhibition of growth. The percentage of arachidonate drops after transformation and a roughly equivalent increase occurs in oleate, but the ratio of total saturated to unsaturated fatty acids—a rough indication of fluidity—remains approximately constant. These results argue against a general increase in lipid fluidity after transformation. Electron spin resonance experiments have confirmed the lack of change in fluidity. Buckman and Weber (1975) used stearic acid nitroxide analogues to show that plasma membranes of Rous sarcoma virus transformed chick cells are slightly less fluid than those of exponentially growing normal cells, and Gaffney (1975) did not find differences in fluidity between normal and transformed mouse and chick cell plasma membranes.

There is some evidence, however, suggesting that lectin receptors are modified after cell transformation. Jansons and Burger (1973) isolated and partially purified a lectin binding receptor for wheat germ agglutinin (WGA) from L-1210 mouse leukemia cells and found that antisera made against the WGA receptor reacted with the L-1210 leukemia, but not with normal lymphocytes. The antisera also reacted with polyoma virus transformed BHK and 3T3 cells, but the nontransformed BHK and 3T3 were not examined. The failure of normal lymphocytes to agglutinate with WGA after trypsinization is in contrast with the behavior of several other cell types, so it is not clear to what extent the antiserum observations may be applied to other systems. Dievard and Bourrillon (1974) purified the *Robinia* lectin receptor released from normal and transformed hepatic cells by trypsin treatment. The glycoprotein lectin receptors from the tumor cells differed from those of normal cells.

Substantial data exist for the proposal that peripheral membrane components interfere with the mobility of specific surface receptors. Yin *et al.* (1972) found that microtubule-disrupting drugs, such as colchicine and vinblastine, affect Con A mediated agglutinability of fibroblasts and also of polymorphonuclear leukocytes (Berlin and Ukena, 1972). At the concentration used (10^{-6} M), these drugs should not have drastic effects directly on the lipid bilayer (Seaman *et al.*, 1973), but this point has to be carefully ruled out. When Ukena *et al.* (1974) examined the topography of Con A receptors on 3T3 and SV40-transformed 3T3 (SV3T3) cells by the Con A–hemocyanin replica technique, they found that colchicine treatment causes changes in cell shape (rounding) and leads to the formation of lectin-induced caplike aggregates of Con A receptors near the center of the rounded cell body. These drug-induced alterations in cell morphology are linked to cytoplasmic microtubules.

Maintenance of membrane shape and topography and the role of cytoplasmic peripheral and membrane-associated components in this process are not well defined, but available morphological and biochemical data support the hypothesis that a cell-membrane-associated microfilament–microtubule system is involved. McNutt *et al.* (1967) found that growing, sparse 3T3 cells do not have as extensive a microfilament–microtubule system associated with the plasma membrane as confluent 3T3 cells. SV3T3 cells had less membrane-associated filament network than either sparse of confluent 3T3, but a flat revertant of the transformed cells was morphologically similar to 3T3. In this system, microfilament–microtubule proteins may restrain the mobility of surface receptors that are linked to peripheral components across the membrane (transmembrane control). Recently it was noted that Con A receptor sites in confluent 3T3 cell membranes are less easily aggregated by ferritin-Con A in regions of high submembrane density of microfilaments than are sites in other regions (Nicolson, 1975). This observation may, in part, explain the decrease in lectin-mediated agglutinability of 3T3 cells at confluency (Nicolson, 1974*b*).

Evidence for microfilament–microtubule involvement in transmembrane control of surface topography also comes from experiments with drugs such as dibutyryl cAMP and cytochalasin B. Hsie *et al.* (1971) found that dibutyryl cAMP treatment converts CHO cells to fibroblastic morphology and lowers WGA-mediated agglutination (similar results were reported by Willingham and Pastan, 1974, for 3T3 and L-929 cells); these effects are reversed by microtubule-disrupting drugs (Hsie and Puck, 1971), implicating their involvement in cell surface regulation. Similarly, Kram and Tomkins (1973) found that dibutyryl cAMP inhibits transport of uridine, leucine, and 2-deoxyglucose in 3T3 cells, and colcemid and vinblastine, but not cytochalasin B, counteract these effects. Cytochalasin B is reported to break up cell microfilament systems (Wessells *et al.*, 1971; Schroeder, 1968) and to modify the lectin-mediated agglutination of some types of cells (Loor, 1973, Kaneko *et al.*, 1973). However, results of cytochalasin B

disruption of cell microfilament systems and alteration of the surface display of
membrane components will have to be verified by alternate means due to recent
findings that cytochalasin B also modifies certain membrane transport systems
(Kletzien and Perdue, 1973).

Changes in lectin-mediated tumor cell agglutinability do not necessarily correlate with tumorigenicity. Dent and Hillcoat (1972) found no difference in agglutinability among three murine lymphomas of differing malignant potential when assayed with Con A or *Phaseolus vulgaris* lectin, and Gantt *et al.* (1969) found no correlation between WGA-mediated agglutination and malignancy of several ascites tumor cells. These results indicate that there are presently no set rules or criteria by which cells can be unambiguously assayed for tumorigenicity by their lectin agglutinability. This lack is understandable, since the survival of a tumor *in vivo* depends on many factors which are undoubtedly different for each type of tumor. Also, host immunological pressures may select for certain cell types during *in vivo* tumor growth which may or may not be related to specific lectin binding sites at the cell surface.

3.4.3. Adhesiveness

Adhesion is the attachment of cells to each other to form small groups of cells in the simplest case, or tissues and organs in more complex cases (reviewed by Curtis, 1967). Little is known about the cell surface structures involved in mammalian cell adhesion, but evidence suggests the involvement of cell surface carbohydrates. Oppenheimer *et al.* (1969) found *in vitro* aggregation of an ascites-grown teratoma to be dependent on the cellular utilization of saccharide precursors. Oppenheimer (1973) has extended this work to several different types of tumor cells and found requirements for complex cell surface oligosaccharides in adhesion. Chipowsky *et al.* (1973) recently showed that SV40-transformed mouse fibroblasts adhere *in vitro* to D-galactose attached covalently to Sephadex beads, but not to D-glucose or N-acetyl-D-glucosamine similarly derivatized. Adhesion of cells to the sugar-coated beads causes changes in the cells which promote cell–cell adhesion, forming large aggregates containing cells and beads. Nontransformed 3T3 cells also bind to the galactose-derivatized beads, although somewhat less well than the transformed cells.

It might be supposed that successful cancer cells should have reduced self-attachment (homotypic adhesion), for an easy release and spread of cells from the primary tumor, and increased attachment to other kinds of cells (heterotypic adhesion) to promote the attachment and growth of secondary tumors (Nicolson and Winkelhake, 1975*a,b*). It seems likely that differing degrees of adhesion may be more important in determining rates of spread of cancer, rather than determining malignancy vs. normality, but some evidence does suggest differences in adhesion between normal and neoplastic cells.

The first experimental evidence for malignancy-related differences in adhesive properties came from Coman (1944), who proposed that malignant cells are less adhesive than their normal counterparts. Coman (1944) studied adhesion by mechanically separating normal and tumor cells using glass micro-needles—adhesion forces could be estimated by the curvatures produced in the calibrated needles during cell separation. When malignant skin and cervix cells were compared to benign skin papillomas, normal skin, and normal cervix uteri cells, the separation forces estimated by needle curvatures were 3–5 times higher for normal cells than for malignant cells. Benign tumor cells were intermediate in adhesion between the normal and malignant cells. Using an approach which measured the mechanical force required to disaggregate cells from cell clumps suspended in physiological buffers, McCutcheon *et al.* (1948) found that malignant cell masses were dispersed more easily and more quickly than normal cell aggregates.

Dorsey and Roth (1973) have tested the decreased-adhesiveness hypothesis with mouse fibroblasts grown in culture, using the aggregate-cell capture assay of Roth *et al.* (1971). This assay measures the number of cells in a single-cell suspension which adhere to aggregates of the same (homotypic) or different (heterotypic) cells circulating in the suspension. The interactions of mouse 3T3 fibroblasts and two malignant derivatives transformed spontaneously (3T12) and by SV40 virus (SV3T3) were studied. The aggregate-cell capture assay showed the malignant SV3T3 cells to be more adhesive, both homo- and heterotypically, than normal 3T3 cells, but the 3T12 malignant line to be somewhat less adhesive than 3T3. Nonmalignant revertants of SV3T3 resembled 3T3 cells rather than SV3T3. However, Dorsey and Roth (1973) also found that another assay for adhesion (Curtis and Greaves, 1965)—the loss of single cells from a homogeneous suspension—showed no difference in the homotypic adhesion of 3T3, 3T12, and SV3T3 cells. This discrepancy implies that the two assays for adhesiveness measure somewhat different phenomena. The authors conclude that adhesiveness does not correlate with malignancy. Unfortunately, the cells studied had been harvested by trypsin treatment—a questionable technique for adhesion assays because of the proteolytic removal of cell surface material (Weiss, 1958).

Dorsey and Roth (1973) also found that single 3T3 cells from sparse cultures were collected significantly better by 3T3 aggregates than were 3T3 cells from confluent cultures, indicating cell density differences in the surface properties of 3T3 cells. Aggregates of 3T12 or SV3T3 cells seemed less able to recognize the differences in these properties, and the authors suggest the malignant cells to be defective, not in intercellular adhesion, but in intercellular recognition. The change in adhesive properties of 3T3 cells with cell density (after cell contact) in tissue culture may be related to several other surface changes seen in culture after contact of normal but not malignant cells. These changes include decrease in transport activity (Section 3.3), accumulation of specific proteins (Pfieffer *et al.*, 1971), extension of glycolipids (Section 3.1.2), loss of antigen reactivity (Hakomori and Kijimoto, 1972), changes in glycosyltransferase activity (Section 3.2.1; Roth and White, 1972) and increases in certain lectin receptors (Nicolson and Lacorbiere, 1973).

Adhesion properties of metastatic tumor cells are most likely important in determining where they will spread *in vivo* (see Chapter 3). When Winkelhake and Nicolson (1975) studied the adhesive properties of low, intermediate, and

high metastatic B16 melanoma variant cell lines selected for pulmonary lung
metastasis by Fidler (1973), they found that the high metastatic B16 variants that
possessed enhanced metastatic behavior *in vivo* had increased homotypic and
heterotypic adhesive properties. Thus the proposal of Coman (1944) that
decreased homotypic adhesion accompanies tumor spread may not be correct as a
general proposal. The increased heterotypic adhesion of the metastatic
melanoma variants appears to be important in determining the target site for
secondary tumor implantation and subsequent growth. Nicolson and Winkelhake
(1975a,b) found that the high metastatic B16 variants adhered much more
strongly to lung cells (target organ) than intermediate or low metastatic variants,
but did not adhere well to non-target-organ cells (liver, spleen, kidney, heart, etc.).
Cell adhesion may be one of the most important factors in determining the organ
specificity of pulmonary tumor spread.

Roseman (1970) has proposed that cell adhesion is dependent on the noncovalent binding of cell surface glycosyltransferase molecules (Section 3.2.1) to the
complementary acceptor molecules on adjacent cells. A large number of these
weak interactions would, on the average, be needed to hold cells together,
although the individual enzyme–substrate complexes might be constantly forming and dissociating. If the affinity of the transferase for acceptor is reduced upon
glycosylation of the acceptor, the adhesive bonds would tend to be broken by this
glycosylation. In that case, adhesion could be maintained by a restricted supply of
sugar donor (Roth, 1973) or by glycosidase restoration of the higher-affinity
acceptor. Freshly aggregated cells could be dissociated, then, by a mixture of
several sugar nucleotides in high concentration, although adhesion might still be
maintained if a limited supply of lipid sugar donors functions between the sugar
nucleotides and the acceptors (Section 3.2.1) or if additional kinds of cell–cell
bonds are formed in the process of adhesion. There is, however, no *a priori* reason
to assume that a transferase has a lower affinity for its glycosyl acceptor after
glycosylation than before, so that catalysis of the sugar transfer might not make a
difference in the cell–cell bond at all. There is evidence for involvement of cell
surface glycosyltransferases in the adhesion of embryonic neural retina cells to
each other and of blood platelets to collagen (reviewed by Roth, 1973). Glycosyltransferases and their changes in cancer are discussed in Section 3.2.1. If
malignant cells have reduced adhesiveness, this theory might explain the reduction by an increased binding of glycosyltransferase molecules to sugar acceptors
on the same cell surface (Roth and White, 1972). The proposal of Roseman (1970)
that cell surface glycosyltransferases play a key role in cellular adhesion has not yet
been proven or disproven, but it has stimulated the study of cell surface
enzymology.

Another approach to the study of mammalian cell adhesion has been the
isolation from cells of specific macromolecules that mediate adhesion in defined
assays. For example, Garber and Moscona (1972; see also Hausman and Moscona,
1973) have isolated a mouse cerebrum factor which specifically causes aggregation
of suspended mouse and chick cerebrum cells, but not of cells from other brain

regions or from nonnervous tissue. Modifications in the abundance or availability of such adhesion factors on the cell surface might alter cell recognition and adhesion of cancer cells.

4. Conclusion

Several cell surface changes have been suggested to accompany the transformation of normal cells to malignancy: varying changes in glycosaminoglycans, proteins, and enzyme activities; decreases in complex glycolipids and possibly adhesiveness; increases in exposure of glycolipids, mobilities of some membrane components, cell agglutinability by lectins, and transport activities. None of these changes has been shown to be the primary distinction of all cancer cells; indeed, no such single primary distinction may exist.

Much success has been realized in the past from the use of model systems which are rather easy to grow *in vitro* such as fibroblasts transformed by tumor virus. However, relatively few human tumors are fibroblastic, and further progress would no doubt be aided by refinements in the culture of other types of tissue. The use of primary cultures with and without high-efficiency transformation by certain tumor viruses avoids some problems found in the past with changes in established cell lines over many generations in culture. Some other relatively new approaches which we feel will be very productive in the future are the isolation of variant tumor cell lines with definable surface alterations and the use of temperature-sensitive cell and virus (transformation) variants.

We have described in this chapter current ideas of normal animal cell surface structure and function, and many of the surface changes which have been suggested to be related to neoplasia. We hope that gathering this information will encourage the integration of it and subsequent data into a more coherent understanding of the complexities of cancer.

ACKNOWLEDGMENTS

We are grateful to Drs. R. Brady, P. Fishman, B. Gaffney, C. G. Gahmberg, S. Hakomori, G. Lipkin, M. J. Weber, and T. M. Yau, who sent us data prior to publication. We would also like to thank our colleagues for helpful discussions, and particularly Ms. Adele Brodginski for extensive help with the manuscript.

5. References

ABELL, C. W., AND MONAHAN, T. M., 1973, The role of adenosine 3′,5′-cyclic monophosphate in the regulation of mammalian cell division, *J. Cell Biol.* **59**:549.

AMBROSE, E. J., JAMES, A. M., AND LOWICK, J. H. B., 1956, Differences between the electrical charge carried by normal and homologous tumour cells, *Nature (London)* **177**:576.

ARNDT-JOVIN, D. J., AND BERG, P., 1971, Quantitative binding of ^{125}I-concanavalin A to normal and transformed cells, *J. Virol.* **8**:716.

AUB, J. C., TIESLAU, C., AND LANKESTER, A., 1963, Reaction of normal and tumor cell surfaces to enzymes. I. Wheat-germ lipase and associated mucopolysaccharides, *Proc. Natl. Acad. Sci. U.S.A.* **50:**613.

AUB, J. C., SANFORD, B. H., AND COTE, M. N., 1965a, Studies on reactivity of tumor and normal cells to a wheat germ agglutinin, *Proc. Natl. Acad. Sci. U.S.A.* **54:**396.

AUB, J. C., SANFORD, B. H., AND WANG, L., 1965b, Reactions of normal and leukemic cell surfaces to a wheat germ agglutinin, *Proc. Natl. Acad. Sci. U.S.A.* **54:**400.

AVRUCH, J., AND FAIRBANKS, G., 1972, Demonstration of a phosphopeptide intermediate in the Mg^{++}-dependent, Na^+- and K^+-stimulated adenosine triphosphate reaction of the erythrocyte membrane, *Proc. Natl. Acad. Sci. U.S.A.* **69:**1216.

BAKER, J. B., AND HUMPHREYS, T., 1972, Turnover of molecules which maintain the normal surfaces of contact-inhibited cells, *Science* **175:**905.

BANNAI, S., AND SHEPPARD, J. R., 1974, Cyclic AMP, ATP and cell contact, *Nature (London)* **250:**62.

BARBARESE, E., SAUERWEIN, H., AND SIMKINS, H., 1973, Alteration in the surface glycoproteins of chick erythrocytes following transformation with erythroblastosis strain R virus, *J. Membr. Biol.* **13:**129.

BARKER, S. A., STACEY, M., TIPPER, D. J., AND KIRKHAM, J. H., 1959, Some observations on certain mucoproteins containing neuraminic acid, *Nature (London)* **184:**BA68.

BENDER, W. W., GARAN, H., AND BERG, H. C., 1971, Proteins of the human erythrocyte membrane as modified by pronase, *J. Mol. Biol.* **58:**783.

BENEDETTI, E. L., AND EMMELOT, P., 1967, Studies on plasma membranes. IV. The ultrastructural localization and content of sialic acid in plasma membranes isolated from rat liver and hepatoma, *J. Cell Sci.* **2:**499.

BERLIN, R. D., 1972, Effect of concanavalin A on phagocytosis, *Nature New Biol.* **235:**44.

BERLIN, R. D., AND UKENA, T. E., 1972, Effect of colchicine and vinblastine on the agglutination of polymorphonuclear leucocytes by concanavalin A, *Nature New Biol.* **238:**120.

BLACK, P. N., 1968, The oncogenic DNA viruses: A review of *in vitro* transformation studies, *Ann. Rev. Microbiol.* **22:**391.

BLASIE, J. K., AND WORTHINGTON, C. R., 1969, Planar liquid-like arrangement of photopigment molecules in frog retinal receptor disk membrane, *J. Mol. Biol.* **39:**417.

BLAUROCK, A. E., 1971, Structure of the nerve myelin membrane: Proof of the low-resolution profile, *J. Mol. Biol.* **56:**35.

BOREK, C., GROB, M., AND BURGER, M. M., 1973, Surface alterations in transformed epithelial and fibroblastic cells in culture: A disturbance of membrane degradation versus biosynthesis? *Exp. Cell Res.* **77:**207.

BOSMANN, H. B., 1972a, Elevated glycosidases and proteolytic enzymes in cells transformed by RNA tumor virus, *Biochim. Biophys. Acta* **264:**339.

BOSMANN, H. B., 1972b, Cell surface glycosyl transferases and acceptors in normal and RNA- and DNA-virus transformed fibroblasts, *Biochem. Biophys. Res. Commun.* **48:**523.

BOSMANN, H. B., 1972c, Sialyl transferase activity in normal and RNA- and DNA-virus transformed cells utilizing desialyzed, trypsinized cell plasma membrane external surface glycoproteins as exogenous acceptors, *Biochem. Biophys. Res. Commun.* **49:**1256.

BOSMANN, H. B., AND HALL, T. C., 1974, Enzyme activity in invasive tumors of human breast and colon, *Proc. Natl. Acad. Sci. U.S.A.* **71:**1833.

BOSMANN, H. B., CASE, K. R., AND MORGAN, H. R., 1974a, Surface biochemical changes accompanying primary infection with Rous sarcoma virus. I. Electrokinetic properties of cells and cell surface glycoprotein: glycosyltransferase activities, *Exp. Cell Res.* **83:**15.

BOSMANN, H. B., LOCKWOOD, T., AND MORGAN, H. R., 1974b, Surface biochemical changes accompanying primary infection with Rous sarcoma virus. II. Proteolytic and glycosidase activity and sublethal autolysis, *Exp. Cell Res.* **83:**25.

BOYSE, E., 1973, Immunogenetics in the study of cell surfaces: Some implications for morphogenesis and cancer, in: *Current Research in Oncology* (C. Anfinsen, M. Potter, and A. Schechter, eds.), pp. 57–94, Academic Press, New York.

BRADY, R. O., AND FISHMAN, P. H., 1974, Biosynthesis of glycolipids in virus-transformed cells, *Biochim. Biophys. Acta* **355:**121.

BRADY, R. O., FISHMAN, P. H., AND MORA, P. T., 1973, Membrane components and enzymes in virally transformed cells, *Fed. Proc.* **32:**102.

BRETSCHER, M. S., 1971a, Human erythrocyte membranes: Specific labeling of surface proteins, *J. Mol. Biol.* **58:**775.

BRETSCHER, M. S., 1971*b*, Major protein which spans the human erythrocyte membrane, *J. Mol. Biol.* **59**:351.

BRETSCHER, M. S., 1971*c*, Major human erythrocyte glycoprotein spans the cell membrane, *Nature New Biol.* **231**:229.

BRETSCHER, M. S., 1972, Phosphatidyl-ethanolamine: Differential labeling in intact cells of human erythrocytes by a membrane impermeable reagent, *J. Mol. Biol.* **71**:523.

BRETSCHER, M. S., 1973, Membrane structure: Some general principles. Membranes are asymmetric lipid bilayers in which cytoplasmically synthesized proteins are dissolved, *Science* **181**:622.

BRETTON, R., WICKER, R., AND BERNHARD, W., 1972, Ultrastructural localization of concanavalin A receptors in normal and SV40-transformed hamster and rat cells, *Int. J. Cancer* **10**:397.

BRYANT, M. L., STONER, G. D., AND METZGER, R. P., 1974, Protein-bound carbohydrate content of normal and tumorous human lung tissue, *Biochim. Biophys. Acta* **343**:226.

BUCK, C. A., GLICK, M. C., AND WARREN, L., 1970, A comparative study of glycoproteins from the surface of control and Rous sarcoma virus transformed hamster cells, *Biochemistry* **9**:4567.

BUCKMAN, T., AND WEBER, M. J., 1975, Spin labeling investigations of membrane alterations in chick embryo fibroblasts transformed by Rous sarcoma virus, *Proc. Natl. Acad. Sci. U.S.A.* (in press).

BURGER, M. M., 1969, A difference in the architecture of the surface membrane of normal and virally transformed cells, *Proc. Natl. Acad. Sci. U.S.A.* **62**:994.

BURGER, M. M., 1970, Proteolytic enzymes initiating cell division and escape from contact inhibition of growth, *Nature (London)* **227**:170.

BURGER, M. M., 1971, Forssman antigen exposed on surface membrane after viral transformation, *Nature New Biol.* **231**:125.

BURGER, M. M., 1973, Surface changes in transformed cells detected by lectins, *Fed. Proc.* **32**:91.

BURGER, M. M., AND GOLDBERG, A. R., 1967, Identification of a tumor specific determinant on neoplastic cell surfaces, *Proc. Natl. Acad. Sci. U.S.A.* **57**:359.

BUSSELL, R. H., AND ROBINSON, W. S., 1973, Membrane proteins of uninfected and Rous sarcoma virus-transformed avian cells, *J. Virol.* **12**:320.

BUTEL, J. S., TEVETHIA, S. S., AND MELNICK, J. L., 1972, Oncogenicity and cell transformation by papovavirus SV40: The role of the viral genome, *Adv. Cancer Res.* **15**:1.

CABANTCHIK, Z. I., AND ROTHSTEIN, A., 1972, The nature of the membrane sites controlling anion permeability of human red blood cells as determined by studies with disulfonic stilbene derivatives, *J. Membr. Biol.* **10**:311.

CAPALDI, R. A., AND GREEN, D. E., 1972, Membrane proteins and membrane structure, *FEBS Lett.* **25**:205.

CARTER, J. R., JR., AVRUCH, J., AND MARTIN, D. B., 1973, Glucose transport by trypsin-treated red blood cell ghosts, *Biochim. Biophys. Acta* **291**:506.

CHEN, L. B., AND BUCHANAN, J. M., 1975, Plasminogen-independent fibrinolysis by proteases produced by transformed chick embryo fibroblasts, *Proc. Natl. Acad. Sci. U.S.A.* **72**:1132.

CHIARUGI, V. P., AND URBANO, P., 1972, Electrophoretic analysis of membrane glycoproteins in normal and polyoma virus transformed BHK$_{21}$ cells, *J. Gen. Virol.* **14**:133.

CHIARUGI, V. P., VANNUCCHI, S., AND URBANO, P., 1974, Exposure of trypsin-removable sulphated polyanions on the surface of normal and virally transformed BHK$^{21/c13}$ cells, *Biochim. Biophys. Acta* **345**:283.

CHIPOWSKY, S., LEE, Y. C., AND ROSEMAN, S., 1973, Adhesion of cultured fibroblasts to insoluble analogues of cell-surface carbohydrates, *Proc. Natl. Acad. Sci. U.S.A.* **70**:2309.

CHOU, I.-N., BLACK, P. H., AND ROBLIN, R. O., 1974*a*, Non-selective inhibition of transformed cell growth by a protease inhibitor, *Proc. Natl. Acad. Sci. U.S.A.* **71**:1748.

CHOU, I.-N., BLACK, P. H., AND ROBLIN, R. O., 1974*b*, Suppression of fibrinolysin T activity fails to restore density-dependent growth inhibition to SV3T3 cells, *Nature (London)* **250**:739.

CHOU, I.-N., BLACK, P. H., AND ROBLIN, R. O., 1974*c*, Effects of protease inhibitors on growth of 3T3 and SV3T3 cells, in: *Control of Proliferation in Animal Cells* (B. Clarkson and R. Baserga, eds.), pp. 339–350, Cold Spring Harbor Laboratory, Cold Spring Harbor, N.Y.

CHRISTENSEN LOU, H. O., CLAUSEN, J., AND BIERRING, F., 1965, Phospholipids and glycolipids of tumours in the central nervous system, *J. Neurochem.* **12**:619.

CHRISTMAN, J. K., AND ACS, G., 1974, Purification and characterization of a cellular fibrinolytic factor associated with oncogenic transformation: The plasminogen activator from SV-40-transformed hamster cells, *Biochim. Biophys. Acta* **340**:339.

CLARKE, M., 1971, Isolation and characterization of a water-soluble protein from bovine erythrocyte membranes, *Biochem. Biophys. Res. Commun.* **45**:1063.

CLARKSON, B., AND BASERGA, R., eds., 1974, *Control of Proliferation in Animal Cells*, Cold Spring Harbor Laboratory, Cold Spring Harbor, N.Y.

CLINE, M. J., AND LIVINGSTON, D. C., 1971, Binding of ^{3}H-concanavalin A by normal and transformed cells, *Nature New Biol.* **232:**155.

COGGIN, J. H., AND ANDERSON, N. G., 1974, Cancer, differentiation and embryonic antigens: Some central problems, *Adv. Cancer Res.* **19:**105.

COMAN, D. R., 1944, Decreased mutual adhesiveness, a property of cells from squamous cell carcinomas, *Cancer Res.* **4:**625.

COMOGLIO, P. M., AND FILOGAMO, G., 1973, Plasma membrane fluidity and surface motility of mouse C-1300 neuroblastoma cells, *J. Cell Sci.* **13:**415.

COMOGLIO, P. M., AND GUGLIELMONE, R., 1972, Two dimensional distribution of concanavalin A receptor molecules on fibroblast and lymphocyte plasma membranes, *FEBS Lett.* **27:**256.

COOPER, A. G., CODINGTON, J. F., AND BROWN, M. C., 1974, *In vivo* release of glycoprotein I from the Ha subline of TA$_3$ murine tumor into ascites fluid and serum, *Proc. Natl. Acad. Sci. U.S.A.* **71:**1224.

CRITCHLEY, D. R., 1974, Cell surface proteins of NIL 1 hamster fibroblasts labeled by a galactose oxidase, tritrated borohydride method, *Cell* **3:**121.

CRITCHLEY, D. R., AND MACPHERSON, I., 1973, Cell density dependent glycolipids in NIL$_2$ hamster cells, derived malignant and transformed cell lines, *Biochim. Biophys. Acta* **296:**145.

CUATRECASAS, P., 1973, Interaction of wheat germ agglutinin and concanavalin A with isolated fat cells, *Biochemistry* **12:**1312.

CUMAR, F. A., BRADY, R. O., KOLODNY, E. H., MCFARLAND, V. W., AND MORA, P. T., 1970, Enzymatic block in the synthesis of gangliosides in DNA virus-transformed tumorigenic mouse cell lines, *Proc. Natl. Acad. Sci. U.S.A.* **67:**757.

CUNNINGHAM, D. D., AND PARDEE, A. B., 1969, Transport changes rapidly initiated by serum addition to "contact inhibited" 3T3 cells, *Proc. Natl. Acad. Sci. U.S.A.* **64:**1049.

CURTIS, A. S. G., 1967, *The Cell Surface*, Academic Press, New York.

CURTIS, A. S. G., AND GREAVES, M. F., 1965, The inhibition of cell aggregation by a pure serum protein, *J. Embryol. Exp. Morphol.* **13:**309.

DANIELLI, J. F., AND DAVSON, H., 1935, A contribution to the theory of permeability of thin films, *J. Cell. Comp. Physiol.* **5:**495.

DAVIS, W. C., 1972, H-2 antigen on cell membranes: An explanation for the alternation of distribution by indirect labeling techniques, *Science* **175:**1006.

DEFENDI, V., AND GASIC, G., 1963, Surface mucopolysaccharides of polyoma virus transformed cells, *J. Cell Comp. Physiol.* **62:**23.

DEN, H., SCHULTZ, A. M., BASU, M., AND ROSEMAN, S., 1971, Glycosyl transferase activities in normal and polyoma-transformed BHK cells, *J. Biol. Chem.* **246:**2721.

DEN, H., SELA, B.-A., ROSEMAN, S., AND SACHS, L., 1974, Blocks in ganglioside synthesis in transformed hamster cells and their revertants, *J. Biol. Chem.* **249:**659.

DENT, P. B., AND HILLCOAT, B. L., 1972, Interaction of phytohemagglutinins and concanavalin A with transplantable mouse lymphomas of differing malignant potential, *J. Natl. Cancer Inst.* **49:**373.

DE PETRIS, S., AND RAFF, M. C., 1972, Distribution of immunoglobulin on the surface of mouse lymphoid cells as determined by immunoferritin electron microscopy: Antibody-induced, temperature-dependent redistribution and its implications for membrane structure, *Eur. J. Immunol.* **2:**523.

DE PETRIS, S., AND RAFF, M. C., 1973, Normal distribution, patching and capping of lymphocyte surface immunoglobulin studied by electron microscopy, *Nature New Biol.* **241:**257.

DEPPERT, W., WERCHAU, H., AND WALTER, G., 1974, Differentiation between intracellular and cell surface glycosyl transferases: Galactosyl transferase activity in intact cells and in cell homogenate, *Proc. Natl. Acad. Sci. U.S.A.* **71:**3068.

DIEVARD, J. C., AND BOURRILLON, R., 1974, Séparation et purification des sites récepteurs de la lectine del Robinia et le concanavaline A, présents á la surface des cellules hépatiques normales et tumorales (hépatome de zajdéla), *Biochim. Biophys. Acta* **345:**198.

DIRINGER, H., STRÖBEL, G., AND KOCH, M. A., 1972, Glycolipids of mouse fibroblasts and virus-transformed mouse cell lines, *Hopp-Seylers Z. Physiol. Chem.* **353:**1769.

DOLJANSKI, F., AND EISENBERG, S., 1963, The action of neuraminidase on the electrophoretic mobility of liver cells, in: *Cell Electrophoresis* (E. J. Ambrose, ed.), pp. 78–84, Churchill, London.

DORSEY, J. K., AND ROTH, S., 1973, Adhesive specificity of normal and transformed mouse fibroblasts, *Dev. Biol.* **33:**249.

DORSEY, J. K., AND ROTH, S., 1974, The effect of polyprenols on cell surface galactosyltransferase activity, in: *Control of Proliferation in Animal Cells* (B. Clarkson and R. Baserga, eds.), pp. 533–539, Cold Spring Harbor Laboratory, Cold Spring Harbor, N.Y.

DRESDEN, M. H., HEILMAN, S. A., AND SCHMIDT, J. D., 1972, Collagenolytic enzymes in human neoplasms, *Cancer Res.* **32:**993.

EDELMAN, G. M., YAHARA, I., AND WANG, J. L., 1973, Receptor mobility and receptor-cytoplasmic interactions in lymphocytes, *Proc. Natl. Acad. Sci. U.S.A.* **70:**1442.

EDIDIN, M., AND FAMBROUGH, D., 1973, Fluidity of the surface of cultured cell muscle fibers: Rapid lateral diffusion of marked surface antigens, *J. Cell Biol.* **57:**27.

EDIDIN, M., AND WEISS, A., 1972, Antigen cap formation in cultured fibroblasts: A reflection of membrane fluidity and of cell motility, *Proc. Natl. Acad. Sci. U.S.A.* **69:**2456.

EDIDIN, M., AND WEISS, A., 1974, Restriction of antigen mobility in the plasma membranes of some cultured fibroblasts, in: *Control of Proliferation in Animal Cells* (B. Clarkson and R. Baserga, eds.), pp. 213–220, Cold Spring Harbor Laboratory, Cold Spring Harbor, N.Y.

ELGSAETER, A., AND BRANTON, G., 1974, Intramembrane particle aggregation in erythrocyte ghosts. I. The effect of protein removal, *J. Cell Biol.* **63:**1018.

ENGELMAN, D. M., 1970, X-ray diffraction studies of phase transitions in the membrane of *Mycoplasma laidlawaii*, *J. Mol. Biol.* **47:**115.

EYLAR, E. H., MADOFF, M. A., BRODY, O. V., AND ONCLEY, J. L., 1962, The contribution of sialic acid to the surface charge of the erythrocyte, *J. Biol. Chem.* **237:**1992.

FAIRBANKS, G., STECK, T. L., AND WALLACH, D. F. H., 1971, Electrophoretic analysis of the major polypeptides of the human erythrocyte membrane, *Biochemistry* **10:**2606.

FIDLER, I. J., 1973, Selection of successive tumor lines for metastasis, *Nature New Biol.* **242:**148.

FIGARD, P. H., AND LEVINE, A. S., 1966, Incorporation of labeled precursors into lipids of tumors induced by Rous sarcoma virus, *Biochim. Biophys. Acta* **125:**428.

FINDLAY, J. B. C., 1974, The receptor proteins for concanavalin A and *Lens culinaris* phytohemagglutinin in the membrane of the human erythrocyte, *J. Biol. Chem.* **249:**4398.

FISHMAN, P. H., BRADY, R. O., BRADLEY, R. M., AARONSON, S. A., AND TODARO, G. J., 1974, Absence of a specific ganglioside galactosyltransferase in mouse cells transformed by murine sarcoma virus, *Proc. Natl. Acad. Sci. U.S.A.* **71:**298.

FORRESTER, J. A., 1963, Microelectrophoresis of normal and polyoma virus transformed hamster kidney fibroblasts, in: *Cell Electrophoresis* (E. J. Ambrose, ed.), pp. 115–124, Churchill, London.

FOSTER, D. O., AND PARDEE, A. B., 1969, Transport of amino acids by confluent and nonconfluent 3T3 and polyoma virus-transformed 3T3 cells growing on glass cover slips, *J. Biol. Chem.* **244:**2675.

FOX, C. F., 1975, Phase transitions in model systems and membranes, *MTP Int. Rev. Sci. Biochem.* **2:**279.

FRANCOIS, D., VU-VAN, T., FEBVRE, H., AND HAGUENAU, F., 1972, Electron microscope study of the fixation of lectins labelled with Raifort peroxidase on human embryonic cells transformed *in vitro* by the Rous sarcoma virus (RSV), Bryan strain, *C. R. Acad. Sci. Ser. D* **274:**1981.

FRYE, L. D., AND EDIDIN, M., 1970, The rapid inter-mixing of cell surface antigens after formation of mouse–human heterokaryons, *J. Cell Sci.* **7:**319.

FUHRMANN, G. F., 1963, Selective effects of neuraminidase on cell surfaces, in: *Cell Electrophoresis* (E. J. Ambrose, ed.), pp. 85–91, Churchill, London.

GAFFNEY, B. J., 1975, Fatty acid chain flexibility in membranes of normal and transformed fibroblasts, *Proc. Natl. Acad. Sci. U.S.A.* **72:**664.

GAHMBERG, C. G., AND HAKOMORI, S., 1973*a*, Altered growth behavior of malignant cells associated with changes in externally labeled glycoprotein and glycolipid, *Proc. Natl. Acad. Sci. U.S.A.* **70:**3329.

GAHMBERG, C. G., AND HAKOMORI, S., 1973*b*, External labeling of cell surface galactose and galactosamine in glycolipid and glycoprotein of human erythrocytes, *J. Biol. Chem.* **248:**4311.

GAHMBERG, C. G., AND HAKOMORI, S., 1974, Organization of glycolipid and glycoprotein in surface membranes dependency on cell cycle and on transformation, *Biochem. Biophys. Res. Commun.* **59:**283.

GAHMBERG, C. G., AND HAKOMORI, S., 1975*a*, Surface carbohydrates of hamster fibroblasts. I. Chemical characterization of surface-labelled glycosphingolipids and a specific ceramide tetrasaccharide for transformants, *J. Biol. Chem.* **250:**2438.

GAHMBERG, C. G., AND HAKOMORI, S., 1975*b*, Surface carbohydrates of hamster fibroblasts. II. Interaction of hamster NIL cell surfaces with *Ricinus communis* lectin and concanavalin A as revealed by surface galactosyllabel, *J. Biol. Chem.* **250:**2447.

GAHMBERG, C. G., UTERMANN, G., AND SIMONS, K., 1972, The membrane proteins of Semliki Forest virus have a hydrophobic part attached to the viral membrane, *FEBS Lett.* **28:**179.

GAHMBERG, C. G., KIEHN, D., AND HAKOMORI, S., 1974, Changes in a surface-labeled galactoprotein and in glycolipid concentrations in cells transformed by a temperature-sensitive polyoma virus mutant, *Nature (London)* **248:**413.

GANTT, R. R., MARTIN, J. R., AND EVANS, V. J., 1969, Agglutination of *in vitro* cultured neoplastic cell lines by a wheat germ agglutinin, *J. Natl. Cancer Inst.* **42:**369.

GARBER, B. B., AND MOSCONA, A. A., 1972, Reconstruction of brain tissue from cell suspensions. II. Specific enhancement of aggregation of embryonic cerebral cells by supernatant from homologous cell cultures, *Dev. Biol.* **27:**235.

GARRIDO, J., BURGLEN, M., SAMOLYK, D., WICKER, R., AND BERNHARD, W., 1974, Ultrastructural comparison between the distribution of concanavalin A and wheat germ agglutinin cell surface receptors of normal and transformed hamster and rat cell lines, *Cancer Res.* **34:**230.

GLASER, M., AND SINGER, S. J., 1971, Circular dichroism and the conformations of membrane proteins: Studies with RBC membranes, *Biochemistry* **10:**1780.

GLASER, M., SIMPKINS, H., SINGER, S. J., SHEETZ, M., AND CHAN, S. I., 1970, On the interaction of lipids and proteins in the red blood cell membrane, *Proc. Natl. Acad. Sci. U.S.A.* **65:**721.

GLICK, M. C., AND BUCK, C. A., 1973, Glycoproteins from the surface of metaphase cells, *Biochemistry* **12:**85.

GLICK, M. C., RABINOWITZ, Z., AND SACHS, L., 1973, Surface membrane glycopeptides correlated with tumorigenesis, *Biochemistry* **12:**4864.

GLICK, M. C., RABINOWITZ, Z., AND SACHS, L., 1974, Surface membrane glycopeptides which coincide with virus transformation and tumorigenesis, *J. Virol.* **13:**967.

GLYNN, R. D., THRASH, C. R., AND CUNNINGHAM, D. D., 1973, Maximal concanavalin A-specific agglutinability without loss of density-dependent growth control, *Proc. Natl. Acad. Sci. U.S.A.* **70:**2676.

GOETZ, I. E., WEINSTEIN, C., AND ROBERTS, E., 1972, Effects of protease inhibitors on growth of hamster tumor cells in culture, *Cancer Res.* **32:**2469.

GOLDBERG, A. R., 1974, Increased protease levels in transformed cells: A casein overlay assay for the detection of plasminogen activator production, *Cell* **2:**95.

GOTO, M., KATAOKA, Y., GOTO, K., YODOYAMA, T., AND SATO, H., 1972, Decrease in agglutinability of cultured tumor cells to concanavalin A at the plateau of cell growth, *Gann* **63:**505.

GRAHAM, J. M., HYNES, R. O., DAVIDSON, E. A., AND BAINTON, D. F., 1975, The location of proteins labeled by the ^{125}I-lactoperoxidase system in the NIL 8 hamster fibroblast, *Cell* **4:**353.

GREEN, D. E., JI, S., AND BRUCKER, R. F., 1973, Structure–function unitization model of biological membranes, *Bioenergetics* **4:**253.

GREENBERG, C. S., AND GLICK, M. C., 1972, Electrophoretic study of the polypeptides from surface membranes of mammalian cells, *Biochemistry* **11:**3680.

GRIMES, W. J., 1973, Glycosyl transferase and sialic acid levels of normal and transformed cells, *Biochemistry* **12:**990.

GRIMES, W. J., 1974, Biological and biochemical characterization of surface changes in normal, MSV- and SV40-transformed, and spontaneously transformed clones of Balb/c cells, in: *Control of Proliferation in Animal Cells* (B. Clarkson and R. Baserga, eds.), pp. 517–531, Cold Spring Harbor Laboratory, Cold Spring Harbor, N.Y.

GRIMES, W. J., AND SCHROEDER, J. L., 1973, Dibutyryl cyclic adenosine 3′ 5′ monophosphate, sugar transport, and regulatory control of cell division in normal and transformed cells, *J. Cell Biol.* **56:**487.

GUIDOTTI, G., 1972, Membrane proteins, *Ann. Rev. Biochem.* **41:**731.

GUIDOTTI, G., 1973, personal communication.

HAKOMORI, S., 1970, Cell-density dependent changes of glycolipids in fibroblasts and loss of this response in the transformed cells, *Proc. Natl. Acad. Sci. U.S.A.* **67:**1741.

HAKOMORI, S., 1973, Glycolipids of tumor cell membrane, *Adv. Cancer Res.* **18:**265.

HAKOMORI, S., 1975a, Structures and organization of cell surface glycolipids. Dependency on cell growth and malignant transformation, *Biochim. Biophys. Acta* **417:**55.

HAKOMORI, S., 1975b, Fucolipids and blood group glycolipids in normal and tumor tissue, *Prog. Biochem. Pharmacol.* (in press).

HAKOMORI, S., AND KIJIMOTO, S., 1972, Forssman reactivity and cell contacts in cultured hamster cells, *Nature New Biol.* **239:**87.

HAKOMORI, S., KOSCIELAK, J., BLOCH, K. J., AND JEANLOZ, R. W., 1967, Immunologic relationship between blood group substances and a fucose-containing glycolipid of human adenocarcinoma, *J. Immunol.* **98:**31.

HAKOMORI, S., TEATHER, C., AND ANDREWS, H., 1968, Organizational difference of cell surface "hematoside" in normal and virally transformed cells, *Biochem. Biophys. Res. Commun.* **33:**563.

HAKOMORI, S., SAITO, T., AND VOGT, P. K., 1971, Transformation by Rous sarcoma virus; effects on cellular glycolipids, *Virology* **44:**609.

HAKOMORI, S., KIJIMOTO, S., AND SIDDIQUI, B., 1972, Glycolipids of normal and transformed cells. A difference in structure and dynamic behavior, in: *Membrane Research* (C. F. Fox, ed.), pp. 253–277, Academic Press, New York.

HAMMARSTRÖM, S., AND BJURSELL, G., 1973, Glycolipid synthesis in baby-hamster-kidney fibroblasts transformed by a thermosensitive mutant of polyoma virus, *FEBS Lett.* **32:**69.

HARTMANN, J. F., BUCK, C. A., DEFENDI, V., GLICK, M. C., AND WARREN, L., 1972, The carbohydrate content of control and virus-transformed cells, *J. Cell Physiol.* **80:**159.

HATANAKA, M., 1974, Transport of sugars in tumor cell membranes, *Biochim. Biophys. Acta* **355:**77.

HAUSMAN, R. E., AND MOSCONA, A. A., 1973, Cell-surface interactions: Differential inhibition by proflavine of embryonic cell aggregation and production of specific cell-aggregating factor, *Proc. Natl. Acad. Sci. U.S.A.* **70:**3111.

HAVEN, F. L., AND BLOOR, W. R., 1956, Lipids in cancer, *Adv. Cancer Res.* **4:**237.

HERSCHMAN, H. R., 1972, Alterations in membranes of cultured cells as a result of transformation by DNA-containing viruses, in: *Membrane Molecular Biology* (C. F. Fox and A. D. Keith, eds.), pp. 471–502, Sinauer Associates, Stamford, Conn.

HOGG, N. M., 1974, A comparison of membrane proteins of normal and transformed cells by lactoperoxidase labeling, *Proc. Natl. Acad. Sci. U.S.A.* **71:**489.

HOLLEY, R. W., 1972, A unifying hypothesis concerning the nature of malignant growth, *Proc. Natl. Acad. Sci. U.S.A.* **69:**2840.

HOLLEY, R. W., 1974, Serum factors and growth control, in: *Control of Proliferation in Animal Cells* (B. Clarkson and R. Baserga, eds.), pp. 13–18, Cold Spring Harbor Laboratory, Cold Spring Harbor, N.Y.

HOVI, T., KESKI-OJA, J., AND VAHERI, A., 1974, Growth control in chick embryo fibroblasts; no evidence for a specific role for cyclic purine nucleotides, *Cell* **2:**235.

HSIE, A. W., AND PUCK, T. T., 1971, Morphological transformation of Chinese hamster cells by dibutryl adenosine cyclic 3′:5′-monophosphate and testosterone, *Proc. Natl. Acad. Sci. U.S.A.* **68:**358.

HSIE, A. W., JONES, C., AND PUCK, T. T., 1971, Further changes in differentiation state accompanying the conversion of Chinese hamster cells of fibroblastic form by dibutyryl adenosine cyclic 3′:5′-monophosphate and hormones, *Proc. Natl. Acad. Sci. U.S.A.* **68:**1648.

HSU, A.-F., BAYNES, J. W., AND HEATH, E. C., 1974, The role of a dolichololigosaccharide as an intermediate in glycoprotein biosynthesis, *Proc. Natl. Acad. Sci. U.S.A.* **71:**2391.

HUANG, C.-C., TSAI, C.-M., AND CANELLAKIS, E. S., 1974, Iodination of cell membranes. II. Characterization of HeLa cell membrane surface proteins, *Biochim. Biophys. Acta* **332:**59.

HUBBARD, A. L., AND COHN, Z., 1972, Enzymatic iodination of the red cell membrane, *J. Cell Biol.* **55:**390.

HUBBELL, W. L., AND McCONNELL, H. M., 1968, Spin-label studies of the excitable membranes of nerve and muscle, *Proc. Natl. Acad. Sci. U.S.A.* **61:**12.

HUET, C., AND BERNHARD, W., 1974, Differences in the surface mobility between normal and SV40-, polyoma- and adenovirus-transformed hamster cells, *Int. J. Cancer* **13:**227.

HYNES, R. O., 1973, Alteration of cell-surface proteins by viral transformation and by proteolysis, *Proc. Natl. Acad. Sci. U.S.A.* **70:**3170.

HYNES, R. O., 1974, Role of surface alterations in cell transformation: The importance of proteases and surface proteins, *Cell* **1:**147.

HYNES, R. O., AND BYE, J. M., 1974, Density and cell cycle dependence of cell surface proteins in hamster fibroblasts, *Cell* **3:**113.

HYNES, R. O., AND HUMPHREYS, K. C., 1974, Characterization of the external proteins of hamster fibroblasts, *J. Cell Biol.* **62:**438.

INBAR, M., AND SACHS, L., 1973, Mobility of carbohydrate containing sites on the surface membrane in relation to the control of cell growth, *FEBS Lett.* **32:**124.

INBAR, M., AND SHINITZKY, M., 1974, Increase of cholesterol level in the surface membrane of lymphoma cells and its inhibitory effect on ascites tumor development, *Proc. Natl. Acad. Sci. U.S.A.* **71:**2128.

INBAR, M., BEN-BASSAT, H., AND SACHS, L., 1971, A specific metabolic activity on the surface membrane in malignant cell-transformation, *Proc. Natl. Acad. Sci. U.S.A.* **68:**2748.

INBAR, M., BEN-BASSAT, H., AND SACHS, L., 1972, Membrane changes associated with malignancy, *Nature New Biol.* **236:**3.

INBAR, M., BEN-BASSAT, H., HUET, C., OSEROFF, A. R., AND SACHS, L., 1973, Inhibition of lectin agglutinability by fixation of the cell surface membrane, *Biochim. Biophys. Acta* **311:**594.

ISHIMOTO, N., TEMIN, H. M., AND STROMINGER, J. L., 1966, Studies of carcinogenesis by avian sarcoma viruses. II. Virus-induced increase in hyaluronic acid synthetase in chicken fibroblasts, *J. Biol. Chem.* **241:**2052.

ISSELBACHER, K. J., 1972, Increased uptake of amino acids and 2-deoxy-D-glucose by virus-transformed cells in culture, *Proc. Natl. Acad. Sci. U.S.A.* **69:**585.

ITO, A., AND SATO, R., 1968, Purification by means of detergents and properties of cytochrome b_5 from liver microsomes, *J. Biol. Chem.* **243:**4922.

JANSONS, V. K., AND BURGER, M. M., 1973, Isolation and characterization of agglutinin receptor sites. II. Isolation and partial purification of a surface membrane receptor for wheat germ agglutinin, *Biochim. Biophys. Acta* **291:**127.

JI, T. H., 1973, Crosslinking sialoglycoproteins of human erythrocyte membranes, *Biochem. Biophys. Res. Commun.* **53:**508.

JI, T. H., 1974, Cross-linking of the glycoproteins in human erythrocyte, *Proc. Natl. Acad. Sci. U.S.A.* **71:**93.

JI, T. H., AND NICOLSON, G. L., 1974, Lectin binding and perturbation of the cell membrane outer surface induces a transmembrane organizational alteration at the inner surface, *Proc. Natl. Acad. Sci. U.S.A.* **71:**2212.

JIMÉNEZ DE ASUÁ, L., ROZENGURT, E., AND DULBECCO, R., 1974, Kinetics of early changes in phosphate and uridine transport and cyclic AMP levels stimulated by serum in density-inhibited 3T3 cells, *Proc. Natl. Acad. Sci. U.S.A.* **71:**96.

JOST, P. C., GRIFFITH, O. H., CAPALDI, R. A., AND VANDERKOOI, G., 1973, Evidence for boundary lipid in membranes, *Proc. Natl. Acad. Sci. U.S.A.* **70:**480.

KANEKO, I., SATOH, H., AND UKITA, T., 1973, Effect of metabolic inhibitors on the agglutination of tumor cells by concanavalin A and *Ricinus communis* agglutinin, *Biochem. Biophys. Res. Commun.* **50:**1087.

KANT, J. A., AND STECK, T. L., 1973, Specifitity in the association of glyceraldehyde 3-phosphate dehydrogenase with isolated human erythrocyte membranes, *J. Biol. Chem.* **248:**8457.

KARNOVSKY, M. J., UNANUE, E. R., AND LEVENTHAL, M., 1972, Ligand-induced movement of lymphocyte membrane macromolecules. II. Mapping of surface moieties, *J. Exp. Med.* **136:**907.

KASÄROV, L. B., AND FRIEDMAN, H., 1974, Enhanced Na^+-K^+-activated adenosine triphosphatase activity in transformed fibroblasts, *Cancer Res.* **34:**1862.

KEITH, A. D., WAGGONER, A. S., AND GRIFFITH, O. H., 1970, Spin labeled mitochrondrial lipids in *Neurospora crassa, Proc. Natl. Acad. Sci. U.S.A.* **61:**819.

KHERA, K. S., ASHKENAZI, A., RAPP, F., AND MELNICK, J. L., 1963, Immunity in hamsters to cells transformed *in vitro* and *in vivo* by SV40: Tests for antigenic relationship among the papovaviruses, *J. Immunol.* **91:**604.

KIJIMOTO, S., AND HAKOMORI, S., 1971, Enhanced glycolipid: α-galactosyltransferase activity in contact-inhibited hamster cells, and loss of this response in polyoma transformants, *Biochem. Biophys. Res. Commun.* **44:**557.

KIMELBERG, H. K., AND MAYHEW, E., 1975, Increased ovabain-sensitive $^{86}Rb^+$ uptake and sodium and potassium ion-activated adenosine triphosphatase activity in transformed cell lines, *J. Biol. Chem.* **250:**100.

KLEEMANN, W., AND MCCONNELL, H. M., 1974, Lateral phase separations in *Escherichia coli* membranes, *Biochim. Biophys. Acta* **345:**220.

KLEIN, G., 1973, Tumor immunology, *Transplant. Proc.* **5:**31.

KLETZIEN, R. F., AND PERDUE, J. F., 1973, Inhibition of sugar transport in chick embryo fibroblasts by cytochalasin B: Evidence for a membrane-specific effect, *J. Biol. Chem.* **248:**711.

KLETZIEN, R. F., AND PERDUE, J. F., 1974a, Sugar transport in chick embryo fibroblasts. II. Alterations in transport following transformation by a temperature-sensitive mutant of the Rous sarcoma virus, *J. Biol. Chem.* **249:**3375.

KLETZIEN, R. F., AND PERDUE, J. F., 1974b, Sugar transport in chick embryo fibroblasts. III. Evidence for post-transcriptional and post-translational regulation of transport following serum addition, *J. Biol. Chem.* **249:**3383.

KORNBERG, R. D., AND MCCONNELL, H. M., 1971a, Lateral diffusion of phopsholipids in a vesicle membrane, *Proc. Natl. Acad. Sci. U.S.A.* **68**:2564.

KORNBERG, R. D., AND MCCONNELL, H. M., 1971b, Inside-outside transitions of phospholipids in vesicle membranes, *Biochemistry* **10**:1111.

KOURILSKY, F. M., SILVESTRE, C., NEAUPORT-SAUTES, C., LOOSFELT, Y., AND DAUSSET, J., 1972, Antibody-induced redistribution of HL-A antigens at the cell surface, *Eur. J. Immunol.* **2**:249.

KRAM, R., AND TOMKINS, G. M., 1973, Pleiotypic control by cyclic AMP: Interaction with cyclic GMP and possible role of microtubules, *Proc. Natl. Acad. Sci. U.S.A.* **70**:1659.

LAI, M. M., AND DUESBERG, P. H., 1972, Differences between the envelope glycoproteins and glycopeptides of avian tumor viruses released from transformed and from nontransformed cells, *Virology* **50**:359.

LEE, A. G., BIRDSALL, N. J. M., AND METCALFE, J. C., 1972, Measurement of fast lateral diffusion of lipids in vesicles and in biological membranes by ^{1}H nuclear magnetic resonance, *Biochemistry* **12**:1650.

LENGEROVÁ, A., 1972, The expression of normal histocompatibility antigens in tumor cells, *Adv. Cancer Res.* **16**:235.

LICHTMAN, M. A., AND WEED, R. I., 1970, Electrophoretic mobility and N-acetyl neuraminic acid content of human normal and leukemic lymphocytes and granulocytes, *Blood* **35**:12.

LIPKIN, G., 1974, personal communication.

LIPKIN, G., AND KNECHT, M. E., 1974, A diffusible factor restoring contact inhibition of growth to malignant melanocytes, *Proc. Natl. Acad. Sci. U.S.A.* **71**:849.

LIS, H., AND SHARON, N., 1973, The biochemistry of plant lectins (phytohemagglutinins), *Ann. Rev. Biochem.* **43**:541.

LOEWENSTEIN, W. R., 1969, Transfer of information through cell junctions and growth control, *Can. Cancer Conf.* **8**:162.

LOOR, F., 1973, Lectin-induced lymphocyte agglutination: An active cellular process? *Exp. Cell Res.* **82**:415.

LOOR, F., FORNI, L., AND PERNIS, G., 1972, The dynamic state of the lymphocyte membrane factor affecting the distribution and turnover of surface immunoglobulins, *Eur. J. Immunol.* **2**:203.

LOWICK, J. H. B., PURDOM, L., JAMES, A. M., AND AMBROSE, E. J., 1961, Some microelectrophoretic studies of normal and tumour cells, *J. R. Microsc. Soc.* **80**:47.

MABRY, E. W., AND CARUBELLI, R., 1972, Sialic acid in human cancer, *Experentia* **28**:182.

MAIZEL, J. V., JR., 1971, Polyacrylamide gel electrophoresis of viral protein, *Methods in Virology*, Vol. 5 (K. Maramorosch and H. Koprowski, eds.), pp. 179–276, Academic Press, New York.

MAKITA, A., AND SEYAMA, Y., 1971, Alterations of Forssman-antigenic reactivity and of monosaccharide composition in plasma membrane from polyoma-transformed hamster cells, *Biochim. Biophys. Acta* **241**:403.

MAKITA, A., AND SHIMOJO, H., 1973, Polysaccharides of SV40-transformed green monkey kidney cells, *Biochim. Biophys. Acta* **304**:571.

MALLUCCI, L., 1971, Binding of concanavalin A to normal and transformed cells as detected by immunofluorescence, *Nature New Biol.* **233**:241.

MARCHELONIS, J. J., CONE, R. E., AND SANTER, V., 1971, Enzymic iodination: A probe for accessible surface proteins of normal and neoplastic lymphocytes, *Biochem. J.* **124**:921.

MARCHESI, V. T., AND STEERS, E., JR., 1968, Selective solubilization of a protein component of the red cell membrane, *Science* **159**:203.

MARCHESI, V. T., STEERS, E., JR., TILLACK, T. W., AND MARCHESI, S. L., 1969, Some properties of spectrin: A fibrous protein isolated from red cell membranes, in: *The Red Cell Membrane, Structure and Function* (G. A. Jamieson and T. J. Greenwalt, eds.), pp. 117–130, Lippincott, Phila.

MÅRTENSSON, E., ÖHMAN, R., GRAVES, M., AND SVENNERHOLM, L., 1974, Galactosyltransferases catalyzing the formation of the galactosyl-galactosyl linkage in glycosphingolipids, *J. Biol. Chem.* **249**:4132.

MARTINEZ-PALOMO, A., 1970, The surface coats of animal cells, *Int. Rev. Cytol.* **29**:29.

MARTINEZ-PALOMO, A., BRAISLOVSKY, C., AND BERNHARD, W., 1969, Ultrastructural modifications of the cell surface and intercellular contacts of some transformed cell strains, *Cancer Res.* **29**:925.

MARTINEZ-PALOMO, A., WICKER, R., AND BERNHARD, W., 1972, Ultrastructural detection of concanavalin surface receptors in normal and in polyoma-transformed cells, *Int. J. Cancer* **9**:676.

MAYHEW, E., 1966, Cellular electrophoretic mobility and the mitotic cycle, *J. Gen. Physiol.* **49**:717.

MAZIA, D., AND RUBY, A., 1968, Dissolution of erythrocyte membranes in water and comparison of the membrane protein with other structural proteins, *Proc. Natl. Acad. Sci. U.S.A.* **61**:1005.

McCLELLAND, D. A., AND BRIDGES, J. M., 1973, The total N-acetyl neuraminic acid content of human normal and lymphatic leukaemic lymphocytes, *Br. J. Cancer* **27**:114.

McCUTCHEON, M., COMAN, D. R., AND MOORE, F. B., 1948, Studies on invasiveness of cancer: Adhesiveness of malignant cells in various human adenocarcinomas, *Cancer* **1**:460.

McNUTT, N. S., CULP, L. A., AND BLACK, P. H., 1971, Contact-inhibited revertant cell lines isolated from SV40-transformed cells. II. Ultrastructural study, *J. Cell Biol.* **50**:691.

McNUTT, N. S., AND WEINSTEIN, R. S., 1973, Membrane ultrastructure at mammalian intercellular junctions, *Prog. Biophys. Mol. Biol.* **26**:45.

MEEZAN, E., WU, H. C., BLACK, P. H., AND ROBBINS, P. W., 1969, Comparative studies on the carbohydrate-containing membrane components of normal and virus-transformed mouse fibroblasts. II. Separation of glycoproteins and glycopeptides by Sephadex chromatography, *Biochemistry* **8**:2518.

MEHRISHI, J. N., 1972, Molecular aspects of the mammalian cell surface, *Prog. Biophys. Mol. Biol.* **25**:1.

MEHRISHI, J. N., AND THOMSON, A. E. R., 1968, Relationship between pH and eletrophoretic mobility for lymphocytes circulating in chronic lymphocytic leukaemia, *Nature (London)* **219**:1080.

MELTZER, M. S., LEONARD, E. J., RAPP, H. J., AND BORSOS, T., 1971, Tumor-specific antigen solubilized by hypertonic potassium chloride, *J. Natl. Cancer Inst.* **47**:703.

MORA, P. T., FISHMAN, P. H., BASSIN, R. H., BRADY, R. O., AND McFARLAND, V. W., 1973, Transformation of Swiss 3T3 cells by murine sarcoma virus is followed by decrease in a glycolipid glycosyltransferase, *Nature New Biol.* **245**:226.

MORAWIECKI, A., 1964, Dissociation of M- and N-group mucoproteins into subunits in detergent solution, *Biochim. Biophys. Acta* **83**:339.

MORRISON, M., MUELLER, T. J., AND HUBER, C. T., 1974, Transmembrane orientation of the glycoproteins in normal human erythrocytes, *J. Biol. Chem.* **249**:2658.

MOYER, S. A., AND SUMMERS, D. F., 1974, Vesicular stomatitis virus envelope glycoprotein alterations induced by host cell transformation, *Cell* **2**:63.

MURAMATSU, T., ATKINSON, P. H., NATHENSON, S. G., AND CECCARINI, C., 1973, Cell-surface glycopeptides: Growth-dependent changes in the carbohydtrate–peptide linkage region, *J. Mol. Biol.* **80**:781.

NICOLSON, G. L., 1971, Difference in the topology of normal and tumor cell membranes as shown by different distributions of ferritin-conjugated concanavalin A on their surfaces, *Nature New Biol.* **233**:244.

NICOLSON, G. L., 1972, Topography of cell membrane concanavalin A-sites modified by proteolysis, *Nature New Biol.* **239**:193.

NICOLSON, G. L., 1973a, Neuraminidase "unmasking" and the failure of trypsin to "unmask" β-D-galactose-like sites on erythrocyte, lymphoma and normal and SV40-transformed 3T3 fibroblast cell membranes, *J. Natl. Cancer Inst.* **50**:1443.

NICOLSON G. L., 1973b, Temperature-dependent mobility of concanavalin A sites on tumour cell surfaces, *Nature New Biol.* **243**:218.

NICOLSON, G. L., 1974a, The interactions of lectins with animal cell surfaces, *Int. Rev. Cytol.* **39**:89.

NICOLSON, G. L., 1974b, Factors influencing the dynamic display of lectin-binding sites on normal and transformed cell surfaces, in: *Control of Proliferation in Animal Cell Surfaces* (B. Clarkson and R. Baserga, eds.), pp. 251–270, Cold Spring Harbor Laboratory, Cold Spring Harbor, N.Y.

NICOLSON, G. L., 1975, Concanavalin A as a quantitative and ultrastructural probe for normal and neoplastic cell surfaces, in: *Concanavalin A* (T. K. Chowdhury, ed.), pp. 153–172, Plenum Press, New York.

NICOLSON, G. L., AND LACORBIERE, M., 1973, Cell contact-dependent increase in membrane D-galactopyranosyl-like residues on normal, but not virus- or spontaneously-transformed murine fibroblasts, *Proc. Natl. Acad. Sci. U.S.A.* **70**:1672.

NICOLSON, G. L., AND PAINTER, R. G., 1973, Anionic sites of human erythrocyte membranes. II. Transmembrane effects of anti-spectrin on the topography of bound positively charged colloidal particles, *J. Cell Biol.* **59**:395.

NICOLSON, G. L., AND SINGER, S. J., 1971, Ferritin-conjugated plant agglutinins as specific saccharide stains for electron microscopy: Application to saccharides bound to cell membranes, *Proc. Natl. Acad. Sci. U.S.A.* **68**:942.

NICOLSON, G. L., AND SINGER, S. J., 1974, The distribution and asymmetry of mammalian cell surface saccharides utilizing ferritin-conjugated plant agglutinins as specific saccharide stains, *J. Cell Biol.* **60**:236.

NICOLSON, G. L., AND WINKELHAKE, J. L., 1975a, An experimental approach to studying organ specificity of pulmonary tumor metastasis, in: *Cell Surfaces and Malignancy* (P. Mora, ed.), Fogarty International Center, Government Printing Office, Washington, D.C.

NICOLSON, G. L., AND WINKELHAKE, J. L., 1975b, Organ specificity of blood-borne metastasis determined by cell adhesion? *Nature* **255**:230.

NICOLSON, G. L., MARCHESI, V. T., AND SINGER, S. J., 1971, The localization of spectrin on the inner surface of human red blood cell membranes with ferritin-conjugated antibodies, *J. Cell Biol.* **51**:265.

NICOLSON, G. L., BLAUSTEIN, J., AND ETZLER, M. E., 1974, Characterization of two plant lectins from *Ricinus communis* and their quantitative interaction with a murine lymphoma, *Biochemistry* **13**:196.

NICOLSON, G. L., LACORBIERE, M., AND ECKHART, W., 1975, Qualitative and quantitative interactions of lectins with untreated and neuraminidase-treated normal, wild-type and temperature-sensitive polyoma-transformed fibroblasts, *Biochemistry* **14**:172.

NIGAM, V. N., AND CANTERO, A., 1972, Polysaccharides in cancer, *Adv. Cancer Res.* **16**:1.

OHTA, N., PARDEE, A. B., MCAUSLAN, B. R., AND BURGER, M. M., 1968, Sialic acid contents and controls of normal and malignant cells, *Biochim. Biophys. Acta* **158**:98.

OLD, L. J., AND BOYSE, E., 1973, Current enigmas in cancer research, *Harvey Lect.* **67**:273.

OPPENHEIMER, S. B., 1973, Utilization of L-glutamine in intercellular adhesion: Ascites tumor and embryonic cells, *Exp. Cell Res.* **77**:175.

OPPENHEIMER, S. B., EDIDIN, M., ORR, C. W., AND ROSEMAN, S., 1969, An L-glutamine requirement for intercellular adhesion, *Proc. Natl. Acad. Sci. U.S.A.* **63**:1395.

OSSOWSKI, L., UNKELESS, J. C., TOBIA, A., QUIGLEY, J. P., RIFKIN, D. B., AND REICH, E., 1973a, An enzymatic function associated with transformation of fibroblasts by oncogenic viruses. II. Mammalian fibroblast cultures transformed by DNA and RNA tumor viruses, *J. Exp. Med.* **137**:112.

OSSOWSKI, L., QUIGLEY, J. P., KELLERMAN, G. M., AND REICH, E., 1973b, Fibrinolysis associated with oncogenic transformation: Requirement of plasminogen for correlated changes in cellular morphology, colony formation in agar, and cell migration, *J. Exp. Med.* **138**:1056.

OSSOWSKI, L., QUIGLEY, J. P., AND REICH, E., 1974, Fibrinolysis associated with oncogenic transformation: Morphological correlates, *J. Biol. Chem.* **249**:4312.

OXENDER, D. L., 1972, Membrane transport, *Ann. Rev. Biochem.* **41**:777.

OZANNE, B., AND SAMBROOK, J., 1971, Binding of radioactively labeled concanavalin A and wheat germ agglutinin to normal and virus-transformed cells, *Nature New Biol.* **232**:156.

PAPAHADJOPOULOS, D., POSTE, G., AND SCHAEFFER, B. E., 1973, Fusion of mammalian cells by unilamellar lipid vesicles: Influence of lipid surface charge, fluidity and cholesterol, *Biochim. Biophys. Acta* **232**:23.

PARDEE, A. B., 1964, Cell division and a hypothesis of cancer, *Natl. Cancer Inst. Monogr.* **14**:7.

PARDEE, A. B., 1974, A restriction point for control of normal animal cell proliferation, *Proc. Natl. Acad. Sci. U.S.A.* **71**:1286.

PARDEE, A. B., JIMÉNEZ DE ASÚA, L., AND ROZENGURT, E., 1974, Functional membrane changes and cell growth: Significance and mechanism, in: *Control of Proliferation in Animal Cells* (B. Clarkson and R. Baserga, eds.), pp. 547–561, Cold Spring Harbor Laboratory, Cold Spring Harbor, N.Y.

PATINKIN, D., SCHLESINGER, M., AND DOLJANSKI, R., 1970, A study ionogenic groups of different types of normal and leukemic cells, *Cancer Res.* **30**:489.

PATT, L. M., AND GRIMES, W. J., 1974, Cell surface glycolipid and glycoprotein glycosyltransferases of normal and transformed cells, *J. Biol. Chem.* **249**:4157.

PAUL, D., 1973, Quiescent SV40 virus transformed 3T3 cells in culture, *Biochem. Biophys. Res. Commun.* **53**:745.

PEARLSTEIN, E., AND WATERFIELD, M. D., 1974, Metabolic studies on ^{125}I-labeled baby hamster kidney cell plasma membranes, *Biochim. Biophys. Acta* **362**:1.

PECK, S. D., AND REIQUAM, C. W., 1973, Disseminated intravascular coagulation in cancer patients: Supportive evidence, *Cancer* **31**:1114.

PERDUE, J. F., 1973, The distribution, ultrastructure, and chemistry of microfilaments in cultured chick embryo fibroblasts, *J. Cell Biol.* **58**:265.

PERDUE, J. F., KLETZIEN, R., AND WRAY, V. L., 1972, The isolation and characterization of plasma membrane from cultured cells. IV. The carbohydrate composition of membranes isolated from oncogenic RNA virus-converted chick embryo fibroblasts, *Biochim. Biophys. Acta* **266**:505.

PFEIFFER, S. E., HERSCHMAN, H. R., LIGHTBODY, J. E., SATO, G., AND LEVINE, L., 1971, Modification of cell surface antigenicity as a function of cell culture conditions, *J. Cell Physiol.* **78**:145.

PHILLIPS, D. R., AND MORRISON, M., 1971, Exposed protein on the intact human erythrocyte, *Biochemistry* **10**:1766.

PHILLIPS, P. G., FURMANSKI, P., AND LUBIN, M., 1974, Cell surface interactions with concanavalin A: Location of bound radiolabeled lectin, *Exp. Cell Res.* **86**:301.

PINTO DA SILVA, P., 1972, Translational mobility of the membrane intercalated particles of human erythrocyte ghosts, pH-dependent, reversible aggregation, *J. Cell Biol.* **53**:777.

PINTO DA SILVA, P., AND NICOLSON, G. L., 1974, Freeze-etch localization of concanavalin A receptors to the membrane intercalated particles on human erythrocyte membranes, *Biochim. Biophys. Acta* **363**:311.

PODUSLO, J. F., GREENBERG, C. S., AND GLICK, M. C., 1972, Proteins exposed on the surface of mammalian membranes, *Biochemistry* **11**:2616.

POSTE, G., 1972, Mechanisms of virus-induced cell fusion, *Int. Rev. Cytol.* **33**:157.

POSTE, G., GREENHAM, L. W., MALLUCCI, L., REEVE, P., AND ALEXANDER, D. J., 1973, The study of cellular "microexudates" by ellipsometry and their relationship to the cell coat, *Exp. Cell Res.* **78**:303.

QUIGLEY, J. P., RIFKIN, D. B., AND REICH, E., 1971, Phospholipid composition of Rous sarcoma virus, host cell membranes and other enveloped RNA viruses, *Virology* **46**:106.

QUIGLEY, J. P., RIFKIN, D. B., AND REICH, E., 1972, Lipid studies of Rous sarcoma virus and host cell membranes, *Virology* **50**:550.

QUIGLEY, J. P., OSSOWSKI, L., AND REICH, E., 1974, Plasminogen, the serum proenzyme activated by factors from cells transformed by oncogenic viruses, *J. Biol. Chem.* **249**:4306.

RIFKIN, D. B., LOEB, J. N., MOORE, G., AND REICH, E., 1974, Properties of plasminogen activators formed by neoplastic human cell cultures, *J. Exp. Med.* **139**:1317.

ROMANO, A. H., AND COLBY, C., 1973, SV40 virus transformation of mouse 3T3 cells does not specifically enhance sugar transport, *Science* **179**:1238.

ROSEMAN, S., 1970, The synthesis of complex carbohydrates by multi-glycosyl-transferase systems and their potential function in intercellular adhesion, *Chem. Phys. Lipids* **5**:270.

ROSENBLITH, J. Z., UKENA, T. E., YIN, H. H., BERLIN, R. D., AND KARNOVSKY, M. J., 1973, A comparative evaluation of the distribution of concanavalin A-binding sites on the surfaces of normal, virally-transformed, and protease-treated fibroblasts, *Proc. Natl. Acad. Sci. U.S.A.* **70**:1625.

ROTH, S., 1973, A molecular model for cell interations, *Quart. Rev. Biol.* **48**:541.

ROTH, S., AND WHITE, D., 1972, Intercellular contact and cell-surface galactosyltransferase activity, *Proc. Natl. Acad. Sci. U.S.A.* **69**:485.

ROTH, S., McGUIRE, E. J., AND ROSEMAN, S., 1971, An assay for intercellular adhesive specificity, *J. Cell Biol.* **51**:525.

ROTH, J., MEYER, H. W., AND BOLCK, F., 1973, Concanavalin A binding sites in the plasma membrane of normal cells, spontaneously transformed cells and tumor cells as visualized by electron microscopy, *Exp. Pathol.* **8**:19.

ROWLATT, C., WICKER, R., AND BERNHARD, W., 1973, Ultrastructural distribution of concanavalin A receptors on hamster embryo and adenovirus tumour cell cultures, *Int. J. Cancer* **11**:314.

ROZENGURT, E., AND JIMÉNEZ DE ASUÁ, L., 1973, Role of cyclic AMP in the early transport changes induced by serum and insulin in quiescent fibroblasts, *Proc. Natl. Acad. Sci. U.S.A.* **70**:3609.

RUBIN, H., AND FODGE, D., 1974, Interrelationships of glycolysis, sugar transport and the initiation of DNA synthesis in chick embryo cells, in: *Control of Proliferation in Animal Cells* (B. Clarkson and R. Baserga, eds.), pp. 801–816, Cold Spring Harbor Laboratory, Cold Spring Harbor, N.Y.

RUDLAND, P. S., GOSPODAROWICZ, D., AND SEIFERT, W., 1974, Activation of guanyl cyclase and intracellular cyclic GMP by fibroblast growth factor, *Nature (London)* **250**:741.

RUOSLAHTI, E., AND VAHERI, A., 1974, Novel human serum protein from fibroblast plasma membrane, *Nature (London)* **248**:789.

SAKIYAMA, H., AND BURGE, B. W., 1972, Comparative studies of the carbohydrate-containing components of 3T3 and simian virus 40-transformed 3T3 mouse fibroblasts, *Biochemistry* **11**:1366.

SAKIYAMA, H., GROSS, S. K., AND ROBBINS, P. W., 1972, Glycolipid synthesis in normal and virus-transformed hamster cell lines, *Proc. Natl. Acad. Sci. U.S.A.* **69**:872.

SATOH, C., DUFF, R., RAPP, F., AND DAVIDSON, E. A., 1973, Production of mucopolysaccharides by normal and transformed cells, *Proc. Natl. Acad. Sci. U.S.A.* **70**:54.

SCANDELLA, C. J., DEVAUX, P., AND McCONNELL, H. M., 1972, Rapid lateral diffusion of phospholipids in rabbit sarcoplasmic reticulum, *Proc. Natl. Acad. Sci. U.S.A.* **69**:2056.

SCHENGRUND, C.-L., LAUSCH, R. N., AND ROSENBERG, A., 1973, Sialidase activity in transformed cells, *J. Biol. Chem.* **248**:4424.

SCHNEBLI, H. P., 1972, A protease-like activity associated with malignant cells, *Schweiz. Med. Wochenschr.* **102**:1194.

SCHNEBLI, H. P., 1974, Growth inhibition of tumor cells by protease inhibitors: Consideration of the mechanisms involved, in: *Control of Proliferation in Animal Cells* (B. Clarkson and R. Baserga, eds.), pp. 327–337, Cold Spring Harbor Laboratory, Cold Spring Harbor, N.Y.

SCHNEBLI, H. P., AND BURGER, M. M., 1972, Selective inhibition of growth of transformed cells by protease inhibitors, *Proc. Natl. Acad. Sci. U.S.A.* **69**:3825.

SCHROEDER, T. E., 1968, Cytokinesis: Filaments in the cleavage furrow, *Exp. Cell Res.* **53**:272.

SCHUBERT, J. C. F., WALTHER, F., HOLZBERG, E., PASCHER, G., AND ZEILLER, K., 1973, Preparative electrophoretic separation of normal and neoplastic human bone marrow cells, *Klin. Wochenschr.* **51**:327.

SEAMAN, P., CHAU-WONG, M., AND MOYYEN, S., 1973, Membrane expansion by vinblastine and strychnine, *Nature New Biol.* **241**:22.

SEFTON, B. M., AND RUBIN, H., 1970, Release from density-dependent growth inhibition by proteolytic enzymes, *Nature (London)* **227**:843.

SEFTON, B. M., AND RUBIN, H., 1971, Stimulation of glucose transport in cultures of density-inhibited chick embryo cells, *Proc. Natl. Acad. Sci. U.S.A.* **68**:3154.

SEGREST, J. P., AND JACKSON, R. L., 1972, Molecular weight determination of glycoproteins by polyacrylamide gel electrophoresis in sodium dodecyl sulfate, *Meth. Enzymol.* **28**:54.

SEGREST, J. P., KAHNE, I., JACKSON, R. L., AND MARCHESI, V. T., 1973, Major glycoprotein of the human erythrocyte membrane: Evidence for an amphipathic molecular structure, *Arch. Biochem. Biophys.* **155**:167.

SEIFERT, W. E., AND RUDLAND, P. S., 1974, Possible involvement of cyclic GMP in growth control of cultured mouse cells, *Nature (London)* **248**:138.

SELA, B., LIS, H., SHARON, N., AND SACHS, L., 1971, Quantitation of N-acetyl-D-galactosamine-like sites on the surface membrane of normal and transformed mammalian cells, *Biochim. Biophys. Acta* **249**:564.

SHEININ, R., AND ONODERA, K., 1972, Studies of the plasma membrane of normal and virus-transformed 3T3 mouse cells, *Biochim. Biophys. Acta* **274**:49.

SHIN, B. C., AND CARRAWAY, K. L., 1973, Cell surface constituents of sarcoma 180 ascites tumor cells, *Biochim. Biophys. Acta* **330**:254.

SHOHAM, J., AND SACHS, L., 1972, Differences in the binding of fluorescent concanavalin A to the surface membrane of normal and transformed cells, *Proc. Natl. Acad. Sci. U.S.A.* **69**:2479.

SIMON-REUSS, I., COOK, G. M. W., SEAMAN, G. V. F., AND HEARD, D. H., 1964, Electrophoretic studies on some types of mammalian tissue cell, *Cancer Res.* **24**:2038.

SINGER, S. J., 1971, The molecular organization of biological membranes, in: *Structure and Function of Biological Membranes* (L. E. Rothfield, ed.), pp. 145–222, Academic Press, New York.

SINGER, S. J., 1974, The molecular organization of membranes, *Ann. Rev. Biochem.* **43**:805.

SINGER, S. J., AND NICOLSON, G. L., 1972, The fluid mosaic model of the structure of cell membranes, *Science* **175**:720.

SMITH, S. B., AND REVEL, J.-P., 1972, Mapping of concanavalin A binding sites on the surface of several cell types, *Dev. Biol.* **27**:434.

STAEHELIN, L. A., 1974, Structure and function of intercellular junctions, *Int. Rev. Cytol.* **39**:191.

STECK, T. L., 1972a, The organization of proteins in human erythrocyte membranes, in: *Membrane Research* (C. F. Fox, ed.), pp. 71–93, Academic Press, New York.

STECK, T. L., 1972b, Crosslinking the major proteins of the isolated erythrocyte membrane, *J. Mol. Biol.* **66**:295.

STECK, T. L., 1974, The organization of proteins in the human red blood cell membrane: A review, *J. Cell Biol.* **62**:1.

STECK, T. L., AND YU, J., 1973, Selective solubilization of proteins from red blood cell membranes by protein perturbants, *J. Supramol. Struct.* **1**:220.

STEIM, J. M., TOURTELLOTTE, M. E., REINERT, J. C., McELHANEY, R. N., AND RADER, R. L., 1969, Calorimetric evidence for the liquid-crystalline state of lipids in a biomembrane, *Proc. Natl. Acad. Sci. U.S.A.* **63**:104.

STEIN, S. M., AND BERESTECKY, J. M., 1975, Exposure of an arginine-rich protein at surface of cells in S, G_2 and M phases of the cell cycle, *J. Cell Physiol.* **85**:243.

STEINER, S., AND MELNICK, J. L., 1974, Altered fucolipid patterns in cultured human cancer cells, *Nature (London)* **251**:717.

STEINER, S., BRENNAN, P. J., AND MELNICK, J. L., 1973a, Fucosylglycolipid metabolism in oncornavirus-transformed cell lines, *Nature New Biol.* **245**:19.

STEINER, S., COURTNEY, R. J., AND MELNICK, J. L., 1973b, Incorporation of 2–deoxy-D-glucose into glycoproteins of normal and SV40-transformed hamster cells, *Cancer* **33**:2402.

STONE, K. R., SMITH, R. E., AND JOKLIK, W. K., 1974, Changes in membrane polypeptides that occur when chick embryo fibroblasts and NRK cells are transformed with avian sarcoma viruses, *Virology* **58**:86.

SUNDQVIST, K. G., 1972, Redistribution of surface antigens—A general property of animal cells? *Nature New Biol.* **239**:147.

TALMADGE, K. W., NOONAN, K. D., AND BURGER, M. M., 1974, The transformed cell surface: An analysis of the increased lectin agglutinability and the concept of growth control by surface proteases, in: *Conntrol of Proliferation in Animal Cells* (B. Clarkson and R. Baserga, eds.), pp. 313–325, Cold Spring Harbor Laboratory, Cold Spring Harbor, N.Y.

TAYLOR, R. B., DUFFUS, W. P. H., RAFF, M. C., AND DE PETRIS, S., 1971, Redistribution and pinocytosis of lymphocyte surface immunoglobulin molecules induced by anti-immunoglobulin antibody, *Nature New Biol.* **233**:225.

TERRY, A. H., AND CULP, L. A., 1974, Substrate-attached glycoproteins from normal and virus-transformed cells, *Biochemistry* **13**:414

THOMSON, A. E. R., AND MEHRISHI, H. N., 1969, Surface properties of normal human circulating small lymphocytes and lymphocytes in chronic lymphocytic leukaemia: Separation, adhesiveness and electrokinetic properties, *Eur. J. Cancer* **5**:195.

TOOZE, J., ed., 1973, *The Molecular Biology of Tumour Viruses*, Cold Spring Harbor Laboratory, Cold Spring Harbor, N.Y.

TOURTELLOTTE, M. E., BRANTON, D., AND KEITH, A., 1970, Membrane structure: Spin labeling and freeze-etching of *Mycoplasma laidlawaii*, *Proc. Natl. Acad. Sci. U.S.A.* **66**:909.

UKENA, T. E., BORYSENKO, J. Z., KARNOVSKY, M. J., AND BERLIN, R. D., 1974, Effects of colchicine, cytochalasin B and 2-deoxyglucose on the topographical organization of surface-bound concanavalin A in normal and transformed fibroblasts, *J. Cell Biol.* **61**:70.

UNKELESS, J. C., GORDON, S., AND REICH, E., 1974a, Secretion of plasminogen activator by stimulated macrophages, *J. Exp. Med.* **139**:834.

UNKELESS, J., DANØ, K., KELLERMAN, G. M., AND REICH, E., 1974b, Fibrinolysis associated with oncogenic transformation. Partial purification and characterization of the cell factor, a plasminogen activator, *J. Biol. Chem.* **249**:4295.

VAHERI, A., AND RUOSLAHTI, E., 1974, Disappearance of a major cell-type specific surface glycoprotein antigen (SF) after transformation of fibroblasts by Rous sarcoma virus, *Int. J. Cancer* **13**:579.

VAHERI, A., RUOSLAHTI, E., AND NORDLING, S., 1972, Neuraminidase stimulates division and sugar uptake in density-inhibited cell cultures, *Nature New Biol.* **238**:211.

VAN BEEK, W. P., SMETS, L. A., AND EMMELOT, P., 1973, Increased sialic acid density in surface glycoprotein of transformed and malignant cells—A general phenomenon? *Cancer Res.* **33**:2913.

VANDERKOOI, G., 1972, Part I: Models of membrane structure. Molecular architecture of biological membranes, *Ann. N.Y. Acad. Sci.* **195**:6.

VASSAR, P. S., 1963, The electric charge density of human tumor cell surfaces, *Lab. Invest.* **12**:1072.

VIDAL, R., TARONE, G., PERONI, F., AND COMOGLIO, P. M., 1974, A comparative study of SV40-transformed fibroblast plasma membrane proteins labeled by enzymatic iodination or with trinitrobenzene sulfonate, *FEBS Lett.* **47**:107.

VLODAVSKY, I., AND SACHS, L., 1974, Difference in the cellular cholesterol to phospholipid ratio in normal lymphocytes and lymphocytic leukaemic cells, *Nature (London)* **250**:67.

VOYLES, B. A., AND MOSKOWITZ, M., 1974, Polyacrylamide gel electrophoresis of glycoproteins on single concentration and gradient gels, *Biochim. Biophys. Acta* **351**:178.

WALLACH, D. F. H., 1969, Cellular membrane alterations in neoplasia: A review and a unifying hypothesis, *Curr. Topics Microbiol. Immunol.* **47**:152.

WALLACH, D. F. H., AND ZAHLER, P. H., 1966, Protein conformation in cellular membranes, *Proc. Natl. Acad. Sci. U.S.A.* **56**:1552.

WARREN, L., CRITCHLEY, D., AND MACPHERSON, I., 1972a, Surface glycoproteins and glycolipids of chicken embryo cells transformed by a temperature-sensitive mutant of Rous sarcoma virus, *Nature (London)* **235**:275.

WARREN, L., FUHRER, J. P., AND BUCK, C. A., 1972b, Surface glycoproteins of normal and transformed cells: A difference determined by sialic acid and a growth-dependent sialyl transferase, *Proc. Natl. Acad. Sci. U.S.A.* **69**:1838.

WARREN, L., FUHRER, J. P., AND BUCK, C. A., 1973, Surface glycoproteins of cells before and after transformation by oncogenic viruses, *Fed. Proc.* **32**:80.

WEBER, M. J., HALE, A. H., AND ROLL, D. E., 1975, Role of protease activity in malignant transformation by Rous sarcoma virus, in: *Proteases in Biological Control* (E. Shaw, E. Reich, and D. Rifkin, eds.), Cold Spring Harbor Laboratory, Cold Spring Harbor, N.Y.

WEINSTEIN, R. S., AND McNUTT, N. S., 1972, Current concepts—Cell junctions, *N. Engl. J. Med.* **286**:521.

WEISS, L., 1958, The effects of trypsin on the size, viability and dry mass of sarcoma 37 cells, *Exp. Cell Res.* **14**:80.

WEISS, L., 1967, *The Cell Periphery, Metastasis and Other Contact Phenomena*, North-Holland, Amsterdam.

WEISS, L., 1973, Neuraminidase, sialic acids, and cell interactions, *J. Natl. Cancer Inst.* **50**:3.

WESSELLS, N. K., SPOONER, B. S., ASH, J. F., BRADLY, M. O., LUDUENA, M. A., TAYLOR, E. L., WRENN, J. T., AND YAMADA, K. M., 1971, Microfilaments in cellular and developmental processes, *Science* **171**:135.

WICKUS, G. G., AND ROBBINS, P. W., 1973, Plasma membrane proteins of normal and Rous sarcoma virus-transformed chick embryo fibroblasts, *Nature New Biol.* **245**:65.

WICKUS, G. G., BRANTON, P. E., AND ROBBINS, P. W., 1974, Rous sarcoma virus transformation of the chick cell surface, in: *Control of Proliferation in Animal Cells* (B. Clarkson and R. Baserga, eds.), pp. 541–546, Cold Spring Harbor Laboratory, Cold Spring Harbor, N.Y.

WILKINS, M. H. F., BLAUROCK, A. E., AND ENGELMAN, D. M., 1971, Bilayer structure in membranes, *Nature New Biol.* **230**:72.

WILLINGHAM, M. C., AND PASTAN, I., 1974, Cyclic AMP mediates the concanavalin A agglutinability of mouse fibroblasts, *J. Cell Biol.* **63**:288.

WINKELHAKE, J. L., AND NICOLSON, G. L., 1975, Adhesion of variant metastatic melanoma cells to BALB/3T3 cells and their virus-transformed derivatives, *J. Natl. Cancer Inst.* (in press).

WINZLER, R. J., 1970, Carbohydrates in cell surfaces, *Int. Rev. Cytol.* **29**:77.

WINZLER, R. J., HARRIS, E. D., PEKAS, D. J., JOHNSON, C. A., AND WEBER, P., 1967, Studies on glycopeptides released by trypsin from intact human erythrocytes, *Biochemistry* **6**:2195.

WOOLLEN, W., AND TURNER, P., 1965, Plasma N-acetyl-β-glucosaminidase and β-glucuronidase in health and disease, *Clin. Chim. Acta* **12**:671.

WU, H. C., MEEZAN, E., BLACK, P. H., AND ROBBINS, P. W., 1969, Comparative studies on the carbohydrate-containing membrane components of normal and virus-transformed mouse fibroblasts. I. Glucosamine-labeling patterns in 3T3, spontaneously transformed 3T3, and SV40-transformed 3T3 cells, *Biochemistry* **8**:2509.

YAHARA, I., AND EDELMAN, G. M., 1972, Restriction of the mobility of lymphocyte immunoglobulin receptors by concanavalin A, *Proc. Natl. Acad. Sci. U.S.A.* **69**:608.

YAHARA, I., AND EDELMAN, G. M., 1973a, Modulation of lymphocyte receptor redistribution by concanavalin A, anti-mitotic agents and alterations of pH, *Nature (London)* **236**:152.

YAHARA, I., AND EDELMAN, G. M., 1973b, The effects of concanavalin A on the mobility of lymphocyte surface receptors, *Exp. Cell Res.* **81**:143.

YAMADA, K. M., AND WESTON, J. A., 1974, Isolation of a major cell surface glycoprotein from fibroblasts, *Proc. Natl. Acad. Sci. U.S.A.* **71**:3492.

YAMAMOTO, K., AND TERAYAMA, H., 1973, Comparison of cell coat acid mucopolysaccharides of normal liver and various ascites hepatoma cells, *Cancer Res.* **33**:2257.

YAU, T. M., AND WEBER, M. J., 1972, Changes in acyl group composition of phospholipids from chicken embryonic fibroblasts after transformation by Rous sarcoma virus, *Biochem. Biophys. Res. Commun.* **49**:114.

YAU, T. M., AND WEBER, M. J., 1974, personal communication.

YIN, H. H., UKENA, T. E., AND BERLIN, R. D., 1972, Effect of colchicine, colccmid and vinblastine on the agglutination by concanavalin A, of transformed cells, *Science* **178**:867.

YOGEESWARAN, G., SHEININ, R., WHERRETT, J. R., AND MURRAY, R. K., 1972, Studies on the glycosphingolipids of normal and virally transformed 3T3 mouse fibroblasts, *J. Biol. Chem.* **247**:5146.

YOGEESWARAN, G., LAINE, R. A., AND HAKOMORI, S., 1974, Mechanism of cell contact-dependent glycolipid synthesis: Further studies with glycolipid–glass complex, *Biochem. Biophys. Res. Commun.* **59**:591.

ZWALL, R. F. A., ROELOFSEN, B., AND COLLEY, C. M., 1973, Localization of red cell membrane constituents, *Biochim. Biophys. Acta* **300**:159.

2

Contact Inhibition

Jan Pontén

1. Introduction

Cells which grow attached to a solid substrate can ordinarily both migrate and divide. Normally the two processes can be inhibited by close cell-to-cell contact. The term "contact inhibition," originally coined to mean only a restraint of locomotion imposed on cells which make contact with each other (Abercrombie and Heaysman, 1954), has also been employed to denote inhibition of mitosis (*cf.* Stoker and Rubin, 1967). There is no indication that spread of tumors is in any direct way dependent on cell division; however, it seems reasonable to assume that capacity to metastasize is related to the migratory behavior of cells *in vitro* (*cf.* Abercrombie and Ambrose, 1962). This chapter will describe contact-dependent control of locomotion of normal and neoplastic cells *in vitro* and attempt to analyze whether lack of such control mechanisms is related to spread of tumor cells as seen in the living organism.

One of the major advantages of tissue culture methods is the possibility of making comparisons between different categories of cells. Based on their growth pattern and cytology, cells from nonneoplastic sources may broadly be divided into four categories: epithelium, glia, fibroblasts, and wandering cells (Table 1). The criteria of Table 1 apply primarily to dense cultures where the cells have interacted with each other to produce the characteristic patterns. Single isolated cells may be difficult to place in their right categories. All four categories are similar to the respective *in vivo* counterparts. Epithelium, for instance, grows as continuous sheets or cords sharply separated from the mesenchyme, a pattern also seen *in vitro*. Fibroblasts form a connective tissue stroma *in vivo* highly reminiscent of the structures which the same cells may form in petri dishes (Hayflick and Moorhead, 1961).

Jan Pontén • The Wallenberg Laboratory, University of Uppsala, Uppsala, Sweden.

TABLE 1

Four Categories of Normal Cells in Vitro

	Prototype source	Growth pattern
Epithelium	Embryonic kidney tubules Embryonic pigment retina	Two-dimensional sheets of tightly interconnected flat polygonal cells with straight borders and little or no cytoplasmic overlapping
Glia	Adult astrocytes	Two-dimensional layers of star-shaped cells with many tightly interwoven cytoplasmic extensions but no nuclear overlapping
Fibroblasts	Embryonic connective tissue	Parallel, often three-dimensional bundles or whorls of bipolar cells
Wandering cells (amebocytes)	Peritoneal macrophages, lymphocytes	Growth as isolated units or cell clumps; highly mobile cells with capacity for survival in suspension

The presence of these large differences between the cell categories (Table 1) makes it necessary to consider the contact behavior of each separately.

Since contact inhibition may be of relevance in distinguishing neoplastic from nonneoplastic cells, it is desirable to have a clear concept of how to distinguish between "normal" and neoplastic cells in culture. This subject has been very confusingly treated and there is still no unequivocal definition of a nonneoplastic cell *in vitro*.

All systems considered adequate representatives of a normal nonneoplastic state have been listed in Table 2. Criteria for making such a selection have been discussed extensively (Pontén, 1971). In essence, the criteria for judging a cell as normal and nonneoplastic are as follows: (1) the cell should be derived from nontumor tissue, (2) it should preserve its characteristic histiotypic differentiation and have a diploid karyotype, (3) it should have a finite life span, and (4) it should not give rise to neoplastic growth after animal implantation. The only exceptions from the requirement of a finite life span are the human lymphoblastoid lines, where considerable indirect evidence favors a nonneoplastic character in spite of

TABLE 2

Culture Systems Considered Good Examples of Normal Nonneoplastic Cells

Epithelium	Early passage embryonic epidermis	DiPasquale (1973)
	Early passage pigmented chick retina	Middleton (1972, 1973)
Glia	Adult human astrocytes (stable diploid strains)	Pontén *et al.* (1969)
	Primary ganglion explants	Weiss (1934), Dunn (1973)
Fibroblasts	Early passage embryonic connective tissue	Abercrombie (1967)
	Embryonic human lung (stable diploid strains, e.g., WI-38)	Elsdale and Foley (1969)
	Adult human skin (stable diploid strains)	Westermark (1973*b*)
Wandering cells	Early passage macrophages	Jacoby (1965)
	Established human lymphoblastoid lines	Nilsson and Pontén (1975)

the infinite life span, which may be due to a peculiar association with Epstein–Barr (mononucleosis) virus (*cf.* Nilsson and Pontén, 1975).

The normal cell systems of Table 2 suffer from certain drawbacks. Early passage populations are often partly composed of an undefined and unstable mixture of many cell types. Stable diploid strains are better defined and probably uniform. Their main disadvantage is that they represent a sample of cell types which have been selected on the basis of rapid growth in serial cultivation *in vitro*. It is possible that the selected cells are not representative for the majority of the normal somatic cells and that their contact behavior is therefore irrelevant. Established lymphoblastoid lines are peculiar because of their unexplained infinite life span and obligate association with Epstein–Barr virus. Contact inhibition studies of these cells may not be representative for nonneoplastic lymphoid cells in general.

Another important factor which influences normal cellular growth patterns *in vitro* is the age of the donor. Human embryonic lung or skin fibroblasts will, for instance, grow to a higher density than those of adult origin (Westermark, 1973*a*).

Neoplastic cells in culture may be produced either by explantation of malignant tumors or by transformation *in vitro*. Transformation can be accomplished spontaneously or by oncogenic virus, chemical carcinogens, or radiation (*cf.* Pontén, 1971). Table 3 lists some of the few neoplastic systems whose contact behavior has been studied in any depth. The common criterion is that these cells either are of proven tumor origin or produce tumors after implantation *in vivo*.

Certain widely employed established cell lines like 3T3, BHK, and NIL occupy an intermediate position between a nonneoplastic and a neoplastic state. These will be referred to as "pseudonormal" lines.

Mouse cells have an unexplained high tendency to undergo a spontaneous change into heteroploid established and usually tumorigenic lines with an infinite life span *in vitro* (Gey *et al.*, 1949; Earle, 1943; Sanford *et al.*, 1954). From such a system, Todaro and Green (1963) managed to select the 3T3 line. It shows well-regulated density-dependent proliferation control in common with many normal cells (Todaro *et al.*, 1965) and is not tumorigenic after transplantation, at least not if moderate numbers of cells are implanted (Aaronson and Todaro, 1968). It is, however, not fully normal because of its heteroploid karyotype, its tendency to throw off tumorigenic variants, and the ease by which it can be transformed by polyoma virus, SV40 (Todaro and Green, 1965, 1966), and

TABLE 3
Examples of Neoplastic Populations Used for Contact Inhibition Studies in Vitro

Carcinoma cells	HeLa cells (Miranda *et al.*, 1974)
Glioma cells	Derived from spontaneous human glioblastoma grade III–IV (Pontén and Macintyre, 1968)
Sarcoma cells	Mouse S-180 (highly malignant "old" transplantable tumor) (Abercrombie *et al.*, 1957), Py3T3, and Sv3T3, mouse cells tranformed by polyoma virus (Bell, 1974) or SV40 (McNutt *et al.*, 1973)
Wandering cells	Human established malignant lymphoma lines (Nilsson and Pontén, 1975)

chemical carcinogens (DiPaolo *et al.*, 1972). The last tendency is in sharp contrast to the case of diploid normal fibroblasts, which so far have resisted chemical transformation *in vitro* (*cf.* Heidelberger, 1973). The 3T3 cells have been used extensively in contact inhibition studies (e.g., Todaro *et al.*, 1965; Holley and Kiernan, 1968; Stoker, 1973; Bell, 1974).

Another established "pseudonormal" line, the BHK Syrian baby hamster kidney line (Macpherson and Stoker, 1962), has been widely used as the "normal" counterpart of polyoma virus transformed hamster cells (Stoker, 1962). The same principal considerations as for 3T3 cells are applicable to the BHK as well as other established rodent lines.

2. The Normal Nonneoplastic Cell at Rest

2.1. Glia Cells and Fibroblasts

Glia cells and fibroblasts in a resting state have sufficient similarities to be usefully incorporated under the same heading. After adherence to a solid substratum, they assume a flattened shape with the nucleus near the center. The upper, relatively smooth fibroblast surface is probably nonadhesive (Carter, 1967) with a moderate number of microvilli. The lower adhesive surface of glia and fibroblasts is, on the other hand, provided with defined attachment points where the cell membrane makes intimate contacts with the proteinaceous microprecipitate which is laid down between the solid glass or plastic and the cell surface proper (Brunk *et al.*, 1971; Eguchi and Okada, 1971). Between the points of attachment, the ventral cell membrane forms a system of interconnected shallow vaults with small invaginations as a sign of active endocytosis (Fig. 1).

It is not known in detail how this specialized and rather complicated morphology is maintained. It is, however, clear that many forces cooperate. Crudely, one

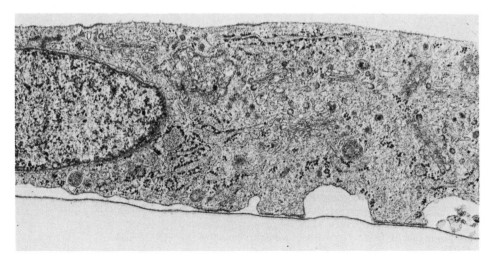

FIGURE 1. Section of a normal glia cell which demonstrates well-developed "feet" attached to a microprecipitate. Courtesy of Dr. Ulf Brunk, Uppsala.

can think of the cell shape as the resultant of two opposite classes of forces: stretching, which is mainly exerted from the attachment points, and contraction, where intracytoplasmatic fiber systems seem to play an essential role.

According to modern views, the cell membrane should be regarded as a fluid viscous structure (Singer and Nicholson, 1972) where phospholipids intermingled with cholesterol and other lipids are basic structural elements. The hydrophobic ends of the lipid molecules meet in the central parts of the membrane, whereas the hydrophilic parts align themselves toward the exterior of the cell and toward the cytoplasm inside of the membrane, giving rise to the bilayered appearance of the membrane seen by electron microscopy. The proteins, which may constitute as much as half of the membrane dry mass (Neville and Kahn, 1974), are either inserted into the membrane (integral proteins) or attached to it as molecules stretched out laterally along the lipid bilayer either on its inside or outside (peripheral proteins). The integral globular proteins may either be inserted into only the outer or the inner portion of the lipid bilayer or may penetrate the lipid bilayer all the way from the inside to the outside. Integral proteins are capable of undergoing fairly rapid lateral movements (Aoki *et al.*, 1969) in the plane of the membrane according to the "fluid mosaic membrane" model (Singer and Nicholson, 1972; also see Chapter 1).

Some of the proteins which reach the outer cell surface have branched polysaccharide parts which stretch out beyond the plane of the bilayer (Bretscher, 1972). The polysaccharide parts of the membrane glycoproteins have a complex chemical structure and intermingle with certain pure polysaccharides and "glyco" parts of membrane glycolipids. In this way, a polysaccharide-rich stratum is formed on the outer cell surface. It is often referred to as the "cell coat" (Gasic and Berwick, 1962) or "glycocalyx" (Bennett, 1963).

Integral and peripheral proteins seem to participate in determining cell shape. In erythrocytes, for instance, an actomyosinlike protein complex, spectrin, is found as a peripheral protein on the cytoplasmic side of the cell membrane. The spectrin complex appears to be attached to intramembraneous particles and has been suggested to be responsible for the asymmetrical shape of the erythrocyte (Weed *et al.*, 1969; Nicholson and Painter, 1973). It has not been shown that membrane proteins by themselves govern locomotion of the whole cell only that they participate in determining the *in situ* shape, notably of erythrocytes.

The cell membrane including its peripheral proteins is not an autonomously mobile skin. Several lines of evidence suggest that cytoplasmic structures influence both the shape and mobility of the cell membrane. Only a beginning has been made to elucidate how this may be possible.

Three major fiber systems which influence cell shape have been identified: microtubules, microfilaments, and 10-nm filaments (Porter, 1966; Behnke, 1970; Goldman and Follett, 1969).

2.1.1. Microtubuli

Microtubuli are thin pipelike structures with a diameter of about 22 nm. In highly ordered fashion, they take part in the formation of cilia and the mitotic spindle. In a less ordered array, they are also found in the cytoplasm of interphase cells. In the latter situation, their arrangement seems to determine (or is determined by) the general cell shape. A bipolar cell such as a fibroblast will have microtubules disposed along the long axis of the cell (Porter, 1966) within the cytoplasm.

The microtubules are formed by aggregation of subunits of a protein called tubulin. Colchicine and vinblastin are two alkaloids which bind to tubulin and have been found to prevent formation of microtubules (*cf.* Allison, 1973).

The microtubules in a stretched out cell at rest are regarded by most observers as a flexible and elastic cytoskeleton which can be disassembled and reassembled via its soluble tubulin subunits. It influences the basic cell shape and cell polarity and is, because of its dynamic structure, capable of reorganization when the cell changes its shape (Goldman *et al.*, 1973). A drastic example is provided by the rounded mitotic cell, where apparently all microtubules are relocated to the spindle from their previous places in the "cytoskeleton," which is thus totally dissolved. Microtubuli are particularly common in such long cell extensions as axons and dendrites of nerve cells (Daniels, 1968, 1972; Yamada *et al.*, 1970; Yamada and Wessells, 1971).

Since all cells including ganglion cells with their long extensions assume a more or less rounded shape when brought into suspension, one must conclude either that the "cytoskeleton" is not rigid enough to support a highly asymmetrical shape or that it is disassembled when a cell loses its solid attachment. The correct alternative should be possible to determine experimentally.

Recent evidence indicates that microtubules are functionally linked to surface membrane glycoproteins (Berlin and Ukena, 1972; Yahara and Edelman, 1972, 1974). Concanavalin A (Con A), which is a protein showing strong binding to certain sugar residues of the cell coat, will inhibit the local clustering of receptor sites normally seen if lymphocytes are exposed to a divalent antibody against a surface protein. The interpretation is that Con A restricts lateral motion of the receptor proteins. This inhibition by Con A can be reversed by drugs which destroy microtubules. Therefore, apparently a link exists between the micro-tubules inside the cell and the proteins in the cell membrane, which in an important manner may regulate the movement of the latter. The link is probably not a direct physicochemical contact, because microtubules have never been observed in close proximity to the inner part of the cell membrane. It has been suggested that microfilaments link microtubules to membrane protein (Yahara and Edelman, 1974).

2.1.2. Microfilaments

The microfilaments are a class of thin fibers without any substructure resolved in the electron microscope. Their diameter is about 6 nm. They occur either singly or packed together in bundles.

The linear bundles of microfilaments found in fibroblasts or glia cells generally lie in the direction of the long axis of a bipolar cell (Spooner *et al.*, 1971). In a polygonal cell, they form parallel arrays, often at sharp angles (Fig. 2). The

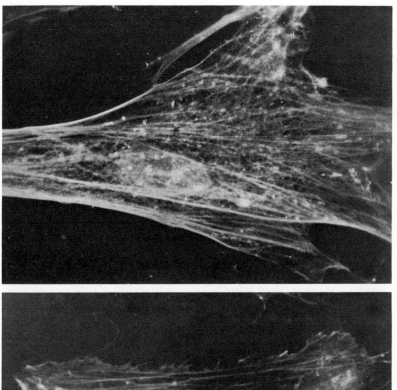

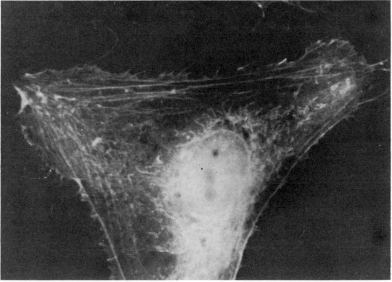

FIGURE 2. Two glia cells stained with fluorescent antiserum against actin. Bundles of microfilaments in parallel to the long axis of the cell (upper panel). In the triangular cell (lower panel), which is less extended, the microfilament bundles are thinner and predominantly located in the submembraneous part of the lateral edge of the cytoplasm. This lamellipodia extend beyond the area delineated by microfilament bundles, particularly around the two visible corners of the cell. Courtesy of Dr. Uno Lindberg, Uppsala.

bundled filaments may run very close (6 nm) to the inside of the cell membrane (Goldman *et al.*, 1973; Wessells *et al.*, 1973). Microfilament bundles are particularly well developed in patches along the dorsal surface of a resting cell (Fig. 3). There is no definite evidence of a whole bundle of microfilaments directly attached to the cell membrane. Their submembraneous location and apparently obligate association with elongated or branched cell shapes under a variety of

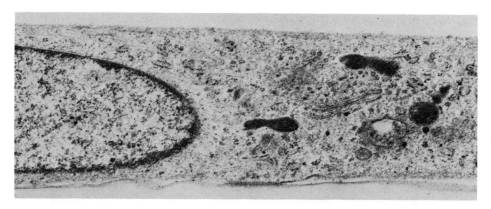

FIGURE 3. Section of a normal glia cell. Note patches of condensed microfilaments along the dorsal cell membrane. One attachment device is connected to the microprecipitate near the middle of the ventral part of the cell membrane. Courtesy of Dr. Ulf Brunk, Uppsala.

conditions suggest that these bundles play an important role in maintaining the shape of attached cells (Wessels *et al.*, 1973). Since asymmetrical cell shape is lost after cell detachment, the microfilament bundles cannot maintain a highly stretched cell form in the absence of a solid cell attachment.

Single "nonbundled" microfilaments are common in all cells. In a resting cell, they may be seen to accumulate near the attachment devices (Fig. 4), perhaps connecting these with the microfilament bundles of the cell's interior. Apart from this, they appear as rather randomly distributed cytoplasmic elements which sometimes merge into the linear bundles.

One important chemical constituent of the microfilaments is an actinlike material which can be visualized by its characteristic reaction with heavy meromyosin (Ishikawa *et al.*, 1969; Spooner *et al.*, 1973). Bundles of microfilaments resolved in the light microscope stain with fluorescent antibodies against actin (Lazarides and Weber, 1974). Myosin, which in common with actin seems to be an obligate component of all eukaryotic cells (Groeschel-Stewart, 1971; Stossel and Pollard, 1973), appears to be predominantly located in submembraneous positions along or within the microfilament bundles (Weber and Groeschel-Stewart, 1974).

Microfilament function is severely but reversibly sensitive to cytochalasin (Carter, 1967; Schroeder, 1970; Wessells *et al.*, 1971).

Because of their content of actin, myosin, and tropomyosin (Lazarides, 1975), their distribution, and the effects of cytochalasin, it has been proposed that the microfilaments are the contractile system of cells (Bernfield and Wessells, 1970; Ishikawa *et al.*, 1969). Strictly speaking, the arguments mainly apply to the bundles, and it is still possible that single microfilaments have other properties than the bundle microfilaments. If the microfilaments are contractile, which presently seems the most likely alternative, they should be regarded as analogues of the actinomyosin filaments of skeletal muscle. It should, however, be pointed out that the analogy is not complete, because the microfilaments in nonmuscle cells seem less stable, with a capacity to be broken down, reassembled, and reoriented in connection with changes in cell shape (Wessells *et al.*, 1973).

2.1.3. The 10-nm Filaments

The so-called 10-nm filaments have been seen only in the cell's interior; i.e., they do not seem to occupy a submembraneous position. They are typically found in colchicine-treated cells in a rather well-defined zone adjacent to the nucleus (Goldman *et al.*, 1973). In non-drug-treated cells, their distribution has been less well defined, however, they have been described in connection with moving organelles (Buckley, 1974). The function of the 10-nm filaments is unknown. An actin content has not been proven. It is possible that they relate in some as yet unknown fashion to the microtubules because of their easy visualization after colchicine treatment.

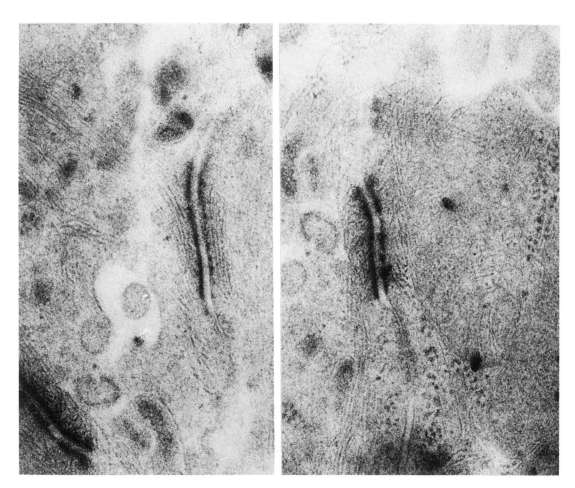

FIGURE 4. Three intracellular attachment points between adjacent glia cells. Note condensation of unidentified material at the cell membrane and relatively regularly spaced microfilaments which run toward and in very close proximity to the specialized attachment areas. Courtesy of Dr. Nils Forsby, Uppsala.

2.1.4. The Combined Arrangement of Microtubules, Microfilaments, and Filaments

It is still too early to give a detailed three-dimensional picture of the arrangement of the musculo-selected system of the nonmuscle cell. It is probably very different from cell type to cell type. It seems clear however, that at least cells of the general morphology of fibroblasts have a submembraneous matrix of actin-containing (Buckley and Porter, 1967; Ambrose et al., 1970; Goldman and Knipe, 1972) microfilaments just under the cell membrane (Spooner et al., 1971). This matrix may not be diffusely spread but concentrated in certain regions, notably the plaques by which the cell attaches to the solid support and its neighbors, but also to other morphologically less well-defined patches. Whether this matrix also contains myosin is unknown. Well-defined parallel bundles of actin, myosin (Weber and Groeschel-Stewart, 1974), and tropomyosin (Lazarides, 1974) of a width of about 1 μm and thus resolved in the light microscope run roughly parallel to the long axis of the cell or in asymmetrical polygonal cells parallel to the sides of the cell (Harris, 1973a; McNutt et al., 1971, 1973). These fibers are particularly prominent in all cell extensions, where they may become closely packed. Myosin and tropomyosin are arranged in striated structures. At least the bundles but perhaps also isolated microfilaments are in all probability contractile, but the mechanism responsible for contraction (see review by Pollard and Weihing, 1974) and relaxation has not been elucidated. The 100-nm filaments do not seem to contain actin and may serve to transmit mechanical forces within the cell. Microtubules are concentrated to the deeper part of the cytoplasm, where they may form an elastic cytoskeleton which takes part in forming the cell shape and possibly also governs the intracytoplasmatic motion of mitochondria and other organelles. How this very complicated and highly dynamic three dimensional structure takes part in cellular locomotion via links to the cell membrane and indirectly to the attachment points of a cell is still largely unresolved.

2.2. Epithelium

Resting epithelial cells have not been studied to the same extent as fibroblasts and glia. The cell membrane presumably has the same fluid mosaic structure, but the conditions under which the proteins move have hardly been studied. The most essential property of epithelial membranes is their capacity to form strong intercellular contacts in the form of junctions of different electron microscopic appearance (Crawford et al., 1972; Middleton, 1973). The dorsal surface is nonadhesive to other cells, latex particles, and Con A coated erythrocytes (DiPasquale and Bell, 1974). Details about presence and distribution of microtubules and filaments in cultivated normal epithelia remain to be elucidated.

2.3. Wandering Cells

Wandering cells, as their name implies, do not rest in culture under physiological conditions and are therefore more properly treated in a subsequent part of this chapter.

In summary, a resting attached cell has an extended, flattened, and asymmetrical shape which is energetically unfavorable and thus requires chemical energy for its maintenance. Attachment to the solid substrate via specialized attachment devices and the presence of a dynamic system of microtubules and microfilaments are two important determinants of gross cell shape. The microtubules and/or the microfilaments appear to be indirectly or directly linked to peripheral and/or integral membrane proteins. The surface of the cell at rest seems to be specialized into a dorsal, ventral, and lateral part, each with its own characteristic microstructure. The extent to which molecules within the membrane of the resting cell are free to move laterally within the plane of the membrane according to the fluid mosaic membrane model is not known. It is also not known how the individual protein and lipid molecules of the membrane are distributed in the dorsal, ventral, or lateral cell surface.

3. Normal Cells in Motion

Cellular movements may be classified according to Table 4, modified after Edelman and Wang (1974).

All the elements of Table 4 may be involved in contact inhibition phenomena; however, only elements 3 and 5 have been extensively studied.

Correlative studies on normal locomotion of different cell types have been rare. The literature contains abundant references to each of the cell types of Table 2, but the studies have always been performed under different conditions.

However, it seems clear that fibroblasts, glia, epithelium, and the two types of wandering cells (macrophages and lymphoblastoids) can be distinguished from each other on the basis of their locomotory pattern.

3.1. Locomotion of Fibroblasts and Glia

Fibroblasts and glia cells have sufficient similarities to be treated under the same heading. The principal locomotory organ is the so-called leading lamella (Ingram, 1969). This is a flat sheet of cytoplasm about 200 nm thick which, often from a broad base, extrudes like a fan from the cells along the solid substrate (Fig. 5). It is fastened to this via an estimated number (in embryonic fibroblasts) of 10–100 "attachment devices" (Abercrombie *et al.*, 1971). The leading lamella is not sharply demarcated from the rest of the cell body. It may stretch out as far as 20–40 μm.

From its edge the leading lamella extrudes lamellipodia (Abercrombie *et al.*, 1970*b*). These can be described as thin projections of rather strikingly uniform thickness (110–60 nm). This makes them morphologically distinct from the remainder of the leading lamella. The lamellipodia either project horizontally along the substrate or more commonly upward into the fluid medium at varying

TABLE 4

Classification and Examples of Cellular Movement

1. Local movement of cell surface receptors	Patch formation in lymphocytes (Aoki *et al.*, 1969). The main driving force is diffusion and/or lipid–protein phase separation. Slowed down by low temperature but not by inhibition of energy production. Abolished by fixation.
2. Global movement of cell surface	Cap formation is only unequivocal example (Edidin and Weiss, 1972; Taylor *et al.*, 1971), but nucleopetal streaming of membrane components in fibroblasts (Abercrombie *et al.*, 1970*c*; Harris and Dunn, 1972) may be of the same nature. Requires energy and intact microfilament–microtubular function (de Petris and Raff, 1973; Edelman *et al.*, 1973). Cap formation may be directed to a certain area, e.g., the antipod to the attachment site of a lymphocyte to a nylon fiber (Rutishauser *et al.*, 1974).
3. Local morphological changes, e.g., extrusion of leading lamellae and ruffling	Actin-containing microfilaments may be the essential driving force (Buckley and Porter, 1967; Allison *et al.*, 1971; Spooner *et al.*, 1971; Buckley, 1974).
4. Global morphological changes— alteration in cell shapes	Requires complex alterations in the microfilament– microtubular system including cycles of depolymerization/ polymerization of its respective subunits.
5. Translocation of cells	Complex series of events which require highly coordinated interactions among microtubules, microfilaments, and cell membrane components. Well-ordered formation and lysis of attachment sites to solid substrata and/or other cells required.
6. Translocation of cell sheets	Apparently characteristic only of epithelium. Requires supracellular organization of forces of locomotion and strong intercellular adhesions.

angles with the solid substrate (Fig. 6). In the latter capacity, they are referred to as "ruffles" (Abercrombie and Ambrose, 1958). Lamellipodia start from the dorsal surface of the leading lamella at or very near its edge and bend backward around their base, which at the same time moves toward the nucleus, giving highly characteristic phase-contrast time-lapse pictures of wavelike transversal bands (Fig. 5). Ruffles are transient: about two-thirds of them have been estimated to disappear within 1 min (Abercrombie *et al.*, 1970*b*). Figure 7 shows how ruffles arise from a fan-shaped leading lamella of a normal glia cell and form a complicated system of mostly vertical thin veils extending rather far out and upward from their site of origin.

The formation of a lamellipodium is rapid; time-lapse movies show that maximal extension may be reached within a few minutes. Its edge constantly moves fairly rapidly back and forth: 4 min has been given as the average interval between one maximal protrusion and the next (Abercrombie *et al.*, 1970*a*). The maximal distance covered by the edge in this time interval may be of the order of 20 μm. These movements are irregular, with interposed periods of standstill.

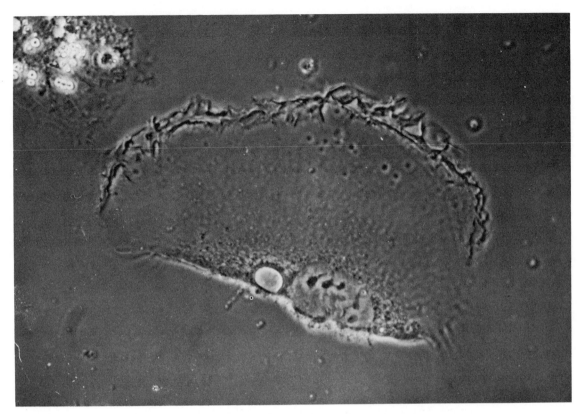

FIGURE 5. A cell with an unusually well-developed "ruffled membrane." The nucleus and an adjacent large vacuole are at the lower end of the cell. Upward a wide leading lamella is spread from a broad indistinct base. Along its entire periphery lamellipodia extend. A few spread along the solid substrate but most form complicated arrays of roughly vertical "ruffles" which extend toward the observer into the fluid medium. In the lower right corner of the cell, the bases of a few retraction fibers may be discerned. Phase-contrast microscopy.

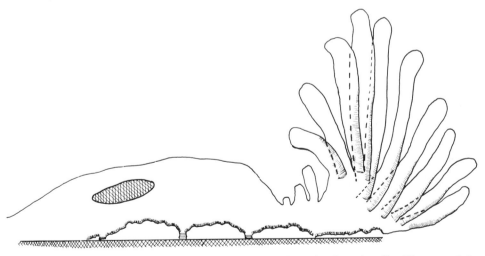

FIGURE 6. Possible sequence in glia cells of the formation of a lateral ruffle. The extended lamellipodium swings backward. At the same time, its base moves a short distance inward. The ruffle disappears relatively close to the lateral edge where it was originally formed. Note that the cell is attached to the solid substrate via specialized attachment devices.

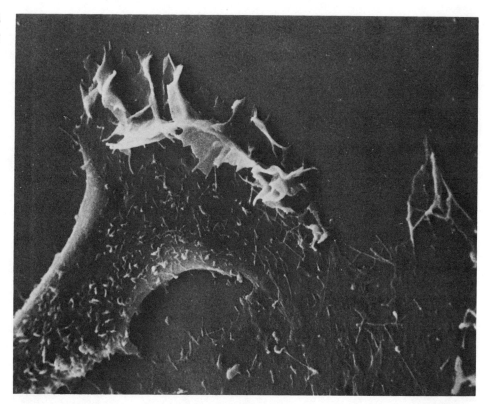

FIGURE 7. Scanning picture of the ruffling margin of a normal human glia cell. Ruffling is confined to a distinct fan-shaped broad segment of the lateral edge. Lamellipodia which extend horizontally along the solid substratum can be seen in all stages of transformation into a complicated array of thin ruffles. Courtesy of Dr. Nils Forsby, Uppsala.

Segments of the leading edge separated by only some 6 μm may move independently of each other. In a cell in locomotion, the forward extensions cover a larger distance than the retractions (Abercrombie *et al.*, 1970*b*).

How lamellipodia disappear is not completely clear. Part of the membrane in the ruffles takes part in pinocytosis. The characteristic vesicles are formed via complex infoldings of the ruffles which are sequestered from the plasma membrane and internalized into the cytoplasm (Abercrombie *et al.*, 1970*c*). Other parts are either resorbed back into the cell or remain as microvilli.

A leading lamella is also provided with so-called microspikes. These are thin, apparently rather rigid extensions from the edge of the ruffled membrane. Microspikes stretch out close to the solid substrate and may move about a "hinge" at their base (Fig. 8).

The membrane of the leading lamella is subject to a further type of movement. This was revealed by observation of small particles brought into contact with moving fibroblasts (Abercrombie *et al.*, 1970*c*; Harris, 1973*a*). They were seen to be transported on the dorsal surface at a steady speed toward the nucleus. The movement seemed independent of the ruffling and oscillation of the leading edge.

The internal structure of the fibroblastic locomotory organ has been studied by Abercrombie *et al.* (1971) in chick heart explants. The cytoplasm of the bulk part

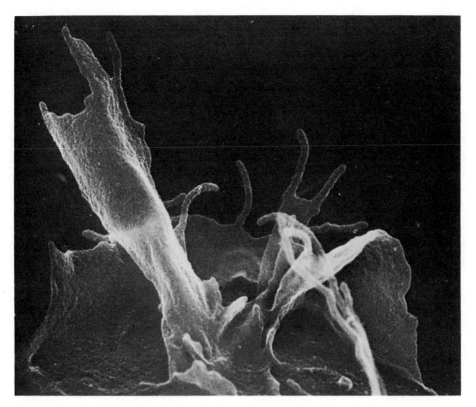

FIGURE 8. Details of marginal lamellipodia ruffles and microspikes. The latter extend from the most peripheral parts of a lamellipodium. Courtesy of Dr. Nils Forsby, Uppsala.

of the leading lamella has the usual set up of organelles. It contains microfilaments basically arranged as in the cell at rest. Sheaths of microfilaments tend to extend only halfway toward the edge of the leading lamella. Some of the dorsal tracts of microfilaments may extend obliquely forward to the ventral surface, where they may connect with the "attachment devices" (Abercrombie *et al.*, 1971).

Lamellipodia, including their appearance as ruffles, do not contain mitochondria, microtubules, or polysomes (Abercrombie *et al.*, 1971). The most conspicuous ultrastructural feature of the lamellipodium is its content of microfilaments, which are arranged in an irregular lattice. Bundles of microfilaments extend into the base of the leading lamella and are possibly in connection with the lattice microfilaments (Wessells *et al.*, 1973; Buckley, 1974).

Locomotion is carried out by the leading lamella. The most compelling evidence is that such a lamella is invariably present at the forward end of a moving cell.

The mechanism by which a leading lamella is formed and by which it pulls the cell in a certain direction are still far from clear and have been subject of much debate. For the formation of the leading lamella and its lamellipodia, at least four alternatives have been suggested. One is that new membrane is preferentially assembled at a segment of the cell periphery, which then gradually extends to become the leading lamella (Abercrombie *et al.*, 1970*c*); a second is that the mechanical strength of the cell membrane is weakened, thus permitting the development of a sheetlike aneurysm. A third possibility is that the microfilament–microtubular apparatus contracts locally, whereby part of the cytoplasm is actively thrust forward (Allison, 1973). One could also conceive of a fourth mechanism based on local osmotic inhibition of water, which would create a volumetric expansion.

The pull which the leading lamella exerts is generally believed to be exerted by microfilaments which take their origin from the attachment points between the substrate and the ventral cell surface. Accompanying this contraction, attachment points at the rear end of the cell loosen up, thus permitting gross translocation in the direction of the leading lamella with its newly formed "feet." The relative lack of attachment points under the tail of a moving cell supports the idea that loosening of attachment to a support is instrumental in converting the energy of internal cellular contraction to net cellular locomotion (Boyde *et al.*, 1969; Revel *et al.*, 1974; Revel, 1974).

When the rear of the cells is displaced forward, long, thin, so-called retraction fibers are formed behind (Fig. 5). They run from a few remaining attachment points as straight threads of cytoplasm into the cell body proper (*cf.* Revel, 1974).

3.2. Locomotion of Epithelial Cells

In common with fibroblasts and glia, epithelial cells move by way of leading lamellae and lamellipodia which they extend along the solid substrate. In contrast to fibroblasts and also to glia cells, there is usually no clear polarity of the epithelial cell shape. This in conjunction with rather feeble extension of lamellipodia (Middleton, 1973) could explain why isolated chick pigment epithelium was found to move at a speed of only 7 μm/h, i.e., more than 10 times slower than chick fibroblasts.

3.3. Locomotion of Wandering Cells

3.3.1. Macrophages

A macrophage is distinguished by (1) a pronounced tendency to attach to solid substrates, (2) an extreme capacity for assuming a large variety of shapes, and (3) a strong capacity for phagocytosis. Such cells are found in virtually all tissue explants, particularly from embryos, but are most conveniently obtained in almost pure form from either sterile peritoneal exudates or blood monocytes (Jacoby, 1965).

The macrophage membrane is highly motile, with numerous extrusions of varying form. Most are thin lamellipodia with ruffles (Fig. 9). Pinocytosis and phagocytosis are both intimately connected with this membrane activity (*cf.* Berry and Spies, 1949).

In dense cultures, macrophages will assume a flat, polygonal, rather uniform shape with a centrally placed nucleus (Lewis and Webster, 1921). Multinucleation is common, presumably caused by cell fusion (Goldstein, 1954).

Macrophages move faster (100 μm/h) than fibroblasts. When in isolation, their
walk is essentially random, with frequent changes of direction. Positive chemotaxis has been repeatedly suggested (Jacoby, 1938; Lasfargues and Delaunay, 1947; Harris, 1953), but it has never been satisfactorily clarified whether this is reinforced "contact guidance" (Weiss, 1961) caused by oriented strings of the material used to "lure" the cells, availability of unoccupied solid surface when dying cells have been used as "baits," or true chemical diffusible signals (see Jacoby, 1965). The locomotory organs of macrophages in culture do not seem to have been as thoroughly studied as those of fibroblasts, and their ultrastructure remains largely unknown.

3.3.2. Lymphoblastoid Cells

Lymphoblastoid cell lines of human origin are composed of modified lymphocytes (B cells) with capacity for immunoglobulin synthesis (Benyesh-Melnick *et al.*, 1963; Moore and Minowada, 1969; Tanigaki *et al.*, 1966; Philipson and Pontén, 1967). Irrespective of their source, these cells have identical properties and are therefore assumed to represent a cell type present in normal lymphoid tissue or blood which is unusually easy to select for prolonged *in vitro* passage (Nilsson, 1971; Nilsson and Pontén, 1975).

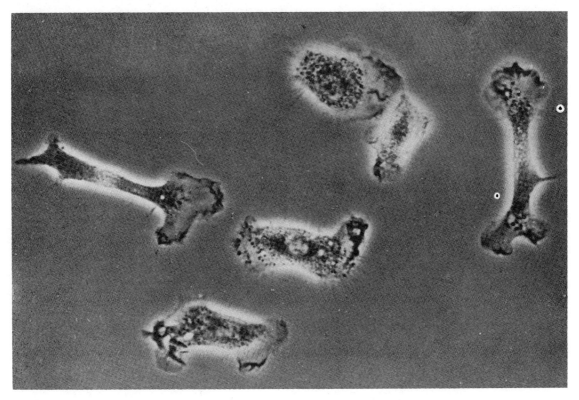

FIGURE 9. Phase-contrast photomicrograph of normal mouse peritoneal macrophages in culture showing the granule-free peripheral cytoplasm and ruffle membranes. From Allison (1973).

The motility pattern of lymphoblastoid cells is complex (Clarkson *et al.*, 1967). They may interchangeably exist in suspension or as attached elements. Attached lymphoblastoid cells have a great preference for other cell surfaces (fibroblasts, glia, etc.) but may also migrate in isolation on plastic or glass (Nilsson *et al.*, 1970).

When associated with other normal cells in culture, lymphoblastoids exhibit a characteristic phenomenon—peripolesis (Pulvertaft, 1959). This means that the lymphoblasts exist in intimate contact with the outside of the cell membrane. Here the lymphoblasts extend lamellipodia from their lateral surface which form, contract, and withdraw faster than the corresponding fibroblastic structures. Another striking difference from fibroblasts, glia, epithelium, and macrophages is that the lively activity of lymphoblasts is never associated with formation of dorsal (or ventral) ruffles. The lamellipodia are located in the front end of the cell and are able to move a lymphoblast with considerable speed (> 2000 μm/h). A common peripoletic pattern is that of a cluster of lymphoblasts within which the individual cells move about randomly in one plane outside the cell membrane but confined to a rather stationary groove between the ventral surface of a "feeder" fibroblast and its solid support (Fig. 10). Movement is violent enough to push the feeder cell nucleus around. The ameboid, very flexible peripoletic lymphoblastoid cells

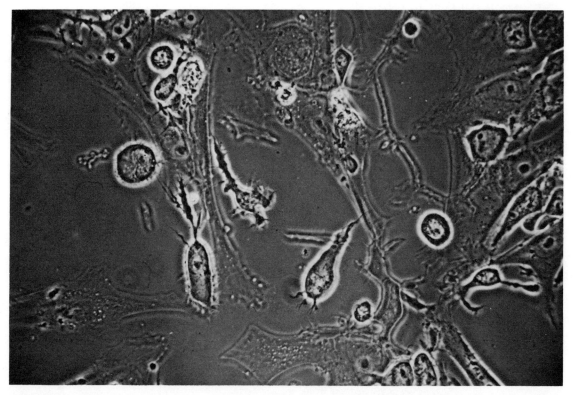

FIGURE 10. Lymphoblastoid cells interacting with a feeder layer of normal human glia attached to a solid plastic substrate. Lymphoblastoid cells are rounded, with a large variety of cell shapes. Note pear-shaped cell below center with three tiny extensions in its forward end and a single retraction fiber as its tail. In the right part of the picture are about half a dozen lymphoblastoid cells engaged in peripolesis.

sometimes sever a sufficient number of attachment points to loosen the feeder cell from the solid substrate. More commonly, however, peripolesis goes on without any visible mutual disturbance of the feeder cell or the lymphoblasts.

Another frequent type of lymphoblastoid movement may be labeled "ping-pong" locomotion. Here one end of the cell extends a leading lamella with lamellipodia, which contract and drag the cell forward. The rear end then loses its grip on the substratum except for five to ten long retraction fibers which remain attached. After a while, these may contract and lamellipodia may be formed at the antipod of the first leading lamella. These will contract, pulling the cell back to its former position. The new rear end will now be the site of retraction fibers, apparently the only remnants of the original lamellipodia. Many such cycles may occur in rapid succession and the cell nucleus will travel like a ping-pong ball over a distance of 30–50 μm (Nilsson *et al.*, 1970). Sometimes the leading lamella will persist at the front end, which will then be the site of cycles of extrusions and contractions which rapidly pull the whole cell in one direction.

In suspension, the lymphoblastoid cells do not extend any thin veil-like lamellipodia. Instead, numerous thin rods protrude from the entire cell surface. These move randomly and will usually not produce any net cellular movement. Sometimes, however, they arise from a rather broad base, giving the cell a polarized appearance. In this case, the cells can move in the direction of the protruding highly mobile rodlike extensions or even reverse. How these extensions propel the cell forward or backward has not been systematically analyzed. When lymphoblastoid cells form clumps, which they readily do, the cytoplasmic extensions are always directed away from the center of the clump (Nilsson and Pontén, 1975).

3.4. Comparison Between Movements of Different Normal Cell Types

Available evidence strongly supports that the basic locomotory mechanism is the same for all eukaryotic cells. The most compelling evidence is the finding of actomyosinlike proteins in all thoroughly investigated nonmuscle cells (Bettex-Galland and Lüscher, 1965; Adelstein *et al.*, 1971; Bray, 1973).

Morphological time-lapse observations strongly suggest that all attached cells move by means of leading lamellae, i.e., cytoplasmic extensions provided with specialized portions which generally either manifest themselves as lamellipodia or microspikes. Sometimes cytoplasmic blebbing is intermingled with lamellipodial activities (Harris, 1973*a*). Lamellipodia and microspikes are confined to the lateral edges.

Table 5 summarizes the differences in locomotory pattern between the cell types that can be distinguished *in vitro*. The most important feature is the enormous differences in the speed by which the cells can move. The reasons for these variations are obscure. At the morphological level, a rough direct correlation seems to exist between the relative size of a front-end lamellipodium and the rest of cell body on the one hand and the speed of translocation on the other. In

TABLE 5

Locomotory Pattern of Cultivated Normal Cells

	Approximate speed (μm/h)	Ruffles	Marginal lamellipodia
Epithelium	70	Sparse	Sparse
Glia	20	Common	Moderately common
Fibroblasts	70	Common	Moderately common
Macrophages	100	Common	Abundant
Lymphoblastoids	1,200	Absent	Abundant

epithelium only a minor fraction of the cytoplasm is even "transformed" into a lamellipodium, whereas a very substantial part of a macrophage or lymphoblast cytoplasm acts as a locomotory organ at any given instant.

This cannot be the only (or even the major?) explanation, because there are clear signs that organized formation of attachment areas is of great importance. Ruffles, which probably arise only when a lamellipodium fails to attach to the solid support (Revel, 1974), are nonexistent in lymphoblastoids but common in all the other more slowly moving cell types. This suggests that either the newly formed front-end attachments are too weak or the loosening of aft attachments does not occur efficiently enough to permit net movement each time a lamellipodium is formed. On the other hand, lymphoblastoid cells seem always successful since a contraction of the leading lamella will lead to some net displacement of the cell body even if this is again reversed.

Obviously other factors would also enter into the picture. The arrangement of the combined microfilament–microtubular system in the different cell types has not been critically compared. Physiological studies of contractility within individual cells seem hardly possible to perform with present techniques but would be highly illuminating. Fluidity within the cell membrane may differ from cell type to cell type and so on.

It is a comforting fact that the speed and mobility of the different cell types *in vitro* are distributed in the same fashion as they are *in vivo*.

3.5. Summary of Normal Cell Locomotion

A still very speculative and incomplete general model of normal cell locomotion would be as follows:

A stretched cell attached to a solid substrate has a tendency to throw out lamellipodia. The process is limited to the lateral cell margins, where it engages only part of the circumference at any one time, usually from a thinned portion of the cytoplasm (the leading lamella). External agents have not been shown to induce formation of lamellipodia. Instead, they apparently arise at random.

Microfilaments are obligate components of lamellipodia. They may arise by polymerization from preexisting soluble subunits. A sol–gel transition may be part

of this process. The principal movement of the lamellipodium is a forward
extension along the solid substrate.

Usually the ventral surface does not form any lasting adhesions with the solid substratum. Sometimes, however, such adhesions are formed either near the base of a lamellipodium or via tips of the microspikes. The contraction of the microfilaments will then pull the cell forward. Forward locomotion probably requires directed loosening of attachment sites in the rear end of the cell.

In all cell types except lymphoblastoid cells, contraction of the lamellipodium may also lead to an upward lift of its edge and body which then as a thin ruffle travel slowly a short way toward the nucleus before being resorbed back into the cell usually as a pinocytotic vesicle.

The intracellular signal for the assumed polymerization of actin, which would be the essential feature of formation of lamellipodia, is unknown, and neither is the trigger for the assumed contraction of the newly polymerized microfilaments, but it may be caused by local depolarization of the cell membrane in analogy with the contraction in striated muscle.

In muscle, an obligate association exists between actin and myosin. The latter protein carries ATPase activity and is instrumental in triggering contractile activity (Stracher and Dreizen, 1966; Huxley, 1969). According to the sliding filament model, shortening of a muscle fiber is caused by creation of new links between actin and myosin which cause the ends of the actin filaments to approach each other. In the electron microscope, no regular array of myosin/actin has been seen in nonmuscle cells. There are, however, indications of myosin molecules inside of the cytoplasm. How these molecules govern contraction of a microfilament system and if this is feasible according to the sliding filament model are presently wholly unclear (*cf.* Allison, 1973).

Intense membrane fluidity accompanies formation of leading lamellae. So far, only movement inward ("receptor sites" for carbon pigment) has been noted. Whether this means that new membrane is assembled at high speed at the tip of the lamellipodium (Abercrombie *et al.*, 1972) or whether the inward motion is counterbalanced by outward movement of other portions of the membrane (de Petris and Raff, 1973) is unsettled.

Microtubules play an indirect role in cell locomotion. In their absence, lamellipodia are formed almost normally but the cell does not move in any direction. No cell tail is formed under these circumstances. Therefore, the required ordered loosening of trailing attachment points may not be possible, making microfilament contraction ineffective (Vasiliev *et al.*, 1969, 1970) for locomotion (but not for ruffling).

4. Locomotion of Isolated Neoplastic Cells

In view of the enormous differences between normal cells, predominantly depending on their histogenetic type (Table 5) and also on the age of the donor, a search for a general locomotion pattern specifically "neoplastic" seems futile. Only in situations (and it is doubtful if they ever have existed in any experiments) where precisely the same cell type is compared in a nonneoplastic and a neoplastic state will it be possible to get decisive data on locomotory deviations characteristic of neoplastic cells. Such a study calls for "minimal-deviation" neoplasia *in vitro*—an ideal not yet achieved.

4.1. Locomotion of Spontaneously Transformed (Tumorigenic) Cells or Cells Derived from Tumors in Vivo

4.1.1. Carcinoma Cells

Carcinoma cells have often been described as more mobile and flexible than normal epithelium, but this impression has never been documented in any depth. Certain carcinoma cells (HeLa, etc.) may grow in suspension. This stands in sharp contrast to normal epithelium which always requires a solid support for survival. This fact—which also applies to sarcoma cells vs. fibroblasts—shows that at least some neoplastic cells have profoundly altered surfaces compared to their normal counterparts. The nature of this "loss of anchorage dependence" (Montagnier and Macpherson, 1964) is obscure, although an increased net negative electric charge often has been proposed (Weiss, 1967). The commonly made observation that carcinoma cells—in contrast to normal epithelium—move in isolation, is probably another aspect of a decreased cohesiveness.

4.1.2. Glioma Cells

Locomotion of human glioma cells has been studied in our laboratory (Westermark, 1973a; Bell, Westermark and Pontén, unpublished). Preliminary observations suggest that their lamellipodia are more prominent than in normal human adult glia. Many glioma lines show "vertical" ruffles not seen in control cells (Westermark, 1973a). These appear as complicated arrays of thin veils extruding upward in to the fluid medium from the perinuclear region (Fig. 11). How these ruffles arise is somewhat obscure, but observation of living cells suggests that they build up *in situ* and are not the result of a transport of an original lateral lamellipodium over the dorsal cell surface. The increased formation of lamellipodia is accompanied by increased pinocytosis. Individual glioma lines differ considerably from each other and it has not yet been possible to discern a common abnormal "glioma pattern" of locomotion (Forsby, unpublished).

4.1.3. Sarcoma Cells

The original observations of a disturbed social behavior of tumor cells were made on a transplantable mouse sarcoma S-180 (Abercrombie *et al.*, 1957). In general the sarcoma cells had more active surface movements than normal fibroblasts. Individual sarcoma cells could assume a variety of interchangeable shapes and were thus more plastic than normal fibroblasts. Similar observation were made by Barski and Belehradek (1965, 1966) on other murine sarcomas.

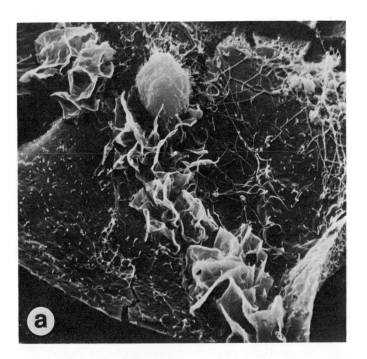

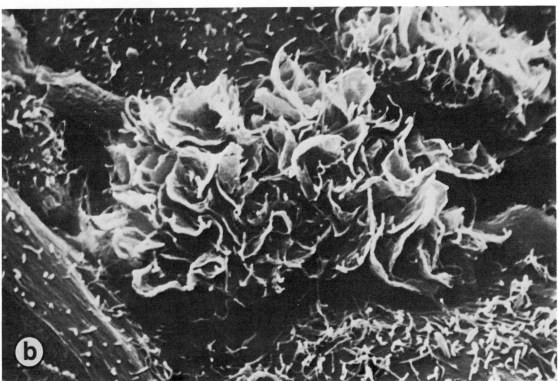

FIGURE 11. Human malignant glioma cells. In panel A, the contact line between two cells is filled with ruffles, indicating a failure of the contact between the cells to paralyze lamellipodia. Panel B shows a large number of thin vertical ruffles from the dorsal surface of a glioma cell.

Spontaneously transformed tumorigenic rat fibroblasts (sarcoma cells) were studied by Veselý and Weiss (1973). There was possibly more active ruffling in the transformed cells compared to normal rat fibroblasts; otherwise, no significant differences were reported.

4.1.4. Lymphoblastoid Cells

Lymphoblastoid cells have been rather well compared with malignant human hematopoietic cells (Nilsson *et al.*, 1970; Nilsson and Pontén, 1975). The overriding principle which emerges is the individuality of the neoplastic cells. By scanning electron microscopy and time-lapse photography, it was possible among a sample of about ten different lines to sort out each as unique with respect to details in surface structure and dynamic morphology. A second finding was that, contrary to expectations, the neoplastic cells were morphologically less flexible than normal lymphoblastoid cells. The latter could vary their behavior over an extremely wide pattern. The lymphoma or myeloma cells studied were, on the other hand, comparatively rigid. Their pattern of locomotion seemed more predictable and stereotypic. This may be an example of how neoplastic cells follow a general rule of "dedifferentiation," i.e., inability to perform highly specialized functions, since lymphoblastoid cells may be thought of as differentiated for high well-coordinated motility.

In summary, spontaneously neoplastic lines show a much wider spectrum of individuality than the corresponding normal prototype cells. Quantitative differences in amount of ruffling, speed of locomotion, etc., have been reported but have not been consistent enough to permit any conclusions about a neoplasia-specific aberration of locomotion of isolated cells.

4.2. Locomotion of Virally Transformed Cells

4.2.1. Polyoma Virus

A very detailed and illuminating study has been performed by Bell (1974) on 3T3 mouse cells (Todaro and Green, 1963) and a polyoma-transformed derivative (Py3T3) (Todaro *et al.*, 1964). It was basically designed to study contact behavior and this aspect will be referred to later.

Isolated 3T3 and Py3T3 were found to move with about the same speed (Medium values about 10 μm/h). Both types formed lamellipodia or lamellipodia-like cytoplasmic extensions. These differed morphologically. In 3T3 cells the lamellipodia were usually broad and fan-shaped and essentially similar to the normal pattern shown in Fig. 5. The Py3T3 sites of locomotory cell margin activity differed by being composed of small sites of ruffling, often at the tips of long cytoplasmic extensions. Sequences were filmed (Bell, 1974) where an originally broad lamellipodium was broken up into smaller units—a phenomenon only rarely observed among 3T3 cells.

3T3 as well as Py3T3 advanced by similar cycles of protrusion and withdrawal of   79
a lamellipodium at the front-end, where the distance covered by the protruding   CONTACT
edge is longer than that of the retraction phase.   INHIBITION

4.2.2. C-Type RNA Viruses

C-type RNA virsues transform fibroblasts and other cells of various species. In the process the cells undergo characteristic morphological changes. Two common transformed cell types are (1) a bipolar elongated cell with pointed ends and (2) a large, round, loosely attached basophilic cell (Tenenbaum and Doljanski, 1943; Temin, 1960). These highly typical effects are most clearly seen when normal fibroblasts are used as targets. In spite of the tremendous virological and cell biological interest shown in Rous sarcoma virus induced transformation of chicken fibroblasts—a system which would seem ideally suited for studies of cell locomotion—no systematic studies seem to have been published. The large number of pinocytotic vesicles often seen suggests hyperactive ruffling but quantification of this impression seems to be lacking.

Spontaneously transformed rat cells already referred to (Veselý and Weiss, 1973) have been "supertransformed" by RSV (Veselý *et al.*, 1968). Such cells lack broad lamellipodia. Instead, they have a few narrow protrusions with a ruffling edge (Veselý and Weiss, 1973) apparently similar to the structures described in Py3T3 by Bell (1974). In addition, vertical ruffles were seen. In spite of marked membrane motility, cell translocation was slow or absent. Movement into a wound was sluggish and disorganized as if the RSV-transformed cells had lost the capacity to become polarized with a defined front and rear end (Veselý and Weiss, 1973). In this respect they resembled normal cells whose microtubules have been destroyed by colchicine (Vasiliev *et al.*, 1970; Gail and Boone, 1971).

Thus all studies on virally transformed cells suggest that they have very profound disturbances of the locomotion and cell membrane behavior which exceed what is usually seen among spontaneously transformed cells. Lamellipodia are often narrow and do not work in coordination so that directed migration may become ineffective.

5. Social Behavior of Normal Cells in Culture

From the very beginning of the tissue culture era, it became apparent (Congdon, 1915; Uhlenhuth, 1915; Loeb, 1921; Lewis and Lewis, 1924) that cells in culture do not behave as autonomous units but interact with each other to form patterns.

Abercrombie and collaborators (see reviews by Abercrombie 1965, 1967, 1970) introduced systematic studies of social behavior of normal and neoplastic cell populations. The basic proposal has been that normal cells interact in such a way that they are prevented from crawling over each other. By this mechanism they will be confined to a monolayer with all cells in extensive contact with their solid substrate (Abercrombie and Heaysman, 1954). Malignant cells, on the other hand, have (at least partly) lost this property and are able to mount normal adjacent cells (Abercrombie *et al.*, 1957). The idea of a neoplastic "loss of contact inhibition" received strong support when it was shown that virally transformed cells (Rubin, 1960, 1962; Vogt and Dulbecco, 1962) layered themselves in three-dimensional piles and thus did not obey the command to remain as a monolayer.

Subsequent work has shown this dichotomy between "contact inhibition" in normal cells and "loss of contact inhibition" in neoplastic cells to be an oversimplication.

5.1. Definition and Assay of Contact Inhibition

A collision between two cells on a plane surface will usually lead to some kind of interaction. Contact inhibition (CI) is said to have occurred if the locomotion of the colliding cells in its original direction is reduced or stopped (Abercrobie, 1970).

The definition of CI is purely operational. It does not say anything about its mechanism. In very general terms, the inability of one cell to continue its migration without any disturbance, if it finds another cell in its way, may depend on either or both of two factors: (1) nonspecific mechanical or physicochemical hindrance or (2) a specific cell-to-cell interaction.

A nonspecific locomotion restraint could be due to a failure of the colliding cell to move under or over the other cell, which would then function as a mechanical obstacle. Another variant is the so-called differential adhesion theory (Abercrombie, 1967; Carter, 1965), which in essence says that a moving cell will stay on the most adhesive surface available. If the upper cell surface of the contacted cell is less adhesive than the solid substratum, the colliding cell will prefer not to climb the back of its neighbor and thus register as contact inhibited.

The specific cell-to-cell interaction idea postulates that CI depends on paralysis of locomotion induced by membrane-to-membrane interactions upon collision.

Obviously, both types of mechanisms will result in monolayering but for quite different reasons.

The simplest estimate of presence of CI is based on the morphology of a fixed culture. If no multilayered areas are found, CI is presumed to exist. This "assay" does not say anything about the nature of the CI. The same holds true for quantifications based on the number of overlapping nuclei (Abercrombie and Heaysman, 1954; Curtis, 1961; Oldfield, 1963; Weston and Hendricks, 1972; Martz, 1973).

Low-power filming permits determination of whether a population is essentially monolayered. It also resolves whether cells remain in fixed positions after collision or continue to move about. The latter finding suggests that specific cell-to-cell binding is not very prominent, but otherwise this method does not tell us very much about the details of cellular interaction.

The only way by which the mechanisms for CI can be reliably observed is by high-resolution time-lapse filming and direct microscopy of living cells (Abercrombie *et al.*, 1970a). There are not many such studies and it is not surprising in view of the extremely varied locomotory pattern for normal cells that we still have rather vague ideas even about the morphological events after cell collision. Filming may with advantage be complemented with ultrastructural studies (Bell and Brunk, unpublished).

"Lack of contact inhibition" may basically depend on (1) nonspecific causes and (2) a defunct specific cell to cell interaction.

Many of the nonspecific reasons for multilayering as a sign of lost contact inhibition are obvious from the considerations above. To this can be added that piles and multiple sheets can be nonspecifically formed by cell division (the new daughter cells may not find any empty space on the solid substrate), by local retractions within a cell sheet (not uncommonly misinterpreted as foci of virally transformed cells), and by interposition of secreted collagen. The last situation has been shown for human lung fibroblasts, where "pancake" after "pancake" of well-ordered fibroblasts can be layered on top of each other provided that the cells are permitted to produce interposed collagen (Elsdale and Foley, 1969; Elsdale and Bard, 1972).

Again it is obvious that valid observations on the mechanism behind multilayering and other abnormal patterns interpreted as "loss of contact inhibition" can be made only from time-lapse films or direct visual inspection under high optical resolution, preferably supplemented with ultrastructural studies.

5.2. Contact Inhibition Among Normal Cells

5.2.1. Fibroblasts

The original (Abercrombie and Heaysman, 1953) as well as most subsequent work on colliding cells in culture has concerned early passage embryonic fibroblasts usually of rat or chicken origin.

Abercrombie and Heaysman (1953, 1954) observed the velocity and direction of cell migration in chick tissue explants in plasma clot cultures. When cells from the circular outgrowth zones of two explants met, it was noted that the mean velocity in the junction area decreased by a factor of about 4 and that the direction of locomotion changed. Before the two zones of outgrowth made contact, the fibroblasts moved radially outward from the center of the explant. After junction, no directional preference existed. From these observations it is clear that embryonic fibroblasts show CI, however, its mechanism was not elucidated by these low-power time-lapse movies.

Subsequent studies under higher optical resolution have attempted to determine the mechanism for CI among fibroblasts. It is important to recognize that three types of collisions may occur: front to front (F-F), front to side (F-S), and side to side (S-S) (Fig. 12).

F-F or F-S contacts often resulted in cessation of ruffling and apparent adhesion between the two colliding cells (Abercrombie and Ambrose, 1958). This led the authors to conclude that CI is caused by a type of specific cell-to-cell interaction, involving the locomotory organ of at least one of the colliding cells: "The adhesion and cessation of activity of a leading ruffled membrane appears to be the visible expression of ... contact inhibition ..."

A detailed analysis mainly of F-F encounters has shown that there is first a delay of some 10–20 min during which the undulating movements of the edge and the push forward of a lamellipodium may continue. At this stage the lamellipodium will be placed under the contracted cell, particularly if F-S collisions are observed (Boyde *et al.*, 1969; Weston and Roth, 1969; Harris, 1973*b*).

The first clear light microscopic reaction on contact seems to be a contraction within the leading lamella (Abercrombie and Heaysman, 1954). This occurs without any severance of its underlying adhesion plaques to the solid substratum (Abercrombie and Dunn, 1975). After contraction, the lamella ceases to move and does not extend any new lamellipodia in the original direction. Pinocytosis and ruffling disappear. The contraction of the leading lamella leads to a shortening of the cell which mainly concerns its tail. Its rearmost part may be loosened from the substratum, leaving a few retraction fibers behind.

After these events, the colliding cell can follow different courses (Fig. 13). It may remain in firm attachment with or without formation of new lamellipodia. If such are formed, they may pull the cell away from its new associate. This is accompanied by formation of intercellular retraction fibers ("snap-back" in Fig. 13). A new

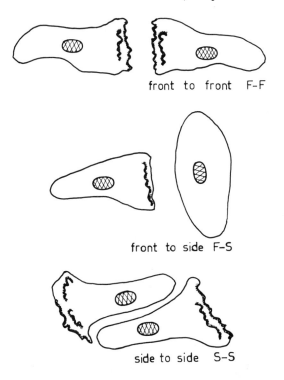

front to front   F-F

front to side F-S

side to side   S-S

FIGURE 12. Schematic drawing of three types of cell collisions.

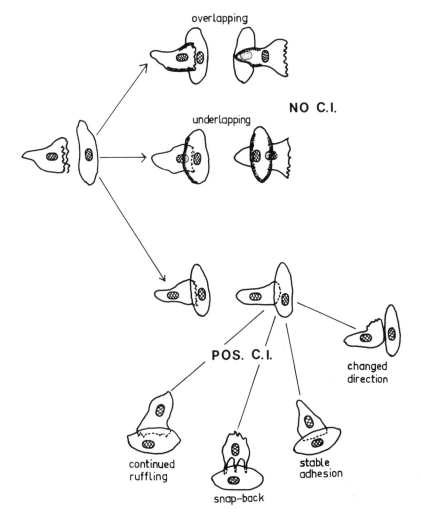

FIGURE 13. Different results of collisions between two cells. In the upper part, absence of contact inhibition is shown as overlapping or underlapping. The lower part of the figure shows four different possibilities of intercellular reactions when contact inhibition is present. Cells can remain in close apposition either with formation of a stable adhesion or with continued ruffling of the leading lamella of the colliding cell. If the cell leaves its position at impact, it may either snap back or veer off along the side of the contacted cell.

lamellipodium may form at the original site, and on this second attempt a lasting contact is usually formed.

Sometimes no lasting adhesion is built up. In that case, the cell or its leading lamella may either back away or more commonly move along the side of the contacted fibroblast. S-S contacts among fibroblasts do not usually lead to adhesion of inhibition of locomotion.

Ultrastructural studies (Heaysman and Pegrun, 1973) have documented that within 20 s after collisions areas of submembraneous specialization can be visualized. After 2 min, very well-developed microfilaments can be seen to converge toward the attachment plaques (Heaysman and Pegrum, 1973).

The overall effect of these events will be a tendency of cells to stick together rather than to move around as bumping cars. If cell division occurs simultaneously, available solid substrate will soon be filled by fibroblasts which—at least before collagenization becomes important—are confined to a monolayer (Abercrombie and Heaysman, 1954). Within this, the cells are clearly bipolar and capable of a slow sliding S-S motion (Elsdale and Foley, 1969).

5.2.2. Glia Cells

The most noteworthy difference between fibroblasts and glia is that only the latter have been shown to become essentially stationary, i.e., remain in fixed positions when a monolayer has been formed. In this layer there is a moderate amount of cytoplasmic (but no nuclear) overlapping. Ruffling has disappeared, but it is not known whether this is a sign of paralysis of lamellipodia and creation of extensive cell-to-cell adhesions or mechanical blocking of ruffling in the presence of continued lamellipodial activity (Pontén et al., 1969).

5.2.3. Epithelium

Contacting epithelia are particularly likely to establish lasting contacts with each other on collision. These cells show no distinct polarity and every type of collision has a high probability of ending as a permanent junction between the two colliding elements. This is shown indirectly by the great cohesion among epithelial cells, which tend to move as large multicellular sheets with little or no reshuffling of their constituent cell units. Extrusion of lamellipodia is confined to the free borders of these cells which are not in complete lateral contact with each other.

5.2.4. Macrophages

Interactions among macrophages have not been very widely studied. They tend strongly to remain as a monolayer even when they are dense. Whether this is caused by paralysis of lamellipodia or perhaps more likely by a strong adhesion to the solid substrate does not seem to have been critically studied.

5.2.5. Lymphoblastoid Cells

Collisions between lymphoblastoid cells have not been quantitatively studied. One very obvious impression from high-resolution films is, however, that they quickly change direction after a collision and that they never form stable associations with each other as long as there is a solid substrate available (a feeder cell, plastic, glass, etc.) to crawl on.

Lymphoblasts in suspension have a strong tendency to agglutinate. This phenomenon is very poorly understood, but may not be of the same nature as, for instance, the adhesion of a fibroblast to a solid substratum or another cell. Only the latter is sensitive to proteolytic enzymes and removal of calcium, two procedures which have no effect on clumps of lymphoblasts (unpublished).

5.2.6. Interactions Between Different Types of Normal Cells

a. Epithelium vs. Fibroblasts. In encounters between epithelial cells and fibroblasts, as reviewed by Abercrombie and Middleton (1968), epithelial sheets remain intact. Approaching fibroblasts are strongly contact inhibited and veer off sideways along the margin of the epithelial sheet. Only occasionally do they migrate under an intact sheet of epithelium. Fibroblasts cannot attach to the upper surface of epithelial cells and do not move over contacted epithelia (DiPasquale and Bell, 1974). In a random mixture of fibroblasts and epithelia, the two kinds of cells will eventually arrange themselves as epithelial islands well kept together and separated from each other by a sea of dense bundles of fibroblasts. Strong interepithelial adhesion in combination with mutual contact inhibition of locomotion would explain such a pattern. Histiotypic reassortment (*cf.* Moscona, 1974) has not been extensively studied in monolayer cultures. It is by no means excluded that, for instance, epithelial cells migrating on a solid surface attach to each other specifically by way of surface-located cell-to-cell ligands in a fashion similar to what occurs in suspensions of embryonic cells (*cf.* Moscona, 1974).

b. Lymphoblastoid Cells vs. Fibroblasts or Glia. Lymphoblastoid cells prefer to move around on a fibroblast and glia cell surface rather than an artificial solid support. Their characteristic peripolesis between the ventral surface of a "feeder" cell and its solid support has already been referred to.

Peripolesis may eventually lead to detachment and death of the feeder cells, presumably because attachment plaques are severed. Apart from this nonimmunological and apparently altogether nonspecific effect, lymphoblastoid cells do not inhibit the locomotion of the feeder cells, which continue to extrude lamellipodia, to ruffle, and to migrate as if they did not carry any lymphoblastoid cells with them. Conversely, lymphoblastoid cells show no signs of contact inhibition when they encounter a glia cell or a fibroblast but move freely across the contacted cell, usually along its ventral surface.

The social behavior of different normal cell types shows a strong resemblance to the *in vivo* situation, where epithelia and glia remain relatively stationary, whereas fibroblasts move about slowly. The wandering cells *in vivo* perform extensive migrations and do not seem to be stopped by a variety of cells and tissue barriers. They are, for instance, capable of migration through vessel walls.

5.3. Mechanism of Normal Contact Inhibition

The only unequivocal common denominator of several types of normal cells is that contact inhibition, defined as a restraint on directional locomotion, exists in all normal cell systems studied. However, the mechanisms may be entirely different. Epithelium shows the strongest indications that specific events (paralysis,

adhesion, contraction) in a contacting lamellipodium are of overriding importance. In fibroblasts, such events are also important but differential adhesion and
other "nonspecific" mechanisms probably also play a role. On the other end of the
scale, macrophages and lymphblastoid cells have no demonstrated signs of
specific membrane-to-membrane interactions. Their CI may be totally "nonspecific" and particularly for the lymphoblastoid cells a pure "bumping-car"
situation.

In his highly illuminating study of 3T3 cells, Bell (1974) showed that CI, in these
cells at least, can be explained by a combination of factors. In all F-F or F-S
encounters, the lamellipodium practically always extended in close apposition to
the solid substratum and not onto the dorsal surface of the contacted cells,
"underlapping." Two factors combine to make this extension inefficient in terms
of continued locomotion. One is that 3T3 cells move by broad lamellipodia and
the other is that they are equipped with densely and evenly distributed ventral
attachment plaques. This "mismatch" makes it almost impossible for one cell to
undermine its neighbor and thus continue migration in the original direction. It
seems beyond experimental reach at present to analyze why certain cells have a
specific shape and a defined number of attachment plaques. Not until more of the
fundamental biology of the cellular musculoskeletal system and its linkage to the
cell membrane is understood does it seem possible to resolve how "nonspecific"
hindrance of locomotion dependent on specializations within the individual cell of
the type described can arise.

For the lamellipodial cycle paralysis–adhesion–contraction, which also was part
of the CI in 3T3, it seems necessary to invoke special interactions between
molecules of the cell coat. The process is rather well described in morphological
terms but its biochemistry remains unresolved. No successful experiment has
been reported where specific movement inhibition or contraction or a lamellipodium has been elicited by isolated molecules or cell fractions. The triggering
mechanism is therefore unknown. The formation of submembraneous microfilaments within only 20 s (Heaysman and Pegrum, 1973) suggests polymerization of
actin from subunits, but new synthesis or even transport within the cell to the
contacting membrane is not excluded. The contraction which occurs in a
lamellipodium upon contact suggests that actinomyosinlike complexes are triggered into a tonic contraction within this specialized locomotory organ. Actinlike
material is quantitatively a major protein estimated at about 10–20% of all cell
proteins (cf. Pollard and Weihing, 1974). It would be most important for an
understanding of contact inhibition to analyze the intracellular distribution of
soluble and insoluble actin in relation to the specific morphology of contact
inhibition. It would be surprising if contractility in nonmuscle cells were not found
to be governed by the same principles as in the well-studied actomyosin complex
of muscle.

Primary specific intercellular attachment at least in F-F situations in 3T3 seems
to be initiated at discrete points along the contacting lamellipodium. Underlapping by further extension of the lamellipodium from the contacting cell will then
continue, but the contacted lamellipodium which no longer is in contact with a

solid substrate will become immobile (Bell, 1974). Such precise behavior suggests   87
the presence of a unidirectional signal with very local effects, presumably   CONTACT
involving coordinated movements and interaction of intramembraneous   INHIBITION
molecules within the contact area of two cells.

6. Social Behavior Among Malignant Cells

6.1. Carcinoma Cells

Interactions between demonstrably malignant cells of epithelial origin have been
only rather cursorily studied. Santesson (1935) noted a diminished coherence and
an irregular growth pattern among mouse mammary carcinoma cells. Trevan and
Roberts (1960) and Wilbanks and Richart (1966) made similar observations on
other types of carcinoma. As pointed out by Abercrombie *et al.* (1970a), these early
studies cannot easily be interpreted in terms of contact inhibition.

6.2. Glioma Cells

Only preliminary studies of glioma cells have been made, which suggest that these
malignant cells, in contrast to normal glia, tend to continue to migrate even under
crowded conditions (unpublished). Contact inhibition in a strict sense has not
been studied.

6.3. Sarcoma Cells

6.3.1. Spontaneous Tumors

The original observations (Abercrombie *et al.*, 1957) *in vitro* with two "old"
transplantable mouse sarcomas concerned their interactions with normal mouse
or chick fibroblasts. Upon collision, the sarcoma cells showed no CI but continued
along their previous paths without any diminished speed. Thus sarcoma cells
migrated over the normal cells apparently without sensing any interference from
them.

    Barski and Belehradek (1965), using another mouse sarcoma, modified the
original conclusions. When their malignant cells encountered coherent sheets of
normal cells identified as endothelium, migration stopped for the majority of the
malignant cells. Only a few isolated "sentinel cells" penetrated the territory
occupied by normal cells. This indicates that the "loss of contact inhibition"
claimed for sarcoma cells may not be absolute.

    Bell (1974) later reinterpreted the results of Abercrombie *et al.* (1957). He
points out that the sarcoma cells were contained in a plasma clot and that their
migration past the normal cells may not have depended on lack of contact
inhibition but rather an artificial passage may have been created by the experimental design, with fibrin fibers precipitated on top of and over the normal cells.

A disordered criss-cross array of fibroblasts has for more than a decade been used in focus-forming assays of different oncogenic viruses (Vogt and Dulbecco, 1962; Stoker and Macpherson, 1961; Todaro and Green, 1964; Temin and Rubin, 1958). The mechanism behind this easily scored morphological change has not been very much studied in terms of contact inhibition.

Veselý and Weiss (1973) studied a spontaneously neoplastic rat line before and after infection by RSV. The RSV-infected variant had acquired a high cloning efficiency in soft agar and was also more polygonal compared to the bipolar shape of the noninfected cells. The cells altered by RSV had largely lost their capacity of directed growth into an empty space. A wound of a cell layer was only slowly filled by cells which appeared to get there more by random migration than by directional locomotion. After mutual contact, the cells did not cross over each other, but membrane activity continued and pinocytosis, which may be considered an indirect sign of ruffling, was uninhibited even under dense conditions.

Careful analysis of collisions between normal embryonic rat fibroblasts and the established fibroblast line before and after infection by RSV (Table 6) revealed that all homotypic collisions lead to arrest of forward displacement and thus by definition to contact inhibition. Paralysis and contraction of the lamellipodium were rare in the RSV-exposed cultures but common in the two other types. Adhesion between colliding cells was more common among the RSV-treated fibroblasts than among the other two types of cells (Table 6). In terms of Fig. 13, the normal fibroblasts showed positive CI with formation of adhesions, the established line showed positive CI but usually with continued ruffling, and the RSV-treated sarcoma cells showed positive CI commonly with formation of adhesions. This similarity between normal and RSV-exposed cells disappeared when collisions with embryonic fibroblasts were considered. As shown under the heading "No contact inhibition" in Table 6, no mutual over- or underlapping was recorded in homotypic interactions between embryonic fibroblasts. When RSV-infected (and uninfected) sarcoma cells met embryonic fibroblasts, there was, on the other hand, very significant over- and underlapping.

One main conclusion by Veselý and Weiss (1973) was that malignant cells may show a high degree of homotypic CI, which also results in monolayering, but that the same cells may reveal lack of CI when cocultivated with normal cells. Another important principle is that CI may not be reciprocal. Whereas normal fibroblasts were inhibited and their leading lamellae contracted after collision with sarcoma cells, the reverse was not true. This confirmed a previous observation by Heaysman (1970).

The social behavior of 3T3 cells transformed by polyoma virus (Py3T3) was followed with time-lapse cinematography by Bell (1974). As already stated, there was only a moderate quantitative difference in the contact behavior of the two cell types. When crossing over occurred, it practically always had the form of underlapping by the contacting cell. In spite of this, Py3T3, in contrast to control 3T3, form thick irregular multilayers. Bell (1974) considered three possibilities to

TABLE 6

Contact Inhibition in Homotypic and Heterotypic Collisions Between Rat Cells[a]

	Tumori-genicity	Soft agar colonies	Contact inhibition (arrest of forward movement)		Formation of adhesions		No contact inhibition (against embryonic fibroblasts)		
			Homotypic	Heterotypic (against embryonic fibroblasts)	Homotypic	Heterotypic (against embryonic fibroblasts)	Overlapping		Underlapping
Embryonic fibroblasts	−	−	100		62		0	0	0
Established fibroblast line (sarcoma cells)	+	−	100	12	48	12	64	88	24
Established fibroblast line (sarcoma cells infected by RSV)	+	+	92	72	88	100	82	92	10

[a] The figures denote the percentage of collisions which result in the tabulated responses. Modified after Veselý and Weiss (1973).

explain this apparent paradox: (1) dense Py3T3, which are difficult to film in detail, could change from a predominant underlapping to an overlapping behavior; (2) Py3T3 could produce collagen and thus form interposed layers of a solid substrate; (3) Py3T3 could continue to divide irrespective of cell density and the new daughter cells would settle on top of underlying PY3T3. Of these possibilities, the last seemed most likely because it would explain all observations in this system in the most simple manner.

6.4. Social Behavior of Lymphoma and Leukemia Cells

Only a few preliminary observations have been made (see Nilsson and Pontén, 1975, and unpublished) on the social behavior of lymphoma and leukemia cells. These suggest that differences between lymphoma lines are considerable. One common factor may be that they are less adhesive against each other and against any feeder cells present. Their locomotion does not seem to be specifically influenced by the presence of other cells.

6.5. Significance of Contact Inhibition for Tumor Dissemination in Vivo

Contact inhibition among normal cells potentially involves all the possibilities of Fig. 13. The degree to which each one is realized is predominantly determined by the cell types directly involved in collisions but also by other factors such as presence of adjoining cells (Veselý and Weiss, 1973) and probably the nature of the solid substrate (Carter, 1965).

Epithelial cells almost always form stable contacts on their first contact with each other. Glia cells change direction, snap back, or form stable adhesions as one of their first choices but only rarely continue to ruffle (Fig. 13) after collision. The most likely alternative seems to be adhesion, and after several encounters the glia cells will eventually arrange themselves as a stable monolayer with specialized attachment areas between over- and underlapping parts of extended cytoplasm. The intercellular adhesions between glia seem less strong than between epithelia. Epithelium therefore tends to move as coherent sheets into a wound, whereas glia cells move in isolation. Fibroblasts may show all four types of "positive CI" illustrated in Fig. 13 and also "no CI" in the form of underlapping. Eventually, stable adhesions become most prominent but never to the exclusion of the other possible outcomes of close cellular interactions. Fibroblasts therefore remain in slow motion relative to each other even in dense cultures. Wandering cells finally show extensive cytoplasmic underlapping, no stable adhesions, and frequent changes of direction of movement after mutual contacts. Their migration pattern is largely independent of the cell density and they are in constant motion, perhaps with the exception of dense macrophage cultures where locomotion may become somewhat restricted.

Heterotypic interactions between normal cells show one well-established feature: epithelial sheets are not broken up by any other approaching normal cells.

Apart from this, different combinations have not been well-enough studied to permit firm conclusions.

The pattern just described is exactly that expected from what is known about the respective cell types *in vivo*. Epithelium is distinguished by its coherence and tendency to occupy defined territories without any intermingling with other cells. In the repair of wounds it tends to move as coherent sheets. Glia cells are probably stationary in the undisturbed adult brain but may be induced to move short distances after brain damage without apparently being able to penetrate into mesenchyme (meninges, vessels). Fibroblasts will migrate extensively in wound repair and penetrate deeply into muscle, vessel walls, tendons, articular cartilage, glia, and other tissue to form a connective tissue scar. Wandering cells, as the name implies, move freely in and out of vessels, within the mesenchyme, across epitheliomesenchymal borders, and between epithelial cells.

Very little is understood about the factors which regulate these behaviors. The parallelism between *in vivo* and *in vitro* should encourage studies of cultivated cells. It would be most interesting to find out the mechanism which determines the path (see Fig. 13) that any given cell type will follow after a homotypic or heterotypic collision. In all likelihood, the cell coat and the adjacent cell membrane are of overriding importance. The mere fact that F-F-, F-S, and S-S collisions (Fig. 12) have different effects shows that the outer cell surface presumably is highly specialized and differentiated with respect to capacity to react to cellular contact. With the rapidly accumulating knowledge about the internal organization of the cell's musculoskeletal system and locomotory organs and the availability of well-defined cocultivation systems, it seems within reach to analyze normal contact inhibition *in vitro* in at least crude molecular terms.

Normal cells *in vivo* have extensive capacity for invasion, i.e., translocation from one place to another through a territory occupied by a foreign cell species. This is called into action during embryonic life (extension of nerve cells, outward migration of neuroectodermal cells, etc.) but is also at work in adult life ("homing" by lymphocytes, formation of inflammatory exudates, scar formation, implantation of trophoblasts including migration through vessel walls, etc.). The essential feature of this scheme is that it is regulated so that certain paths are forbidden. Adult epithelium does not invade mesenchyme, glia cells do not trespass into meninges, fibroblasts do not penetrate through vessel walls, trophoblasts do not invade the deeper parts of the uterus, and so on. The social behavior of normal cells *in vitro* looks like a simplified but principally faithful reproduction of this complicated scheme.

Local and distant spread of malignant tumors can be thought of as a deviation from the normal pattern outlined above. This means that all histiotypically recognizable kinds of cells have their special criteria for pathological invasive behavior. For adult epithelium, then, any encroachment on mesenchymal territory is pathological and signifies acquisition of infiltrating properties. This becomes very clear in the progression of carcinoma *in situ* to invasive carcinoma. For fibroblasts, the situation is different. Penetration into muscle is, for instance, not *per se* pathological; however, if fibroblasts are found in vessel lumina this can be taken as a sign of malignant infiltration. For leukocytes, which normally do not respect any tissue borders, invasive growth is a meaningless criterion of malignancy.

Viewed in this light, it is not unexpected that studies of the social behavior of malignant cells *in vitro* have failed to shed much light on the mechanism of tumor invasion and metastasis. "Lack of contact inhibition" is far too crude to be a biologically meaningful counterpart of malignant invasion. The emphasis in experiments on sarcoma cells may have been misleading. Observed shifts in the frequency of different collision events (Fig. 13) do not follow the same pattern in different systems. The recording of these events may at best have only an indirect bearing on how sarcoma cells may spread as distinct from normal fibroblasts. It is not unlikely that malignancy in this particular class of cells primarily depends on a failure to stop proliferating rather than any qualitative disturbance in locomotion capability.

It is difficult to predict how studies on contact inhibition will aid in understanding and preventing metastasis. Cell culture methods are very powerful tools for attacking difficult problems in cell biology. A much better understanding of normal cell interaction seems a likely possibility. An important but unresolved problem is whether contact inhibition is related to proliferation control. In normal glia, a precise correlation seems to exist between regulation of cell locomotion and proliferation (Pontén *et al.*, 1969). To a large extent this also seems true for fibroblasts. Still, however, critical high-resolution comparisons have not been made. It would not be surprising if regulation of proliferation and movement turned out to operate independently. *In vivo* the two are apparently often dissociated, as indicated by classes of cells (e.g., wandering macrophages) that migrate extensively but do not divide much and intestinal crypt epithelium, which proliferates continuously but only slides passively toward the tips of the villi to be shed into the lumen of the gut. Another example is squamous cell carcinoma *in situ*, which shows all the hallmarks of malignancy including unregulated proliferation but in spite of this does not invade its stroma.

A very obvious fact which has never been much discussed and which should not be regarded as self-evident is that malignant cell populations almost always will acquire the potential for infiltrative growth, i.e., enter a path which normally is forbidden. This suggests that a deficient proliferation control is very likely to develop into a deficient locomotion control. Since the former as well as the latter can be quantified *in vitro*, it would be of significance to know how strong the correlation between the two variables is. Locomotion *per se* may not be the important parameter but rather a certain aspect such as the capacity of forming specific adhesions to a lamellipodium. It is possible that elucidation of the nature of the locomotion control may also shed light on the important problem of why malignant cells do not submit to physiological growth control.

A very interesting avenue would be to try to recapitulate embryonic and other regulated types of cell translocations *in vitro* to attempt to isolate the signals responsible for these phenomena. Which cells can respond by chemotaxis? When are cell contacts necessary? Which molecules function in chemotaxis and contact-regulated locomotion and adhesion? How are signals from the exterior received and translated into a certain locomotory behavior?

Not until these and other questions have been answered does it seem likely that one could profitably start to understand the abnormal migration patterns which so often follow a malignant transformation.

Metastasis is in all probability not a nonspecific mechanistic result of invasion and transport via vessels. It probably reflects aberrations in cell behavior which in turn depend on more or less subtle disturbances in a biological system for cell and tissue recognition that we are deplorably ignorant about (see Chapter 3).

7. Conclusion

Contact inhibition can be defined as a restraint of directional locomotion of a cell after contact with another object, usually a cell. Contact inhibition can lead to either (1) a changed direction of locomotion without formation of intercellular adhesions, (2) reversed locomotion with retention of intercellular contact fibers, (3) a standstill with continued activity of the locomotory organ of the contacting cell (extension of lamellipodia, ruffling), or (4) a standstill with formation of lasting intercellular adhesion, tonic contraction, and paralysis of the locomotory organ of the contacting cell. If no contact inhibition exists, the contacting cell usually moves under the contacted cell.

All normal cells show strong contact inhibition but by different mechanisms. Epithelium preferentially reacts according to (4). Glia cells may show all four types of contact inhibition but eventually alternative (4) becomes predominant. Fibroblasts show all four types but eventually (1) and (4) become dominant. Macrophages prefer (1) and (3) and lymphoblastoid cells (1). The end result will be that epithelium and glia cells form monolayers with no movement of the individual cells. Fibroblasts grow into three-dimensional sheets, bundles, or whorls where individual bipolar cells, often in a cohort, slide slowly past each other. Macrophages move around within a monolayer without any fixed positions for the individual cells. Lymphoblastoid cells migrate rapidly only on the outside of other ("feeder") cells, where they never form a stable array.

Only alternative (4)—i.e., adhesion–contraction–paralysis of a lamellipodium—seems to be a highly specific event. It may reflect an important control mechanism for locomotion *in vivo* as well as *in vitro*. The molecular mechanism behind its triggering and execution is unknown.

After malignant transformation, cells have always shown some departure from the normal pattern described above. Malignant epithelium shows diminished tendency for intercellular adhesion. Malignant glia cells also seem to be less likely to form stable cell-to-cell adhesions. Malignant fibroblasts have shown variable patterns, with increased underlapping, decreased tendency to establishment of adhesions, and extensive continued ruffling in dense layers. Malignant macrophages have not been studied, and malignant lymphoma cells have been less mobile than normal lymphoblastoid cells.

The aberrations in malignant cells cannot indiscriminately be described as "lack of contact inhibition." Instead, they reflect a more or less subtle deviation from a normal migration pattern which only sometimes conforms to criteria for a loss of contact inhibition. It is possible that the normal adhesion–contraction–paralysis cycle of lamellipodia may always be disturbed in malignancy, but too few precise studies have been made to permit any generalizations.

A disturbed contact behavior among malignant cells *in vitro* has often been assumed to reflect infiltrative growth *in vivo*. Infiltration *in vivo* relates to very specific situations involving malignant cells against normal cells. Few attempts have been made to simulate these conditions *in vitro* and analyze the results in terms of contact inhibition. It is still unknown if and how a disturbed contact behavior *in vitro* relates to tumor cell invasion *in vivo*, but it does not seem unlikely that the two in some as yet undetermined fashion reflect a membrane change characteristic of the malignant state.

A promising start has been made in the elucidation of the function and structure of the cell's musculoskeletal system and its connection with specific molecules in the cell membrane. Links between this and putative cell recognition sites on the outer cell surface need to be identified in order to understand normal and pathological regulation of cell locomotion.

ACKNOWLEDGMENTS

Dr. Uno Lindberg at the Wallenberg Laboratory in Uppsala has kindly read the manuscript and given much constructive advice. Mrs. Kerstin Lindberg is gratefully thanked for excellent secretarial help and support. Published and unpublished experiments from our group have almost exclusively been aided by grants from the Swedish Cancer Society.

8. References

AARONSON, S. A., AND TODARO, G. J., 1968, Basis for the acquisition of malignant potential by mouse cells cultivated in vitro, *Science* **162**:1024.

ABERCROMBIE, M., 1965, The locomotory behavior of cells, in: *Cells and Tissues in Culture* (E. N. Willmer, ed.), pp. 177–202, Academic Press, New York.

ABERCROMBIE, M., 1967, Contact inhibition: The phenomenon and its biological implications for orientation of cell movements *Natl. Cancer Inst. Monogr.* **26**:249.

ABERCROMBIE, M., 1970, Contact inhibition in tissue culture, *In Vitro* **6**:128.

ABERCROMBIE, M., AND AMBROSE, E. J., 1958, Interference microscope studies of cell contacts in tissue culture, *Exp. Cell Res.* **15**:332.

ABERCROMBIE, M., AND AMBROSE, E. J., 1962, The surface properties of cancer cells: A review, *Cancer Res.* **22**:525.

ABERCROMBIE, M., AND DUNN, G., 1975, Adhesions of fibroblasts to substratum during contact inhibition observed by interference reflection microscopy, *Exptl. Cell Res.* **92**:57.

ABERCROMBIE, M., AND HEAYSMAN, J. E. M., 1953, Observations on the social behavior of cells in tissue culture. I. Speed of movement of chick heart fibroblasts in relation to their mutual contacts, *Exp. Cell Res.* **5**:111.

ABERCROMBIE, M., AND HEAYSMAN, J. E. M., 1954, Social behavior of cells in tissue culture. II. "monolayering" of fibroblasts, *Exp. Cell Res.* **6**:293.

ABERCROMBIE, M., AND MIDDLETON, C. A., 1968, Epithelial-mesenchymal interactions affecting locomotion of cells in culture, in: *Epithelial-Mesenchymal Interactions* (R. Fleischmajer and R. E. Billingham, eds.), p. 56, Williams and Wilkins, Baltimore.

ABERCROMBIE, M., HEAYSMAN, J. E. M., AND KARTHAUSER, H. M., 1957, Social behavior of cells in tissue culture. III. Mutual influences of sarcoma cells and fibroblasts, *Exp. Cell Res.* **13**:276.

ABERCROMBIE, M., HEAYSMAN, E. M., AND PEGRUM, S. M., 1970a, Locomotion of fibroblasts in culture. I. Movements of the leading edge, *Exp. Cell Res.* **59**:393.

ABERCROMBIE, M., HEAYSMAN, J. E. M., AND PEGRUM, S. M., 1970b, The locomotion of fibroblasts in culture. II. "Ruffling," *Exp. Cell Res.* **60**:437.

ABERCROMBIE, M., HEAYSMAN, J. E. M., AND PEGRUM, S. M., 1970c, The locomotion of fibroblasts in culture. III. Movements of particles on the dorsal surface of the leading lamella, *Exp. Cell Res.* **62**:389.

ABERCROMBIE, M., HEAYSMAN, J. E. M., AND PEGRUM, S. M., 1971, The locomotion of fibroblasts in culture. IV. Electron microscopy of the leading lamella, *Exp. Cell Res.* **67**:359.

ABERCROMBIE, M., HEAYSMAN, J. E. M., AND PEGRUM, S. M., 1972, The locomotion of fibroblasts in culture. V. Surface marking with concanavalin A, *Exp. Cell Res.* **73**:536.

ADELSTEIN, R. S., POLLARD, T. D., AND KUEHL, W. M., 1971, Isolation and characterization of myosin and two myosin fragments from human blood platelets, *Proc. Natl. Acad. Sci. U.S.A.* **68**:2703.

ALBRECHT-BÜHLER, G., 1973, A quantitative difference in the movement of marker particles in the plasma membrane of 3T3 mouse fibroblasts and their polyoma transformants, *Exp. Cell Res.* **78**:67.

ALLISON, A. C., 1973, The role of microfilaments and microtubules in cell movement, endocytosis and exocytosis, in: *Locomotion of Tissue Cells* (R. Porter and D. W. Fitzsimmons, eds.), Ciba Foundation Symposium 14, pp. 109–148, Elsevier, Excerpta Medica, North-Holland, Amsterdam.

ALLISON, A. C., DAVIES, P., AND DE PETRIS, S., 1971, Role of contractile microfilaments in macrophage movement and endocytosis, *Nature New Biol.* **232**:153.

AMBROSE, E. J., BATZDORF, U., OSBORN, J. S., AND STUART, P. R., 1970, Sub-surface structures in normal and malignant cells, *Nature (London)* **227**:397.

AOKI, T., HÄMMERLING, V., DE HARVEN, E., BOYSE, E. A., AND OLD, L. J., 1969, Antigenic structure of cell surfaces: An immunoferritin study of the occurrence and topography of H-21, and TL alloantigens on mouse cells, *J. Exp. Med.* **130**:979.

BARSKI, G., AND BELEHRADEK, J., 1965, Étude microinématographique du méchanisme d'invasion cancéreuse en cultures de tissu normal associé aux cellules malignes, *Exp. Cell Res.* **37**:464.

BARSKI, G., AND BELEHRADEK, J., 1965, Étude microinématographique du méchanisme d'invasion cancéreuse en cultures de tissu normal associé aux cellules malignes, *Exp. Cell Res.* **37**:464.

BEHNKE, O., 1970, Microtubules in disk-shaped blood cells, *Int. Rev. Exp. Pathol.* **9**:1.

BELL, P. B., 1974, Movement, contact behavior and morphology of 3T3 and polyoma-transformed 3T3 mouse fibroblasts in culture—A comparative study, doctoral dissertation, Yale University.

BENNETT, H. S., 1963, Morphological aspects of extracellular polysaccharides, *J. Histochem. Cytochem.* **11**:14.

BENYESH-MELNICK, M., FERNBACH, D. J., AND LEWIS, R. T., 1963, Studies on human leukemia. I. Spontaneous lymphoblastoid transformation of fibroblastic bone marrow cultures derived from leukemic and nonleukemic children, *J. Natl. Cancer Inst.* **31**:1311.

BERLIN, R. D., AND UKENA, T. E., 1972, Effect of colchicine and vinblastine on the agglutination of polymorphonuclear leucocytes by concanavalin A, *Nature New Biol.* **238**:120.

BERNFIELD, M. R. AND WESSELLS, N. K., 1970, Intra- and extracellular control of epithelial morphogenesis, *Devl. Biol. Suppl.* **4**:195.

BERRY, L. J., AND SPIES, T. D., 1949, Phagocytosis, *Medicine* **28**:239.

BETTEX-GALLAND, M., AND LÜSCHER, E. F., 1965, Thrombosthenin, the contractile protein from blood platelets and its relation to other contractile proteins, *Adv. Protein Chem.* **20**:1.

BOYDE, A., GRAINGER, F., AND JONES, D. W., 1969, Scanning electron microscopic observations of chick embryo fibroblasts *in vitro*, with particular reference to the movement of cells under others, *Z. Zellforsch. Mikrosk. Anat.* **94**:46.

BRAY, D., 1973, Cytoplasmic actin: A comparative study, *Cold Spring Harbor Symp. Quant. Biol.* **37**:567.

BRETSCHER, M., 1972, Major human erythrocyte glycoprotein spans the cell membrane, *Nature New Biol.* **231**:229.

BRUNK, U., ERICSSON, J., PONTÉN, J., AND WESTERMARK, B., 1971, Specialization of cell surfaces in contact inhibited, human glia-like cells *in vitro, Exp. Cell Res.* **67**:407.

BUCKLEY, I. K., 1974, Subcellular motility: A correlated light and electron microscopic study using cultured cells, *Tissue Cell* **6**:1.

BUCKLEY, I. K., AND PORTER, K. R., 1967, Cytoplasmic fibrils in living cultured cells: A light and electron microscope study, *Protoplasma* **64**:349.

CARTER, S. B., 1965, Principles of cell motility: The direction of cell movement and cancer invasion, *Nature (London)* **208**:1183.

CARTER, S. B., 1967, Haptotaxis and the mechanism of cell motility, *Nature (London)* **213**:256.

CLARKSON, B., STRIFE, A., AND DE HARVEN, E., 1967, Continuous culture of seven new cell lines (SK-L1 to 7) from patients with acute leukemia, *Cancer* **20**:926.

CONGDON, E. D., 1915, The identification of tissues in artificial cultures, *Anat. Rec.* **9**:343.

CRAWFORD, B., CLONEY, R. A., AND CAHN, R. D., 1972, Cloned pigmented retinal cells: The effects of cytochalasin B on ultrastructure and behavior, *Z. Zellforsch. Mikrosk. Anat.* **130**:135.

CURTIS, A. S. G., 1961, Control of some cell-contact reactions in tissue culture, *J. Natl. Cancer Inst.* **26**:253.

DANIELS, M. P., 1968, Colchicine inhibition of nerve process elongation *in vitro, J. Cell Biol.* **39**:31.

DANIELS, M. P., 1972, Colchicine inhibition of nerve fiber formation *in vitro, J. Cell Biol.* **53**:164.

DE PETRIS, S., AND RAFF, M. C., 1973, Fluidity of the plasma membrane and its implications for cell movement, in: *Locomotion of Tissue Cells* (R. Porter and D. W. Fitzsimons, ed.), pp. 27–52, Ciba Foundation Symposium, Associated Scientific Publishers, Amsterdam.

DERMER, G. D., LUE, J., AND NEUSTEIN, H. B., 1974, Comparison of surface material, cytoplasmic filaments, and intercellular junctions from untransformed and two mouse sarcoma virus-transformed cell lines, *Cancer Res.* **34**:31.

DIPAOLO, J. A., TAKANO, K., AND POPESCU, N. C., 1972, Quantitation of chemically induced neoplastic transformation of BALB/3T3 cloned cell lines, *Cancer Res.* **32**:2686.

DIPASQUALE, A., 1973, An analysis of the contact behavior and locomotion of epithelial cells in vitro, doctoral dissertation, Yale University.

DIPASQUALE, A., AND BELL, P. B., 1974, The upper cell surface: Its inability to support active cell movement in culture, *J. Cell Biol.* **62**:198.

DUNN, G. A., 1973, Extension of nerve fibres, their mutual interaction and direction of growth in tissue culture, in: *Locomotion of Tissue Cells* (R. Porter and D. W. Fitzsimons, eds.), pp. 211–232, Associated Scientific Publishers, Amsterdam.

EARLE, W. R., 1943, Production of malignancy *in vitro*. IV. The mouse fibroblasts, cultures and changes seen in the living cells, *J. Natl. Cancer Inst.* **4**:165.

EDELMAN, G. M., AND WANG, J. L., 1974, The cell surface–membrane complex in cell interactions, International Workshop on Cell Surfaces and Malignancy, Fogarthy International Center, National Institute of Health, Bethesda, Md., September 11–13.

EDELMAN, G. M., YAHARA, I., AND WANG, J. L., 1973, Receptor mobility and receptor cytoplasmic, interactions in lymphocytes, *Proc. Natl. Acad. Sci. U.S.A.* **70**:1442.

EDIDIN, M., AND WEISS, A., 1972, Antigen cap formation in cultured fibroblasts: a reflection of membrane fluidity and of cell motility, *Proc. Natl. Acad. Sci. U.S.A.* **69**:2456.

EGUCHI, G., AND OKADA, T. S., 1971, Ultrastructure of the differentiated cell colony derived from a singly isolated chondrocyte in *in vitro* culture, *Dev. Growth Differ.* **12**:297.

ELSDALE, T., AND BARD, J., 1972, Collagen substrata for studies on cell behavior, *J. Cell Biol.* **54**:626.

ELSDALE, T., AND FOLEY, R., 1969, Morphogenetic aspects of multilayering in Petri dish cultures of human fetal lung fibroblasts, *J. Cell Biol.* **41**:298.

GAIL, M. H., AND BOONE, C. W., 1971, Effect of colcemid on fibroblast motility, *Exp. Cell Res.* **65**:221.

GASIC, G., AND BERWICK, L., 1962, Hela stain for acid containing mucins: Adaptation to electron microscopy, *J. Cell Biol.* **19**:223.

GEY, G. O., GEY, M. K., FIROR, W. M., AND SELF, W. O., 1949, Cultural and cytologic studies on autologous normal and malignant cells of specific *in vitro* origin, *Acta Unio Int. Contra Cancrum* **6**:706.

GOLDMAN, R. D., AND FOLLETT, E. A.C., 1969, The structure of the major cell processes of isolated BHK-21 fibroblasts. *Exp. Cell Res.* **57**:263.

GOLDMAN, R., AND KNIPE, D., 1972, Functions of cytoplasmic fibers in non-muscle cell motility, *Cold Spring Harbor Symp. Quant. Biol.* **37**:523.

GOLDMAN, R. D., BERG, G., BUSHNELL, A., CHANG, C.-M., DICKERMAN, L., HOPKINS, N., MILLER, M. L., POLLACK, R., AND WANG, E., 1973, Fibrillar systems in cell motility, in: *Locomotion of Tissue Cells* (R. Porter and D. W. Fitzsimmons, eds.), pp. 83–107, Associated Scientific Publishers, Amsterdam.

GOLDSTEIN, M. N., 1954, Formation of giant cells from human mono-cytes cultivated on cellophane, *Anat. Rec.* **118**:577.

GROESCHEL-STEWART, U., 1971, Comparative studies of human smooth and striated muscle myosins, *Biochem. Biophys. Acta* **229**:322.

HARRIS, H., 1953, Chemotaxis of monocytes, *Br. J. Exp. Pathol.* **34**:276.

HARRIS, A. K., 1973a, Cell surface movements related to cell locomotion, in: *Locomotion of Tissue Cells* (R. Porter and D. W. Fitzsimons, eds.), pp. 3–26, Associated Scientific Publishers, Amsterdam.

HARRIS, A. K., 1973b, Location of cellular adhesions to solid substrata, *Dev. Biol.* **35**:97.

HARRIS, A. K., AND DUNN, G., 1972, Centripetal transport of attached particles on both surfaces of moving fibroblasts, *Exp. Cell Res.* **73**:519.

HARRISON, R. G., 1910, The outgrowth of nerve fiber as a mode of protoplasmic movement, *J. Exp. Zool.* **9**:787.

HAYFLICK, L., AND MOORHEAD, P. S., 1961, The serial cultivation of human diploid cell strains, *Exp. Cell Res.* **25**:585.

HEAYSMAN, J. E. M., 1970, Non-reciprocal contact inhibition, *Experientia* **26**:1344.

HEAYSMAN, J. E. M., AND PEGRUM, S. M., 1973, Early contacts between fibroblasts, *Exp. Cell Res.* **78**:71.

HEIDELBERGER, C., 1973, Chemical oncogenesis in culture, *Adv. Cancer Res.* **18**:317.

HOLLEY, R. W., AND KIERNAN, J. A., 1968, "Contact inhibition" of cell division in 3T3 cells, *Proc. Natl. Acad. Sci. U.S.A.* **60**:300.

HUXLEY, H. E., 1969, The mechanism of muscular contraction, *Science* **164**:1356.

INGRAM, V. M., 1969, A side view of moving fibroblasts, *Nature (London)* **222**:641.

ISHIKAWA, H., BISCHOFF, R., AND HOLTZER, H., 1969, Formation of arrowhead complexes with heavy meromyosin in a variety of cell types, *J. Cell Biol.* **43**:312.

JACOBY, F., 1938, On the identity of blood monocytes and tissue macrophages; their growth rates *in vitro*, *J. Physiol. (London)* **93**:48.

JACOBY, F., 1965, Macrophages, in: *Cells and Tissues in Culture* (E. N. Willmer, ed.), pp. 1–93, Academic Press, New York.

LASFARGI E., AND DELAUNAY, A., 1947, Nouvelles recherches sur le tactisme des macrophages *in vitro*, *Ann. Inst. Pasteur* **73**:14.

LAZARIDES, E., 1975, Tropomyosin antibody: The specific localization of tropomyosin in nonmuscle cells, *J. Cell Biol.* **65**:549.

LAZARIDES, E., AND WEBER, K., 1974, Actin antibody: The specific visualization of actin fibers in nonmuscle cells, *Proc. Natl. Acad. Sci U.S.A.* **71**:2268.

LEWIS, C. T., AND LEWIS, M. R., 1924, Behavior of cells in tissue cultures, in: *General Cytology* (E. W. Cowdry, ed.), pp. 383–447, University of Chicago Press, Chicago.

LEWIS, W. H., AND WEBSTER, L. T., 1921, Wandering cells, endothelial cells, and fibroblasts in cultures from human lymph nodes, *J. Exp. Med.* **34**:397.

LOEB, L., 1921, Ameboid movement, tissue formation and consistency of protoplasm, *Am. J. Physiol.* **56**:140.

MACPHERSON, I., AND STOKER, M., 1962, Polyoma transformation of hamster cell clones—An investigation of genetic factors affecting cell competence, *Virology* **16**:147.

MARTZ, E., 1973, Contact inhibition of speed in 3T3 and its independence from postconfluence inhibition of cell division, *J. Cell. Physiol.* **81**:39.

MCNUTT, N. S., CULP, L. A., AND BLACK, P. H., 1971, Contact-inhibited revertant cell lines isolated from SV40-transformed cells. II. Ultrastructural study, *J. Cell Biol.* **50**:691.

MCNUTT, N. S., CULP, L. A., AND BLACK, P. H., 1973, Contact-inhibited revertant cell lines isolated from SV40-transformed cells. IV. Microfilament distribution and cell shape in untransformed, transformed, and revertant Balb/c 3T3 cells, *J. Cell Biol.* **56**:412.

MIDDLETON, C. A., 1972, Contact inhibition of locomotion in cultures of pigmented retina epithelium, *Exp. Cell Res.* **70**:91.

MIDDLETON, C. A., 1973, The control of epithelial cell locomotion in tissue culture, in: *Locomotion of Tissue Cells* (R. Porter and D. W. Fitzsimons, eds.), pp. 251–270, Associated Scientific Publishers, Amsterdam.

MIRANDA, A. F., GODMAN, G. C., AND TANENBAUM, S., 1974, Action of cytochalasin D on cells of established lines. II. Cortex and microfilaments, *J. Cell Biol.* **62:**406.

MONTAGNIER, L., AND MACPHERSON, I., 1964, Croissance sélective en gélose de cellules de hamster transformées par le virus du polyome, *C. R. Acad. Sci.* **258:**4171.

MOORE, G. E., AND MINOWADA, J., 1969, Human hemapoietic cell lines: A progress report, *Hemic Cells in Vitro* **4:**100.

MOSCONA, A. A., 1974, Surface specification of embryonic cells: Lectin receptors, cell recognition, and specific cell ligands, in: *The Cell Surface in Development* (A. A. Moscona, ed.), pp. 67–99, Wiley, New York.

NEVILLE, D. M., JR., AND KAHN, C. R., 1974, Isolation of plasma membranes for cell surface membrane receptor studies, in: *Methods in Molecular Biology*, Vol. 5: *Subcellular Particles Structures and Organelles* (A. I. Laskin and J. A. Last, eds.), pp. 57–88, Dekker, New York.

NICHOLSON, G. L., AND PAINTER, R. G., 1973, Anionic sites of human erythrocyte membranes. II. Antispectrin-induced transmembrane aggregation of the binding sites for positively charged colloidal particles, *J. Cell Biol.* **59:**395.

NILSSON, K., 1971, High frequency establishment of immunoglobulin producing lymphoblastoid cell lines from normal and malignant lymphoid tissue and peripheral blood, *Int. J. Cancer* **8:**432.

NILSSON, K., AND PONTÉN, J., 1975, Classification and biological nature of established human hematopoietic cell lines, *Int. J. Cancer* (in press).

NILSSON, K., NILSSON, L., AND PONTÉN, J., 1970, Lymphocytes are mobile (film), Third International Conference on Lymphatic Tissue and Germinal Centers in Immune Reactions, Uppsala.

OLDFIELD, F. E., 1963, Orientation behavior of chick leucocytes in tissue culture and their interactions with fibroblasts, *Exp. Cell Res.* **30:**125.

PHILIPSON, L., AND PONTÉN, J., 1967, Immunoglobulin synthesis in long term cultures of lymph nodes from Hodgkin's disease, *Life Sci.* **6:**2635.

POLLACK, R., OSBORN, M., AND WEVER, K., 1974, Patterns of organization of actin and myosin in normal and transformed nonmuscle cells: Immunofluorescence—contraction/SV40/achorage/microfilaments, *J. Cell Biol.* (in press).

POLLARD, T. D., AND WEIHING, R. R., 1974, Cytoplasmic actin and myosin and cell movement, in: *Critical Reviews in Biochemistry*, Vol. 2, pp. 1–65, (G. D. Fasman, ed.), CRC Press, Cleveland.

PONTÉN, J., 1971, *Spontaneous and Virus Induced Transformation in Cell Culture* (S. Gard, C. Hallauer, and K. F. Meyer, eds.), Springer, New York.

PONTÉN, J., AND MACINTYRE, E. H., 1968, Long term culture of normal and neoplastic human glia, *Acta Pathol. Microbiol. Scand.* **74:**465.

PONTÉN, J., WESTERMARK, B., AND HUGOSSON, R., 1969, Regulation of proliferation and movement of human glia-like cells in culture, *Exp. Cell Res.* **58:**393.

PORTER, K. R., 1966, Cytoplasmic microtubules and their functions, in: *Principles of Biomolecular Organization* (G. E. W. Wolstenholme, and M. O'Connor, eds.), pp. 308–345, Churchill, London.

PULVERTAFT, R. J., 1959, Cellular associations in normal and abnormal lymphocytes, *Proc. R. Soc. Med.* **52:**315.

REVEL, J. P., 1974, Scanning electron microscope studies of cell surface morphology and labeling, *in situ* and *in vitro*, in: *Scanning Electron Microscopy* (O. Johari and I. Corvin, eds.), pp. 542–548.

REVEL, J. P., HOCH, P., AND HO, D., 1974, Adhesion of culture cells to their substratum, *Exptl. Cell Res.* **84:**207.

RUBIN, H., 1960, The suppression of morphological alterations in cells infected with Rouse sarcoma virus, *Virology* **12:**14.

RUBIN, H., 1962, Response of cell and organism to infection with avian tumor viruses, *Bacteriol. Rev.* **26:**1.

RUTISHAUSER, U., YAHARA, I., AND EDELMAN, G. M., 1974, Morphology, motility and surface behavior of lymphocytes bound to nylon fibers, *Proc. Natl. Acad. Sci. U.S.A.* **71;**1149.

SANFORD, K. K., LIKELY, G. D., AND EARLE, W. R., 1954, The development of variations in transplantability and morphology within a clone of mouse fibroblasts transformed to sarcoma-producing cells *in vitro*, *J. Natl. Cancer Inst.* **15:**215.

SANTESSON, L., 1935, Characteristics of epithelial mouse tumour cells *in vitro* and tumour strains *in vivo*, *Acta Pathol. Microbiol. Scand. Suppl.* **24:**1.

SCHROEDER, T. E., 1970, The contractile ring. 1. Fine structure of dividing mammalian (HeLa) cells and the effects of cytochalasin B, *Z. Zellforsch. Mikrosk. Anat.* **109:**431.

SINGER, S. J., AND NICHOLSON, G. L., 1972, The fluid mosaic model of the structure of cell membranes, *Science* **175:**720.

SPOONER, B. S., YAMADA, K. M., AND WESSELLS, N. K., 1971, Microfilaments and cell locomotion, *J. Cell Biol.* **49**:595.

SPOONER, B. S., ASH, J. F., WRENN, J. T., FRATER, R. B., AND WESSELLS, N. K., 1973, Heavy meromyosin binding to microfilaments involved in cell and morphogenetic movements, *Tissue Cell* **5**:37.

STOKER, M., 1962, Characteristics of normal and transformed clones arising from BHK21 cells exposed to polyoma virus, *Virology* **18**:649.

STOKER, M., 1973, Role of diffusion boundary layer in contact inhibition of growth, *Nature (London)* **246**:200.

STOKER, M., AND MACPHERSON, I., 1961, Studies on transformation of hamster cells by polyoma virus *in vitro*, *Virology* **14**:359.

STOKER, M., AND RUBIN, H., 1967, Density dependent inhibition of cell growth in culture, *Nature (London)* **215**:171.

STOSSEL, T. P., AND POLLARD, T. D., 1973, Myosin in polymorphnuclear leukocytes, *J. Biol. Chem.* **248**:8288.

STRACHER, A., AND DREIZEN, P., 1966, Structure and function of the contractile protein myosin, in: *Current Topics in Bioenergetics*, Vol. 1 (D. R. Sandai, ed.), p. 154, Academic Press, New York.

TANIGAKI, N., YAGI, Y., MOORE, G. E., AND PRESSMAN, D., 1966, Immunoglobulin production in human leukemia cell lines, *J. Immunol.* **97**:634.

TAYLOR, R. G., DUFFUS, P. H., RAFF, M. C., AND DE PETRIS, S., 1971, Redistribution and pinocytosis of lymphocyte surface immunoglobulin molecules induced by anti-immunoglobulin antibody, *Nature New Biol.* **233**:225.

TEMIN, H. M., 1960, The control of cellular morphology in embryonic cells infected with Rous sarcoma virus *in vitro*, *Virology* **10**:182.

TEMIN, H. M., AND RUBIN, H., 1958, Characteristics of an assay of Rous sarcoma virus and Rous sarcoma cells in tissue culture, *Virology* **6**:669.

TENENBAUM, E., AND DOLJANSKI, L., 1943, Studies on Rous sarcoma cells cultivated in vitro: Morphological properties of Rous sarcoma cells, *Cancer Res.* **3**:585.

TODARO, G. J., AND GREEN, H., 1963, Quantitative studies of the growth of mouse embryo cells in culture and their development into established lines, *J. Cell Biol.* **17**:299.

TODARO, G. J., AND GREEN, H., 1964, An assay for cellular transformation by SV40, *Virology* **23**:117.

TODARO, G. J., AND GREEN, H., 1965, Successive transformations of an established cell line by polyoma virus and SV40, *Science* **14**:513.

TODARO, G. J., AND GREEN, H., 1966, High frequency of SV40 transformation of mouse cell line 3T3, *Virology* **28**:756.

TODARO, G. J., GREEN, H., AND GOLDBERG, B. D., 1964, Transformation of properties of an established cell line by SV40 and polyoma virus, *Proc. Natl. Acad. Sci. U.S.A.* **51**:66.

TODARO, G. J., LAZAR, G. K., AND GREEN, H., 1965, The initiation of cell division in a contact inhibited mammalian cell line, *J. Cell. Comp. Physiol.* **66**:325.

TREVAN, D. J., AND ROBERTS, D. C., 1960, Sheet information by cells of an ascites tumour *in vitro*, *Br. J. Cancer* **14**:724.

UHLENHUTH, E., 1915, The form of the epithelial cells in culture of frog skin, and its relation to the consistency of the medium, *J. Exp. Med.* **22**:76.

VASILIEV, J. M., GELFAND, I. M., DOMNINA, L. V., AND RAPPOPORT, R. I., 1969, Wound healing processes in cell cultures, *Exp. Cell Res.* **54**:83.

VASILIEV, J. M., GELFAND, I. M., DOMNINA, L. V., IVANOVA, O. Y., KOMM, S. G., AND OLSHEVSKAJA, L. V., 1970, Effect of colcemic on the locomotory behaviour of fibroblasts, *J. Embryol. Morphol.* **24**:625.

VAUGHAN, R. B., AND TRINKAUS, J. P., 1966, Movements of epithelial cell sheets *in vitro*, *J. Cell Sci.* **1**:407.

VESELÝ, P., AND WEISS, A., 1973, Cell locomotion and contact inhibition of normal and neoplastic rat cells, *Int. J. Cancer* **11**:64.

VESELÝ, P., DONNER, L., CINATI, J., AND SOVOVA, V., 1968, Interaction of Rous sarcoma virus with rat embryo fibroblasts of inbred Lewis strain *in vitro*, *Folia Biol.* **14**:457.

VOGT, M., AND DULBECCO, R., 1962, Properties of cells transformed by polyoma virus, *Cold Spring Harbor Symp. Quant.* **27**:367.

WEBER, K., AND GROESCHEL-STEWART, U., 1974, Myosin antibody: The specific visualization of myosin containing filaments in nonmuscle cells, *Proc. Natl. Acad. Sci. U.S.A.* **71**:4561.

WEED, R. L., LACELLE, P. L., AND MERRILL, E. W., 1969, Metabolic dependence of red cell deformability, *J. Clin. Invest.* **48**:795.

WEISS, P., 1934, *In vitro* experiments on the factors determining the course of the outgrowing nerve fibre, *J. Exp. Zool.* **68**:393.

WEISS, L., 1961, The measurement of cell adhesion, *Exp. Cell Res. Suppl.* **8**:141.

WEISS, L., 1967, *The Cell Periphery: Metastasis and Other Contact Phenomena*, North-Holland, Amsterdam.

WESSELLS, N. K., SPOONER, D. S., ASH, J. F., BRADLEY, M. O., LUDUENA, M. A., TAYLOR, E. L., WRENN, J. T., AND YAMADA, K. M., 1971, Microfilaments in cellular and developmental processes, *Science* **171**:135.

WESSELLS, N. K., SPOONER, B. S., AND LUDUENA, M. A., 1973, Surface movements, microfilaments and cell locomotion, in: *Locomotion of Tissue Cells* (R. Porter and D. W. Fitzsimons, eds.), pp. 53–82, Ciba Foundation Symposium 14, Associated Scientific Publishers, Amsterdam.

WESTERMARK, B., 1973a, Growth control of normal and neoplastic human glia-like cells in culture Acta Universitatis Upsaliensis, Abstracts of Uppsala Dissertations in Medicine, 164.

WESTERMARK, B., 1973b, Growth regulatory interactions between stationary human glia-like cells and normal and neoplastic cells in culture. I. Normal cells, *Exp. Cell Res.* **81**:195.

WESTON, J. A., AND HENDRICKS, K. L., 1972, Reversible transformation by urea of contact-inhibited fibroblasts, *Proc. Natl. Acad. Sci. U.S.A.* **69**:3727.

WESTON, J. A., AND ROTH, S. A., 1969, Contact inhibition: Behavioral manifestation of cellular adhesive properties *in vitro*, in: *Cellular Recognition* (R. T. Smith and R. A. Good, eds.), Appleton-Century-Crofts, New York.

WILBANKS, G. D., AND RICHART, R. M., 1966, The *in vitro* interaction of intraepithelial neoplasia, normal epithelium and fibroblasts from the adult human uterine cervix, *Cancer Res.* **26**:1641.

YAHARA, I., AND EDELMAN, G. M., 1972, Restriction of the mobility of lymphocyte immunoglobulin receptors by concanavalin A, *Proc. Natl. Acad. Sci. U.S.A.* **69**:608.

YAHARA, I., AND EDELMAN, G. M., 1974, Modulation of lymphocyte receptor mobility by concanavalin A and colchicine, *Ann. N.Y. Acad. Sci.* (in press).

YAMADA, K. M., AND WESSELLS, N. K., 1971, Axon elongation: Effect of nerve growth factor on microtubule protein, *Exp. Cell Res.* **49**:614.

YAMADA, K. M., SPOONER, B. S., AND WESSELLS, N. K., 1970, Axon growth: Roles of microfilaments and microtubules, *Proc. Natl. Acad. Sci. U.S.A.* **66**:1206.

3

Mechanisms of Cancer Invasion and Metastasis

Isaiah J. Fidler

1. Introduction

The spread of cancer cells from a primary site to a distant organ is called metastasis. It is one of the most intriguing phases in the pathogenesis of the disease; indeed, cancer metastasis is responsible for most therapeutic failures, as patients succumb to the multiple tumor growths. It would seem that, short of the complete prevention of cancer, the most urgent goal of oncologists should be the arrest and/or prevention of such tumor spread. In this regard, it is remarkable that current theories of the mechanisms responsible for cancer metastasis are fragmented and controversial. The following discussion is not intended to be totally inclusive or an exhaustive review of the literature. The prime intent is to summarize and consolidate early findings, hypotheses, and suggestions, and to describe some recent experiments. It is hoped that this presentation will promote further collaborative efforts to clarify and elucidate the mechanisms responsible for the pathogenesis of metastasis.

Neoplasms can be conveniently categorized into two major groups. Highly differentiated tumors that grow slowly, are usually encapsulated, and differ only minimally from their normal precursors are classified as benign. In the second group, malignant neoplasms ordinarily consist of fast-growing cells that may have a variety of abnormal chromosomes and usually are pleomorphic, with various degrees of anaplasia (Prehn, 1972). This morphological classification of neoplasms is based on the supposition that microscopic examination can be used to

Isaiah J. Fidler•Department of Pathology, University School of Medicine, University of Pennsylvania, Philadelphia, Pennsylvania. Present address: Basic Research Program, Frederick Cancer Research Center, Frederick, Maryland.

predict the biological behavior of the tumors *in vivo* and thus serve as a prognostic tool. Unfortunately, although the cellular structure of a tumor may give a rough guide to its potential clinical course, attempts at prognosis by morphological grading of tumors are at best arbitrary. The morphological and histological features of a malignant tumor should be considered as only one of several parameters on which the outcome of the disease depends. In the final analysis, the only two major characteristics unique to malignant cells are their invasive and metastatic properties.

The development of tumor metastasis involves five major steps: (1) invasion of cells from the primary tumor into surrounding tissue and penetration of blood and/or lymph vessels; (2) release of tumor cell emboli into the circulation; (3) arrest of the emboli in small vascular channels of distinct organs; (4) tumor cell invasion of the wall of the arresting vessel, infiltration into adjacent tissue, and multiplication; and (5) growth of vascularized stroma into the new tumor as proliferating tumor cells invade the distant organ (Zeidman, 1957). The final development of arrested tumor emboli leads to the formation of secondary tumor growths, or metastases. The process of invasion, embolization, arrest, and development of emboli can then commence once again.

2. Invasion

The first and most crucial step in the pathogenesis of metastasis is the invasion of normal host tissues by malignant cells. The mechanisms responsible for the phenomenon are complicated and controversial, and they depend on many tumor and/or host factors. Tumor cell invasion could be caused by tumor multiplication and growth leading to increased tissue pressure and mechanical expansion, by loss of tumor cell adhesiveness and increased or excessive motility, by destruction of host stroma by tumor cell products, or by the effects of the host response to tumor cell invasion. In fact, it is conceivable that all of these processes could be involved in the invasive phenomenon, and that the importance of each could differ from one tumor system to another, making comparisons and generalized conclusions unnecessary if not impossible.

2.1. Cellular Multiplication and Mechanical Expansion

By histological criteria, malignant invasive neoplasms are frequently found to be anaplastic, with many mitotic figures, indicating rapid cell multiplication. Such rapidly dividing anaplastic tumors are more invasive and lead to a higher incidence of metastasis than more differentiated tumors (Franks, 1973). Clearly, a continuous and progressive multiplication of tumor cells within a restricted space could bring about an increase in tissue pressure, leading first to disruption in blood supply and later to pressure atrophy, and the latter could easily account for destruction of otherwise normal tissues. Eaves (1973) has expanded and supported the hypothesis by Young (1959) that the invasion of host tissue by malignant tumor cells can be accounted for by purely mechanical factors. They suggested that the invasive properties of malignant neoplasms stem from the increased hydrostatic pressure in tumor cells as compared with adjacent normal cells, the higher intracellular osmotic pressure causing an increase in tissue pressure. Thus they maintained that tumor cells penetrating normal tissues are comparable to plant roots penetrating the soil, exerting mechanical hydrostatic pressures to move along lines of lesser resistance.

Although tumor cell proliferation usually precedes invasion, it is probably not essential to invasion *per se*. Generally speaking, the rate of cell multiplication does not correlate well with invasive properties. It is well known that normal leukocytes can invade tissues with great ease, yet they do not divide at the site of invasion. On the other hand, many rapidly dividing normal cells that participate in wound healing or organ regeneration have no invasive characteristics. Similarly, the rates at which tumor cells proliferate *in vivo* do not necessarily correlate with their invasive properties. Some rapidly growing tumors, such as breast fibroadenomas, do not invade host tissues, whereas breast carcinomas grow very slowly and are highly invasive (Willis, 1960). Therefore, although mechanical forces may aid tumor cell invasion, their influence on the outcome of the phenomenon probably is minimal.

2.2. Characteristics of Tumor Cell Growth in Vitro

There are clear differences between the *in vitro* growth characteristics of normal and neoplastic cells. Normal cells grown in culture generally migrate on the surface of the vessel until they form an organized monolayer, and, upon cell-to-cell contact, cell movement is stalled and division ceases. This property, which is called "contact inhibition" (Abercrombie and Heaysman, 1954; Abercrombie and Ambrose, 1962) or "density-dependent inhibition" (Stoker and Rubin, 1967), appears to be a general property of normal cells. In contrast, neoplastic cells *in vitro* are less inhibited by cell-to-cell contact, and their locomotion and division continue unabated, leading to multilayered, randomly oriented cultures. Aaronson and Todaro (1968) found a direct relationship between loss of growth inhibition upon cell-to-cell contact *in vitro* and tumorigenicity *in vivo*.

Abercrombie and Heaysman (1954) originally suggested that *in vitro* contact inhibition of division could be due either to restraint of cellular locomotion in the direction of cell contact or to inhibition of overlapping with another cell of the same type. Steinberg (1973) demonstrated that the latter mechanism is in fact responsible for the phenomenon. His data show that the locomotion of contact-inhibited cells is not decreased but that the cells, which adhere strongly to the surface of culture vessels, do not accept the relatively weak adhesive forces offered by other cells as a substitute for the stronger forces, and this lack of "adhesion substitution" results in an avoidance of overlapping. Presumably, then, either cancer cells do not adhere strongly to the substratum or they prefer overlapping, leading to the formation of multilayered cultures.

ISAIAH J.
FIDLER

The invasive properties of malignant tumor cells have also been attributed, at least in part, to their reduced adhesiveness (Coman, 1944, 1953; deLong *et al.*, 1950; Zeidman, 1957). Coman defined "adhesiveness" as the tendency of a cell to attach to another cell of the same type, and he showed that loss of adhesiveness was accompanied by an increase in "stickiness," which he defined as the tendency to attach to a histologically different cell. Reduced adhesiveness of tumor cells would facilitate their separation from each other and allow for cells with increased motility to invade normal tissues. Indeed, Coman (1953) found that a variety of human tumor cells attach only loosely to one another and separate easily to migrate into surrounding normal tissues. The loss of adhesiveness was attributed to a deficiency of calcium bound to the cell surface, due not to lack of available exogenous calcium but rather to a defect in calcium binding (Coman, 1953; Zeidman, 1957). Perfusion of livers with a chelating agent alters the structural integrity of the membranes of normal cells, which form tight intercellular junctions (Coman, 1954, 1961). Thus if a calcium bridge is important for intercellular adhesion (Steinberg, 1958; Lilien and Moscona, 1967), cancer cells could become detached and migrate from the primary site.

However, the hypothesis that the invasiveness of neoplastic cells is directly related to their reduced adhesive properties has been questioned. Dorsey and Roth (1973) demonstrated that malignant tumor cells of different types behave differently in cell aggregate capture assays, indicating that malignancy or invasiveness *per se* is not necessarily determined by decreased intercellular adhesiveness. Instead, they proposed that tumor cell invasiveness results from a decrease in intercellular recognition and in adhesion between tumor cells.

Several investigators have reported that the degree of cell adhesion *in vitro* does not regulate the rate of cell locomotion. Curtis and Buultjens (1973) showed that changes in cell adhesiveness induced by alteration of cell surface lipid composition do not affect the average speed of motility or the rate of pseudopod initiation and, moreover, that changes in cell adhesion do not alter contact inhibition of growth, confirming studies by Steinberg (1973). Similarly, Easty and Easty (1974), investigating the relationship of tumor cell locomotion to invasive properties, found that neither colcemid, which inhibits the formation of cell processes and presumably affects locomotion, nor dibutyryl cyclic AMP, which might restore certain aspects of normal behavior to tumor cells *in vitro*, has any effect on the invasion of biological membranes by mouse tumor cells.

The importance of increased tumor cell motility *in vivo* to invasiveness was recognized by many early investigators. Willis (1960) cited the findings of Virchow in 1863 and Grohe in 1865, who demonstrated the *in vitro* migration and motility of cells from tumor explants. Those findings have been questioned repeatedly, since the migrating cells could have been normal host leukocytes or fibroblasts; nevertheless, their significance is obvious.

Clearly, increased motility *in vivo* is not unique to tumor cells. Some normal cells are quite motile. During embryogenesis there is a mass organized migration of normal differentiating cells; and in the adult, although cell locomotion is restricted mostly to white blood cells, some parenchymal and stromal cells are potentially motile, as is evident from their behavior during wound healing, regeneration, and repair processes. One interesting case of apparent invasive properties or normal adult cells has been reported by Taptiklis (1968). In his experiments, dissociated thyroid cells of mice injected intravenously into syngeneic animals were able to survive in the lungs in a dormant state and proliferate up to a year later in response to stimulation by thyrotropic hormone. It was clear from the data that the normal adult thyroid cells were able to penetrate endothelial walls and migrate to the extravascular tissues.

In general, however, increased or excessive motility *in vivo* is one of several common characteristics of malignant cells. Unfortunately, motility of tumor cells *in vivo* has not been investigated in such minute detail as in *in vitro* systems, and several questions remain unanswered. Wood *et al.* (1967) used microcinematographic techniques to investigate the *in vivo* motility of V × 2 carcinoma cells in rabbit tissues. Their studies confirmed many *in vitro* observations and suggested that the locomotion of tumor cells *in vivo* is nondirectional and lacks chemotaxis. The latter finding was contradicted, however, in studies by Ozaki *et al.* (1971), who used a different tumor system. They reported the isolation of a tumor cell product that is chemotactic for other tumor cells. The factor, isolated from some tumor tissues of animal and human origin, is a highly purified protein free of nucleoproteins and proteolytic activities. It induces extravascular migration of circulating tumor cells but has no effects on vascular permeability or leukocyte migration. On the other hand, a chemotactic factor isolated from inflamed sites attracts leukocytes but has no effect on tumor cells. These data suggest that a chemotactic factor secreted by some tumor cells may influence their motility and subsequent invasiveness.

2.4. Destruction or Modification of Host Tissues

Disruption or destruction of the normal tissues around a tumor would weaken the natural barriers to its growth, invasion, and spread. Increased tissue pressure could be responsible for such pathology, as discussed above. However, most data suggest that destruction of surrounding tissues is probably due to lytic enzymes or toxic substances produced by, stored in, and secreted from invasive tumor cells. The evidence is compelling. Direct observations of tumor cell invasion *in vivo* were reported by Franks (1973), and there have been many ultrastructural studies of tumor invasion in epithelial systems, since the basal lamina provides a clear demarcating line between neoplastic and normal tissues. Sequential studies have demonstrated that tumor cell infiltration is always preceded by lysis and damage to the basal lamina. Hashimoto *et al.* (1973) reported, on the basis of electron microscopic and physiochemical studies of squamous cell carcinoma of human skin, that a tumor-specific collagenolytic enzyme facilitates the breakdown of the collagen-containing basal lamina, which allows for the subsequent migration of tumor cells into underlying tissues.

One major biochemical prerequisite of an invasive tumor could be its ability to synthesize, store, and secrete high levels of proteolytic enzymes that disrupt host stroma and facilitate invasion by tumor cells. Recently, Unkeless *et al.* (1973) and Ossowski *et al.* (1973) described an apparent general enzymatic change accompanying malignant transformation. They found the fibrinolytic or proteolytic activities in a wide variety of tumor cells to be much higher than those in normal cells. Proteolytic enzymes have been demonstrated in many animal and human tumors, such as human squamous cell carcinoma, basal cell epithelioma of skin, and malignant melanoma (for review, see Hashimoto *et al.*, 1973). In addition, Daniel (1970) reported that malignant mouse fibroblasts produce two substances, one affecting differentiation of embryonic chick epidermis and the other causing toxicity. Increased levels of proteolytic enzymes in and around invading tumor cells were reported by Sylvan (1973), who found cathepsin B, a lysosomal proteinase similar to trypsin and papain, at the cell surface in isolated tumor cells but not in normal cells. Cathepsin B brings about detachment of cells growing firmly on glass. Obviously, the findings suggest that increased levels of such proteolytic enzymes active at physiological pH could provide the means for the separation of tumor cells from one another, facilitating their locomotion and subsequent penetration into normal host tissues.

2.5. Effects of Host Factors on Tumor Invasion

Susceptibility to tumor cell invasion varies with tissue type: cartilage, tendons, ligaments, and arteries are relatively resistant, whereas veins, lymphatics, soft tissues, and muscles are easily invaded. It appears that tissues rich in ground substance or in elastic or dense collagen fibers provide a successful barrier to malignant cells. *In vitro*, tumor cells can actively penetrate normal tissue, but their invasion stops when they are confronted by cells from another tumor (Schleich, 1973). Prior to invasion, tumor cells must adhere to normal tissues, but they are not able to penetrate all tissues to which they adhere. For example, adult rat scrotal sac was found to be completely resistant to infiltration by tumor cells that easily invaded the rat omentum, and invasion of the scrotal sac was not facilitated even after a week of intimate contact with tumor cells, apparently because of the dense layers of collagen and elastic fibers in the sac (Easty and Easty, 1973).

Interestingly, a normal host response to injury, the inflammatory response, may actually aid the invasion of malignant neoplasms. Actively growing tumors may induce a localized inflammatory reaction and accumulation of neutrophils, lymphocytes, and/or macrophages. It is well known that leukocytes contain a large number of proteolytic enzymes, and if neutrophils accumulate in an area and their emigration is slow they may begin to break down, discharging enzymes such as lysozymes, which are destructive to autochthonous tissues. There are many enzymes associated with lysozymes, including collagenases, elastases and other hydrolytic enzymes (Ward, 1971), all of which can destroy host tissues and, as a result, enhance tumor cell invasion.

3. Metastasis

107

MECHANISMS
OF CANCER
INVASION AND
METASTASIS

Invasion and metastasis are the only reliable criteria that distinguish malignant neoplasms from benign. Although all tumors that metastasize are malignant, not all malignant tumors develop clinical metastases. The most common examples of the latter are the basal cell carcinoma of skin and glioma of the brain. Both are highly invasive but almost never produce clinical metastases. Whether these tumors do not invade blood vessels or lymphatics, or whether their cells cannot survive in the circulation (as discussed below), is unclear. Most other malignant neoplasms will, in time, spread to distant organs, with the number, size, and distribution of secondary tumor growths dependent on the clinical duration of the disease. The spread of tumor cells could take place by three major routes: by direct extension or transplantation, through the lymphatic system, and through the bloodstream.

3.1. Metastasis by Direct Extension

Tumors that grow in or invade body cavities could release cells or fragments that would travel in the cavity to seed on serosal and/or mucosal surfaces and develop into new growths. Primary or metastatic cancers of the ovary often shed many cells into the peritoneal cavity, where they subsequently grow to cover all peritoneal surfaces. It is interesting to note, however, that with primary ovarian tumors the shed tumor cells rarely infiltrate the parenchyma of organs, although they firmly adhere to their surfaces. Apparently, initial adherence and invasion are two properties that are not interchangeable.

Primary tumors of the central nervous system, although highly invasive, rarely develop metastases in organs outside the nervous system. Their mode of spread appears to be by direct extension or via the cerebrospinal fluid. Batzdorf (1973) reported that tumor cells shed from primary malignant neoplasms can gain entrance into the cerebrospinal fluid and in time attach to meningeal surfaces and develop into new tumor foci. Such invasive cells from brain tumors have a decreased cell-to-cell adhesiveness *in vitro*, a characteristic associated with malignancy.

3.2. Lymphatic Metastasis

The lymphatic system provides the most common pathway for the initial spread of many carcinomas. The pattern of lymph node involvement depends on the site of the primary tumor and its lymphatic drainage. Lymphatic spread represents the infiltration of a draining regional lymph node (RLN) by tumor cells, with metastasis to distant lymph nodes occurring later. Alternatively, tumor cells may bypass the chain of regional lymph nodes due to obstruction of RLNs by proliferating tumor cells, acute inflammatory changes, or fibrosis following preventive local X-irradiation.

In 1860, Virchow stated that within the lymph node "the elements lie crowded together like a charcoal filter." This basic concept, that the lymph node acts as a purely mechanical organ, has since been expanded. The role of lymph nodes in initiation and maintenance of host immune response, in addition to their role as a barrier to infections, is well established. That carcinomas frequently metastasize to the lymphatic system has been recognized almost from the beginning of investigative studies of tumors. However, the role of the lymph, lymph nodes, and lymphatics in the biology of metastasis is still controversial and unclear and lacks unifying concepts. It should be pointed out that many investigations performed to study experimental lymphatic spread of tumors have used normal animals inoculated with transplantable or induced tumors. In these essentially artificial models, an otherwise normal lymph node or lymphatic system is suddenly confronted with a large number of tumor cells. Whether the results of such studies are totally relevant to clinical oncology is questionable. Animal models paralleling clinical situations are rare, especially for the late events of clinical lymphatic spread.

3.2.1. The Lymphatic System

The lymph represents a collection of tissue fluids in lymphatic capillaries, which merge into larger lymphatic vessels. These connect and pass through the lymph nodes, where the lymph becomes enriched with lymphocytes. The lymph empties into the bloodstream via the thoracic duct at the venular angles in the neck at the region of the supraclavicular lymph nodes.

The lymph node is surrounded with a thick connective tissue capsule, from which trabeculae are extended internally, and reticular fibers extend from these trabeculae into the substance of the node. The cortex of the node consists of large numbers of lymphocytes organized into nodules with distinct germinal centers. Deeper cortical zones contain the postcapillary venules. The medulla contains phagocytic cells in addition to lymphoid elements. The anatomy of lymph nodes helps convert the lymph flow to percolation. The lymph entering a node passes through the subcapsular, intermediary, and medullary sinuses to reach the efferent lymphatics. As discussed below, the growth of tumor in lymph nodes tends to follow this direction of flow. There are two major functions attributed to the lymph nodes—filtration of foreign matter and production of immune cells, the lymphocytes.

3.2.2. Spread of Cancer in the Lymphatic System

Theoretically, there are two mechanisms by which cancer spreads in the lymphatic system. The first and probably least frequent was advanced by Handley (1922), who claimed that metastasis did not occur by embolism but rather by permeation of lymphatics. Some carcinomas do tend to permeate the lymphatic vessels of nerves, where direct extension of tumor from primary site to lymph nodes was suspected to occur, but subsequent pathological studies of many tumor systems failed to substantiate Handley's suggestion. Microscopic examination of serial blocks of tissues between a primary tumor and the regional lymph nodes failed to

demonstrate the presence of "extending" tumor growth. It is no longer questioned that the initial spread of tumor in lymphatics takes place by tumor
embolism in lymph vessels. Tumor emboli may be trapped in the first lymph node
encountered on their route; alternatively, they may transverse lymph nodes or
even bypass them to form distant nodal metastases (the "skip" metastasis).

Originally, it was thought that the only lymphatic–venous communication
occurred at the venular angles in the neck; however, several studies established
that the vascular and lymphatic systems have numerous communications. In the
rat, lymph can reach the venous circulation without passing through any lymph
nodes (Engeset, 1959). There are many nodal bypasses in the paracapsular tissue
which directly connect afferent lymphatics. Once in the lymphatic vessels leading
to the thoracic duct, emboli can reach the neck veins to enter the circulation. Other
pathways for tumor dissemination in the lymphatic system have been shown to
exist. When Zeidman (1965) injected V × 2 carcinoma into the thoracic duct in
rabbits, he observed direct lymphatic pathways from the thoracic duct to the
mediastinal, intercostal, and supraclavicular lymph nodes. This finding indicates
that metastases from a primary gastric carcinoma that are found in supraclavicular lymph nodes may be due to tumor emboli from the thoracic duct that reach the
node via direct pathways, and not to obstruction and retrograde extension of
tumor from the duct. The great interest in bloodborne metastases has tended to
minimize the role of the lymphatics in metastasis. Tumor cells can readily pass
from blood to lymphatic channels and back again (Fisher and Fisher, 1966),
indicating that the two systems are probably inseparable in the pathogenesis of the
disease.

3.2.3. Tumor Growth in Lymph Nodes

Lymph nodes in the area of a primary neoplasm often are enlarged and clinically
palpable. Histologically, the increase in their size may be due to active growth of
tumor cells or to hyperplasia of follicles accompanied by proliferation of
reticulum cells and sinus endothelium. Often, lymph node sinuses may be filled
with histiocytes. Lymph node hyperplasia and sinus histiocytosis may indicate a
host reactivity to autochthonous tumors. Berg *et al.* (1973) suggested that the
presence of any enlarged, nontumorous, apical (regional) lymph node in patients
with breast cancer could be taken as a sign for better prognosis than if the nodes
were small or clinically absent. In their studies, reactive nodes (better prognosis)
exhibited a high degree of germinal center hyperplasia rather than sinus
histiocytosis. A more favorable prognosis has also been described for patients
demonstrating lymphocytic infiltration into tumor, since Lane *et al.* (1961)
observed that such infiltrations were more frequent in tumors from patients who
lived at least 10 years after surgical removal than in those from patients who were
not cured by surgery.

Lymph nodes are immunologically reactive in patients with neoplasms. The
presence of a tumor may stimulate the production and release of immunocompetent cells (Alexander *et al.*, 1972) in the lymphoreticular system. The reaction
commences in the RLNs but later extends to distant nodes and even the spleen.

Proliferative changes in the RLNs may therefore precede the spread and subsequent growth of tumor emboli therein.

Tumor emboli reaching a lymph node are usually arrested in the subcapsular sinus of one or more lobules, where initial growth takes place. Subsequently, tumor cells may grow toward the hilum of the node to reach the efferent channels. Ludwig and Titus (1967) studied such progressive tumor growth of the Walker 256 carcinoma in normal lymph nodes of rats. Two hours after intralymphatic injection, tumor cells began to infiltrate the cortical pulp from the marginal sinus, and 0.2% of the injected cells reached the medullary sinus 24 h later. Growth of tumor cells began under the limiting membrane of the marginal sinus, and by 2 wk after the intralymphatic injection there was evidence for some tumor cell death within the node.

Zeidman (1965) injected small doses of tumor cells intravenously and intralymphatically into different groups of rabbits and found that metastases were always more numerous in the lungs than in the nodes. The difference was thought to be due to different levels of local immune response; that is, tumor cells arrested in lymph nodes were subjected to a large number of immunocompetent cells. In subsequent studies (Zeidman and Fidler, 1970), rabbits were exposed to either total-body X-irradiation or local nodal irradiation. The effectiveness of the dose was monitored by sequential peripheral blood cell counts. No increase in nodal metastases was noted after irradiation; however, lung metastases increased significantly. Moreover, deLong and Coman (1950) studied the growth rate of the $V \times 2$ carcinoma implanted directly into various organs. The largest growths appeared in the spleen, an organ of great importance for a viable immune system. The success of lymph node metastasis may depend on the relative number of arrested tumor emboli. Injection of large numbers of cells may lead to 100% takes in nodes, although small numbers of emboli may indeed be destroyed, as suggested by Zeidman and Buss (1954), who proposed that lymph *per se* may be a relatively noxious milieu for the growth of tumor cells.

3.2.4. The Barrier Function of Lymph Nodes

Lymph nodes may act as an efficient filter for early circulating tumor emboli. Strauli (1970) reviewed the experimental models utilized to study the barrier (complete) vs. filter (incomplete) function of the lymph node. He pointed out that many experiments are conducted with *normal* nodes, which may not resemble the reactive RLNs in cancer patients. Furthermore, in many studies the lymph nodes are challenged by intralymphatic injection of carbon particles, bacteria, or erythrocytes, the relevance to circulating malignant cells being at best questionable. It seems that the lymph node can act as an effective filter for small quantities of intralymphatically injected red blood cells. Injection of larger quantities of erythrocytes leads to a marked reduction in filtration efficiency.

The lymph nodes (of normal animals) can be an effective but temporary barrier to tumor spread. Zeidman and Buss (1954) injected Brown–Pearce or $V \times 2$ carcinoma cells into the afferent popliteal lymphatics of rabbits and removed the lymph nodes 1–42 days after injection. Later, only two of 30 animals developed distant metastases. This was taken as evidence for the effectiveness of the lymph node as a temporary barrier to tumor spread for at least 6 wk after the initial arrest of the tumor emboli. Conversely, Fisher and Fisher (1965) reported that the lymph node is not an effective barrier to the spread of cancer. Their evidence was based in part on studies of tumor cells labeled with ^{51}Cr and injected into the afferent popliteal lymphatics of rabbits. When efferent popliteal lymph was collected and monitored for radioactivity, high radioactive counts in the lymph were found, which were interpreted to be direct proof of the ineffectiveness of the lymph node as a barrier to the spread of cancer. These seemingly conflicting findings are not mutually exclusive. A new study might determine that tumor cells which easily traverse the lymph node fail to develop into metastases. Tumor cells trapped in the node may be the ones with the potential to develop into secondary growths. On the other hand, it is conceivable that the unreliability of the ^{51}Cr labeling technique is responsible for the conflicting results, as discussed below.

The filtration capacity of a lymph node can be altered by several mechanisms. Tumor proliferation and acute or chronic inflammatory reactions can lead to a decreased efficiency. Local X-irradiation, which is common in radiotherapy of neoplasms, could lead to fibrosis of the node and thus to cessation of filtration. In experimental studies, local X-irradiation of a lymph node has been shown to decrease its filtration for erythrocytes but not for tumor cells (Fisher and Fisher, 1967b). In contrast, Herman et al. (1968), who perfused the popliteal node of a dog with a small number of autologous erythrocytes, observed that the primary filtration mechanism was phagocytosis, and that local irradiation with 1000–3000 R in a single dose had no detectable effect on the filtering function. These opposite findings indicate that the unique properties of malignant tumor cells rather than the functional characteristics of lymph nodes may determine whether tumor cells traverse the structure or are arrested.

3.2.5. The Role of the Regional Lymph Node in Neoplasia

It is unquestionable that the RLN is immunologically involved in the host response to neoplasms. The importance of the RLN to the initiation of systemic immunity has been established in various systems. Billingham et al. (1956) demonstrated that skin allografts lacking lymphatic connections are tolerated until there is a restoration of the lymphatic system. Apparently, either soluble products or lymphocytes from the graft must reach the RLN by afferent lymphatics to initiate proliferation of immunocompetent cells responsible for the rejection. Numerous reports by Fisher and coworkers (for review, see Fisher et al., 1974) have demonstrated that, in mice, initiation and maintenance of immunity and reactivity to tumor reside within the draining RLN. Specifically, they reported that immune cells from the RLN are more cytotoxic in vitro to tumor cells than are immune cells obtained from other sources. This suggests that the RLN contains immune cytotoxic mechanisms, so that the histological absence of growing tumor cells should not be interpreted as evidence for lack of lymphatic metastases.

There are several limitations inherent in experimental studies of the RLN that use transplantable tumors in rodents. Since the animals in such models are essentially normal and die shortly after tumor challenge, at best only early events in the reaction of the RLN to transplantable neoplasms can be investigated, whereas clinical oncology is concerned with later stages of the disease, which are not approximated by such experimental models. Studies from our laboratories (Fidler *et al.*, 1974) have attempted to overcome these limitations. We investigated the *in vitro* cell-mediated reactivity of non-glass-adherent lymphocytes to autochthonous spontaneous neoplasms of dogs, and for each test we used lymphocytes obtained from RLNs, distant lymph nodes, and peripheral blood. Our data are preliminary, but so far we have found that the reactivities mediated by lymphocytes from the three sources are very similar. Spontaneous tumors of dogs are probably a good animal model for investigations of neoplasia, since the biological behavior of many dog tumors parallels that of human tumors. Thus our findings may be more relevant to human disease than findings obtained in experimental rodent systems. It must be pointed out that *in vitro* studies of cell-mediated reactivity do not always correlate with the extent of the disease *in vivo*. *In vitro* lymphocyte-mediated destruction of autochthonous or allogeneic human breast tumor cells can almost always be detected, whether the donor of the lymphocytes has been free of tumor for some time or has an actively growing tumor (Hellström *et al.*, 1971).

Perhaps the conclusions of Crile (1969) may serve as an appropriate summary for the dilemma of how to deal with RLNs in cancer patients. He suggested that *early* in the course of breast cancer development, when the primary tumor is small and the RLNs are not involved grossly, their removal may lead to an increase in the incidence of metastasis. However, *late* in the course of the disease, or when tumor is already growing in the RLNs, they are probably of no importance to host immunity and should be removed.

3.3. Hematogenous Metastasis

3.3.1. Tumor Cell Embolism

Prior to their embolization, malignant tumor cells must invade blood vessels. The thin-walled veins (and lymphatics), in contrast to arteries, whose walls contain elastic and collagen fibers, offer little resistance to penetration and thus provide the most common pathways for bloodborne tumor emboli. After infiltrating the vessels, tumor cells may be carried away passively in the bloodstream, or they may remain localized and proliferate at the site of invasion. Frequently, a thrombus may form around the actively growing tumor cells. A direct association between the growth potential of a malignant tumor and the formation of fibrin around it has been suggested by many investigators. Initially, O'Meara (1958) demonstrated that fibrin is always found around the growing edge of a cancer. He suggested that the growth of the tumor actually depends on the formation of a nearby fibrin lattice meshwork, and that the formation of such fibrin is maintained by the tumor cells themselves. Later studies established that the factor secreted by tumor cells is

thromboplastic in nature, and it was called "cancer coagulative factor" (O'Meara, 1964). Many observers have noted that patients with advanced cancer show increased blood coagulability and increased levels of fibrinogen. Indeed, it is not uncommon to diagnose thrombophlebitis of the legs in patients with either pancreatic or ovarian carcinomas. Also, some patients with terminal lung cancer could develop extensive venous thrombosis (Cliffton and Grossi, 1974).

Once a thrombus is formed around single or clustered tumor cells, pieces may break off and be carried away in the venous circulation. Although thrombus formation is frequent, it does not represent a constant feature of metastasis. Evidence presented below suggests that the tumor cells themselves may have unique properties which determine their fate. In either case, embolization of tumor cells is probably a continuous process. Most malignant tumors have a well-established blood supply with multiple thin-walled vessels. Franks (1973) suggested that the pathogenesis of metastasis begins immediately with the development of primary cancers. In support, he cited the large number of clinical cases in which primary tumors have been surgically removed, yet the patient has succumbed to metastatic lesions many years later; and there is some evidence from experimental studies to support his hypothesis. Romsdahl *et al.* (1961) demonstrated that tumor emboli can be isolated from the circulatory system long before metastases are formed. Cytological analysis of blood from animals implanted with tumors by intramuscular injection revealed the presence of tumor cells as early as 24 h after injection. However, if the leg of the animal was amputated up to 6 days after tumor injection, metastasis was completely prevented, suggesting that although the tumor cells circulated they failed to form metastases. Obviously, not all tumor emboli represent metastases. Some years ago, Lubarsch (1912) suggested that tumor cells which arrive at the microvascular system of distant organs die to release a toxin that prepares the vascular endothelium for implantation of subsequently arriving emboli. Alternatively, multiple tumor cell emboli may be released rapidly. Zeidman (1957), in a review of the mechanisms of metastasis, suggested that a sudden change in venous pressure, such as may occur during a cough, could lead to a sudden blood turbulence, releasing a large number of emboli. Diagnostic procedures, surgical trauma, or general manipulation of primary invasive neoplasms can also cause a sudden increase in the number of tumor cells circulating in the blood of patients (Griffiths, 1960; Fisher and Fisher, 1967c). And once in the bloodstream the tumor cells can be transported passively to be arrested in the capillary beds of distant organs.

3.3.2. Tumor Cell Arrest

The mere presence of tumor emboli in the blood does not constitute metastasis. Whether a tumor will metastasize is determined by the ability of circulating tumor cells to survive the turbulence of the bloodstream, evade possible host defense mechanisms, attach firmly to the endothelium of distant small vessels, and gain entrance to the extravascular tissues. Therefore, the prognostic value of the presence or absence of circulating tumor cells in cancer patients is unclear. The number of tumor emboli does seem to correlate well with the clinical duration and size of the primary tumor and whether there are areas of necrosis present that cause blood vessels to hemorrhage and provide easy access for tumor cells. Malmgren (1967) reported no correlation between the presence of tumor emboli and prognosis, since the incidence of later metastases in patients without evidence of circulating emboli did not differ from that in patients found to have tumor cells in their blood. In addition, it is well known that many patients exhibiting high numbers of circulating tumor cells have survived for many years after their primary neoplasms have been surgically removed.

Warren (1973), in a review of the mechanisms by which tumor cells are arrested in the microcirculation and begin to grow, divided the process into several steps. The survival of tumor cells in the circulation is probably related to unique surface properties. Tumor emboli have to attach firmly (as contrasted with passive lodgement) to the internal layer of the intima of a vessel, and after attachment the successful tumor cells must penetrate the vessel wall to reach and grow in the extravascular tissues.

The importance of tumor cell surface characteristics to their survival and growth cannot be overemphasized. Indeed, the subject has been reviewed repeatedly (Abercrombie and Ambrose, 1962) and is discussed in great detail in another chapter in this volume. Among the many unique surface characteristics of tumor cells are decreased adhesiveness and increased stickiness. The latter and cell surface charge could determine the degree of initial interaction with the endothelium of distant microvasculature. Berwick and Coman (1962) demonstrated that calcium, which is deficient in tumor cells, is not involved in the property of stickiness, which was reduced by treatment of tumor cells with neuraminidase. This suggested that tumor cell surface mucopolysaccharides may be associated with the degree of *in vivo* tumor cell arrest. The sialomucin coat of transformed fibroblasts was demonstrated to govern their loss of contact inhibition of growth, light cellular junctions, and stable cell contacts (Martinez-Palomo *et al.*, 1969; Ambrose, 1967).

Cell surface charge, as reflected by the mobility of cancer cells and related to formation of metastases, has been the subject of several investigations. Abercrombie and Ambrose (1962) demonstrated that tumor cells migrate further in an electric field than do normal cells. Increased electrophoretic mobility is related to an increase in the net negative charge per unit area of the tumor cell membrane (Purdam *et al.*, 1958), and surface charge differences are correlated with a reduction in mutual adhesiveness. For example, ascitic sarcoma cells capable of metastasis have been shown to possess a greater net negative charge than cells from solid tumors that rarely metastasize (Klein and Klein, 1956).

The electrophoretic mobility of tumor cells *in vitro* does not appear to reflect their degree of malignancy. Weiss and Hauschka (1970) transplanted TA3 mouse ascites carcinoma cells into six different strains of mice. Despite obvious differences in "malignancy," defined as the mean survival time of recipient animals, of various strains, the excised tumors from any mouse strain retained the same electrophoretic mobility as TA3 cells (syngeneic to the A/HeHa). Neuraminidase treatment of the different tumors reduced their electrophoretic mobilities to the same degree, suggesting that their surface sialic acid contents were similar. In other studies of metastasis, Hagmar (1972a,b) investigated the effects of substituted dextran- and heparin-treated tumor cells on experimental metastasis. Polyanions such as heparin, dextran, and dextran sulfate increased the tumor cell net negative surface charge, but the polycation DEAE-dextran reduced it, as determined by cell electrophoresis. Little is known of the nature of cell surface receptor sites for these polymers, nor is it clear how polyelectrolytes bound to cells affect host–tumor interaction *in vivo*.

Several investigators have studied the enzymatic modifications of cell surface residues as reflected in cell surface charge. Hagmar and Norrby (1973) demonstrated that reduction of the electrophoretic mobility after trypsinization of B-16 melanoma cells altered their behavior *in vivo* to bring about an unusual increase in extrapulmonary metastases. Membrane changes related to plant lectin binding sites, sugar content, and ultrastructural details are discussed elsewhere (see Robbins and Nicolson, Chap. 1). Any or all of these changes may lead to alteration in the net cell surface charge. The arrest of tumor cells may be due to such negative cell surface charge, stemming from tumor cell membrane sialic acid residues. Increased metastatic capabilities of tumor cells *in vivo* have correlated well with increased sialic acid contents (Bosmann *et al.*, 1973), but the observation is not necessarily applicable to all tumor systems.

Gasic and Gasic (1962) reported that pretreatment of mice with *Vibrio cholerae* neuraminidase brought about a dramatic reduction in metastases after intravenous injections of tumor cells. The effects of the injected neuraminidase were attributed to induction of profound thrombocytopenia. Metastasis was also inhibited by pretreatment of recipient mice with heterologous antiplatelet serum, and transfusion of platelets easily reversed this inhibition (Gasic *et al.*, 1968). Later studies (Gasic *et al.*, 1973) correlated the ability of tumor cells to aggregate platelets *in vitro* with their ability to produce thrombocytopenia *in vivo*, which corresponds to a low yield of metastases. When thrombocytopenia followed the intravenous injection of tumor cells, platelets concentrated in the lung capillary bed, the site of embolic lodgement.

Active attachment of tumor cells to vascular endothelium must be distinguished from passive lodgement. The attachment of tumor cells could be facilitated by several factors. The relationship of fibrin formation in the microvasculature and its effects on tumor cell arrest and survival have been studied extensively. Patients with advanced cancer may be hypercoagulable, demonstrating increased levels of clotting factors II, V, VII, and VIII. Increased levels of fibrinolysin inhibitors have also been found in cancer patients who developed venous thrombosis. Formation of fibrinogen and fibrin clot enhances tumor cell attachment and survival in the microvasculature (Cliffton and Grossi, 1974). The exact event *in vivo* is still unclear, but some information has been gained. Wood (1958) used direct microscopic observation of an ear chamber to study the arrest, attachment, and emigration of V × 2 carcinoma cells injected into the vessels of a rabbit.

Infused tumor cells became fixed in a clump with fibrin and then penetrated the vessel wall to reach the extravascular tissues. A selective localization of radioactively labeled plasmin and fibrinogen was found around arrested tumor cells. Moreover, fibrinolysin injected locally reversed the sequential tumor cell clumping, attachment, and penetration of the vessel wall (Wood, 1964). Anticoagulants in general, and heparin or fibrinolysin in particular, administered before intravenous injection of tumor cells can reduce the incidence of experimental metastases. Indeed, fibrinolytic agents were found to be effective in reducing metastasis in several animal models and clinical trials in man (Cliffton and Grossi, 1974; Thornes, 1972).

The adhesion of tumor cells to endothelium may lead to damage in vessel wall and subsequent accumulation of neutrophils. Tumor cells may then gain access to the extravascular tissues by following the pathway set by leukocytes that have traversed the vessel wall (Zeidman, 1961; Wood *et al.*, 1961). As mentioned above, platelets may aggregate at the site of tumor cell lodgement and release mediators that contribute to vascular spasm, increased permeability, and, perhaps, increased motility of tumor cells (Gasic *et al.*, 1973). The release of histamine may cause interendothelial gaps and increased vascular permeability (Majno *et al.*, 1969). However, Ozaki *et al.* (1971) demonstrated that neither histamine nor bradykinin enhances endothelial adhesion or emigration of tumor cells. On the other hand, they isolated a specific tumor cell product that influences the extent of tumor cell adhesion and penetration through vascular endothelium, although the purified protein has no effect on normal leukocytes.

The degree of tumor cell attachment in the microvasculature can be enhanced by localized trauma. Fisher *et al.* (1967) reviewed the mechanisms that could be responsible for localization of tumor cells at sites of trauma. They suggested that tissue damaged physically, chemically, or even by reduction of oxygen tension provides a better environment for the development of bloodborne tumor cells. Hepatic metastases could be enhanced by direct trauma, altered blood flow, or conditions resulting in liver cirrhosis. Moreover, tumor cells dormant in the liver were stimulated to proliferate by manipulation of organs. Apparently, trauma may lead to endothelial damage and increased adherence of tumor cells. In addition, general repair mechanisms or stimuli of proliferation or normal regeneration may directly aid the growth of the tumor. Since manipulation and diagnostic procedures have been shown to result in an increase of circulating tumor emboli and also might enhance tumor growth, they should be kept to a minimum.

3.3.3. The Fate of Circulating Tumor Emboli

The frequency of circulating tumor cells in patients with malignancies does not correspond with development of metastases. For many years, the fate of such emboli has been unclear. The inability to correlate the presence of emboli in the blood to metastasis or to explain the appearance of secondary growth in organs past the capillary bed of the lungs led Virchow to suggest that tumor spread was actually due to the circulation of tumor juices rather than viable cells (Fisher and Fisher, 1967c). Indeed, only in 1952 did Zeidman and Buss conclusively demonstrate that viable tumor cells could traverse the capillary beds of organs encountered and thus yield metastases in other parts of the body.

Early studies in experimental metastasis dealt largely with the problem of explaining the unusual distribution of bloodborne metastases. Both in man and in experimental animals, metastases are frequent in some organs, such as the lung and liver, and relatively rare in the spleen, skeletal muscle, and thyroid. Coman *et al.* (1951) found that direct intravascular injection of tumor cells was followed by cell arrest in the capillaries of organs in which metastases are more frequent, and that no tumor cells were arrested in the arterioles of organs where metastases are rare. This observation suggested that the distribution of metastases depends primarily on mechanical factors, such as the arrest of emboli in capillaries of secondary organs. Local host factors were not eliminated entirely, as explanations were lacking for arteriolar arrest in some organs without the establishment of metastases after such arrest. Further evidence for the importance of local "soil" factors can be found elsewhere. In 1889, Paget suggested the "soil" hypothesis, which attributed to various tissues different metabolic or biological properties that could either enhance or inhibit the growth of arrested tumor cells. Lucké *et al.* (1952) compared experimental metastases of V × 2 carcinoma in the liver and lung of rabbits; liver metastases were larger and more numerous. Also, mitotic counts in liver metastases in man are higher than counts in lung metastases (Willis, 1960). Collectively, the evidence suggests that both mechanical and local "soil" factors determine whether metastases will develop after the arrest of tumor emboli.

In other experiments, the fate of circulating tumor cells was followed by direct observation. Wood (1958) made microcinematographic studies of the development of a metastasis following arrest of V × 2 carcinoma emboli in the rabbit ear chamber. In similar microcinematographic studies, Zeidman (1961) observed the incidence of arrested emboli in mesenteric capillaries of rabbits. Some tumor cells could distort and pass through the narrow capillary tube, but others appeared more rigid and were arrested. The incidence of arrest varied with the type of tumor used. This work established the morphological foundation for previous indirect demonstrations that some tumor cell emboli could pass immediately through the vascular bed of the lung (Zeidman and Buss, 1952), liver, and kidney (Zeidman *et al.*, 1956).

The above experiments yielded rather qualitative information in the fate of circulating tumor cells. Some cells pass through the narrow vessels of an organ immediately. Of those cells arrested, some yield metastases, others die. It would be of obvious importance to obtain quantitative information relating to these observations. Is recirculation of tumor cells emboli a short-lived phenomenon? How many tumor cells die, and what is their death rate? How many surviving cells are needed to produce a metastasis? These and related questions can only be answered with more precise quantitative methods permitting easy identification and counting of tumor cell emboli.

Some quantitative studies of various phases of metastasis have been made. Zeidman *et al.* (1950) demonstrated that the number of metastases is directly proportional to the number of tumor cells injected intravenously, and that the great majority of injected tumor cells fail to form tumors. Others have used morphological identification to study the fate of circulating tumor cells. Greene and Harvey (1964) injected tumor cell suspensions intravenously into recipient animals, the animals were killed, and attempts were made to identify and count the arrested tumor emboli by routine microscopy. Indeed, morphological identification of tumor cells has been used extensively as an experimental tool; however, such identification is considered unreliable. Often, isolated tumor cells cannot be identified with certainty, and inflammatory cells may be mistaken for tumor cells (Joansson, 1958).

Goldie *et al.* (1953) used a different approach to study the fate of circulating tumor cells. After intravenous injection of tumor cells, blood or organ brei from the recipient was injected intraperitoneally into normal animals, and the rate of peritoneal growth indicated the number of tumor cells in the original inoculum. Wexler *et al.* (1969) collected the venous blood draining a primary tumor, injected this blood intravenously into normal animals, and then counted the number of lung metastases. The lung counts were used as an index of the number of tumor cell emboli released from the primary growth. Although this approach yields a rough idea about the number of tumor cell emboli released into the circulation, "the sensitivity in detecting the presence of circulating tumor cells and the ability to quantitate the numbers of cells remain to be established" (Wexler *et al.*, 1969). Agostino and Cliffton (1965), in related studies, inoculated normal rats with samples of organ brei taken from animals that had received tumor cells intravenously. Their results, which agree with those of Greene and Harvey (1964), indicate that tumor cells may lodge in organs and yet fail to develop into metastases.

The search for quantitative information dealing with tumor cell arrest and dissemination was considerably advanced with the advent of radioactive labeling of living cells. Several conditions must be satisfied if labeled cells are to be used for the study of metastasis. The radioactive label should be firmly bound to the cell while it is viable. Upon cell death, the label must not be reutilized but rapidly excreted from the body. The label must not alter the biological behavior of the tumor cell, yet must be of sufficient radioactivity to allow *in vivo* detection of relatively few cells. Injected tumor cells must be homogeneous and test animals syngeneic.

Tumor cells labeled with [^{3}H]thymidine or ^{51}Cr have been used in several studies of dissemination (Baserga *et al.*, 1960; Fisher and Fisher, 1967a), but the results obtained were controversial because the techniques failed to meet one or more of the above criteria. Experiments in our laboratory have been carried out with a homogeneous population of tumor cells labeled *in vitro* with ^{125}IdUrd, an analogue of thymidine that is incorporated exclusively into the DNA of proliferating cells. The label is released only after cell DNA breaks down after cell death, and in contrast to tritium from labeled thymidine it is reutilized very little. After

cell death the label is released mostly as ^{125}I, and most of the free radioiodine is
excreted. The data obtained in our experiment (Fidler, 1970) demonstrated that
the majority of the cells injected intravenously were arrested in the narrow
capillary bed of the first organ encountered. After this initial arrest, some of the
cells were released back into the circulation and recirculated, depending on their
viability. The phenomenon was not observed when dead labeled tumor cells were
injected into another set of mice.

It has long been recognized that the majority of intravenously injected tumor
cells fail to form metastases. Such findings have reinforced a widespread opinion
that most tumor cell emboli die. The data seem to rule out the possibility that the
emboli remain alive but dormant. Death probably begins shortly after injection,
and in our system only 1% of the cells survived for 24 h. The majority of the cells
were arrested in the lungs, where 14 days later gross metastases were observed.
The metastases were derived from very few surviving tumor cells, and it is
conceivable that even a single tumor cell could suffice (Fidler, 1970).

3.3.4. Development and Growth of Arrested Tumor Emboli

As discussed above, tumor cells arrested in the microcirculation may traverse the
vessel wall to reach the extravascular tissues. The process may be facilitated by a
specific tumor cell product that is chemotactic to other tumor cells but not to
normal cells. Such a factor, which has been isolated from tumors of human and
animals as a purified protein free of proteolytic activity (Ozaki *et al.*, 1971), causes
endothelial adhesion and emigration of tumor cells of extravascular tissues. The
tumor cells may also reach the perivascular connective tissue. Multiplication of
tumor cells starts soon after new blood vessels begin to grow to supply the
developing tumor colony, and recent studies suggest that tumor cells are able to
initiate and maintain vascular proliferation in the host. A diffusible factor called
"tumor angiogenesis factor" has been isolated from several tumors of humans and
animals. The characteristics of the factor and its possible relationship to the
development of primary and secondary neoplasms are discussed in detail
elsewhere (Folkman, Chap. 13, Vol. 3).

The most frequent sites for metastases are the lung and liver (Willis, 1960),
possibly because most of the venous blood drains into these organs. All the
systemic venous circulation returns through the right side of the heart to be
filtered through the capillary bed of the lung. Similarly, the portal circulation
passes through the liver. Metastases are also commonly seen in the bones of many
cancer patients. Cancer cells in the venous system could reach the bones via the
paravertebral plexus of veins. Numerous interconnections to the plexus from the
inferior vena cava, pelvic veins, internal mammaries, and intercostal veins have
been found. Alternatively, tumor emboli could reach the bones directly via
Batson's plexus, possibly under conditions of increased intraabdominal pressure,
which tend to reflux blood towards the plexus (Sandberg and Moore, 1957).
Infrequent sites of metastasis are organs such as muscle, spleen, thyroid, and
cartilage. Coman *et al.* (1951) suggested that the number of metastases is

proportional to the number of tumor emboli arrested within the capillary bed of an organ. In muscles, spleen and thyroid, tumor cells are arrested in arterioles that present an effective barrier to extravascular invasion. The mechanisms responsible for the latency and organ selectivity of metastasis are unclear. Do tumor cells home to particular organs, or are they arrested in many organs but develop only in selective ones? Although in our quantitative analysis of the fate of circulating tumor cells (Fidler, 1970) metastatic growths of mouse melanoma were observed only in the lungs, the lask of metastases elsewhere could not be attributed to the failure of arrest of tumor cells in those sites. Many tumor cells were arrested in the liver, yet no metastases or viable tumor cells were found there 14 days later. Only future studies can clarify the factors responsible for the development and growth of arrested tumor emboli.

3.3.5. Alterations in Tumor–Host Relationship

Many experimental factors have been investigated which significantly affect the outcome of bloodborne metastases. The duration and rate of tumor growth can be related to the incidence of development of metastases. Various hormones, such as growth hormones, adrenocorticotropic hormone, adrenal steroids, and medroxyprogesterone, can bring about an increase in metastases. Physical trauma as well as X-irradiation of the host has been reported to enhance the process. On the other hand, several factors have been reported to have beneficial effects on metastasis, causing a reduction in tumor spread. Among these are chemotherapeutic cytotoxic agents, which act directly on tumor cells, anticoagulants such as heparin, warfarin, and fibrinolytic agents (plasmin), and X-irradiation of primary cancers. Since hormones and X-irradiation are used extensively in clinical oncology, they warrant special consideration.

a. X-Irradiation and Metastasis. The effects of X-irradiation on the outcome of experimental metastasis are well documented. Irradiation of host animals before but not after intravenous injection of tumor cells enhances the incidence of pulmonary metastasis in mice (Fidler and Zeidman, 1972), rats (Dao and Yogo, 1967), and rabbits (Zeidman and Fidler, 1970). Although it is tempting to attribute the observed enhancement of pulmonary metastasis to host immunosuppression as seen in some systems (Vaage *et al.*, 1974), such a generalized relationship is contradicted by results obtained with other tumor systems. Dao and Yogo (1967) irradiated only one side of the chest of rats, the other side being shielded completely; after injection of tumor cells, metastases increased only in the irradiated lobes. We (Zeidman and Fidler, 1970) investigated the effects of X-rays to either the lungs or lymph nodes on experimental metastasis of the V × 2 carcinoma in rabbits. Tumor cells were injected intravenously into one set of rabbits and intralymphatically into another set. X-irradiation prior to tumor cell injection enhanced the incidence of pulmonary metastasis but had no effect on metastasis to lymph nodes. Later quantitative analysis of the enhancement of experimental metastasis by X-irradiation of mice (Fidler and Zeidman, 1972) suggested that irradiation causes an increase in immediate arrest of tumor cell emboli in the pulmonary vascular bed. This effect on trapping action is probably related to endothelial injury such as cellular congestion, increased permeability, or narrowing of small vessel lumina, which leads to slowing of the blood flow (Arena, 1971). The narrowing of vessel lumina, added to the tendency of tumor cell emboli to localize at sites of tissue damage (Fisher *et al.*, 1967), would enhance the trapping of tumor cells in the pulmonary capillary bed. The subsequent appearance of increased lung metastases is probably directly related to the number of initially arrested tumor cells. Since X-irradiation, which leads to enhancement of cancer metastasis in several animal models, is used for therapy in human patients with surgically inoperable cancers, it is of primary importance to attempt to minimize these potentially harmful enhancing effects.

b. Effects of Glucocorticoids (Cortisone) on Metastasis. The enhancement of experimental metastasis by steroid hormones such as cortisone is well documented. Agosin *et al.* (1952) observed that cortisone treatment of mice injected with a transplantable mammary carcinoma led to widespread metastases, while no metastasis was found in control tumor-bearing mice. Later investigators confirmed this finding in different mouse-tumor systems (Albert and Zeidman, 1962; Baserga and Shubik, 1955; Fidler and Lieber, 1972), and similar results have been observed in other tumor systems. Zeidman (1962) reported enhancement of metastasis by cortisone in rabbits inoculated with the Brown-Pearce carcinoma. Enhancement of the growth and spread of spontaneous neoplasms in human patients treated with corticosteroids has also been suspected for a long time (American Medical Association, 1951), and enhancement of metastasis have been directly related to the glucocorticoid activity of the steroid (Albert and Zeidman, 1962). Several explanations have been proposed for the possible mechanism responsible for the phenomenon. Agosin *et al.* (1952) first suggested that cortisone affects connective tissue in a way that allows larger numbers of tumor emboli to be released from the primary tumor into the circulation. However, the work of Baserga and Shubik (1955) demonstrated that cortisone can increase the number of metastases even when it is administered after the transplanted tumor has been removed. Further microcinematographic studies by Zeidman (1962) clearly indicated that, at least within the first 30 min after injection of tumor cells into cortisone-treated rabbits, the arrest of tumor cells within mesenteric capillaries is greatly enhanced. And our studies (Fidler and Lieber, 1972) have demonstrated quantitative differences in initial tumor arrest, circulation, and survival of ^{125}IdUrd-labeled tumor cells between normal and cortisone-treated syngeneic mice. In the latter, initial cell arrest was higher than in control animals, but cell survival did not differ. The result was a net increase in surviving tumor cells, and hence an increase in pulmonary metastases. Glucocorticoids may alter the capillary endothelial surface, which may lead to increased stickiness and arrest of tumor cell emboli. This mechanism was first proposed by Zeidman (1962), who observed Brown–Pearce tumor cells injected into mesenteric arteries of cortisone-treated and normal rabbits. Even though capillary and tumor cell diameters remained constant in both groups, more tumor emboli were arrested in the capillaries of treated rabbits. It is possible that glucocorticoids alter capillary endothelium and increase its adhesive properties in the same manner as was reported for hepatoma cells (Ballard and Tomkins, 1970).

4. Speculations on Tumor–Host Interaction

4.1. Unique Characteristics of Metastatic Tumor Cells

Data suggesting that tumor cell properties may determine the outcome of metastasis have been reported by several investigators. Sugarbaker (1952) injected tumor cell suspensions from different types of tumors into the same site in rats and found that each type established its own unique pattern of metastasis. Fisher and Fisher (1967a) demonstrated that tumor cells can traverse different organs at different rates, and data of Zeidman and Buss (1952) proved that tumor cells from different tumors interact differently with the capillary bed of an organ. Furthermore, the rate at which tumor cells pass through capillaries is not related to their size but rather is attributed to their plasticity and ability to distort their shape (Zeidman, 1961).

In earlier quantitative studies of the fate of tumor cells, we demonstrated that the mere presence of tumor cells in the blood does not constitute a metastasis, since most circulating tumor cells die rapidly, with only about 0.1% surviving to form secondary growths (for review, see Fidler, 1974a). Several questions remain unanswered: What affects the distribution, survival, and fate of circulating tumor cells? Is the process of metastasis dependent mostly on mechanical or "soil" factors in the host, or is the process also determined by qualities unique to malignant tumor cells? Do tumor emboli survive at random to yield metastases, or do the few surviving circulating tumor cells have properties that determine their success? It is well known that the number of experimental pulmonary metastases is proportional to the total number of circulating tumor emboli. Moreover, dead tumor cells or even syngeneic embryo cells injected intravenously along with live tumor cells can significantly increase the incidence of metastasis, and tumor cells in small clumps are more successful in forming metastases than are the same malignant cells suspended singly (Fidler, 1973a).

Evidence supporting the hypothesis that malignant cell properties may determine the outcome of metastasis came from our studies in which B-16 melanoma tumor cell lines were selected for their capacity to form successful artificial metastases in their syngeneic hosts, C57BL/6 mice. Tumor cells were injected intravenously into mice, and 3 wk later pulmonary metastases were harvested and adapted to growth in tissue culture. The cultured tumor cells were then injected intravenously into normal mice, and the subsequent pulmonary metastases were again harvested and placed into new tissue cultures. The procedure was repeated several times, and all such tumor lines were assayed for their ability to form metastases. With each successive line, the incidence of pulmonary metastases increased significantly, suggesting that the survival of tumor cells in the circulation is not a random phenomenon but rather depends on unique tumor cell properties (Fidler, 1973b). The development of B-16 melanoma tumor lines is particularly useful for studying cell properties that render one line highly "metastatic" while another is not. Moreover, since all the lines are tumorigenic, they serve as controls for each other; that is, "normal" controls are not necessary in comparing tumor cell characteristics for malignancy.

Studies with the B-16 lines have confirmed many early hypotheses and observations. Bosmann et al. (1973) reported several major biochemical differences between the two cell lines (low and high metastasis) in electrophoretic mobility and in levels of degradative enzymes, surface glycoproteins, glycosyl transferases, glycosidases, and proteases. Also, the degree of initial arrest of ^{125}IdUrd-labeled tumor cells in the microvasculature is directly proportioned to the subsequent number of pulmonary metastases. Tumor cells that yield high numbers of metastases tend to clump with peripheral blood lymphocytes (Fidler, 1974a) and also cause aggregation of platelets in vivo and in vitro, an event that may directly enhance metastasis (Gasic et al., 1973). Thus the accumulating data strongly suggest that metastatic tumor cells have unique properties that allow for their success.

4.2. Host Immune Response and Metastasis

Immune reactivity to neoplasia is one host factor that could influence metastatic spread (Alexander et al., 1972). For many years, investigators have suspected that some circulating tumor cells were destroyed by specific host immune mechanisms, but evidence for such a hypothesis is still lacking. In fact, some studies actually contradict the view that a patient's resistance to tumor is related to the activity of his reticuloendothelial system (Fisher and Fisher, 1967c). Borberg et al. (1972) reported that intravenous injection of lymphocytes from immunized syngeneic or allogeneic mice or even from sheep inhibits tumor grafts in mice; but, on the other hand, Fisher et al. (1972) did not find injection of sensitized lymphocytes to be inhibitory to the growth of transplanted tumors. It would appear that the outcome of such experiments may be related to the number of lymphocytes transferred (a high number of lymphocytes may be required to inhibit tumor growth in vivo), as well as to the antigenic characteristics of the tumor cell line itself.

When an animal is preimmunized and then challenged with live tumor cells, an acceleration of tumor growth can sometimes be observed. The phenomenon has been termed "tumor enhancement," and it can be transferred by passage of immune lymphocytes (Hutchin et al., 1967). Generally, the mechanism responsible for enhancement of tumor growth in vivo is thought to be related to presence of the so-called blocking factors. These serum factors, which interfere with cell-mediated cytotoxicity, are presumed to be either antibodies, antigen–antibody complexes, antigen alone, or even of nonimmunological nature (for review, see Heppner, 1972). Presence of blocking factors in serum has been correlated to enhancement of metastasis in an experimental system. Duff *et al.* (1973) reported that injection of herpes simplex virus type I or type II or simian virus 40 into weanling golden hamsters failed to induce immunity to transformed hamster cells; on the other hand, prior immunization with type I virus resulted in a marked enhancement of metastatic tumors. The authors proposed that blocking factors to the type I virus prevented cell-mediated cytotoxicity and so enhanced metastasis.

Many experimental and/or spontaneous tumors of animals and some of man are known to possess specific antigens on their cell surfaces that differ from the transplantation antigens of the host's normal cells. The capacity of the host to recognize these tumor-associated antigens as foreign and to react toward their destruction constitutes the immune surveillance mechanism, and it has been suggested that the occasional tumor cell which evades the host's immune surveillance mechanism proliferates to cause clinical cancer. Recently, the generalized concept of immune surveillance to neoplasia has come under critical questioning (Kripke and Borsos, 1974) and challenge (see also Melief and Schwartz, Chap. 5, Vol. 1). Prehn and Lappé (1971) have advanced the theory that the normal immune response to neoplasia might have a dual role: in the early course of the development of cancer or with tumors that are weakly antigenic, the cell-mediated response would directly stimulate rather than inhibit tumor growth; but the tumor would be inhibited at a later stage, when the immune response is strongly active, or if it were highly antigenic.

We have confirmed the hypothesis of Prehn and Lappé (1971) in several experimental tissue culture systems, using transplanted mouse tumors or spontaneous cancers of dogs. Similarly, we reported that immune reactivity to circulating tumor emboli may have a dual function; small numbers of sensitized immune cells (lymphocytes) could actually aid in the successful spread of the neoplasms, whereas high numbers of the same immune cells would dramatically reduce the incidence of pulmonary nodules (Fidler, 1974a). Further experiments comparing various controls with syngeneic mice that were either immunized against the B-16 melanoma or thymectomized and X-irradiated demonstrated a significant decrease in the incidence of experimental pulmonary metastases after intravenous injection of tumor cells. This decrease in pulmonary metastases in immunosuppressed mice was completely reversible by intravenous injection of lymphocytes 24 h prior to tumor cell injection. Again, however, the administration of a high number of lymphocytes 24 h before tumor cell injection brought about a significant decrease in the incidence of metastases.

What is the mechanism by which a low ratio of lymphocytes to tumor cells aids in the survival of the tumor? We observed that after *in vitro* incubation of B-16 melanoma cell with lymphocytes, clumps consisting of tumor cells and lymphocytes were formed. Many studies of the mechanisms of metastasis demonstrated that larger tumor emboli survive better than single cells to yield metastases. If lymphocytes cause tumor cells to clump but do not kill them, the resulting larger emboli may be more readily trapped in the capillary bed of a distant organ, leading to a subsequent increase in metastases; but once a critical ratio of immune cells is exceeded, cytotoxicity to tumor cells may occur.

What is the nature of the reacting immune cells? Why do immune cells stimulate tumor growth when present in small numbers but inhibit growth when present in large numbers? Lymphocytes and macrophages are known to cooperate in the mediation of cellular cytotoxicity (for review, see Alexander *et al.*, 1972), but the role of the normal or activated macrophage in the phenomenon of immune stimulation of tumor growth is unknown. Specifically, do macrophages cooperate in mediation of cytotoxicity only, or do they aid lymphocytes in stimulating tumor growth? Moreover, can normal or activated syngeneic macrophages abrogate the stimulation to tumor growth mediated by low numbers of syngeneic lymphocytes? Our preliminary *in vitro* studies have demonstrated that, although lymphocytes from tumor-bearing animals do indeed have a dual role in their relationship to the cancer cells, macrophages are only cytotoxic, suggesting that macrophages may be important in host defense to neoplasia (Fidler, 1974*a,b*).

Stimulated lymphocytes are known to release a large number of biologically active mediators that participate in the phenomenon of cellular reactivity *in vivo*. *In vitro* investigations of these mediators strongly suggest that some are chemotactic to macrophages, preventing their migration out of the area and, in some cases, activating the macrophages and perhaps rendering them cytotoxic (for review, see David, 1971). Several questions can be raised when host–tumor interactions are scrutinized in a patient with a progressive cancer. Did the tumor escape host defense mechanisms? Did lymphocyte–macrophage interaction take place, or is one of the cell populations functionally defective?

It is well known that the macrophage plays an important role in specific immunity to neoplasia (Alexander *et al.*, 1972) *In vitro* cytotoxicity mediated by macrophages has been demonstrated in a variety of tumor systems after cell-to-cell interaction, and Hibbs *et al.* (1972) have suggested that the selective *in vitro* toxicity mediated by macrophages is directed against abnormal growth characteristics of cells rather than their antigenic composition. Normal macrophages, although not demonstrably cytotoxic to tumor cells, can be "armed" (made specifically cytotoxic) either by exposure to supernatants derived from cultures of syngeneic spleen cells sensitized *in vivo* and mixed with tumor cells or by incubation with sensitized syngeneic thymocytes (Evans and Alexander, 1970; Fidler, 1974*b*). Studies from our laboratories (Fidler, 1974*b*) have dealt with activation of mouse macrophages by a factor released from sensitized xenogeneic lymphocytes obtained from rats sensitized to the mouse B-16 melanoma tumor. Mice with established pulmonary metastases (which untreated would have progressed to kill the host) were inoculated intravenously with syngeneic macrophages that had been activated *in vitro*. Two to three weeks later, treated and untreated mice were killed and examined for pulmonary metastases. Mice treated with activated macrophages showed a dramatic decrease in pulmonary tumor nodules. It appears, then, that the macrophages obtained from tumor-bearing mice were either not cytotoxic *in vivo* or not sufficiently effective, as seen by the constant and rapid progression of tumor growth leading to death of the host. Thus it is most significant that these macrophages could be rendered cytotoxic by xenogeneic lymphocyte supernatants. Indeed, this approach to macrophage activation could be a method of overcoming or even bypassing the possible defect in the syngeneic immune mechanism that permits the growth and spread of cancers.

5. Conclusion

Several major limitations are encountered in attempts to interpret experimental data dealing with mechanisms of tumor metastasis. Many, if not most, studies represent experiences with one tumor–animal or *in vitro* system. Malignant tumor cells in general probably have some common properties, but there are many quantitative and qualitative differences in their biological behavior. It is also well known that host responses to spontaneous and induced tumors differ quantitatively. For one, tumor cells from virally or chemically induced neoplasms in rodents elicit a much stronger host immune reactivity than do cells from spontaneous tumors. The immune response may indeed have a dual role in the response to neoplasia. Enhancement of tumor growth (Prehn and Lappé, 1971) and of growth and metastasis (Fidler, 1974a) has been reported. On the other hand, numerous reports of immune inhibition of cancer metastasis (Vaage, 1973; Milas et al., 1974; Carnaud et al., 1974; Fidler, 1974b) have also been published. These seemingly conflicting findings could simply be due to different properties inherent to the tumor cells in the studies. Ideally, future studies should employ several tumor–animal models simultaneously to indicate whether experimental results are general in scope.

Another major difficulty lies with the selection of an appropriate animal model for investigation. Experimental research should use a model as similar to human cancer as possible, but most investigations have been performed with transplantable or induced tumors and have been carried out in essentially normal animals. Do such experimental data fail to correspond to the clinical situation confronting the oncologist? Is that the reason for the clinical failure of so many agents or therapeutic modalities that are promising at the experimental level? Animals injected with tumor cells may simply not be good models for patients who develop cancer spontaneously. Ideally, future studies of the mechanisms of tumor invasion and spread should be carried out in primary animal hosts, to determine whether results obtained with experimentally induced tumor systems are relevant to clinical oncology.

The data summarized in the preceding sections indicate that the outcome of cancer metastasis depends on the interaction of tumor cells with their host. The phenomenon is complex and is affected by a multitude of factors. The main factor may be the malignant characteristics of cancer cells—including loss of adhesiveness, increased motility, secretion of proteolytic enzymes, and/or presence of surface characteristics that allow for survival in the circulation. Host immune defense mechanisms, involving a possible stimulation and/or inhibition of tumor growth and spread, may also be of great importance. Future studies of animals with primary tumors should include manipulations of both host defense mechanisms and tumor properties. Either or both could determine the ideal therapeutic approach to the arrest and prevention of metastasis.

ACKNOWLEDGMENTS

I would like to express my sincere appreciation to my friend and teacher Irving Zeidman, M.D., for inspiring me to investigate the pathogenesis of cancer metastasis. This work was supported by USPHS grant CA-12456 from the National Cancer Institute.

6. References

AARONSON, S. A., AND TODARO, G. J., 1968, Basis for the acquisition of malignant potential by mouse cells cultivated *in vitro, Science* **162**:1024.

ABERCROMBIE, M., AND AMBROSE, E. J., 1962, The surface properties of cancer cells: A review, *Cancer Res.* **22**:525.

ABERCROMBIE, M., AND HEAYSMAN, J. E. M., 1954, Observations on the social behavior of cells in tissue culture. II. "Monolayering" of fibroblasts, *Exp. Cell Res.* **6**:293.

AGOSIN, M., CHRISTEN, R., BADINEZ, Q., GASIC, G., NEGHME, A., PIZARRO, O., AND JARPA, A., 1952, Cortisone induced metastases of adenocarcinoma in mice, *Proc. Soc. Exp. Biol. Med.* **80**:128.

AGOSTINO, D., AND CLIFFTON, E. E., 1965, Organ localization and effect of trauma on the fate of circulating cancer cells, *Cancer Res.* **25**:1728.

ALBERT, D., AND ZEIDMAN, I., 1962, Relation of glucocorticoid activity of steroids to number of metastases, *Cancer Res.* **22**:1297.

ALEXANDER, P., EVANS, R., AND GRANT, C. K., 1972, The interplay of lymphoid cells and macrophages in tumor immunity, *Ann. Inst. Pasteur* **122**:645.

AMBROSE, E. J., 1967, Biochemical and biophysical properties of cell membranes, in: *Candian Cancer Conference: Proceedings of the Seventh Canadian Cancer Research Conference, Toronto,* p. 247, Academic Press, New York.

AMERICAN MEDICAL ASSOCIATION, 1951, Meeting of the Subcommittee on Steroids and Cancer, *J. Am. Med. Assoc.* **146**:655.

ARENA, V., 1971, *Ionizing Irradiation and Life,* Mosby, St. Louis.

BALLARD, P. L., AND TOMKINS, G. M., 1970, Glucocorticoid induced alterations of the surface membrane of cultured hepatoma cells, *J. Cell. Biol.* **47**:222.

BASERGA, R., AND SHUBIK, P., 1955, Action of cortisone on disseminated tumor cells after removal of the primary growth, *Science* **121**:100.

BASERGA, R., KISIELESKI, W. E., AND HALVERSEN, K., 1960, A study on the establishment and growth of tumor metastases with tritiated thymidine, *Cancer Res.* **20**:910.

BATZDORF, U., 1973, Metastasis of primary central nervous system tumors including tissue culture studies, in: *Chemotherapy of Cancer Dissémination and Metastasis* (S. Garattini and G. Franchi, eds.), pp. 205–211, Raven Press, New York.

BERG, J. W., HUVOS, A. G., AXTELL, L. M., AND ROBBINS, G. Y., 1973, A new sign of favorable prognosis in mammary cancer: Hyperplastic reactive lymph nodes in the apex of the axilla, *Ann. Surg.* **177**:8.

BERWICK, L., AND COMAN, D. R., 1962, Some chemical factors in cellular adhesion and stickiness, *Cancer Res.* **22**:982.

BILLINGHAM, R. E., BRENT, L., AND MEDAWAR, P. B., 1956, Quantitative studies on tissue transplantation immunity, *Philos. Trans. R. Soc. London Ser. B* **239**:357.

BORBERG, H., OETTGEN, H. F., CHOUDRY, K., AND BEATTIE, E. J., JR., 1972, Inhibition of established transplants of chemically induced sarcomas in syngeneic mice by lymphocytes from immunized donors, *Int. J. Cancer* **10**:539.

BOSMANN, H. B., BIEBER, G. F., BROWN, A. E., CASE, K. R., GERSTEN, D. M., KIMMERER, T. W., AND LIONE, A., 1973, Biochemical parameters correlated with tumor cell implantation, *Nature (London)* **246**:487.

CARNAUD, C., HOCH, B., AND TRAININ, N., 1974, Influence of immunologic competence of the host on metastasis induced by the 3LL Lewis tumor in mice, *J. Natl. Cancer Inst.* **52**:395.

CLIFFTON, E. E., AND GROSSI, C. E., 1974, The rationale of anticoagulants in the treatment of cancer, *J. Med.* **5**:107.

COMAN, D. R., 1944, Decreased mutual adhesiveness, a property of cells from squamous cell carcinomas, *Cancer Res.* **4**:625.

COMAN, D. R., 1953, Mechanisms responsible for the origin and distribution of blood-borne tumor metastases: A review, *Cancer Res.* **13**:397.

COMAN, D. R., 1954, Cellular adhesiveness in relation to the invasiveness of cancer: Electron microscopy of liver perfused with a chelating agent, *Cancer Res.* **14**:519.

COMAN, D. R., 1961, Adhesiveness and stickiness: Two independent properties of the cell surface, *Cancer Res.* **21**:1436.

COMAN, D. R., DeLONG, R. P., AND MCCUTCHEON, M., 1951, Studies on the mechanism of metastasis: The distribution of tumors in various organs in relation to the distribution of arterial emboli, *Cancer Res.* **11**:648.

CRILE, G., 1969, Possible role of uninvolved regional nodes in preventing metastasis from breast cancer, *Cancer* **24**:1283.

CURTIS, A. S. G., AND BUULTJENS, T. E. J., 1973, Cell adhesion and locomotion, in: *Locomotion of Tissue Cells*, Ciba Foundation Symposium 14, pp. 171–180, Associated Scientific Publishers, Amsterdam.

DANIEL, M. R., 1970, Diffusible factors from malignant cells which affect epidermal survival and differentiation, *Br. J. Cancer* **54**:712.

DAO, T. L., AND YOGO, H., 1967, Enhancement of pulmonary metastasis by x-irradiation in rats bearing mammary cancer, *Cancer* **20**:2020.

DAVID, J. R., 1971, Migration inhibitory factor and mediators of cellular hypersensitivity *in vitro*, in: *Progress in Immunology* (B. Amos, ed.), pp. 400–412, Academic Press, New York.

DeLONG, R. P., AND COMAN, D. R., 1950, Relative susceptibility of various organs to tumor transplantation, *Cancer Res.* **10**:513.

DeLONG, R. P., COMAN, D. R., AND ZEIDMAN, I., 1950, The significance of low calcium and high potassium content in neoplastic tissue, *Cancer* **3**:718.

DORSEY, J. K., AND ROTH, S., 1973, Adhesive specificity in normal and transformed mouse fibroblasts, *Dev. Biol.* **33**:249.

DUFF, R., DOLLER, E., AND RAPP, F., 1973, Immunologic manipulation of metastases due to herpesvirus transformed cells, *Science* **180**:79.

EASTY, D. M., AND EASTY, G. C., 1974, Measurement of the ability of cells to infiltrate normal tissue *in vitro*, *Br. J. Cancer* **29**:36.

EASTY, G. C., AND EASTY, D. M., 1973, *In vitro* systems for the study of tumor infiltration, in: *Chemotherapy of Cancer Dissemination and Metastasis* (S. Garattini and G. Franchi, eds.), pp. 45–51, Raven Press, New York.

EAVES, G., 1973, The invasive growth of malignant tumors as a purely mechanical process, *J. Pathol.* **109**:233.

ENGESET, A., 1959, Lymphaticovenous communications in the albino rat, *J. Anat.* **93**:380.

EVANS, R., AND ALEXANDER, P., 1970, Cooperation of immune lymphoid cells with macrophages in tumor immunity, *Nature (London)* **228**:620.

FIDLER, I. J., 1970, Metastasis: Quantitative analysis of distribution and fate of tumor emboli labeled with ^{125}I-5-iodo-2′-deoxyuridine, *J. Natl. Cancer Inst.* **45**:775.

FIDLER, I. J., 1973a, The relationship of embolic homogeneity, number, size and viability to the incidence of experimental metastasis, *Eur. J. Cancer* **9**:223.

FIDLER, I. J., 1973b, Selection of successive tumor lines for metastasis, *Nature New Biol.* **242**:148.

FIDLER, I. J., 1974a, Immune stimulation–inhibition of experimental cancer metastasis, *Cancer Res.* **34**:491.

FIDLER, I. J., 1974b, Inhibition of pulmonary metastasis by intravenous injection of specifically activated macrophages, *Cancer Res.* **34**:1074.

FIDLER, I. J., AND LIEBER, S., 1972, Quantitative analysis of the mechanism of glucocorticoid enhancement of experimental metastasis, *Res. Commun. Chem. Pathol. Pharmacol.* **4**:607.

FIDLER, I. J., AND ZEIDMAN, I., 1972, Enhancement of experimental metastasis by x-ray: A possible mechanism, *J. Med.* **3**:172.

FIDLER, I. J., McWILLIAMS, R. W., AND BECK-NIELSEN, S., 1974, Immune reactivity of lymphocytes obtained from original lymph node, distant lymph node, and peripheral blood to autochthonous neoplasms of the dog, *Immunolog. Comm.*, in press, 1975.

FISHER, B., AND FISHER, E. R., 1965, Transmigration of lymph nodes by tumor cells, *Science* **152**:1397.

FISHER, B., AND FISHER, E. R., 1966, The interrelationship of hematogenous and lymphatic tumor cell dissemination, *Surg. Gynecol. Obst.* **122**:791.

FISHER, B., AND FISHER, E. R., 1967*a*, The organ distribution of disseminated ^{51}Cr-labeled tumor cells, *Cancer Res.* **27**:9412.

FISHER, B., AND FISHER, E. R., 1967*b*, Barrier function of lymph node to tumor cells and erythrocytes. I. Normal nodes, *Cancer* **20**:1907.

FISHER, E. R., AND FISHER, B., 1967*c*, Recent observations on the concept of metastasis, *Arch. Pathol.* **83**:321.

FISHER, B., FISHER, E. R., AND FEDUSKA, N., 1967, Trauma and the localization of tumor cells, *Cancer* **20**:23.

FISHER, B., SAFFER, E. A., AND FISHER, E. R., 1972, Experience with lymphocyte immunotherapy in experimental tumor systems, *Cancer* **27**:771.

FISHER, B., SAFFER, E. A., AND FISHER, E. R., 1974, Studies concerning the regional lymph node in cancer. IV. Tumor inhibition by regional lymph node cells, *Cancer* **33**:631.

FRANKS, L. M., 1973, Structure and biological malignancy of tumors, in: *Chemotherapy of Cancer Dissemination and Metastasis* (S. Garattin and G. Franchi, eds.), pp. 71–78, Raven Press, New York.

GASIC, G. J., AND GASIC, T. B., 1962, Removal of sialic acid from the cell coat in tumor cells and vascular endothelium and its effects on metastasis, *Proc. Natl. Acad. Sci. U.S.A.* **48**:1172.

GASIC, G. J., GASIC, T. B., AND STEWART, C. C., 1968, Antimetastatic effects associated with platelet reduction, *Proc. Natl. Acad. Sci. U.S.A.* **61**:46.

GASIC, G. J., GASIC, T. B., GALANTI, N., JOHNSON, T., AND MURPHY, S., 1973, Platelet–tumor cell interaction in mice: The role of platelets in the spread of malignant disease, *Int. J. Cancer* **11**:704.

GOLDIE, H., JEFFRIES, B. R., JONES, A. M., AND WALKER, M., 1953, Detection of metastatic tumor cells by intraperitoneal inoculation of organ brei from tumor bearing mice, *Cancer Res.* **13**:566.

GREENE, H. S. N., AND HARVEY, E. K., 1964, The relationship between the dissemination of tumor cells and the distribution of metastases, *Cancer Res.* **24**:799.

GRIFFITHS, J. F., 1960, The dissemination of cancer cells during operative procedures, *Ann. Roy. Coll. Surg. Engl.* **27**:14.

HAGMAR, B., 1972*a*, Cell surface charge and metastasis formation, *Acta Pathol. Microbiol. Scand. Sect. A* **80**:357.

HAGMAR, B., 1972*b*, Defibrination and metastasis formation: Effects of arvin on experimental metastases in mice, *Eur. J. Cancer* **8**:17.

HAGMAR, B., AND NORRBY, K., 1973, Influence of cultivation, trypsinization and aggregation on the transplantability of melanoma B16 cells, *Int. J. Cancer* **11**:663.

HANDLEY, W. S., 1922, *Cancer of the Breast and Its Treatment,* Harper and Row, New York.

HASHIMOTO, K., YAMANISHI, Y., MAEYENS, E., DABBOUS, M. K., AND KANZAKI, T., 1973, Collagenolytic activities of squamous cell carcinoma of the skin, *Cancer Res.* **33**:2790.

HELLSTRÖM, I., HELLSTRÖM, K. E., SJÖGREN, H. O., AND WARNER, G. A., 1971, Demonstration of cell mediated immunity to human neoplasms of various histological types, *Int. J. Cancer* **7**:1.

HEPPNER, G. H., 1972, Blocking antibodies and enhancement, *Ser. Haematol.* **4**:41.

HERMAN, P. G., BENNINGHOFF, D. L., AND MELLINS, H. Z., 1968, Radiation effect on the barrier function of the lymph node, *Radiology* **91**:698.

HIBBS, L. B., JR., LAMBERT, L. H., JR., AND REMINGTON, J. S., 1972, Control of carcinogenesis: A possible role for the activated macrophage, *Science* **177**:990.

HUTCHIN, P., AMOS, D. B., AND PRIOLEAU, W. H., 1967, Interaction of humoral antibodies and immune lymphocytes, *Transplantation* **5**:68.

JOANSSON, O., 1958, The viability of circulating tumor cells in experimental cancer, *Surg. Forum* **9**:577.

KLEIN, G., AND KLEIN, E., 1956, Conversion of solid neoplasms into ascites tumors, *Ann. N.Y. Acad. Sci.* **63**:640.

KRIPKE, M. L., AND BORSOS, T., 1974, Immune surveillance revisited, *J. Natl. Cancer Inst.* **52**:1393.

LANE, M., GOKSEL, H., SALERNO, R. A., AND HAAGENSEN, C. D., 1961, Clinicopathologic analysis of the surgical curability of breast cancers: A minimum ten-year study of a personal series, *Ann. Surg.* **153**:483.

LILIEN, J. E., AND MOSCONA, A. A., 1967, Cell aggregation: Its enhancement by a supernatant from cultures of homologous cells, *Science* **157**:70.

LUBARSCH, E., 1912, Die Bedeutung des Traumas für Entstehung und Wachstum krankhafter Gewächse, *Med. Klin.* **8**:1651.

LUCKÉ, B., BREEDIS, C., WOO, Z. P., BERWICK, L., AND NOWELL, P., 1952, Differential growth of metastatic tumors in liver and lung: Experiments with rabbit V2 carcinoma, *Cancer Res.* **12**:734.

LUDWIG, J., AND TITUS, J. L., 1967, Experimental tumor cell emboli in lymph nodes, *Arch, Pathol.* **84**:304.

MAJNO, G., SHEA, S. M., AND LEVENTHAL, M., 1969, Endothelial contraction induced by histamine-type mediators, *J. Cell Biol.* **42**:647.

MALMGREN, R. A., 1967, Studies of circulating tumor cells in cancer patients, in: *Mechanisms of Invasion of Cancer* (P. Deroix, ed.), pp. 108–117, Springer, New York.

MARTINEZ-PALOMO, BRAISLOVSKY, C., AND BERNHARD, W., 1969, Ultrastructural modifications of the cell surface and intercellular contacts of some transformed cell strains, *Cancer Res.* **29**:925.

MILAS, L., HUNTER, N., MASON, K., AND WITHERS, H. R., 1974, Immunological resistance to pulmonary metastases in C3Hf/Bu mice bearing syngeneic fibrosarcoma of different sizes, *Cancer Res.* **34**:61.

O'MEARA, R. A. Q., 1958, Coagulative properties of cancers, *Ir. J. Med. Sci.* **394**:474.

O'MEARA, R. A. Q., 1964, Fibrinolytic treatment of cancer, *Lancet* **ii**:963.

OSSOWSKI, L., UNKELESS, J. C., TOBIA, A., QUIGLEY, J. P., RIFKIN, D. B., AND REICH, E., 1973, An enzymatic function associated with transformation of fibroblasts by oncogenic viruses. II. Mammalian fibroblast cultures transformed by DNA and RNA viruses, *J. Exp. Med.* **137**:113.

OZAKI, T., YOSHIDA, K., USHIJIMA, K., AND HAYASHI, H., 1971, Studies on the mechanisms of invasion in cancer. II. *In vivo* effects of a factor chemotactic for cancer cells, *Int. J. Cancer* **7**:93.

PAGET, S., 1889, The distribution of secondary growths in cancer of the breast, *Lancet* **i**:571.

PREHN, R. T., 1972, Neoplasia, in: *Principles of Pathobiology* (M. F. Lavia and R. B. Hill, eds.), pp. 191–232, Oxford University Press, New York.

PREHN, R. T., AND LAPPÉ, M. A., 1971, An immunostimulation theory of tumor development, *Transplant. Rev.* **7**:26.

PURDAM, L., AMBROSE, E. J., AND KLEIN, G., 1958, A correlation between electrical surface charge and some biological characteristics during the stepwise progression of a mouse sarcoma, *Nature (London)* **181**:1586.

ROMSDAHL, M. D., CHU, E. W., HUME, R., AND SMITH, R. R., 1961, The time of metastasis and release of circulating tumor cells as determined in an experimental system, *Cancer* **14**:883.

SANDBERG, A. A., AND MOORE, E. G., 1957, Examination of blood for tumor cells, *J. Natl. Cancer Inst.* **12**:1.

SCHLEICH, A., 1973, The confrontation of normal and malignant cells *in vitro*: An experimental system in tumor invasion studies, in: *Chemotherapy of Cancer Dissemination and Metastasis* (S. Garattini and G. Franchi, eds.), pp. 51–57, Raven Press, New York.

STEINBERG, M. S., 1958, On the chemical bonds between animal cells: A mechanism for tight, specific cell association, *Am. Nat.* **92**:65.

STEINBERG, M. S., 1973, Cell movement in confluent monolayers: A reevaluation of the causes of "contact inhibition" in: *Locomotion of Tissue Cells*, Ciba Foundation Symposium 14, pp. 333–341, Associated Scientific Publishers, Amsterdam.

STOKER, M. P. G., AND RUBIN, H., 1967, Density dependent inhibition of growth in culture, *Nature (London)* **215**:172.

STRAULI, P., 1970, The barrier function of lymph nodes: A review of experimental studies and their implications for cancer surgery, in: *Surgical Oncology* (F. Saegesser, ed.), pp. 161–176, Hans Huber, Bern.

SUGARBAKER, E. D., 1952, The organ selectivity of experimentally induced metastases in rats, *Cancer* **5**:606.

SYLVAN, B., 1973, Biochemical and enzymatic factors involved in cellular detachment, in: *Chemotherapy of Cancer Dissemination and Metastasis* (S. Garattini and G. Franchi, eds.), pp. 129–138, Raven Press, New York.

TAPTIKLIS, N., 1968, Dormancy by dissociated thyroid cells in the lungs of mice, *Eur. J. Cancer* **4**:59.

THORNES, R. D., 1972, Warfarin as maintenance therapy for cancer, *J. Ir. Coll. Physicians Surg.* **2**:2.

UNKELESS, J. C., TOBIA, A., OSSOWSKI, L., QUIGLEY, J. P., RIFKIN, D. B., AND REICH, E., 1973, An enzymatic function associated with transformation of fibroblasts by oncogenic viruses. I. Chick embryo fibroblast cultures transformed by avian RNA tumor viruses, *J. Exp. Med.* **137**:85.

VAAGE, J., 1973, Humoral and cellular immune factors in the systemic control of artificially-induced metastases in C3Hf mice, *Cancer Res.* **33**:1957.

VAAGE, J., DOROSHOW, J. H., AND DuBois, T. T., 1974, Radiation induced changes in established tumor immunity, *Cancer Res.* **34**:129.

VIRCHOW, R., 1860, *Cellular Pathology* (transl. from 2nd ed. by Frank Chance), R. M. DeWitt, New York.

WARD, P. A., 1971, Inflammation, in: *Principles of Pathobiology* (M. F. Lavia and R. B. Hill, eds.), pp. 96–126, Oxford University Press, New York.

WARREN, B. A., 1973, Environment of the blood-borne tumor embolus adherent to vessel wall, *J. Med.* **4**:150.

WEISS, L., AND HAUSCHKA, T. S., 1970, Malignancy, electrophoretic mobilities and sialic acids at the electrokinetic surface of TA3 cells, *Int. J. Cancer* **6**:270.

WEXLER, H., RYAN, J. J., AND KETCHAM, A., 1969, The study of circulating tumor cells by the formation of pulmonary embolic tumor growths in a secondary host, *Cancer* **23**:946.

WILLIS, R. A., 1960, *Pathology of Tumors*, 3rd ed., Butterworths, Washington, D.C.

WOOD, S., JR., 1958, Pathogenesis of metastasis formation observed *in vivo* in the rabbit ear chamber, *Arch. Pathol.* **66**:550.

WOOD, S., JR., 1964, Experimental studies of the intravascular dissemination of ascites V2 carcinoma cells in the rabbit with special reference to fibrinogen and fibrinolytic agents, *Bull. Schweiz. Akad. Med. Wiss.* **20**:12.

WOOD, S., JR., HOLYOKE, E. D., AND YARDLEY, J. H., 1961, Mechanisms of metastasis production by blood-borne cancer cells, *Can. Cancer Conf.* **4**:167.

WOOD, S., JR., BAKER, R. R., AND MARZOCCHI, B., 1967, Locomotion of cancer cells in vivo compared with normal cells, in: *Mechanisms of Invasion in Cancer* (P. Denoix, ed.), pp. 26–30, Springer-Verlag, Berlin.

YOUNG, J. S., 1959, The invasive growth of malignant tumors: An experimental interpretation based on elastic–jelly models, *J. Pathol. Bacteriol.* **77**:321.

ZEIDMAN, I., 1957, Metastasis: A review of recent advances, *Cancer Res.* **17**:157.

ZEIDMAN, I., 1961, The fate of circulating tumor cells. I. Passage of cells through capillaries, *Cancer Res.* **21**:38.

ZEIDMAN, I., 1962, The fate of circulating tumor cells. II. A mechanism of cortisone action in increasing metastases, *Cancer Res.* **22**:501.

ZEIDMAN, I., 1965, Fate of circulating tumor cells. III. Comparison of metastatic growth produced by tumor cell emboli in veins and lymphatics, *Cancer Res.* **3**:324.

ZEIDMAN, I., AND BUSS, J. M., 1952, Transpulmonary passage of tumor cell emboli, *Cancer Res.* **12**:731.

ZEIDMAN, I., AND BUSS, J. M., 1954, Experimental studies on the spread of cancer in the lymphatic system. I. Effectiveness of the lymph node as a barrier to the passage of embolic tumor cells, *Cancer Res.* **14**:403.

ZEIDMAN, I., AND FIDLER, I. J., 1970, Effect of irradiation on experimental metastases via lymph and blood stream, *J. Med.* **1**:9.

ZEIDMAN, I., McCUTCHEON, M., AND COMAN, D. R., 1950, Factors affecting the number of tumor metastases, experiments with a transplantable mouse tumor, *Cancer Res.* **10**:357.

ZEIDMAN, I., GAMBLE, W. J., AND CLOVIS, W. L., 1956, Immediate passage of tumor cell emboli through the liver and kidney, *Cancer Res.* **16**:814.

Immunology

4

Studies of Soluble Transplantation and Tumor Antigens

LLOYD W. LAW and ETTORE APPELLA

1. Introduction

Considerable progress has been made in the last 15 years in solubilizing and purifying transplantation antigens (H-2) of the mouse. Until recently, adequate biological assays for activity of solubilized materials were not performed; thus activity was measured principally in terms of inhibition of complement-dependent cytotoxicity of lymphoid cells or inhibition of hemagglutination using specially prepared antisera against known determinants. Neither assay is a measure of completeness of antigen; haptenic or nonantigenic fragments may be detected as well as definitive determinants. Recently, newer methods—for example, the use of nonionic detergents—have been used to solubilize H–2 antigens; these so far have precluded adequate biological testing because of the nature of the solubilized material.

Our objective in the present chapter is to discuss present knowledge in this field following the use of more intense biological assays of solubilized material and also to discuss the progress achieved in attempts to isolate, solubilize, and purify tumor-associated antigens specifically of the transplantation type, the so-called TSTAs.

LLOYD W. LAW and ETTORE APPELLA • Laboratory of Cell Biology, National Cancer Institute, Bethesda, Maryland.

LLOYD W. LAW
AND
ETTORE
APPELLA

The cell membrane is under the control of a large number of genetic loci. Some of the products of these loci can be detected by immunological methods as alloantigens. In the mouse, about 43 different cell surface alloantigens have been discovered, among which is the H-2 complex, the main locus concerned in transplantation phenomena. Genetically, the H-2 complex appears to contain at least two *H* genes, *H-2D* and *H-2K*, in two genetic regions (*D* and *K*) separated by the *Ss* (Slp) gene (Klein and Shreffler, 1972; Snell *et al.*, 1971). A considerable amount of genetic material which comprises approximately 500 genes lies between *H-2D* and *H-2K* (Shreffler and Klein, 1970). By recombination experiments, three *Ir* loci have been located near the *K* region; genes other than *H-2D* have so far not been assigned to the *D* region (Lieberman *et al.*, 1972; McDevitt and Sela, 1965). A great many different alleles, about 30 in all, have been detected in the H-2 loci. The extent of this polymorphism has surpassed all expectations.

A substantial body of data on the biochemical characteristics of the H-2 antigens has been accumulated (Nathenson, 1970; Mann and Fahey, 1971). The studies so far have involved only two H-2 products but have established the protein nature of H-2 antigens. Little information, however, has been obtained on the chemical structure of any single specificity. Whether there are only two *H*-genes in the H-2 complex remains also an open question. The *H-2K* and *H-2D* genes can actually be clusters of cistrons so closely linked that they have not yet been separated by recombination.

Since H-2 antigens are membrane-bound components, one of the major concerns has been their solubilization. Among various methods, limited papain digestion (Shimada and Nathenson, 1969; Hess and Davies, 1974; Appella *et al.*, 1975) is the best-documented approach. The solubilization followed by monitoring for alloantigenic activity has given reasonable yields, in the range of 20–40% of the total activity of the membrane suspension taken as 100%. The solubilized protein components were purified by ion-exchange chromatography, gel filtration on Sephadex, affinity chromatography on a column of *Lens culinaris* lectin Sepharose, and discontinuous polyacrylamide gel electrophoresis (Hess and Davies, 1974; Appella *et al.*, 1975). The final products were 300–700 times more active than the starting material. No disulfide bonds could be detected after alkaline cleavage, and this has suggested the absence of covalently linked protein subunits in papain-solubilized molecules. An estimate of the molecular weight of these components was of the order of 50,000 (Appella *et al.*, 1975). Highly purified material showed a diffuse staining pattern after electrophoresis; this characteristic appears to be due to an inherent molecular heterogeneity of the molecules, although other factors causing it have not been investigated.

Procedures have been described for solubilizing presumably intact H-2 alloantigen molecules using the nonionic detergent Non-Idet P-40 (NP40). This method has been combined with indirect immunoprecipitation and sodium dodecylsulfate–polyacrylamide gel electrophoresis. The molecular weight was found to be 88,000 when the antigens were treated with sodium dodecylsulfate and electrophoresed, and to be about 45,000 when the same sample was reduced with 2-mercaptoethanol (Schwartz et al., 1973). These results point out that the antigens may exist at least partially as dimers linked by disulfide bonds. When this material was chromatographed on a Biogel A 1.5-m column in buffered 0.5% NP40, the approximate molecular weight of the peak of H-2 activity was calculated to be 380,000. The peak material appears to be an aggregate made of noncovalent bonded units that may represent the actual native form of the antigen; however, this has not been definitely established. Membranes of labeled cells have also been solubilized with 0.5% Triton X-100 (Silver and Hood, 1974). H-2 alloantigenic activity was immunoprecipitated and electrophoresed on sodium dodecylsulfate polyacrylamide. Two polypeptide chains with molecular weights of 47,000 and 11,500, respectively, were obtained. These two chains resemble the large and small fragments of the HL-A molecules (Tanigaki et al., 1974). Besides the molecular weights, further evidence for the high degree of similarity between the small component and human β_2-microglobulin was obtained at the level of the primary structure (Rask et al., 1974). Chymotryptic as well as tryptic digests have revealed a large number of peptides shared by the two proteins. In addition, it could be demonstrated that antibodies against human β_2-microglobulin cocapped FITC-labeled antibodies directed against H-2K^a or H-2D^a, and lysed more than 85% of mouse spleen cells in the presence of complement (Rask et al., 1974).

Evidence has been given that highly purified papain-solubilized HL-A antigens are composed of two polypeptide chains, the smaller of which is identical chemically and immunologically to β_2-microglobulin. It has also been shown that β_2-microglobulin is physically linked to the HL-A antigen on the cell surface. In a similar fashion, highly purified papain H-2 alloantigens have been dissociated by exposure to acid to yield a small polypeptide chain and a larger component. Both H-2K and H-2D molecules are composed of a 11,000–12,000 mol wt component and a 36,000–37,000 mol wt component (Table 1). The large component retains most of the alloantigenic specificities of the parental molecules, while the small component carries the antigenic specificity similar to the small polypeptide isolated with the aid of nonionic detergent or from 3 M NaSCN extracts of liver

TABLE 1

Molecular Weight Estimations of Papain-Solubilized H-2 Alloantigens[a]

	Average mol wt of papain fragment	Mol wt of intact molecule[b]
H-2.4 (H-2^d, *D* gene)	39,000[b]	43,000
H-2.4 (H-2^a, *D* gene)	37,000[c]	
H-2.31 (H-2^d, *K* gene)	44,000[b]	47,000
H-2.23 (H-2^a, *K* gene)	37,000[c]	

[a] Data refer to the large component. The small component was shown to be 11,000 mol wt.
[b] Values taken from Schwartz et al. (1973). The molecular weight for the intact molecule was obtained after solubilization of the alloantigens with NP40.
[c] Values taken from Natori et al. (1975b).

cell membranes (Natori *et al.*, 1974*a,b*). Specificities of the D and K ends of the H-2 complex have been shown by both immunological and immunochemical methods to be separate entities on the cell surface and to be expressed on different molecules (Neaport-Santes *et al.*, 1973; Cullen *et al.*, 1972). This differentiating function appears to reside with the large polypeptide chain; the small component is common to both the K and D products of the H-2 loci. It has been reported that some antigenic specificities are limited to only one or a few H-2 alleles (private), whereas others are shared by several alleles (public). Data have been obtained that show that private and public specificities are located on the same molecule (Cullen *et al.*, 1972; Cullen and Nathenson, 1971; Natori *et al.*, 1975*b*).

3. Biological Properties of H-2 Antigens

Papain-solubilized alloantigens have been subjected in this laboratory to intensive biological studies. The material used for such studies consisted of partially purified preparations obtained after chromatography on a Sephadex G150 column. A fraction designated F2 in the included volume that has a molecular weight of about 50,000 contained all the H-2 serological specificities assayed for by inhibition of immunocytolysis of lymph node cells labeled with ^{51}Cr. However, this assay may be positive for haptenic fragments as well as complete antigens. Fraction F2 accelerated skin graft rejection in congenic strains of mice that differ only at the H-2 locus (Strober *et al.*, 1970). This association strongly suggested that serological specificities and transplantation antigens were located on the same molecules or on molecules of similar molecular weights. However, these studies did not provide critical evidence for the completeness of the antigen. Specific immunological enhancement (protection against rejection of tumor cells) both active and passive was elicited by this F2 fraction (Law *et al.*, 1971). Since in order to achieve enhancement alloantibodies must combine with all the determinants of the transplantation antigens, it was presumed that the F2 fraction of soluble antigen represented a complete molecule containing all the major determinants detected *in situ*.

When the F2 fraction of H-2^a antigen was injected into B10.D2 mice at birth with continuous daily injections through a period of 4–5 wk, antibody tolerance was achieved; however, skin graft rejection of congenic B10.A grafts occurred at the same time as in controls (Law *et al.*, 1972, 1974*b*). GVH, MLR, and CML activity were preserved in lymphoid cells of these humorally tolerant mice (Law *et al.*, 1973). Sera from humorally tolerant animals did not block in an *in vitro* microcytotoxicity assay (Wright *et al.*, 1974). These results are compatible with the concept that serum fractions are required for the induction and maintenance of tolerance to skin grafts. However, sera from B10.D2 made tolerant to H-2^a antigens either by intact cells or by soluble antigens did not interfere with the *in vitro* cytotoxicity of sensitized lymphoid cells when a short-term ^{51}Cr release assay was used, nor did these sera from tolerant mice have capacity to induce specific immunological enhancement of sarcoma I (Law *et al.*, 1974*b*). These

139

STUDIES OF
SOLUBLE
TRANS-
PLANTATION
AND TUMOR
ANTIGENS

TABLE 2
Biological Characterization of F2 Fraction (H-2^a Antigen)

Yield: 65% of crude membrane (CM); specific activity: 32 times that of CM
Specific activities confined to this fraction and peaked in same tube
Activity of all allogeneic specificities assayed = H-2.1, 3,4,5,11,*23*,25,28 (immunologically specific)
Transplantation immunity (skin graft and neonatal heart rejection) elicited in *congenic mice* by F2 and
 not F1 and F3 fractions
Cytotoxic and hemagglutinating antibodies induced by F2 in congenic B10.D2 and B10.B mice
Specific immunological enhancement induced by F2 fraction (A strain tumors in congenic mice)
Humoral tolerance induced in congenic B10.D2 mice (Specific and long lasting)

observations clearly do not support the concept that immunological tolerance
results from an interposed serum factor preventing immunological reactivity.
Our evidence that all biological activities assayed were confined to a single peak
(the F2 fraction) strongly suggests that we are dealing with a single molecular
entity. We have reported that the β_2-microglobulin activity is also confined to our
fraction F2 and therefore resembles what is found *in situ* on the cell membrane
(Natori *et al.*, 1975a). Table 2 summarizes biological activities of H-2^a antigen.

The mechanism responsible for induction by soluble H-2^a antigen of humoral
tolerance (but not complete tolerance) in B10.D2 newborn mice is not understood
but may be related to isoantigenic differences between recipient and donor
(Howard *et al.*, 1962). We have now been able to induce complete operational
tolerance in more than 20% of B10.A mice through the use of soluble H-2^d
antigen obtained by papain digestion of the membrane antigens of B10.D2 spleen
cells (Law, Appella, and Strober, unpublished observations). Multiple H-2
antigenic differences are effective in the donor–recipient pair of congenic strains
B10.A→B10.D2, and complete tolerance in the newborn using spleen or bone
marrow cells is difficult to achieve even with large numbers of cells. In the
reciprocal donor–recipient situation B10.D2→B10.A, only H-2.31 (and possibly
H-2.34) antigenic differences are effective; thus complete tolerance is also
attained more easily and with lower numbers of viable spleen or bone marrow
cells. Also, in contrast to the rather high level of immunogenicity provided by H-2^a
soluble antigen in adult congenic mice as detected by skin graft rejection, H-2^d
soluble antigen is relatively nonimmunogenic. It is likely, therefore, that these
differences in the induction of tolerance in the reciprocal donor–recipient
combinations used are related to factors (for example, differences in combinations of haplotypes used) other than modifications of the antigen as a result of the
solubilization procedures.

4. Tumor Antigens

Tumor-associated antigens (TAAs) are of diverse types and have been detected by
diverse methods *in vivo* or *in vitro*; however, some of these identified antigens are
not strictly tumor specific. These antigens may be found on the cell membrane or

located within the cytoplasm or nucleus. The present discussion will be restricted to those antigens occurring on the membrane of neoplastic cells of experimental animals. Important membrane antigens occurring on many but not all neoplastic cells are those designated TSTAs. They are probably tumor specific and have the capacity to induce a rejection response in the syngeneic animal; they resemble closely in function the histocompatibility antigens (H antigens) in the induction of homograft reactions. There are many other classes of antigens occurring on the cell membrane of both normal and neoplastic cells. These antigenic alterations are accessible to host surveillance and are therefore targets, as are histocompatibility antigens and TSTAs, of cellular and humoral immune reactions. Unlike histocompatibility antigens and TSTAs, they do not usually induce tumor or tissue rejection reactions. The existence of other membrane components, however, should be borne in mind in any studies attempting to characterize TSTAs by *in vitro* methods or in attempts to isolate and solubilize TSTAs. These other membrane antigens may be grouped for convenience into certain categories, as follows (see Hauschka, 1973).

4.1. Tissue Specificity Antigens

Tissue specificity antigens (TIs) are also designated "differentiation antigens" and have been thoroughly analyzed on normal and leukemic mouse thymocytes and lymphocytes. Ly-1,2,3,4, Thy-1 (θ), and Tla (TL) antigens are typical examples. Tla antigen coded by the *Tla* gene is of special interest since it appears to be tumor specific, occurring only on leukemic thymocytes. Although the presence of Tla antigen probably represents gene activation, this antigen is not responsible for the malignant behavior of leukemic cells nor does Tla act as a TSTA. It is detectable only by serological assays, as are the other TIs.

4.2. Species Antigens

Species antigens (SPs) are probably numerous. The best example is the lymphocyte antigen of the mouse *MSLA* detectable by adsorption with heteroantisera.

4.3. Receptor Site Antigens

Receptor sites antigens on the cell membrane were initially viewed as "tumor specific." Some virus-transformed cells showed increased agglutination over normal controls by lectins such as agglutinins of wheat germ (WGA) or the jack bean (Con A). However, it has been shown that normal cells also show agglutinability, particularly during cell division or following protease treatment; nonetheless, these receptor sites may be more commonly expressed on neoplastic cells.

4.4. Fetal and Embryonic Antigens

The recent increasing use of *in vitro* techniques has led to the discovery of tumor-associated antigens expressed on some neoplastic cells; some of these appear embryonic in nature. The exact mechanism for their appearance after malignant transformation is unknown. Derepression of genes responsible for the synthesis of fetal antigens (postulated for the CEA of Gold) or uncovering of binding sites similar to lectin agglutinin reactivity is a likely explanation. Studies by Baldwin *et al.* (1972*a*) and by Ting *et al* (1972) in which isoantigenic differences were controlled reveal that the fetal antigens, at least of certain neoplasms of the rat and mouse, do not function as TSTAs and are distinct entities.

4.5. Tissue- or Organ-Type Specific Antigens

Although there is evidence for the existence of unique antigens existing on neoplastic cells of man, the usual finding employing *in vitro* assays is that of common cross-reacting antigens. Cross-reactions have been reported among histologically similar human tumors of 15 or more types—for example, neoplasms of breast, lung, ovary, and urinary bladder. There is a strong possibility that these are normal organ- or tissue-specific antigens. It remains to be seen what the roles of these antigens are *in vivo*. The existence of organ- or tissue-specific boundaries in neoplasms of experimental animals is not well defined, but recent *in vitro* studies employing colony inhibition and the microcytotoxicity assay indicate cross-reactivities of some nature apparently unrelated to TSTA (Ankerst *et al.*, 1974; Steele and Sjögren, 1974).

4.6. Other Antigens Provided by H Loci

Much attention is given usually only to strong histocompatibility loci (e.g., H-2 of the mouse). It is estimated by Snell (1974), however, that there are probably at least 80 additional *H* loci providing membrane antigens detectable by transplantation rejection, lymphocytotoxicity, and red cell agglutination. To rule out such factors, one must always deal with strictly syngeneic systems.

4.7. Virion and Cellular Antigens of MuLVs

Mice of certain strains infected with or bearing leukemias induced by the FMR group of viruses or by G (Gross) virus have detectable soluble antigens in their plasma. These are of two types: infectious virus antigens and a nonvirion antigen. The latter has the same specificity as a cell surface antigen. These antigens have been detected by adsorption, complement-dependent cytotoxicity, and immunofluorescence. Their relationship to *in vivo* tumor rejection—also specific for the FMR group of leukemias as distinct from G leukemias—remains obscure.

141

STUDIES OF
SOLUBLE
TRANS-
PLANTATION
AND TUMOR
ANTIGENS

LLOYD W. LAW
AND
ETTORE
APPELLA

TSTAs more properly designated tumor rejection antigens, conveniently fall into three distinct groups: (1) membrane of neoplastic cells induced by chemical carcinogens, (2) those on neoplastic cells induced by DNA oncogenic viruses (e.g., polyoma, adeno- and SV40 viruses), and (3) those on cells induced by the RNA-containing oncogenic viruses (e.g., leukemia–sarcoma complex viruses and MTV.

Many spontaneously occurring neoplasms do not induce tumor rejection, and *in vitro* assays also indicate the absence of TSTA; in addition, tumors induced by certain carcinogens—for example, by aminoazofluorene—are not usually detectably antigenic. This finding along with the observation that MCA-transformed fibroblasts in Millipore diffusion chambers lack detectable TSTA indicates a positive role for certain carcinogens in inducing antigenic changes on the cell membrane.

A striking characteristic of TSTAs of chemically induced neoplasms of various histological types and in several species is the lack of cross-immunization against each other—that is, the existence of individually distinct TSTAs. This specificity is known to extend also to other antigenic reactions such as indirect immunofluorescence, delayed cutaneous reactivity, and inhibition of leukocyte migration. It must be admitted, however, that such studies of concordance have not been extensive. As mentioned above, there are reports of cross-reacting antigens of certain carcinogen-induced neoplasms. These studies concern chiefly the results obtained from *in vitro* lymphocytotoxicity assays and appear not to be related directly to TSTA.

In contrast to the diversity of TSTAs expressed on carcinogen-induced neoplasms (principally of sarcomas and hepatomas), tumor cells induced by polyoma virus, the adenoviruses, and SV40 (DNA oncogenic viruses) contain TSTAs that cross-react and are therefore common antigens. This group-specific cross-reactivity extends across species and histological type of neoplasms and strongly suggests viral induction or coding of TSTA. These neoplasms do not as a rule release infectious virus, nevertheless, specific virus fingerprints are detectable. The use of classical serological assays reveals a second group of antigens (neoantigens) confined to the cytoplasm or nucleus; this group bears no close biological relationship to TSTA. Neoantigens of this type may be detectable also in *in vivo* infections and in early *in vitro* lysis.

The TSTAs of DNA-virus-induced neoplastic cells are not identical with the mature virus particle, whereas the distinction between TSTAs and virion antigens is less clear in neoplasms induced by enveloped C-type viruses (RNA oncogenic viruses), where infectious virus is continuously released. Since these viruses, for example, on leukemic cells, mature by budding from the cell surface, this surface localization may represent effective antigen. There are methods available to distinguish between TSTA and virion antigen and these are discussed later. Most identified TSTAs on neoplastic cells induced by RNA-containing viruses show, as do DNA viruses, group-specific cross-reactivity. In addition, however, TSTAs have been identified that are individually distinct (Law and Takemoto, 1973; Morton *et al.*, 1969).

143

STUDIES OF
SOLUBLE
TRANS-
PLANTATION
AND TUMOR
ANTIGENS

6. Characterization of TSTA

Tumor rejection carried out in a completely syngeneic system—that is, one in which genetic differences between host and tumor are eliminated—provides the most critical and convincing evidence for the presence and functioning of TSTAs. This assay is cumbersome and sometimes difficult. As a consequence, other *in vivo* and *in vitro* antigen assays have been used in studies of membrane-expressed tumor antigens and the immune responses they induce. In attempts to demonstrate TSTAs (tumor rejection antigens) by other *in vivo* reactions or by serological reactions *in vitro*, it should be borne in mind that immune reactions may be directed against membrane receptors other than the membrane receptor in question. These other sites detailed previously—fetal antigens, differentiation antigens, tissue-specific antigens, etc.—may be totally irrelevant to the antigen being investigated, or indeed the immune response may be nonspecific. It is therefore necessary to examine the specificity of each reaction very carefully and, more importantly, to obtain a good correspondence between the specificity of the rejection-inducing response and its *in vitro* counterpart. The value of many *in vitro* assays for assessing the rejection potential of an *in vivo* host is not clear; in fact, the recent literature is contradictory on this point. The puzzling findings employing colony inhibition and microcytotoxicity assays and the effects of "blocking" and "deblocking" factors do not have as yet a reliable *in vivo* counterpart. Thus studies restricted to *in vitro* assays must be interpreted with caution as to their relevance to a specific host–tumor immune response.

Although contamination of passaged neoplasms with passenger viruses, particularly type C RNA viruses, has not proved a serious limitation to studies of TSTAs, it may seriously influence interpretations of results based strictly on *in vitro* cytotoxicity assays. Target cells, particularly lymphoid cells, are known to acquire cell surface changes as a result of infections with nononcogenic viruses such as LCM or measles virus that render them vulnerable to cytotoxic antibodies or sensitized lymphoid cells.

7. Isolation, Solubilization, and Purification of Tumor-Associated Membrane Antigens

Numerous attempts have been made to isolate and then solubilize and purify tumor antigens existing on neoplastic cells of several species of animals. The methods used to solubilize and purify histocompatibility antigens have been employed extensively in these investigations. A typical feature of most attempts,

TABLE 3

Biological Effects of Soluble TSTAs (or TAAs)

Tissue source	TSTA (or TAA) present	Methods used	Results	References
Carcinogen-induced sarcomas, hepatomas (inbred rats)	TSTA (specific)	Papain digestion + ion-exchange chromatography	Neutralization with preparations of immunofluorescent antibody and of cytotoxicity in CI and microcytotoxicity assays No tumor rejection Mol wt 55,000	Baldwin et al. (1972b) (see also text)
Carcinogen-induced hepatomas (inbred guinea pigs)	TSTA (specific)	3 M KCl and gel filtration chromatography	Soluble antigen identified by 1. Delayed cutaneous sensitivity 2. Macrophage migration inhibition 3. Lymphocyte transformation No significant tumor rejection Mol wt 75,000–150,000	Meltzer et al. (1971) Leonard et al. (1972)
Spontaneous melanoma (B-16) (inbred mouse)	TAA(?)	Ammonium sulfate precipitation plus Sephadex G-200 fractionation	Soluble antigen identified by antigen-binding radioimmunoassay; activity also with normal fibroblasts Mol wt 150,000–200,000	Bystryn et al. (1974)
Carcinogen-induced sarcoma (inbred mouse)	TSTA	3 M KCl and sonication plus 3 M KCl	Delayed hypersensitivity reaction (foot pad swelling); >1000 μ g/ml antigen was optimal No tumor rejection mentioned	Brannen et al. 1974
Carcinogen-induced sarcoma (inbred guinea pig)	TSTA (specific)	Isotonic saline, ultracentrifugation, and Sephadex G150 fractionation and DEAE-Sephadex chromatography	Activity assayed by skin hypersensitivity and inhibition of macrophage migration Activity not restricted to a single molecular species (Tumor rejection?)	Suter et al. (1972) (see also text)

Tumor	TSTA	Method	Results/Comments	Reference
Carcinogen-induced sarcoma (inbred rat)	TSTA (specific)	3 M KCl or papain digestion plus affinity chromatography	Specific activity detected using ^{125}I labeling of antigen in a radioimmunoassay (Tumor rejection?)	Thomson et al. (1973)
Adenovirus 12 induced sarcomas (hamster)	TSTA (specific)	Sonication, hypotonic lysis plus Sephadex G200 fractionation	Specific fraction protected against tumor in inbred hamsters. Same fraction from embryonic tissue also gave protection. Mol wt of active fraction 70,000	Hollinshead et al. (1972), Hollinshead and Alford (1969)
SV40-induced sarcoma (inbred mouse)	TSTA (specific)	Papain digestion and Sephadex G150 fractionation	Specific inhibition of humoral cytotoxicity in all fractions (Specific tumor rejection even with "crude membrane" questionable)	Smith et al. (1970)
SV40-induced sarcoma (inbred mouse)	TSTA (specific)	3 M KCl	Nonfractionated material provided specific inhibition of macrophage migration (Tumor rejection not studied)	Blasecki and Tevethia (1973)
SV40-induced sarcoma (inbred mouse)	TSTA (specific)	Papain digestion and Sephadex G150 chromatography	Tumor rejection specific for an F fraction and for crude soluble antigen at concentrations as low as 5 μ g protein. Specific inhibition of humoral cytotoxicity not achieved. Mol wt 30,000–40,000	Drapkin et al. (1974), Law et al. (1975)
Lymphoma (mice)	TSTA? (specificity?)	Sonication and Sephadex G200 chromatography	Two fractions provided tumor rejection in a small number of mice. No specificity studies given; rejection also attained with alloantigenic lymphoid tissue (see text)	Prager et al. (1973)

TABLE 3—*continued*

Tissue source	TSTA (or TAA) present	Methods used	Results	References
RLV-induced lymphoma (inbred mice)	TSTA(?)	Hypotonic NaCl plus autodigestion plus electrofocussing	Absorption of cytotoxicity in allogeneic antisera Tumor rejection not mentioned but induction of leukemia by virus was inhibited with preparation (?)	Martyré *et al.* (1973) Jolles *et al.* (1970)
RLV-induced leukemia (inbred mice)	TSTA (specific)	Papain digestion, Sephadex G150 fractionation	Specific tumor rejection related to TSTA and not virion antigens; immunogenicity confined to F2 fraction Specific inhibition of humoral cytotoxicity by soluble antigen Mol wt 30,000—40,000	Law and Appella (1973) Law *et al.* (1975) Chang *et al.* (1974)

however, has been a low yield of antigenic material, heterogeneity of the recovered material, and usually a striking lability. The starting material used by several investigators was a solid tumor mass. It is difficult to envision a distinct separation of membrane materials from internal organelles unless there are included markers for organelle-specific enzymes, for example, or membrane markers of some type, say histocompatibility (transplantation) antigens.

147

STUDIES OF
SOLUBLE
TRANS-
PLANTATION
AND TUMOR
ANTIGENS

Table 3 lists some features of investigations of pertinence to the isolation, solubilization, and in some cases purification of TSTAs, or in instances where TSTAs have not been characterized, to presence of tumor-associated antigens, TAAs. Assays for antigenic activity have been varied, some restricted to a single assay, and in most instances the major function of TSTAs—that is, the capacity to reject a tumor in specific fashion, using host and tumor that are syngeneic—has not been assayed or was found to be nonexistent.

Allegedly solubilized TSTAs have been described from membranes of guinea pig sarcomas (Holmes *et al.*, 1970; Oettgen *et al.*, 1968) and from adenovirus 12 tumors of the hamster and mouse (Potter and Oxford, 1970). Specific tumor rejection was obtained, and in the case of the guinea pig sarcomas specific delayed cutaneous hypersensitivity reactions were striking. These investigators, however, used ultracentrifugation in the range of 100,000g preceded by homogenization, exposure to low-intensity sonic energy, or freeze-thawing. Certainly, alloantigens are known not to be solubilized in this manner and there is no evidence to rule out the existence of membrane fragments in the preparations of these investigators. Investigations have been extended by one of the groups (Suter *et al.*, 1972) using MCA-induced sarcomas of inbred strain 13 guinea pigs; further fractionation was performed by ammonium sulfate precipitation followed by gel filtration on Sephadex G150 and DEAE-Sephadex chromatography. Specific antigenic activity was detectable by delayed cutaneous reactivity and by macrophage migration inhibition; however, antigenic activity was not restricted to a single species of molecule. Apparently, tumor rejection was not studied.

Manson *et al.* (1963) have used decompression in the nitrogen bomb followed by ultracentrifugation in sucrose solutions of different concentrations. They used leukemic cells L-5178Y of DBA/2 mice. Homograft sensitization in C57BL/6 was obtained with the microsomal lipoprotein fraction (MLP). Later, Manson *et al.* (1974) reported that preparations obtained in a similar manner provided immunity against a cell challenge in DBA/2 mice of L-5178Y, thus indicating the existence of a tumor antigen of the transplantation type. The specificity of this response, however, has not been documented. Effective MLP is a particulate material and further studies of its activity following solubilization and fractionation should be pursued.

Turning now to the findings of cell membrane expressed tumor antigens detailed in Table 3, the following are pertinent:

1. Meltzer *et al.* (1971) and Leonard *et al.* (1972, 1974) used 3 M KCl for extraction of antigen (TSA) from guinea pig hepatomas; this was followed by Sephadex G200 fractionation. At least for one line of tumor (line 1), the extracted membrane material is soluble, with an antigen yield of 10% and a molecular

weight in the range of 70,000–100,000. The soluble TSA extracts had positive reactivity, specific for the tumor tested, in delayed cutaneous reactions, inhibition of migration of peritoneal cells, and stimulation of lymphocyte transformation; relatively large amounts of soluble antigen (maximal responses obtained with 1500 μ g/ml) were necessary to elicit these responses. Satisfactory immunogenicity as detected in tumor rejection has not been reported.

2. Baldwin and colleagues report studies of isolation and solubilization of cell membrane expressed antigens from rat hepatomas and sarcomas; their most complete studies deal with a single carcinogen-induced hepatoma, D-23, and membrane fractions (ENMs) of this hepatoma. The ENMs were obtained by nitrogen cavitation followed by centrifugation at 105,000g for 60 min (Baldwin *et al.*, 1973; Baldwin and Moore, 1969). The antigenic activity was detected by the ability of the membrane preparation to specifically adsorb antibody from the sera of rats immunized against tumor cells and to elicit tumor-specific antibody response as measured by indirect immunofluorescence and by specific complement-dependent cytotoxicity for D-23 hepatoma cells in the colony inhibition assay. Relatively large amounts of crude membrane material (16.9 mg protein) were required to elicit detectable levels of antibody. These membrane preparations did not elicit transplantation immunity, however, nor did the soluble antigens of D-23 discussed below.

Later studies used limited papain digestion followed by DEAE-cellulose chromatography to solubilize D-23 antigen (Baldwin *et al.*, 1972*b*). The major antigenic fraction (determined by fluorescent antibody neutralizing activity) was found to be quite heterogeneous as revealed by polyacrylamide gel electrophoresis. Recently this soluble D-23 antigen preparation, stated to have components with molecular weights in the region of 55,000, was shown to neutralize the "blocking" activity of tumor-bearer serum in colony inhibition assays. Further biological studies of this solubilized material are necessary in order to properly identify the material as TSTA distinct from other measurable membrane components (see Chap. 7).

3. Hollinshead *et al.* (1972) reported immunogenic activity in preparations of an Ad12-induced tumor in the inbred PD-4 hamster. Sonication followed by Sephadex gel filtration (G200 column) yielded a fraction that specifically immunized against this tumor. A disturbing feature, however, was that a similar fraction derived from PD-4 embryo membranes was also immunogenic.

4. Smith *et al.* (1970) used papain digestion and fractionation on a Sephadex G150 column to study TSTA on an SV40-induced neoplasm of the AL/N strain mouse. Inhibition of complement-dependent cytotoxicity was observed with soluble material from all three peaks obtained (excluded volume, also); specificity assays were not done with the fractionated material. "Crude membrane" was studied for *in vivo* tumor rejection using small numbers of animals in this system where even after sublethal irradiation control animals seldom develop progressively growing tumors.

5. Several of the studies listed in Table 3 used only a single assay system to detect activity in tumor preparations isolated and solubilized by different procedures: antigen binding radioimmunoassays (Thomson *et al.*, 1973; Bystryn *et al.*,

1974), delayed cutaneous hypersensitivity reaction (Brannen *et al.*, 1974), and
inhibition of macrophage migration (Blasecki and Tevethia, 1973). Strong TSTA
had been previously identified in some of the neoplasms studied and indirect
evidence indicates that the soluble antigen(s) detected may in fact be identical or
similar to TSTA; however, in no case, was there any evidence to indicate that these
soluble preparations had tumor rejection potential. There is ample evidence to
indicate that a number of antigenic systems may be expressed following neoplastic
conversion. Many of these are detectable by *in vitro* assays that may have no
significance to *in vivo* events.

STUDIES OF
SOLUBLE
TRANS-
PLANTATION
AND TUMOR
ANTIGENS

6. Nonvirion TSTAs distinct from virus structural proteins are difficult to
characterize on lymphomas that usually release infectious C-type viruses. There
was no attempt to make this distinction in two studies listed in Table 3 employing
lymphoma tissues as a source of membrane antigens. A soluble fraction obtained
by autodigestion and electrofocusing was observed by Martyré *et al.* (1973) to
adsorb cytotoxic activity from allogeneic antisera specific for FMR. This procedure does not allow distinction from the known serologically detectable virion
structural antigens. Preimmunization with this fraction was stated to inhibit the
induction of leukemia by virus and to facilitate the growth of ascitic grafts of the
leukemia (Jolles *et al.*, 1970). Neither assay specifically characterizes the activity as
that of TSTA. Prager *et al.* (1973) used the long transplantable lymphoma
6C3HED to solubilize membrane material by sonication and Sephadex G200
fractionation. Two fractions of the solubilized material were found capable of
immunizing against the 6C3HED neoplasm. Specificity studies were, however,
not included. Allogeneic lymphoid tissues from many strains of mice are also
capable of providing protection against grafting of 6C3HED cells (see Prager *et
al.*, 1973; Merino *et al.*, 1973). Thus the identity of the component being
solubilized remains to be answered.

8. Isolation, Solubilization, and Partial Purification of Tumor Antigens with Tumor Rejection Activity

In this laboratory, our efforts at solubilizing and purifying tumor antigens have
been directed at those membrane-bound antigens of the transplantation type
specified by the DNA and RNA oncogenic viruses. Tumor-associated cell surface
antigens of the transplantation type (TSTAs) are consistently found on neoplastic
cells transformed by the oncogenic viruses. They are of interest because they
provide targèts for immune repression and also because they may reflect
membrane changes intimately related to the malignant behavior of the cell.
Tumor viruses might induce TSTA by one of several methods: (1) by interfering
metabolically with membrane biosynthesis (but only if this is a permanent
interference), (2) by derepressing cellular (embryonal) genes (this now appears to
be unlikely in view of the more recent functional studies of fetal or embryonal
antigens), (3) by the budding infectious virus acting as antigen, and (4) by coding
for a nonvirion protein component (that is not a structural component of the

virion). The coding may be in the form of altering normal histocompatibility antigens.

8.1. Characteristics of Soluble TSTA on SV40-Induced Neoplasms

mKSA (Tu-5) is an SV40-transformed neoplasm of BALB/c mice. One subline of this undifferentiated sarcoma was adapted into the ascites form (ASC) and another subline was adapted to grow in monolayer tissue culture (TC). Through continuous passage, this latter subline has lost its oncogenic potential so that its TD_{50} is now 2×10^6 to 2×10^7 cells. The ASC line remains virulent with a TD_{50} near 10^3 cells. The SV40 cells will immunize against 2×10^7 ASC neoplastic cells. As shown by Howell *et al.* (1974) the T cell is effective in causing tumor regression in this system.

The method previously used for isolation and solubilization of H-2 antigens was adapted to obtain immunogenic TSTA from this non-virus-producing mKSA neoplasm. Briefly the method was as follows: mKSA–ASC containing $2–6 \times 10^9$ tumor cells was harvested in tris-buffered saline (TBS), usually from 300 animals. Cells were equilibrated in a cell disruption bomb (model 4635, Parr Instrument Company, Moline, Illinois) at 400 psi nitrogen for 30 min and rapidly released to effect disruption of 90% or more of all cells. The resulting cell homogenate was centrifuged at $600g$ for 12 min to remove nuclei and cell debris. The supernatant was centrifuged at $55,000g$ for 90min, and the sediment was suspended in 0.05 M tris, pH 8.4, at approximately 10 mg dry weight/ml. This crude membrane (CM) was either used in experiments or digested with papain (Worthington Biochemical Corporation, Freehold, New Jersey) at a ratio of 1 mg papain to 100 mg protein, at 37°C in the presence of 0.01 M dithiothreitol. The reaction was stopped after 1 h by the addition of iodoacetamide to a final concentration of 0.022 M, and insoluble sediment was removed after centrifugation at $105,000g$ for 90 min.

Soluble supernatant was exhaustively dialyzed against 0.15 M tris, pH 8.2, and was then concentrated by ultrafiltration with use of a UM-2 membrane (Amicon Corporation, Lexington, Massachusetts). The resulting crude soluble material (CS) was either utilized in experiments or applied to Sephadex G150; the eluate was collected and a chromatogram was obtained by measuring its optical density (OD280). F1, F2 and F3 fractions were collected.

The immunogenicity of our various fractions has been given in detail (Drapkin *et al.*, 1974). CM prepared from ASC cells afforded complete protection against challenge with 10^4 and 10^5 cells and partial protection against 10^6 neoplastic cells ($TD_{50} = 10^3$ cells). CS afforded complete protection at 10^4 cells and partial protection at 10^5 cells. CM preparations from both the ASC and TC cell lines were equally immunogenic. Immunization with both the F2 and F3 fractions (Sephadex G150) provided striking resistance to challenge with 10^4 neoplastic cells. This resistance was reflected not only in the "takes" of tumor in syngeneic BALB/c hosts but also in the rate of tumor growth. For example, 50% of the tumor-bearing control mice had died of large tumors at 40 days, whereas none of the F2 and F3 151

STUDIES OF
SOLUBLE
TRANS-
PLANTATION
AND TUMOR
ANTIGENS
fraction recipients was dead at this time.

Poor resolution was obtained in all of our preparations of F2 and F3 fractions and this raises the question of whether F3 carries some F2 activity. To demonstrate specificity of the immune response, animals given mKSA-ASC *CM* were again made strongly immune to challenge with mKSA-ASC but demonstrated no immunity to challenge with Adj-PC-5, a BALB/c plasma cell tumor containing its own strong TSTA, at a dose 5–50 times its TD_{50}. Using additional preparations of our mKSA–CS material, we immunized BALB/c mice with graded doses and challenged with the SV40-induced mKSA. A total immunizing dose of as little as 5.0 μg *CS* material (2.5 μg × 2) provided protection against a challenge of 7×10^3 and 7×10^4 neoplast cells (Law *et al.*, 1975). This protection approximates that provided by immunization with 10^6 intact mKSA (TC) cells. Immunogenic yield is probably therefore close to 20% for this *CS* preparation.

We had initially hoped to develop an appropriate *in vitro* ^{51}Cr-release cytotoxicity assay to monitor TSTA titers at progressive stages in our isolation and purification procedures. Anti-mKSA serum was not cytotoxic for any of the SV40 target cells used, nor could effective antiserum be produced despite the strong immunogenicity observed in our tumor rejection studies. This contrasts with studies in which *in vitro* assays were capable of detecting specific antigenicity but not *in vivo* tumor rejection (Baldwin *et al.*, 1972b, 1973) and should indicate the need for caution in interpreting results with assays other than tumor rejection to indicate the presence of solubilized TSTA. Recently we have observed our CS and F2 fractions to be capable of inhibiting in specific fashion migration of peritoneal exudate cells (Maurer *et al.* 1975) and of eliciting specific lymphocyte stimulation in the mixed lymphocyte–tumor cell assay (Dean *et al.* 1975). In the migration inhibition study 10 μg/ml (3.3 μg/chamber) and in lymphocyte stimulation 0.1 μg/well had significant activity.

8.2. Characteristics of Soluble RBL-5 TSTA

RBL-5, a lymphoblastic leukemia, was induced by Rauscher leukemogenic virus (RLV) in a C57BL/6 mouse. It is routinely passaged in syngeneic mice in the ascitic form. RBL-5 cells are immunogenic and provide immunity against other leukemias of the FMR group. RBL-5 is a good target cell; it is easily and specifically lysed *in vitro* by sensitized syngeneic lymphocytes and by specific cytotoxic antisera in the presence of complement, as discussed later; however, it is not very immunosensitive. As a consequence, our *in vivo* assays have been with a challenge of leukemic cells from LSTRA, an MLV-induced leukemia, and FBL-3, an FLV-induced leukemia. Both are known to contain TSTAs of the FMR group. CBF_1 mice have been used as recipients since LSTRA is of BALB/c origin and FBL-3 of C5B1/6 origin.

The methods used for extraction and further purification of soluble TSTA from RBL-5 membranes were similar to those used and tested for H-2 and for SV40 antigens.

Significant inhibition of growth reflected in tumor "takes" and growth rates was observed for both LSTRA and FBL-3 following immunization with *CM* and the F2 fraction of the chromatographed material. F1 and F3 fractions used at the same concentrations as F2 were found ineffective. Crude soluble (CS) preparations of FBL-3 cells were also found to be immunogenic as assayed in the Winn test (Law *et al.*, 1975). Specificity controls were of two types: (1) C57BL mice immunized with the *CM* and *CS* preparations of RBL-5 at concentrations and schedule providing resistance to leukemic cells did not resist a polyoma-induced neoplasm No. 89, and (2) *CS* and F2 fraction preparations of normal C57BL spleen cells failed to protect against challenge with sensitive FBL-3 leukemic cells.

In contrast to the immunogenic preparations of mKSA, both *CM* and *CS* preparations of RBL-5 membranes induced cytotoxic antisera in syngeneic mice, and inhibition of complement-dependent cytotoxicity, using ^{51}Cr release, has provided a reliable assay for monitoring our solubilization and purification procedure. The *CM* preparation, papain-solubilized *CS*, and pooled F2 fraction (but not F1 and F3) inhibited lysis of the syngeneic antiserum using RBL-5 targets. This antiserum was not cytotoxic for normal lymph node cells nor for SV-AL/N fibroblasts known to contain S40 TSTA (Law and Appella, 1973).

We tried to calculate the overall yield of activity of this TSTA using inhibition of ^{51}Cr release. If inhibition titers obtained with the *CM* antigen preparations are used (titers ranging from 1/64 to 1/128 at 50% inhibition of lysis), the F2 fraction contains 4–6% of the *CM* total activity.

In the pooled F2 fraction as well as in the *CM* preparation, H-2 specificities 2 and 28 were also detected using monospecific alloantisera. The activity we observed in our cytotoxicity assays coincides with the pooled F2 fraction of H-2 specificities.

8.3. Distinction Between New Cellular Antigen (TSTA) and Viral Antigens on RBL-5 Leukemic Cells

TSTAs of neoplasms induced by DNA oncogenic virus (e.g., SV40 and polyoma neoplasms) are easily distinguished from virion antigens. In the case of RNA-virus-induced neoplasms, this distinction is much less clear since most of these neoplastic cells continuously release infectious virus. This is true with RBL-5 leukemic cells, the source of our surface antigen preparations. We have therefore attempted to distinguish whether or not these antigens are virus structural proteins or are of nonvirion origin but nevertheless coded by the virus (Chang *et al.*, 1974). The following findings are pertinent:

1. X-irradiated and freeze-thawed RBL-5 cells released infectious type-C virus as detected by the XC syncytial cell plaque assay; in contrast, none of our antigen preparations, even at concentrations as high as 500 μg/ml (protein), showed infectious virus by this assay.
2. The antiserum prepared in syngeneic C57BL mice by immunization with our RBL-5 *CM* or *CS* preparations was found not to manifest any neutralizing activity against the homologous virus RLV by the XC assay or by focus

reduction assay using MSV(RLV). Thus these antigen preparations were free of virion antigens, at least in concentrations capable of inducing detectable amounts of neutralizing antibody by these assays.

153

STUDIES OF
SOLUBLE
TRANS-
PLANTATION
AND TUMOR
ANTIGENS

3. Through the use of a more sensitive microcomplement fixation (CF) assay, it was found that our *CS* and F2 (but not F3) preparations reacted with syngeneic antiserum. This syngeneic antiserum did not react, however, with high-titered RLV (homologous virus) or with MLV. These results indicate the existence of a component in *CS* and the F2 fraction, both known to be immunogenic (as reflected in tumor rejection), that is not virion antigen. However, all of our antigenic preparations reacted with broad antisera—Fischer rat anti-MSV(MLV) and hamster anti-RLV—in trace amounts, indicating cross-contamination with viron antigen. This differential reactivity of syngeneic antiserum with *CS* and the purified F2 fraction indicates the existence of a detectable component that is not a virion antigen. Further work is necessary to confirm that this detectable component provides the biological activity we have observed, that is, immunogenicity and blocking of cytoxicity, and in fact represents a new cellular antigen of the TSTA type coded by the virus (RLV).

An approach to decisively differentiate TSTA from virion antigens is to utilize "nonproducer" tumor cells. Recently we have studied leukemia RBL-3, which was originally induced in BL/6 mice by RLV in a similar manner to RBL-5 and maintained by *in vitro* culture. This line proved to be immunogenic *in vivo* in BL/6 mice against leukemia FBL-3, which possesses FMR tumor antigen shared by RBL-5, and *vice versa*. Moreover, this lymphocytic neoplasm produced no infectious RLV but was nevertheless MuLV *gs*-antigen positive. Therefore, this can be defined as a "nonproducer" neoplasm in the classical sense. The syngeneic anti-*CM* sera were cytotoxic against RBL-3 cells as well as against RBL-5 cells, suggesting again the dissociation of tumor cell surface antigen (TSTA) from virion antigen.

Thus, in summary, our results show that TSTAs on SV40-induced neoplastic cells (mKSA) were isolated and solubilized. The immunogenic activity (that is, tumor rejection activity) was contained mainly in the peak (F2 fraction) that was positive for alloantigenic activity. This specific activity could be titrated *in vivo* by serial dilutions to as low as 5 μg (protein) per mouse. This represents a yield in terms of immunogenicity of approximately 20%. Tumor-specific antibody was not evoked with the *CM* antigen preparations in syngeneic mice.

TSTA on RLV-induced leukemic cells (RNA oncogenic virus induced) was also isolated and solubilized from RBL-5 leukemic cell membranes. Specific immunogenicity was retained, again in the peak (F2 fraction) containing alloantigenic activity. Cytotoxic antisera were induced by these antigenic preparations. When a micro-CF assay was used, these antisera appeared to detect a specific component that was not related to structural viral proteins. Thus the solubilized antigen of this RNA oncogenic virus-induced neoplasm appears to be a new cellular antigen analogous to the TSTA of DNA oncogenic virus-induced neoplasms.

LLOYD W. LAW
AND
ETTORE
APPELLA

9. Conclusion

The methods used in this laboratory to solubilize and partially purify H-2 antigens are found to preserve biological activity as detected by *in vitro* and *in vivo* assays. All biological activity was confined to a single peak following Sephadex G150 fractionation. This strongly suggests that we are dealing with a single molecular entity that has a molecular weight of approximately 50,000. No evidence was obtained for the existence of separate classes of fragments in our preparations. In addition β_2-microglobulin activity was confined to this same peak and therefore resembles what is found *in situ* on the cell membrane.

Tumor-associated antigens (TAAs) have been solubilized by a variety of methods. Antigenic activities sometimes specific in nature have been detected in these preparations. In many syngeneic systems used, the evidence is neither extensive nor conclusive that it is the TSTAs that have been solubilized and are responsible for the detectable activity. Tumor rejection has not been achieved or attempted in many studies, principally as a result of the low yield of antigenic materials. The relevance of the *in vitro* or indirect *in vivo* assays used to *in vivo* surveillance of tumor growth has not been assessed adequately in many studies.

The H-2 model has provided clues and methodology for solubilization of well-defined TSTAs in this laboratory. The isolated and solubilized TSTAs from a DNA-virus-induced and from an RNA-virus-induced neoplasm were contained in the peak (F2 fraction) that was in each instance positive for alloantigenic activity. Specific tumor rejection was achieved in syngeneic mice by each preparation. Cytotoxic antibodies were also induced by the membrane preparation of RNA-virus-induced neoplastic cells. This activity was apparently not related to structural viral proteins. The fact that TSTA and H-2 cochromatograph on the Sephadex G150 column points to some similarity in molecular size and structure between the two types of antigen.

10. References

ANKERST, J., STEELE, G., JR., AND SJÖGREN, H. O., 1974, Cross-reacting tumor-associated antigen(s) of adenovirus type 9-induced fibroadenomas in rats, *Cancer Res.* **34:**1794.

APPELLA, E., HENRIKSEN, O., NATORI, T., TANIGAKI, N., LAW, L. W., AND PRESSMAN, D., 1975, Basic structure of mouse histocompatibility antigens, *Transplant. Proc.* **VII:**191.

BALDWIN, R. W., AND MOORE, M., 1969, Isolation of membrane-associated tumor-specific antigen from an aminoazo-dye-induced rat hepatoma, *Int. J. Cancer* **4:**753.

BALDWIN, R. W., GLAVES, D., AND VOSE, B. M., 1972a, Embryonic antigen expression in chemically induced rat hepatomas and sarcomas, *Int. J. Cancer* **10:**233.

BALDWIN, R. W., PRICE, M. R., AND ROBINS, R. A., 1972b, Blocking of lymphocyte mediated cytotoxicity for rat hepatoma cells by tumour-specific antigen–antibody complexes, *Nature New Biol.* **238:**185.

BALDWIN, R. W., EMBLETON, M. J., AND MOORE, M., 1973, Immunogenicity of rat hepatoma membrane fractions, *Br. J. Cancer* **28:**389.

BLASECKI, J. W., AND TEVETHIA, S. S., 1973, *In vitro* assay of cellular immunity to tumor-specific antigen(s) of virus-induced tumors by macrophage migration inhibition, *J. Immunol.* **110:**590.

BRANNEN, G. E., ADAMS, J. S., AND SANTOS, G. W., 1974, Tumor-specific immunity in 3-methylcholanthrene-induced murine fibrosarcomas. I. *In vivo* demonstration of immunity with 3 preparations of soluble antigens, *J. Natl. Cancer Inst.* **53:**165.

155

STUDIES OF
SOLUBLE
TRANS-
PLANTATION
AND TUMOR
ANTIGENS

BYSTRYN, J. S., SCHENKEIN, I., BAUR, S., AND UHR, J. W., 1974, Partial isolation and characterization of antigen(s) associated with murine melanoma, *J. Natl. Cancer Inst.* **52**:1263.

CHANG, K. S. S., LAW, L. W., AND APPELLA, E., 1975, Distinction between tumor specific transplantation antigen and virion antigens in solubilized products from membranes of virus-induced leukemic cells, *Int. J. Cancer* **15**:483.

CULLEN, S. E., AND NATHENSON, S. G., 1971, Distribution of H-2 alloantigenic specificities on radiolabeled papain-solubilized antigen fragments, *J. Immunol.* **107**:563.

CULLEN, S. E., SCHWARTZ, B. D., NATHENSON, S. G., AND CHERRY, M., 1972, The molecular basis of codominant expression of the histocompatibility-2 genetic region, *Proc. Natl. Acad. Sci. U.S.A.* **69**:1394.

DEAN, J. H., McCOY, J. L., LEWIS, D., APPELLA, E., AND LAW, L. W. 1975, Studies of lymphocyte stimulation by intact tumor cell and solubilized tumor antigen. *Int. J. Cancer* (in press).

DRAPKIN, M. S., APPELLA, E., AND LAW, L. W., 1974, Immunogenic properties of soluble tumor-specific transplantation antigen induced by simian virus 40, *J. Natl. Cancer Inst.* **52**:259.

HAUSCHKA, T. S., 1973, Tumor immunity, in: *Principles of Immunology* (N. R. Rose, F. Malgrom, and C. J. von Oss, eds.), pp. 417–438, Macmilan, New York.

HESS, M., AND DAVIES, D. A., 1974, Basic structure of mouse histocompatibility antigens, *Eur. J. Biochem.* **41**:1.

HOLLINSHEAD, A., AND ALFORD, T. C., 1969, Identification of a soluble transplantation antigen from the membrane fraction of adenovirus tumour cells, *J. Gen. Virol.* **5**:411.

HOLLINSHEAD, A., McCAMMON, J. R., AND YOHN, D. S., 1972, Immunogenicity of a soluble membrane antigen from adenovirus-12 induced tumor cells demonstrated in inbred hamsters (PD-4), *Can. J. Microbiol.* **18**:1365.

HOLMES, E. C., KAHAN, B. O., AND MORTON, D. L., 1970, Soluble tumor-specific transplantation antigens from induced guinea pig sarcomas, *Cancer* **25**:373.

HOWARD, J. G., MICHIE, D., AND WOODRUFF, M. F. A., 1962, in: *Transplantation* (G. E. W. Wostenholme and M. P. Cameron, eds.), pp. 138–160, Little, Brown, Boston.

HOWELL, S. B., DEAN, J. H., ESBER, E. C., AND LAW, L. W., 1974, Cell interactions in adoptive immune rejection of a syngeneic tumor, *Int. J. Cancer* **14**:662.

JOLLES, P., SCHOENTGEN, F., HALLE-PANNENKO, O., AND MARTYRÉ, M. C., 1970, Purification of soluble transplantation antigens by isoelectric focusing, *FEBS Lett.* **8**:167.

KLEIN, J., AND SCHREFFLER, D. C., 1972, Evidence supporting a two-gene model for the H-2 histocompatibility system of the mouse, *J. Exp. Med.* **135**:924.

LAW, L. W., AND APPELLA, E., 1973, Immunogenic properties of solubilized tumour antigen from an RNA virus transformed neoplasm, *Nature (London)* **243**:83.

LAW, L. W., AND TAKEMOTO, K. K., 1973, Specific transplantation antigens of murine neoplasms induced by visna and progressive pneumonia viruses, *J. Natl. Cancer Inst.* **50**:1075.

LAW, L. W., APPELLA, E., WRIGHT, P. W., AND STROBER, S., 1971, Immunologic enhancement of allogeneic tumor growth with soluble histocompatibility-2 antigens, *Proc. Natl. Acad. Sci. U.S.A.* **68**:3078.

LAW, L. W., APPELLA, E., STROBER, S., WRIGHT, P. W., AND FISCHETTI, T., 1972, Induction of immunological tolerance to soluble histocompatibility-2 antigens of mice, *Proc. Natl. Acad. Sc:. U.S.A.* **69**:1858.

LAW, L. W., APPELLA, E., COHEN, J., AND DEAN, J. H., 1973, Reactivity of lymphoid cells from mice humorally tolerant to histocompatibility antigens, *Nature New Biol.* **246**:174.

LAW, L. W., APPELLA, E., AND CHANG, K. S. S., 1975, Biologic effects of solubilized and tumor specific antigens, *Transplant. Proc.* **VII**:233.

LAW, L. W., APPELLA, E., COHEN, J. M., AND WRIGHT, P. W., 1974, Role of serum factors from tolerant mice in blocking and in immunologic enhancement, *Transplantation* **18**:14.

LAW, L. W., APPELLA, E., STROBER, S., WRIGHT, P. W., AND FISCHETTI, T., 1974b, Soluble transplantation antigens: Further studies of their tolerogenic properties, *Transplantation* **18**:487.

LEONARD, E. J., MELTZER, M. S., BORSOS, T., AND RAPP, H. J., 1972, Properties of tumor-specific antigen solubilized by hypertonic KCl, in: Conference on Immunology of Carcinogenesis, *Natl. Cancer Inst. Monogr.* **35**:129.

LEONARD, E. J., MELTZER, M. S., BORSOS, T., AND RAPP, H. J., 1974, Immunogenicity of soluble tumor-specific antigen, in: *Immunological Aspects of Neoplasia: Proceedings of the 26th Annual Symposium on Fundamental Research*, Vol. 26, Williams and Wilkins, Baltimore.

LIEBERMAN, R., PAUL, W. E., HUMPHREY, W., AND STIMPFLING, J. H., 1972, H-2 linked immune response (*Ir*) genes: Independent loci for *Ir-IrG* and *Ir-IrA* genes, *J. Exp. Med.* **122**:517.

MANN, D. L., AND FAHEY, J. L., 1971, Histocompatibility antigens, *Ann. Rev. Microbiol.* **25**:679.

MANSON, L. A., GOLDSTEIN, L., THORN, R., AND PALMER, J., 1975, Immune response against apparently host compatible transplantable tumors, *Transplant. Proc.* **VII**:161.

MARTYRÉ, M. C., HALLE-PANNENKO, O., AND JOLLES, P., 1973, Characterization and partial purification of normal and tumor associated transplantation antigens of Rauscher leukemia cells, *Eur. J. Cancer* **9**:757.

MAURER, B. A., DEAN, J. H., MCCOY, J. L., APPELLA, E., AND LAW, L. W., Assessment of cell-mediated immunity in mice against PPD, soluble H-2 alloantigens and SV-40 tumor antigens. (Submitted to *Cellular Immunology*).

MCDEVITT, H. O., AND SELA, M., 1965, Genetic control of the antibody response. I. Demonstration of determinant-specific differences in response to synthetic polypeptide antigens, *J. Exp. Med.* **122**:517.

MELTZER, M. S., LEONARD, E. J., RAPP, H. J., AND BOROS, T., 1971, Tumor-specific antigen solubilized by hypertonic KC1, *J. Natl. Cancer Inst.* **47**:703.

MERINO, F., ABEYOUNIS, C. J., AND MILGROM, F., 1973, Theta antigen on a murine lymphosarcoma, *Transplant. Proc.* **5**:975.

MORTON, D. L., MILLER, G. F., AND WOOD, D. A., 1969, Demonstration of tumor-specific immunity against antigens unrelated to the mammary tumor virus, *J. Natl. Cancer Inst.* **42**:290.

NATHENSON, S. G., 1970, Biochemical properties of histocompatibility antigens, *Ann. Rev. Genet.* **4**:69.

NATORI, T., TANIGAKI, N., AND PRESSMAN, D., 1975a, The 11,000-dalton fragment of mouse H-2 antigen: Isolation and identification, *Transplantation* **18**:550.

NATORI, T., TANIGAKI, N., PRESSMAN, D., HENRIKSEN, O., APPELLA, E., LAW, L. W., 1975b, Two components of papain-solubilized H-2 antigen molecules, *Immunogenetics* (submitted).

NEAPORT-SANTES, C., LILLY, F., SILVESTRE, D., AND KOURILSKY, F. M., 1973, Independence of H-2K and H-2D antigenic determinants on the surface of mouse lymphocytes, *J. Exp. Med.* **137**:511.

OETTGEN, H. F., OLD, L. J., MCLEAN, E. P., AND CARSWELL, E. A., 1968, Delayed hypersensitivity and transplantation immunity elicited by soluble antigens of chemically induced tumours in guinea pigs, *Nature (London)* **220**:293.

POTTER, C. W., AND OXFORD, J. S., 1970, Transplantation immunity following immunization with extracts of adenovirus 12 tumour cells, *Int. J. Cancer* **6**:410.

PRAGER, M. D., HOLLINSHEAD, A. C., RIBBLE, R. J., AND DERR, I., 1973, Induction of immunity to a mouse lymphoma by multiple methods, including vaccination with soluble membrane fractions, *J. Natl. Cancer Inst.* **51**:1603.

RASK, L., LINDBLOM, J. B., AND PETERSON, P. A., 1974, Subunit structure of H-2 alloantigens, *Nature (London)* **249**:833.

SCHWARTZ, B. D., KATO, K., CULLEN, S. E., AND NATHENSON, S. G., 1973, H-2 histocompatibility alloantigens: Some biochemical properties of the molecules solubilized by NP-40 detergent, *Biochemistry* **12**:2157.

SHIMADA, A., AND NATHENSON, S. G., 1969, Murine histocompatibility-2 (H-2) alloantigens: Purification and some chemical properties of soluble products from H-2^b and H-2^d genotypes released by papain digestion of membrane fractions, *Biochemistry* **8**:4048.

SHREFFLER, D. C., AND KLEIN, J., 1970, Genetic organization and gene action of mouse H-2 region, *Transplant. Proc.* **2**:5.

SILVER, J., AND HOOD, L., 1974, Detergent-solubilized H-2 alloantigen is associated with a small molecular weight polypeptide, *Nature (London)* **249**:764.

SMITH, R. W., MORGANROTH, J., AND MORA, P. T., 1970, SV40 virus-induced tumour specific transplantation antigen in cultured mouse cells, *Nature (London)* **227**:141.

SNELL, G., 1974, Immunogenetics: Retrospect and prospect, *Immunogenetics* **1**:4.

SNELL, G. D., CHERRY, M., AND DEMANT, P., 1971, Evidence that H-2 private specificities can be arranged in two mutually exclusive systems possibly homologous with two subsystems of HL-A, *Transplant. Proc.* **3**:183.

STEELE, JR., G., AND SJÖGREN, H., 1974, Cross-reacting tumor-associated antigen(s) among chemically induced rat colon carcinomas, *Cancer Res.* **34**:1801.

STROBER, S., APPELLA, E., AND LAW, L. W., 1970, Serologic and immunogenic activity of mouse transplantation antigens controlted by the H-2 locus, *Proc. Natl. Acad. Sci. U.S.A.* **67**:765.

SUTER, L., BLOOM, B. R., WADSWORTH, E. M., AND OETTGEN, H. F., 1972, Use of the macrophage migration inhibition test to monitor fractionation of soluble antigens of chemically induced sarcomas of guinea pigs, *J. Immunol.* **109**:766.

TANIGAKI, N., KATAGIRI, M., NAKAMURO, K., KREITER, V. P., AND PRESSMAN, D., 1974, II. Small fragments derived from papain-solubilized HL-A antigen molecules, *Immunology* **26**:155.

THOMSON, D. M. P., SELLERS, V., ECCLES, S., AND ALEXANDER, P., 1973, Radioimmunoassay of tumour-specific transplantation antigen of a chemically induced rat sarcoma: Circulating soluble tumour antigen tumour bearers, *Br. J. Cancer* **28:**377.

TING, C. C., LAVRIN, D. H., SHIU, G., AND HERBERMAN, R. B., 1972, Expression of fetal antigens in tumor cells, *Proc. Natl. Acad. Sci. U.S.A.* **69:**1664.

WRIGHT, P. W., LAW, L. W., APPELLA, E., AND BERNSTEIN, I. D., 1974, Absence of serum blocking activity in mice immunologically tolerant to soluble histocompatibility-2 antigens, *Transplantation* **17:**524.

157

STUDIES OF
SOLUBLE
TRANS-
PLANTATION
AND TUMOR
ANTIGENS

RNA Oncogenic Virus-Associated Antigens

And Host Immune Response to Them

TADAO AOKI and LOUIS R. SIBAL

1. Introduction

The rapid development of analytical techniques has revealed the complexity of antigens associated with type B and type C RNA viruses. These antigens may be broadly categorized as either viral, cellular, or soluble (Aoki, 1973) (Table 1). Based on the morphological structure of viruses, which consists of an inner nucleoid and an outer shell surrounded by an envelope acquired during budding of the virus from the surface of infected cells (deHarven, 1968), viral antigens can additionally be divided into viral envelope antigens (VEAs) and intraviral antigens. Cell surface antigens (CSAs) induced by viruses and by malignant transformation (mutation of the cellular genome) possess several type specificities (Klein, 1969; Old and Boyse, 1965). To date, while viral antigens have been found intracellularly, no viral-genome-induced cellular antigens have been demonstrated there. Several groups of soluble antigens corresponding to the above specificities have been detected in the circulation and in the kidneys of virus-infected animals (see below).

This chapter will cover the specificities and characteristics of RNA oncogenic virus-associated antigens from the biological, virological, and biochemical points of view, as well as the host immune response to these antigens. The focus of attention will be on mammalian systems, especially the mouse, with occasional

TADAO AOKI AND LOUIS R. SIBAL • Viral Oncology Area, Division of Cancer Cause and Prevention, National Cancer Institute, NIH, Bethesda, Maryland.

TABLE 1
Classification of RNA Oncogenic Virus Associated Antigens

Viral:	a. Envelope antigens (VEAs)[a]
	i. Group-specific VEA
	ii. Subgroup-specific VEAs
	iii. Type-specific VEAs
	iv. Subtype-specific VEAs
	b. Intraviral antigens
	i. gs-1,2,3,4,5 (type C virus)
	ii. S-1,2,3,4,5 (type B virus)
	iii. Reverse transcriptases
Cellular:	a. Cell surface
	i. Several classes identified by serological techniques
	ii. Tumor-associated transplantation antigens (TATAs)
	iii. VEAs (type C virus)
	b. Intracellular—intraviral antigens
Soluble:	a. In circulation—several classes of VEA and cell surface antigens
	b. In kidney—most antigens described above

[a] See Table 2.

reference to the avian system. Because of the ready availability of inbred, recombinant inbred, and congenic strains, studies essential for the definition of antigenic specificities have been possible in the mouse (Snell and Stimpfling, 1966).

2. Virion Antigens

Studies of virion antigens have long focused on well-known murine leukemia viruses (MuLVs) [Gross (G), Graffi, (Gi), Friend (F), Moloney (M), and Rauscher (R)] as representatives of type C viruses and on murine mammary tumor virus (MuMTV) as the only established type B virus (Old and Boyse, 1965). Presently, many as yet uncharacterized endogenous type C viruses are being detected and/or isolated from various transformed as well as nontransformed cells (Todaro, 1972; Lowry *et al.*, 1971; Aaronson *et al.*, 1971b). In both cases, questions of oncogenicity, vertical and/or horizontal transmission, existence of single or multiple viral genes, and relationship between environmental factors and phenotypic expression of these and other viruses remain to be answered.

2.1. Viral Envelope Antigens

2.1.1. Biological Specificities

The unexpected diversity of VEAs in type C virus populations was revealed by immunoelectron microscopy, neutralization tests, and radioimmunoassay (Aoki *et al.*, 1974a; Strand and August, 1974; Eckner and Steeves, 1972; Levy *et al.*, 1969; Geering *et al.*, 1966). Depending on the use of sera from nonimmunized and immunized hosts of different species, four major specificities of VEAs were demonstrated on type C viruses (Aoki, 1974) (Table 2): (1) group-specific VEA (gsVEA) broadly reactive with the sera of selected aged autoimmune NZB mice, includes VEA of type C viruses released from other species; (2) subgroup-specific VEAs (sub-gsVEAs) shared by several virus populations, demonstrable with xenogeneic antisera, also includes VEAs of type C viruses from other species; (3) type-specific VEAs (tsVEAs) detectable specifically on individual virus populations by mouse hyperimmune sera; and (4) subtype-specific VEAs (sub-tsVEAs) consisting of at least two tsVEAs in mixed form on individual viruses of some populations, demonstrable by different mouse hyperimmune sera. A new classification of type C viruses has been made possible by use of these antigenic specificities as markers. This method of categorization may likewise be applied to type B virus.

An important question which needs to be studied pertains to the release of endogenous type C viruses. In particular, different virus populations, in terms of host ranges and VEAs, predominate from time to time during *in vitro* passages of cultured nonmalignant as well as malignant cells and during *in vivo* transplantation of tumors (paper in preparation). Depending on the population(s) of endogenous type C viruses, cells sometimes acquire new cell surface antigens, such as MEV-SA1 (mouse endogenous virus–surface antigen 1: Herberman *et al.*, 1974). This phenomenon may be explained by the following possibilities: (1) alteration or mutation of original endogenous type C viruses, (2) hybridization between different classes of endogenous viruses, and (3) replacement of original type C viruses with other classes of viruses or selection of some special endogenous viruses. Among these hypotheses, replacement or selection seems most likely; that is, individual cells may possess several different genes, each of which produces a respective class of endogenous type C virus as a phenotypic expression. The phenotypic expression of certain types of virus may prevent the simultaneous phenotypic expression of other types of endogenous viruses. When circumstances

161

RNA
ONCOGENIC
VIRUS-
ASSOCIATED
ANTIGENS

TABLE 2
Classification of Type C Virus Envelope Antigens (VEAs)

Designation of VEA	Serum or antiserum used for detection	Description
gsVEA	Serum from selected autoimmune aged NZB mice	A common VEA among most, if not all, type C viruses
sub-gsVEAs	Rat or rabbit anti-MuLV sera[a]	VEAs common to some groups of type C viruses
tsVEAs	Mouse anti-MuLV sera	Specific VEAs of individual type C viruses
sub-tsVEAs[b]	Mouse anti-MuLV sera	Further individually specified tsVEAs

[a] These antisera also recognize some tsVEAs.
[b] One mouse-typing serum reacts occasionally with VEAs of several different type C viruses. In addition, one virus also reacts sometimes with at least two different mouse typing sera.

induce the phenotypic expression of the second type of virus, expression of the first disappears (replacement). If an extremely small number of certain endogenous viruses exist among the predominant virus populations, under special circumstances those few viruses may become the predominant population which suppresses the previously predominant viruses (selection). However, it is difficult to distinguish experimentally between these two possibilities.

2.1.2. Chemically and Physically Purified Viral Envelope Antigens

Polyacrylamide gel electrophoresis of disrupted, purified virions has resolved many molecules ranging from less than 10,000 to more than 100,000 daltons, of which only five to seven are considered major components. These antigenic specificities have been clarified to some extent. A uniform nomenclature for the components of RNA oncogenic virus used in this chapter seems to have been generally accepted by most investigators (August *et al.*, 1974). This designation is based on expressing molecular weight in thousands, e.g., the 30,000 dalton protein of MuLV is referred to as MuLV p30 and the 69,000 dalton glycoprotein as MuLV gp69 (Table 3).

Two glycoproteins, gp69 and gp71, appear to be VEAs and to contain multiple antigenic determinants ranging from tsVEA to gsVEA (Strand and August, 1973, 1974; Nowinski *et al.*, 1972). These glycoproteins are difficult to separate by high-resolution chromatography and their biochemical differences have not yet been fully defined. They seem, however, to be antigenically quite similar, if not identical, since antisera against gp69 and gp71 prepared in rabbits showed strong and similar capacities to neutralize a variety of MuLVs and other type C viruses.

A similar VEA of type B virus has been found to be gp52 (S-1), which can be purified from MuMTV in the milk of all mouse strains with a high incidence of spontaneous mammary tumor (Parks *et al.*, 1974; Teramoto *et al.*, 1974). This glycoprotein is also associated with mouse mammary adenocarcinomas and is antigenically common to all MuMTVs and mammary tumors tested. Recent

TABLE 3
Major Virion Polypeptides Purified by Polyacrylamide Gel Electrophoresis

Mammalian		Avian
Type C virus (R-MuLV)[a]	Type B virus (MuMTV)[a]	Type C virus (AMV)[a]
gp69～71[b]	gp52	gp85
	gp36	gp35
p30	p27(28)	p27
		p19
p15	p14	p15
p12		p12
p10	p10	p10

[a] R-MuLV, Rauscher murine leukemia virus: MuMTV, murine mammary tumor virus; AMV, avian myeloblastoma virus.
[b] gp69, glycoprotein 69,000 daltons; p30, protein 30,000 daltons.

investigations indicate the presence of gp52 on the viral envelope. This new   163
observation is contrary to the previous finding that S-1 exists inside the virion   RNA
(Nowinski *et al.*, 1971). Therefore, gp52 seems to be gsVEA but, as noted before,   ONCOGENIC
the species for immunization should be selected with care so that the specificity of   VIRUS-
the VEA detected can be determined. Although the location of gp52 needs to be   ASSOCIATED
clarified by further studies, its specificity has been found to differ considerably   ANTIGENS
from that of the major polypeptides on the envelope of type C viruses.

2.2. Intraviral Antigens

2.2.1. Biological Specificities

Historically, five intraviral components of type C virus were demonstrated by
Ouchterlony gel immunodiffusion and the specificity of two major antigens, gs1
and gs3, was well defined (Geering *et al.*, 1966, 1970; Gregoriades and Old, 1969).
These were later shown to coexist on a single molecule (Gilden and Oroszlan,
1972; Parks and Scolnick, 1972). One reason for distinguishing between these
antigenic determinants is that gs1 antibody belongs to IgG class and gs3 antibody
to IgM class, resulting in a difference in mobility of the antibodies. While gs1 is
specific for all isolates of type C viruses including endogenous viruses from a given
species, making it possible to determine the species of origin of the virus, the
specificity of gs3 is shared by type C viruses derived from many different species
such as the mouse, rat, hamster, cat, woolly monkey, gibbon, and baboon (Gilden
et al., 1974). Thus gs1 and gs3 are also designated as intraspecies and interspecies
antigens, respectively (Schäfer *et al.*, 1970). When a new type C virus is detected in
a species which has hitherto not been found to produce the virus, it is helpful for
its characterization to examine whether the virus contains gs1 cross-reacting with
known type C virus or only with gs3. The latter case suggests the possibility that a
new type C virus exists in this species.

Specific RNA-directed DNA polymerases (reverse transcriptase) have been
detected in various classes of RNA type C and type B viruses (Green and Gerard,
1974). Humoral antibody to reverse transcriptase was found by its inhibiting effect
on enzyme activity in the serum of rats with MuLV-releasing tumors (Aaronson *et
al.*, 1971*a*). Since antiserum against the reverse transcriptase of some MuLVs
showed a cross-reaction with other groups of MuLVs, it seems most likely that the
reverse transcriptases of several mammalian type C viruses are antigenically
related (Table 4). In fact, although reverse transcriptase is a universal component
of RNA oncogenic viruses, there are distinct classes of reverse transcriptases: (1)
antibodies to the avian enzyme do not inhibit the enzyme activities of other type C
or type B viruses; (2) antibodies to mammalian type C reverse transcriptases do
not inhibit the enzyme activity of type B viruses; and (3) antibodies to the baboon
type C and RD-114 virus reverse transcriptases do not inhibit that of MuLV or
woolly monkey sarcoma SSV-1. Antisera to reverse transcriptases have been
prepared by immunizing rabbits with partially purified reverse transcriptases.
Naturally occurring antibodies to MuLV reverse transcriptases have been

TABLE 4
Antigenic Relatedness of RNA Virus Reverse Transcriptase (RT)

Reverse transcriptase inactivated by antiserum[a]			
Anti-MuLV[b] RT	Anti-RD-114 virus[b] RT	Anti-avian virus[b] RT	Anti-MuMTV[b] RT
RT of MuLV	RT of RD-114 virus	RT of Schmidt–Ruppin strain Rous sarcoma virus[c]	RT of MuMTV
Rat leukemia virus	Baboon type C virus M7	Bryan strain Rous sarcoma virus	
Hamster leukemia virus		Rous-associated leukosis viruses RAV-1 and RAV-2	
Feline leukemia virus[c]			
Simian sarcoma virus SSV-1[c] (woolly monkey virus)		Avian myeloblastosis virus	
Gibbon type C virus			

[a] The RTs of a relatively large group of viruses—viper, Visna, Mason–Pfizer monkey, and simian "foamy" viruses—were not inhibited by antibodies to the RTs of MuLV and avian leukosis virus.
[b] MuLV, murine leukemia virus; RD-114 virus, feline endogenous viruses acquired by human rhabdomyosarcoma 114 cell line during transplantation in fetal cats; MuMTV, murine mammary tumor virus.
[c] Reciprocal cross-reactivity with anti-MuLV demonstrated.

detected as antigen–antibody complexes in the kidney of virus-infected hosts. When homologous antisera to the MuLV reverse transcriptase were used, rat, hamster, cat, woolly monkey, and gibbon reverse transcriptases were only partially inactivated (Parks *et al.*, 1972). These findings suggest antigenic relatedness but not identity among the viral reverse transcriptases of these species. Therefore, it may be stated that reverse transcriptases contain both intraspecies (group) specific and interspecies determinants.

2.2.2. Physical-Chemical Properties

A major intraviral polypeptide of approximately 30,000 daltons, (range 27,000–33,000), referred to as p30, accounts for almost 30% of the virion mass (Oroszlan *et al.*, 1970). The p30 was defined as having gs1 and gs3, which reside on a single molecule as mentioned before. In addition, this protein possesses type-specific antigenic determinants (Strand and August, 1974; Stephenson *et al.*, 1974); competition radioimmunoassays in combination with different murine type C viruses, anti-R-MuLV serum, and labeled R-MuLV p30 demonstrated different antigenic activities in the order of R-MuLV > M-MuLV > F-MuLV > G-MuLV (Strand and August, 1974). In another study using a similar assay, the reactivities of the p30 polypeptides of three MuLV strains were readily distinguishable on the basis of the different slopes of the inhibition curves (Stephenson *et al.*, 1974). The p30 reactivities of two endogenous isolates from BALB/c embryo cells were indistinguishable from AKR-MuLV but were unlike R- or M-MuLV. In both studies, however, the significance of the results remains to some extent questionable, because standard stock viruses were not derived from single clones.

Although the p30 possesses gs1, there are some exceptions, as is the case with RD-114 virus, which arose in the human rhabdomyosarcoma cell line RD-114 after passage through a fetal cat. From hybridization data, however, RD-114 virus has been determined to be of feline origin (Okabe *et al.*, 1973). The p30 molecule does not share reactivity with this FeLV (feline leukemia virus) p30, but does show considerable immunological activity to other endogenous feline type C isolates and to baboon M7 and other endogenous type C viruses (Sherr *et al.*, 1974). Another exception is the recent finding that while group-specific antisera to lower mammalian type C viruses are nonreactive to woolly monkey and gibbon p30, essentially complete cross-reactivity occurs between woolly monkey and gibbon proteins. Thus group-specific (intraspecies) intraviral antigenic determinants can generally be taken to indicate the species of origin, but failure to detect them is not decisive, and the combined utilization of virological, biochemical, and immunological data is usually needed for the identification of new virus isolates.

The p30 also carries common intraspecies reactivities of type C viruses (Gilden and Oroszlan, 1972; Parks and Scolnick, 1972). To date, all mammalian type C viruses contain this protein. This does not imply that each p30 molecule contains a fixed number of identical antigenic determinants, but rather a spectrum of determinants which are common to mammalian type C viruses. In addition, it is worth noting that the p30 of the M7 baboon virus cross-reacts strongly with p30 of the RD-114 virus, suggesting a close relationship but little or no cross-reactivity with woolly monkey sarcoma virus SSV-1 or gibbon viruses isolated from other nonhuman primates. These findings indicate the need for the careful selection of reagents for the detection of viral expression in cells of other primates, including man. Other viruses tested in this system—avian type C, murine type B, Mason–Pfizer monkey, and feline and primate syncytium-forming viruses—had no detectable interspecies reactivity; hence the observations described above appear to be entirely limited to *mammalian type C viruses*. Furthermore, the p27 of MuMTV is antigenically unrelated to the p30 of mammalian type C viruses. Its usefulness as a probe should be clarified by further studies.

Another purified component of type C viruses is p12, which is antigenically distinct from other biochemically defined viral proteins and possesses only type-specific determinants (Tronick *et al.*, 1973, 1974). The high degree of its type specificity is attested to by the fact that differences in antigenic reactivities among type C virus strains, including murine endogenous, woolly monkey, and gibbon type C viruses, can be readily distinguished by radioimmunoassay. The significance of these observations is heightened by the fact that p12 (as well as p30) is fully translated in cells in the absence of detectable virus release and can be concentrated to levels that are measurable by radioimmunoassay (Stephenson *et al.*, 1974). Consequently, this antigenic marker may be extremely useful in identifying closely related type C viruses.

Reverse transcriptases have been solubilized and partially purified from RNA tumor viruses of several animal species. Because of the limited amounts available of some of these viruses and the fact that the enzyme represents only approximately 0.1% of the viral protein moiety, rigorous antigenic characterization of reverse transcriptases has not yet been possible (Green and Gerard, 1974). It appears, however, that the enzymes of type C viruses of mammalian origin have a single subunit of approximately 70,000 daltons, whereas those of type B and Mason–Pfizer monkey viruses are larger, approximately 110,000 daltons. A reverse transcriptase has been isolated from the peripheral blood leukocytes of a patient with acute myelogenous leukemia. This enzyme has a molecular weight of 70,000 daltons and is strongly inhibited by antisera to woolly monkey sarcoma virus SSV-1 and gibbon type C viruses (Gallagher et al., 1974). Although these studies require confirmation, the authors suggest the presence of a common viral protein in this human disease.

3. Virus-Induced Antigens

Virus-induced antigens have been studied extensively in murine leukemias, especially in G, Gi, F, M, and R systems, and in sarcoma systems, by serological and transplantation methods (see below). The analysis of type B virus induced cell surface antigens has been limited to transplantation studies because of the difficulty of preparing suitable cell suspensions from the solid mammary tumor. Although many endogenous type C viruses are being found, the study of virus-induced cellular antigens is still in its initial stages. This section will review mainly the murine leukemia system, particularly the G antigen system.

3.1. Cell Surface Antigens

3.1.1. Biological Specificities

Cell surface antigens were first demonstrated by the rejection of transplanted MuLV-induced tumors. During rejection, the host produced specific antibody which was cytotoxic to the tumor cells in the presence of complement. Rigorous serological studies have demonstrated that leukemias induced by the same strains of MuLV share common antigens while leukemias induced by other strains of MuLV possess antigens with different specificities (Old and Boyse, 1965). These phenomena were also observed in different animal species. This finding is in major contrast to the situation with chemical-carcinogen-induced tumors, in which individual antigen specificities are found (Old et al., 1962). Both shared and individual antigenicities were found in mammary tumors (Dezfulian et al., 1968; Vaage, 1968a,b; Silobreic and Suit, 1967; Suit and Silobreic, 1967; Morton et al., 1965).

In the G leukemia system, G cell surface antigens (GCSAs) demonstrated to date are GCSAa, b, c (Aoki et al., 1972; Herberman, 1972; Geering et al., 1966; Old et

167
RNA
ONCOGENIC
VIRUS-
ASSOCIATED
ANTIGENS

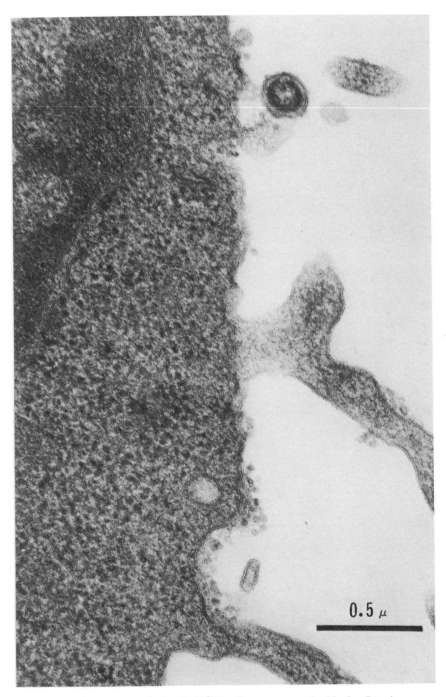

FIGURE 1. C57BL/6 Gross leukemia E♂G2 cells were reacted with the G-typing *mouse* serum; only sectors of the cell surface are labeled with southern bean mosaic virus.

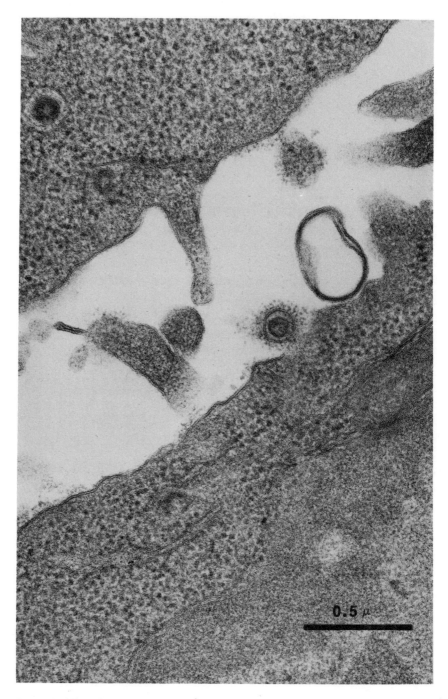

FIGURE 2. C57BL/6 Gross leukemia E♂G2 cells were reacted with the G-typing *rat* serum; the entire viral envelope and sectors of the cell surface are labeled with ferritin.

al., 1965), G_L, G_T (Nowinski and Peters, 1973), and G_{IX} (Stockert et al., 1971). As observed in other tumor systems, different species can recognize different specific antigens in this system; the G-typing *mouse* serum contains antibodies only against GCSAa, c, but the G-typing *rat* serum contains, in addition, antibodies against GCSAb, G_L, G_T, and G_{IX} (Aoki et al., 1972). Among them, G_{IX} is a normal T-cell antigen of certain mouse strains, inherited in Mendelian fashion, but may be induced by G-MuLV in cells of any genotype and in cells of phenotypes other than the T-cell (Ikeda et al., 1973). Immunoelectron microscopy demonstrated that the G-typing *rat* serum reacts with both the viral envelope and the cell surface, whereas the G-typing *mouse* serum reacts only with the cell surface and not with the viral envelope (Aoki, 1971, 1973; Aoki et al., 1970) (Figs. 1 and 2). Moreover, it is well known that G-MuLV is broadly transmitted horizontally as well as vertically to most, if not all, strains of mice and rats (Aoki et al., 1968c; Boyse et al., 1967). Therefore, it is reasonable to detect some G antigens on the surface of Gi, F, M, and R leukemia cells (Levy et al., 1969; Old et al., 1964). F leukemia cells have been shown to possess three classes of CSAs (Ting and Herberman, 1974; Ting et al., 1974): (1) fetal antigen common among F, M, and R leukemias; (2) a CSA common between F and M, and another CSA common between F and R; and (3) F-specific CSA. It has become evident that a common antigen among F, M, and R leukemias previously reported (Old and Boyse, 1965; Old et al., 1964) is a fetal antigen or a combination of common antigens between F and M, and between F and R.

In addition to MuLV-associated CSAs, there are other type C virus-induced CSAs, namely, MSV-induced CSAs. Surprisingly, although MSV has obtained its viral envelope from MuLV and/or endogenous type C viruses, *in vitro* MSV-transformed and subcloned mouse and rat nonproducer cells induce a small amount of common specific CSAs different from MuLV and its induced antigens (Aoki et al., 1973a). No difference is demonstrated in the specificity of Kirsten (Ki)- and M-MSV-induced nonproducer CSAs. It has also been shown that a species other than mouse, the rabbit, is able to recognize at least two MSV-induced CSAs differing from those of mouse and rat nonproducer cells (Aoki et al., 1974c). Furthermore, woolly monkey sarcoma virus SSV-1-transformed mouse and rat nonproducer cells have been found to carry two more CSAs. The latter four different antigen classes are designated sarcoma cell surface antigens SCSAa, b, c, d (Table 5). SCSAa is uniquely conferred by SSV-1, SCSAb is shared with MSV- and SSV-1-transformed rat nonproducer cells, SCSAc is common to MSV-transformed mouse nonproducer cells and SSV-1-transformed rat nonproducer cells, and SCSAd is broadly reactive with the rabbit antiserum against these three nonproducer cell lines.

Besides virus-induced antigens, an antigen common to VEA is present on the cell surface. In the NZB lymphoma system, type C virus producer and non-producer cell lines carry a common glycoprotein on cell surfaces (Kennel et al., 1973). This glycoprotein stimulates the host to produce neutralizing antibody against this type C virus. Additionally, some gs⁺ and cellular helper factor positive avian embryo fibroblasts (nonmalignant) possess an antigen common to VEA of Bryan strain Rous sarcoma virus (B-RSV) on the cell surface (Hanafusa et al.,

TABLE 5

Summary Data of Antigenic Specificities Detected on the Surface of Kirsten Murine Sarcoma Virus (Ki-MSV) and Woolly Monkey Sarcoma Virus (WSV) Transformed Cells

Antigenic specifi-city	Detected on cell surfaces of			Interpretation
	Ki-MSV-transformed BALB/3T3 cell line K-BALB	Ki-MSV-transformed normal rat kidney fibroblast line K-NRK	WSV-trans-formed normal rat kidney fibroblast line W-NRK	
SCSA[a]a	−	−	+	WSV-induced CSA[b] in W-NRK
SCSAb	−	+	+	A common Ki-MSV- and WSV-induced specific CSA in K- and W-NRK
SCSAc	+	−	+	A common Ki-MSV- and WSV-induced specific CSA in K-BALB and W-NRK
SCSAd	+	+	+	A common specific CSA induced by Ki-MSV and WSV in K-BALB, K-NRK and W-NRK

[a] SCSA, sarcoma cell surface antigen.
[b] CSA, cell surface antigen.

1973; Aoki, 1975). This antigen can absorb antibody to VEA of B-RSV from chick anti-B-RSV serum, as detected by immunoelectron microscopy and neutralization tests. These findings may open a way to detect defective human oncogenic type C virus, if it exists in this form.

It is of great interest that during long-term cell culture or long-term transplantation of malignant cells, cell surface antigens apparently associated with endogenous type C viruses and/or their viral genome, as well as VEAs, frequently convert from one specificity to another as described above, and are accompanied by changes in CSAs (paper in preparation). Although many genes seem to be involved in the appearance of various endogenous type C viruses, it remains unclear which of the endogenous viruses are responsible for the conversion of cell surface antigens.

3.1.2. Physical-Chemical Properties

What little is known biochemically about RNA oncogenic virus induced cell surface antigens in the G, F, M, and R leukemia systems contrasts with the more solid information on VEAs. Solubilized G-MuLV-associated surface antigens, following papain digestion and precipitation with ammonium sulfate, were fractionated by chromatography into two peaks of 60,000 and 45,000 daltons on Sephadex G150, sucrose density 1.05 g/ml (Herberman *et al.*, 1973). The antigens were labile, being inactivated by two cycles of freeze-thawing or storage at 4°C for

1 wk. Similar results were obtained with F-, M-, and R-MuLV-associated surface
antigens (Lilly and Nathanson, 1969). The relationship between solubilized
virus-induced surface antigens and circulating free soluble antigens (see below)
has not been established.

A solubilized CSA common to VEA in the NZB lymphoma system was found to
be a glycoprotein with a molecular weight of 70,000 daltons (gp70) (Kennel *et al.*,
1973). This finding is consistent with the presence of VEAs gp69 and gp71 of
MuLV, and provides a better marker for detecting VEAs on nonmalignant as well
as malignant nonproducer cells infected with type C viruses. If indeed certain
human tumors might be induced by type C viruses, the tumor cells could be
nonproducers, because no mature type C viruses have been detected to date.
Pending the detection of mature viruses, CSAs common to VEAs would be very
important markers for the detection of possible human oncogenic type C viruses.

3.1.3. Antigenic Modulation

The phenomenon of antigenic modulation is a special case of progressive tumor
growth. When tumor-specific antigen-positive malignant cells are transplanted
into syngeneic hosts preimmunized with the antigen, host resistance to the tumor
cells is lacking or is extremely weak. As long as the specific antibody is present, the
phenotype of the tumor cells is changed from antigen positive to antigen negative.
When the tumor cells are transplanted back into untreated hosts, the antigen
again become phenotypic. The phenomenon was originally observed *in vitro* as
well as *in vivo* in the murine TL (thymus–leukemia) antigen system (Boyse and
Old, 1969); although the responsible oncogenic viruses have not yet been
discovered, their existence is inferred. Incomplete antigenic modulation also has
been observed in some GCSAa, c of G-MuLV-induced C57BL/6 leukemia (Aoki
and Johnson, 1972) and in fetal antigen of R- and F-MuLV-induced C57BL/6
leukemias (Ortaldo *et al.*, 1974). The MuLV-induced leukemia showed only
incomplete antigenic modulation in animals; the original amount of antigen
diminished markedly but was not entirely abolished. This phenomenon may
occur in other virus-induced tumors, such as MSV-induced sarcoma (Greenberger *et al.*, 1974). Indeed, antigenic modulation could be more general than
initially expected. Further investigation of this problem may provide a means to
analyze the relationship among genes, phenotypic expression of antigen, virus
infection, and tumor growth.

3.2. Intracellular Antigens

It is well known that intraviral antigens including virus-specific reverse transcriptases can be detected intracellularly, sometimes in both cytoplasmic and nuclear
areas (Stephenson *et al.*, 1974; Hilgers *et al.*, 1972). In particular, type B virus
exists in the cytoplasmic area as naked type A particles, which are occasionally
detected in tumors such as Leydig's tumor as an inclusion body under the light
microscope or as a crystal under the electron microscope (Pourrean-Schneider *et*

171
RNA
ONCOGENIC
VIRUS-
ASSOCIATED
ANTIGENS

al., 1968). Consequently, such tumor cells may provide a better source of type B intraviral components than the milk of MuMTV-positive mice, because type B components are often heavily contaminated with type C viruses in the milk (Nowinski *et al.*, 1968).

The presence of gs3 has also been revealed on the surface of type C virus induced and/or associated malignant cells by immunofluorescence and immunoelectron microscopy (Yoshiki *et al.*, 1964, 1973).

3.3. Soluble Antigens

Soluble antigens associated with RNA oncogenic viruses have been demonstrated in the circulation in free form and in the kidney as antigen–antibody complexes. Free soluble antigens were first detected in the plasma of mice infected with F-, M-, and R-MuLV (Stück *et al.*, 1964a), but have not been studied as extensively as the G soluble antigen (GSA) system (Aoki *et al.*, 1968a,b, 1972), which will be taken as the model system in this chapter and described in detail.

3.3.1. Biological Specificities

Based on the knowledge of the diverse classes of G surface antigens, GSAs in the circulation corresponding to GCSAa, b, c, tsVEA, and gsVEA have been demonstrated by inhibition studies using indirect immunofluorescence and immunoelectron microscopy (Aoki *et al.*, 1972). While GSAs corresponding to G_{IX}, G_L, G_T, and intraviral antigens have not yet been detected in the circulation, GCSAs, VEAs, and most known intraviral antigens have been found as antigen–antibody complexes in the kidney (Hollis *et al.*, 1974; Oldstone *et al.*, 1972a; Mellors *et al.*, 1971).

What is the origin of soluble antigens? They may be released into the body fluids (1) during turnover of the cell membrane, including virus budding, and (2) from destroyed cells and virions. However, when GSAs adsorbed on G^- indicator cells were examined by immunoelectron microscopy, neither cellular nor viral fragments were detectable in the labeled areas. This finding suggests that GSAs may be molecules carrying antigenic sites. The situation observed *in vitro* may also occur *in vivo*; that is, after release, soluble antigens may be adsorbed onto the surface of cells and viruses. This is a kind of antigenic conversion in which originally MuLV-associated antigen-negative cells become positive by the adsorption of soluble antigens onto the cell surface (Stück *et al.*, 1964b). In animals, the source of soluble antigens may be nontransformed MuLV-infected cells as well as foci of malignantly transformed cells.

The detection and/or isolation of soluble antigens can aid significantly in (1) the early diagnosis of a given virus infection, (2) the understanding of the relationship among oncogenic viruses, tumors, and hosts, (3) the analysis of genetic influences on virus infection or virus production, and (4) the evaluation of potential methods of therapy, especially immunotherapy.

3.3.2. Physical-Chemical Properties

173

RNA
ONCOGENIC
VIRUS-
ASSOCIATED
ANTIGENS

Although MuLV passes the 200-nm but not the 50-nm Millipore filter, GSAs are filtrable through 50- and 10-nm Millipore filters (Aoki *et al.*, 1968*a*). They are not sedimented by centrifugation of infective plasma at 100,000*g* for 2 h. At this time, the supernatant fluid is free of G-MuLV, as shown by the absence of leukemogenic activity. Most GSAs, however, are sedimentable by centrifugation at 100,000*g* for 18 h. In addition, they have sedimentation coefficients of 6.4 S on sucrose rate zonal centrifugation (unpublished observations). The stability of GSAs is similar to that of solubilized GCSAs; three cycles of freeze-thawing, storage at 4°C for 4–6 days, or heating at 56°C for 30 min inactivates the antigenicity (Herberman *et al.*, 1973; Aoki *et al.*, 1968*a*). Soluble antigens associated with MuMTV have been found to have similar properties (Plata *et al.*, 1973).

4. Host Immune Response

After oncogenic virus infection and activation or the initiation of tumor growth, hosts respond immunologically to tumor- and/or virus-associated antigens, regardless of whether the tumor progresses or regresses. Several pathways of host immune response will be reviewed briefly.

4.1. Protection

When on occasion a tumor patient goes into spontaneous remission without having undergone medical treatment, it is assumed that his condition has been brought about by an appropriate immune response (Southam, 1960). Such host resistance has been studied in experimental animal systems using transplanted instead of spontaneous and/or primary tumors because of convenience and availability (Klein, 1968); although studies with spontaneous tumors might more nearly approximate the human situation, experimental findings to date have been scant.

Investigations of the host immune response to transplanted tumors have proven more promising, especially in the areas of tumor-associated transplantation antigen(s) (TATA)[1] and cell-mediated immunity. When surface antigens derived from tumors are used to transfer adoptive immunity with sensitized lymphocytes and to carry out active immunization, the antigens must be rendered safe from the biohazard standpoint without loss of antigenic activity. Optimum conditions for fixation and stabilization of virus-induced tumor cells by formalin have been found (Kudo *et al.*, 1974); these conditions obviate the oncogenic potential of the cells while retaining antigenicity. Formalin-fixation of antigens

---

[1] The term "tumor-associated transplantation antigen" (TATA) denotes two or more restrictive antigens: (1) tumor-specific transplantation antigen (TSTA) formed by malignant transformation and (2) virus-induced specific transplantation antigen (VSTA) acquired by virus infection.

may become useful in immunotherapy as well as in the diagnosis of tumor patients.

Whenever passive immunization with humoral antibody shows effective results, it has been assumed that humoral antibody has stimulated immunologically competent cells which play a primary role in tumor rejection (Ortez de Landazuri *et al.*, 1974). And since wild-type G-MuLV-induced spontaneous leukemia cells of AKR mice were recently found to be destroyed by transfusion of the fifth component of complement (Kassel *et al.*, 1973), humoral antibody also should be considered as an essential factor in tumor regression. Moreover, the formation of natural antibody to various classes of RNA oncogenic virus-associated antigens is a special host immune response in cases of virus-induced tumor-bearing hosts. Such instances include the G natural antibody production in some mouse strains resistant to G-MuLV (Aoki *et al.*, 1966) and the formation of natural antibody to gsVEA in NZB mice (Aoki *et al.*, 1970) and apparently to tsVEA or sub-gsVEA in other strains of mice (Aaronson and Stephenson, 1974; Batzing *et al.*, 1974). This natural antibody formation is to a certain extent effective in the protection against tumor induction by viruses. In contrast, the production of natural antibody to chemical-carcinogen-induced tumor antigens is rare, if it exists.

4.2. Escapes

Although hosts may respond to antigens associated with virus-induced tumors and produce weak but specific antibodies, the tumors usually grow too fast to regress by host immunity. In this case, antigen and antibody coexist, possibly as antigen–antibody complexes which may constitute one type of serum blocking factor (Baldwin *et al.*, 1974; Sjögren *et al.*, 1971; Hellström *et al.*, 1971). Both the virus infection and the growth of virus-induced tumors suppress the general host immune response, resulting in the acceleration of tumor growth (Wedderburn and Salaman, 1968; Salaman and Wedderburn, 1966; Southam, 1960). Furthermore, phenomena like antigenic modulation and immune suppression are difficult to distinguish from each other in detail, because they may appear simultaneously.

The classic concept of immunological tolerance holds that as a result of the exposure to a large amount of given antigens in embryonic or neonatal stages a host is rendered incapable of producing humoral antibodies against these antigens in the course of his lifetime (Billingham *et al.*, 1956). Immunological tolerance has long been considered to play a role in the growth of RNA oncogenic virus induced tumors. It has been revealed, however, that MuLV-associated antigen–antibody complexes are trapped by glomeruli of the neonatally MuLV-infected mouse kidney while free antibodies are not detectable in the circulation (Hollis *et al.*, 1974; Oldstone *et al.*, 1972a; Mellors *et al.*,1971). Specific neutralizing antibody was isolated from kidney eluates of neonatally M-MuLV-infected BALB/c mice, and several classes of specific antibodies to cell surface as well as intraviral G antigens (including MuLV-specific reverse transcriptase) were found

175

RNA
ONCOGENIC
VIRUS-
ASSOCIATED
ANTIGENS

to exist in the kidney of AKR mice as complexes with antigens, as demonstrated by complement fixation tests, immunofluorescence microscopy, immunoelectron microscopy, and enzymatic assays.

A possible interpretation of these findings is that the excess amount of antigens in the circulation reacts immediately with humoral antibodies produced in extremely small amounts by neonatally infected mice to make antigen–antibody complexes, which are of an appropriate molecular size to be trapped by kidney glomeruli. Consequently, although no antibodies seem to be produced in these mice, they are capable of making a small amount, indicating the lack of the "complete" immunological tolerance described by many investigators. We feel that this concept should be modified to indicate "incomplete" immunological tolerance.

Is a type of incomplete immunological tolerance analogous to that found in humoral antibody formation also present in cell-mediated immunity? When C57BL/6 mice were neonatally infected with M-MuLV, after immunological maturation their spleen cells did not show positive ^{51}Cr-releasing lymphocyte-mediated cytotoxicity against syngeneic M-leukemia cells, although specific humoral antibodies to M-MuLV-associated antigens were detectable as immune complexes in the kidney eluates of these mice (Chieco-Bianchi *et al.*, 1974). In this case, it was found that a state of thymus-derived (T)-cell unresponsiveness occurred in neonatally infected mice. Since only spleen lymphocytes were examined, however, it is possible that active lymphocytes from other organs may be detectable. Nevertheless, partial tolerance to M-MuLV-associated antigens also did occur in this system.

5. Comments

Based on the present discussion of antigens associated with RNA oncogenic viruses, we wish to discuss some related problems and hypotheses.

5.1. Detection of Virus Expression

Mammalian RNA tumor viruses contain major structural proteins and induce a series of cell surface and soluble antigens. Many of these have already been sufficiently well characterized to serve as markers for tumor virus expression (Table 6). At present, the components of a number of mammalian tumor virus, of species ranging from the mouse to the higher primates, are readily detectable by immunological techniques and process broadly cross-reactive determinants (interspecies determinants); these are gsVEA, sub-gsVEA and gp69~71 on the cell surface, as well as, intracellularly, p30 (gs3) and reverse transcriptase. If a human oncogenic virus is found, it may or may not possess these antigens; nonetheless, the probability of contamination of human tumor cells with a known type C virus from other species can be ruled out if the intraspecies antigens of this virus show no cross-reaction with known intraspecies antigens.

TABLE 6
Application of Type C Virus Antigens to Detection of New Viruses

Purified antigen	Characteristics	Application
p12	Type specific; found in cells in absence of mature viruses	Useful for distinguishing closely related viruses; possibly intraviral component(s)
p30	Major intraviral component(s); *intra-* and *inter*species specific; found in cells without mature viruses	*Intraspecies*: Useful in identifying species *Interspecies*: Common among most mammalian species, useful probe for human virus activity
Reverse transcriptase	Minor intraviral component(s); *intra-* and *inter*species specific	*Intraspecies*: Useful in identifying species *Interspecies*: Useful probe for human virus activity with limitations
gp69-71	Major component(s) of viral envelope; group-, subgroup-, type-, subtype-specific; possibly found in absence of mature viruses	Group specific: May be useful probe for human virus activity; not fully evaluated (see Table 3)

Many considerations must be taken into account concerning the use of well-defined viral reagents in test systems. Virus and virus-induced antigens are considerably more complex than expected and may possess antigenic determinants which differ in concentration and affinity. Hence one can expect differences in the populations of antibodies produced against them, depending on the nature of host species and the mode of immunization. For example, antibodies to p30 produced in the goat are predominantly directed to interspecies determinants (gs3) of the molecule, where amino acid sequences are homologous among type C viruses from different species. On the other hand, antibodies produced in the guinea pig may be almost nonreactive to shared sequences reacting preferentially to group-specific (gs1) determinants where amino acid sequences are more variable in different species.

To date, the presence of human RNA oncogenic viruses has not been demonstrated in spite of the efforts of many investigators. However, results obtained from experimental studies strongly suggest the presence of these viruses in human tumors, and it would appear that the antigenic markers found in experimental systems could serve as probes for virus and virus expression in human tumors. Such markers should satisfy the following conditions: (1) be detectable by immunological techniques as a defined viral component, (2) be produced in the absence of detectable mature or budding viruses, and (3) have broad cross-reactivity between possibly human RNA oncogenic viruses and those of other species.

5.2. Host Immune Response

Utilization of the antigens mentioned above makes it possible to study several problems concerning the host immune response to these antigens. In the

177

RNA
ONCOGENIC
VIRUS-
ASSOCIATED
ANTIGENS

prophylaxis and immunotherapy of those human tumors which may have been caused by human RNA oncogenic viruses, the demonstration and characterization of such human viruses represent but one approach to the ultimate goal. The other is to consider the range of host immune responses which might be evoked by the viruses. Recent studies in animals suggest some mechanisms which may be paralleled in humans.

In some mouse strains with a high incidence of spontaneous leukemia such as AKR and C58, it has long been considered that "complete" immunological tolerance applies in the case of vertically transmitted RNA oncogenic viruses and their associated antigens (Gross, 1951). Some new work, on the other hand, has revealed that immunological tolerance to MuLV is "incomplete" in these mice (see above), an encouraging finding which points to the application of immunological methods in the prevention and cure of virus-induced tumors. For instance, in prophylaxis, both active and passive immunizations could be undertaken with gsVEA or sub-gsVEA, because of their broader antigenic spectrum. In contrast, when tsVEAs with their narrower antigenic range are being used for immunizations, multiple tsVEAs must be utilized to cover different classes of viruses. In these approaches, however, we have to consider two important problems: (1) Does reaction with tumor-specific antigens induced by malignant transformation occur? If we take advantage of incomplete immunological tolerance against antigens associated with oncogenic RNA viruses for the prevention and treatment of virus-induced tumors, the enhanced immune response to the antigens may also damage nonmalignant somatic cells infected with the viruses, because the somatic cells carry these antigens. Therefore, in virus-induced tumors, tumor-specific antigens should also be considered, and the method to prevent such a risk must be investigated. (2) Deposit of antigen–antibody complexes sometimes induces autoimmune diseases such as nephritis (Oldstone *et al.*, 1972*b*). We have to pay attention to this risk in cases of incomplete immunological tolerance.

In addition to active and passive immunizations, immunotherapy may be established by the transfer of adoptive immunity against CSAs as well as VEAs; the latter also induce cytolysis with antisera to VEAs in the presence of complement. There is a recent trend toward inducing the rejection of transplanted tumors by using sensitized lymphocytes. It is interesting, moreover, that the intravenous injection of the fifth component of complement alone into leukemic AKR mice destroys many of the leukemia cells (Kassel *et al.*, 1973). This finding seems to indicate (1) the importance of humoral antibody in the treatment of AKR spontaneous leukemias, because complement is not required in cell-mediated immunity, and (2) the retention of antibody activity by humoral antigen–antibody complexes in the circulation either because active antibody sites are incompletely saturated by soluble antigens or because antibodies bind antigens on the surface of malignant cells. Therefore, it would seem that the role of humoral antibody in the treatment of tumors cannot be ignored.

Antigenic modulation presents a problem which, unless it can be overcome or circumvented, would permit some tumors to escape from effective immunotherapy. Demonstration of antigenic modulation has been based on *in vitro* experiments (Old *et al.*, 1968), indicating a humoral immune response;

however, it is still questionable whether this modulation also occurs in cell-mediated immunity.

Ideal tumor treatment might combine immunotherapy with chemotherapy. For this, the chemotherapeutic reagent should have two effects, a direct effect on malignant cells and an indirect effect through the enhancement of host immune response, or at least no suppressive effects. Because of their immunosuppressive effects, conventional antitumor drugs do not satisfy these conditions. Therefore, new reagents are being sought to meet such needs. BCG is one of the candidates (Borsos and Rapp, 1973). In addition, a preparation of dried *Streptococcus hemolyticus* with a low virulence (Okamoto *et al.*, 1972) has been found to satisfy these conditions in experimental and clinical applications (Kurokawa *et al.*, 1972; Okamoto *et al.*, 1966). The cocci showed a direct antitumor effect and induced an increase in the production of natural antibodies (Aoki *et al.*, 1974*b*) both to GCSAs (Aoki *et al.*, 1966) and to a cell surface differentiation antigen PC1; the latter antigen seems most likely to be induced by xVEA$^+$ type C viruses (Aoki *et al.*, 1973*b*; Aoki and Todaro, 1973; Aoki and Takahashi, 1972; Herberman and Aoki, 1972). These new reagents indicate a direction which may become important for the immunotherapy of tumors.

In conclusion, while the results of experimental systems suggest useful immunological approaches to the prevention and treatment of possibly virus-induced human tumors, the demonstration of the existence of human RNA oncogenic viruses is a prime requirement. Because mature or budding viruses have yet to be detected in human tumors, it is considered likely that certain suppressive mechanisms affect the maturation of such oncogenic viruses. Progress in elucidating this problem lies as much in drawing fruitful analogies from model systems as in being aware of possible differences in the human system.

6. References

AARONSON, S. A., AND STEPHENSON, J. R., 1974, Widespread natural occurrence of high titers of neutralizing antibodies to a specific class of endogenous mouse type-C virus, *Proc. Natl. Acad. Sci. U.S.A.* **71**:1957.

AARONSON, S. A., PARKS, W. P., SCOLNICK, E. M., AND TODARO, G. J., 1971*a*, Antibody to the RNA-dependent DNA polymerase of mammalian C-type RNA tumor viruses, *Proc. Natl. Acad. Sci. U.S.A.* **68**:920.

AARONSON, S. A., TODARO, G. J., AND SCOLNICK, E. M., 1971*b*, Induction of murine C-type viruses from clonal lines of virus-free BALB/3T3 cells, *Science* **174**:157.

AOKI, T., 1971, Surface antigens of murine leukemia cells and murine leukemia viruses, *Transplant. Proc.* **3**:1195.

AOKI, T., 1973, An analysis of antigens on the surface of murine leukemia viruses and cells, in: Unifying Concepts of Leukemia (R. M. Dutcher and L. Chieco-Bianchi, eds.), *Bibl. Haematol. (Basel)* **39**:307.

AOKI, T., 1974, Murine type-C RNA viruses: A proposed reclassification, other possible pathogenicities, and a new immunologic function, *J. Natl. Cancer Inst.* **52**:1029.

AOKI, T., 1975, Surface antigens of normal and neoplastic lymphohematopoietic cells, in: *Immunological Aspects of Neoplasia* (E. Hersh, ed.), presented at the 26th Annual Symposium on Fundamental Cancer Research, Houston, Texas, pp. 149–167, Williams & Wilkinson, Baltimore, Md.

AOKI, T., AND JOHNSON, P. A., 1972, Suppression of Gross leukemia cell-surface antigens: A kind of antigenic modulation, *J. Natl. Cancer Inst.* **49**:183.

AOKI, T., AND TAKAHASHI, T., 1972, Viral and cellular surface antigens of murine leukemias and myelomas: Serological analysis by immunoelectron microscopy, *J. Exp. Med.* **135**:443.

AOKI, T., AND TODARO, G. J., 1973, Antigenic properties of endogenous type-C viruses from spontaneously transformed clones of BALB/3T3, *Proc. Natl. Acad. Sci. U.S.A.* **70**:1598.

AOKI, T., BOYSE, E. A., AND OLD, L. J., 1966, Occurrence of natural antibody to the G (Gross) leukemia antigen in mice, *Cancer Res.* **26**:1415.

AOKI, T., BOYSE, E. A., AND OLD, L. J., 1968a, Wild-type Gross leukemia virus. I. Soluble antigen (GSA) in the plasma and tissues of infected mice, *J. Natl. Cancer Inst.* **41**:89.

AOKI, T., BOYSE, E. A., AND OLD, L. J., 1968b, Wild-type Gross leukemia virus. II. Influence of immunogenetic factors on natural transmission and on the consequences of infection, *J. Natl. Cancer Inst.* **41**:97.

AOKI, T., BOYSE, E. A., AND OLD, L. J., 1968c, Wild-type Gross leukemia virus. III. Serological tests as indicators of leukemia risk, *J. Natl. Cancer Inst.* **41**:103.

AOKI, T., BOYSE, E. A., OLD, L. J., deHARVEN, E., HÄMMERLING, U., AND WOOD, H. A., 1970, G (Gross) and H-2 cell surface antigens: Location on Gross leukemia cells by electron microscopy with visually labeled antibody, *Proc. Natl. Acad. Sci. U.S.A.* **65**:569.

AOKI, T., HERBERMAN, R. B., JOHNSON, P. A., LIU, M., AND STURM, M. M., 1972, Wild-type Gross leukemia virus: Classification of soluble antigens (GSAs), *J. Virol.* **10**:1208.

AOKI, T., STEPHENSON, J. R., AND AARONSON, S. A., 1973a, Demonstration of a cell-surface antigen associated with murine sarcoma virus by immunoelectron microscopy, *Proc. Natl. Acad. Sci. U.S.A.* **70**:742.

AOKI, T., POTTER, M., AND STURM, M. M., 1973b, Analysis of type C viruses associated with primary and short-term transplanted mouse plasma cell tumors by immunoelectron microscopy, *J. Natl. Cancer Inst.* **51**:1609.

AOKI, T., HUEBNER, R. J., CHANG, K. S. S., STURM, M. M., AND LIU, M., 1974a, Diversity of envelope antigens on murine type C RNA viruses, *J. Natl. Cancer Inst.* **52**:1189.

AOKI, T., KVEDAR, J. P., KUDO, T., PLATA, E. J., SENDO, F., AND HOLLIS, V. W., JR., 1974b, Enhancement of host immune response to cell surface antigens by the extract of *Streptococcus hemolyticus*, in: *Comparative Leukemia Research, 1973* (Y. Ito and R. M. Dutcher, eds.), pp. 237–240, University of Tokyo Press, Japan.

AOKI, T., STEPHENSON, J. R., AARONSON, S. A., AND HSU, K. C., 1974c, Surface antigens of mammalian sarcoma virus-transformed nonproducer cells, *Proc. Natl. Acad. Sci. U.S.A.* (in press).

AUGUST, J. T., BOLOGNESI, D. P., FLEISSNER, E., GILDEN, R. V., AND NOWINSKI, R. C., 1974, Letter to Editor: A proposed nomenclature for virion proteins of oncogenic RNA viruses, *Virology* **60**:595.

BALDWIN, R. W., BOWEN, J. G., EMBLETON, M. J., PRICE, M. R., AND ROBINS, R. A., 1974, Serum factors modifying lymphocyte cytotoxicity for tumor cells, *Adv. Biosci.* **12**:539.

BATZING, B. L., YURCONIC, M., JR., AND HANNA, M. G., JR., 1974, Autogenous immunity to endogenous RNA tumor virus: Chronic humoral immune response to virus envelope antigens in B6C3F₁ mice, *J. Natl. Cancer Inst.* **52**:117.

BILLINGHAM, R. E., BRENT, L., AND MEDAWAR, P. B., 1956, Quantitative studies on tissue transplantation immunity. III. Actively acquired tolerance, *Philos. Trans. R. Soc. London* **239**:357.

BORSOS, T., AND RAPP, H. J., eds., 1973, Conference on the use of BCG in therapy of cancer, *Natl. Cancer Inst. Monogr.* **39.**

BOYSE, E. A., AND OLD, L. J., 1969, Some aspects of normal and abnormal cell surface genetics, *Ann. Rev. Genet.* **3**:269.

BOYSE, E. A., OLD, L. J., AND AOKI, T., 1967, Immunogenetics of leukemia in the mouse, in: *Treatment of Burkitt's tumor* (J. H. Burchenal and D. P. Burkitt, eds.), UICC Monograph Series, Vol. 8, pp. 248–257, Springer, New York.

CHIECO-BIANCHI, L., SENDO, F., AOKI, T., AND BARRERA, O. L., 1974, Immunologic tolerance to antigens associated with murine leukemia viruses: T-cell unresponsiveness? *J. Natl. Cancer Inst.* **52**:1345.

deHARVEN, E., 1968, Morphology of murine leukemia viruses, in: *Experimental Leukemia* (M. Rich, ed.), pp. 97–129, Appleton-Century-Crofts, New York.

DEZFULIAN, M., ZEE, T., DE OME, K. B., BLAIR, P. B., AND WEISS, D. W., 1968, Role of the mammary tumor virus in the immunogenicity of spontaneous mammary carcinomas of BALB/c mice and in the responsiveness of the hosts, *Cancer Res.* **28**:1759.

179

RNA
ONCOGENIC
VIRUS-
ASSOCIATED
ANTIGENS

ECKNER, R. J., AND STEEVES, R. A., 1972, A classification of the murine leukemia viruses: Neutralization of pseudotype of Friend spleen focus-forming virus by type-specific murine antisera, *J. Exp. Med.* **136:**832.

GALLAGHER, R. E., TODARO, G. J., SMITH, R. G., LIVINGSTON, D. M., AND GALLO, R. C., 1974, Relationship between RNA-directed DNA polymerase (reverse transcriptase) from human acute leukemic blood cells and primate type-C viruses, *Proc. Natl. Acad. Sci. U.S.A.* **71:**1309.

GEERING, G., OLD, L. J., AND BOYSE, E. A., 1966, Antigens of leukemias induced by naturally occurring murine leukemia virus: Their relation to the antigens of Gross virus and other murine leukemia viruses, *J. Exp. Med.* **124:**753.

GEERING, G., AOKI, T., AND OLD, L. J., 1970, Shared viral antigen of mammalian leukemia viruses, *Nature (London)* **226:**265.

GILDEN, R. V., AND OROSZLAN, S., 1972, Group-specific antigens of RNA tumor viruses as markers for subinfectious expression of the RNA virus genome, *Proc. Natl. Acad. Sci. U.S.A.* **69:**1021.

GILDEN, R. V., TONI, R., HANSON, M., BOVA, D., CHARMAN, H. P., AND OROSZLAN, S., 1974, Immunochemical studies of the major internal polypeptide of woolly monkey and gibbon ape type C viruses, *J. Immunol.* **112:**1250.

GREEN, M., AND GERARD, G. F., 1974, RNA-directed DNA polymerase—Properties and functions in oncogenic RNA viruses and cells, in: *Progress in Nucleic Acid Research and Molecular Biology,* Academic Press, New York.

GREENBERGER, J. S., STEPHENSON, J. R., AOKI, T., AND AARONSON, S. A., 1974, Cell surface antigens of murine sarcoma virus transformed nonproducer cells: Further evidence for lack of transplantation immunity, *Int. J. Cancer* **14:**145.

GREGORIADES, A., AND OLD, L. J., 1969, Isolation and some characteristics of a group-specific antigen of the murine leukemia viruses, *Virology* **37:**189.

GROSS, L., 1951, Pathogenic properties, and "vertical" transmission of the mouse leukemia agent, *Proc. Soc. Exp. Bid. Med.* **78:**342.

HANAFUSA, H., AOKI, T., KAWAI, S., MIYAMOTO, T., AND WILSNACK, R. E., 1973, Presence of antigen common to avian tumor viral envelope antigen in normal chick embryo cells, *Virology* **56:**22.

HELLSTRÖM, I., SJÖGREN, H. O., WARNER, G. A., AND HELLSTRÖM, K. E., 1971, Blocking of cell-mediated tumor immunity by sera from patients with growing neoplasms, *Int. J. Cancer* **7:**226.

HERBERMAN, R. B., 1972, Serological analysis of cell surface antigens of tumors induced by murine leukemia virus, *J. Natl. Cancer Inst.* **48:**265.

HERBERMAN, R. B., AND AOKI, T., 1972, Immune and natural antibodies to syngeneic murine plasma cell tumors, *J. Exp. Med.* **136:**94.

HERBERMAN, R. B., AOKI, T., AND NUNN, M. E., 1973, Solubilization of G (Gross) antigens on the surface of G leukemia cells, *J. Natl. Cancer Inst.* **50:**481.

HERBERMAN, R. B., AOKI, T., NUNN, M. E., LAVRIN, D. H., SOARES, N., GAZDAR, A., HOLDEN, H., AND CHANG, K. S. S., 1974, Specificity of ^{51}Cr-release cytotoxicity by lymphocytes immune to murine sarcoma virus, *J. Natl. Cancer Inst.* **53:**1103.

HILGERS, J., NOWINSKI, R. C., GEERING, G., AND HARDY, W., 1972, Detection of avian and mammalian oncogenic RNA viruses (oncornaviruses) by immunofluorescence, *Cancer Res.* **32:**98.

HOLLIS, V. W., JR., AOKI, T., BARRERA, O. L., OLDSTONE, M. B. A., AND DIXON, F. J., 1974, Detection of naturally occurring antibodies to RNA-dependent DNA polymerase of murine leukemia virus in kidney eluates of AKR mice, *J. Virol.* **13:**448.

IKEDA, H., STOCKERT, E., ROWE, W. P., BOYSE, E. A., LILLY, F., SATO, H., JACOBBS, S., AND OLD, L. J., 1973, Relation of chromosome 4 (linkage group VIII) to murine leukemia virus-associated antigens of AKR mice, *J. Exp. Med.* **137:**1103.

KASSEL, R. L., OLD, L. J., CARSWELL, E. A., FIORE, N. C., AND HARDY, W. D., JR., 1973, Serum-mediated leukemia cell destruction in AKR mice: Role of complement in the phenomenon, *J. Exp. Med.* **138:**925.

KENNEL, S. J., DEL VILLANO, B. C., LEVY, R. L., AND LERNER, R. A., 1973, Properties of an oncornavirus glycoprotein: Evidence for its presence on the surface of virions and infected cells, *Virology* **55:**464.

KLEIN, G., 1968, Tumor specific transplantation antigen, *Cancer Res.* **28:**625.

KLEIN, G., 1969, Tumor antigens, *Ann. Rev. Microbiol.* **20:**223.

KUDO, T., AOKI, T., AND MORRISON, J. L., 1974, Stabilization of antigens on surfaces of malignant cells by formalin treatment, *J. Natl. Cancer Inst.* **52:**1553.

KUROKAWA, T., HATTORI, T., AND FURUE, H., 1972, Clinical experiences with the streptococcal anticancer preparation, OK-432 (NSCB116209), *Cancer Chemother. Rep. Part. I* **56:**211.

181

RNA
ONCOGENIC
VIRUS-
ASSOCIATED
ANTIGENS

LEVY, J. P., VARET, B., AND OPPENHEIM, E., 1969, Neutralization of Graffi leukemia virus, *Nature (London)* **224**:606.

LILLY, F., AND NATHANSON, S. G., 1969, Studies on the FMR antigen, *Transplant. Proc.* **1**:85.

LOWRY, D. R., ROWE, W. P., TEICH, N., AND HARTLEY, J. A., 1971, High frequency activation *in vitro* by 5-iododeoxyuridine, *Science* **174**:155.

MCALLISTER, R. M., NELSON-REES, W. A., JOHNSON, E. Y., RONGEY, R. W., AND GARDNER, M. B., 1971, Disseminated rhabdomyosarcoma formed in kittens by cultured human rhabdomyosarcoma cells, *J. Natl. Cancer Inst.* **47**:603.

MELLORS, R. C., SHIRAI, T., AOKI, T., HUEBNER, R. J., AND KRAWCZYNSKI, K., 1971, Wild-type Gross leukemia viruses and the pathogenesis of the glomerulonephritis of New Zealand mice, *J. Exp. Med.* **133**:113.

MORTON, D. L., MILLER, G. F., AND WOOD, D. A., 1965, Demonstration of tumor-specific immunity against antigens unrelated to the mammary tumor virus in spontaneous mammary adenocarcinomas, *J. Natl. Cancer Inst.* **42**:303.

NOWINSKI, R. C., AND PETERS, E. D., 1973, Cell surface antigens associated with murine leukemia virus: Definition of the G_L and G_T antigenic systems, *H. Virol.* **12**:1104.

NOWINSKI, R. C., OLD, L. J., BOYSE, E. A., DEHARVEN, E., AND GEERING, G., 1968, Group-specific viral antigens in the milk and tissues of mice naturally infected with mammary tumor virus or Gross leukemia virus, *Virology* **34**:617.

NOWINSKI, R. C., SARKAR, N. H., OLD, L. J., MOORE, D. H., SCHEER, D. I., AND HILGERS, J., 1971, Characteristics of the structural components of the mouse mammary tumor virus. II. Viral proteins and antigens, *Virology* **46**:1.

NOWINSKI, R. C., FLEISSNER, E., SARKAR, N. H., AND AOKI, T., 1972, Chromatographic separation and antigenic analysis of proteins of the oncornavirus. II. Mammalian leukemia–sarcoma viruses, *J. Virol.* **9**:359.

OKABE, H., GILDEN, R. V., AND HATANAKA, M., 1973, Extensive homology of RD114 virus DNA with RNA of feline cell origin, *Nature New Biol.* **244**:54.

OKAMOTO, H., MINAMI, M., SHOIN, S., KOSHIMURA, S., AND SHIMIZU, R., 1966, Experimental anticancer studies. Part XXXI. On the streptococcal preparation having potent anticancer activity, *Jpn. J. Exp. Med.* **36**:175.

OKAMOTO, H., SHOIN, S., KOSHIMURA, S., AND SHIMIZU, R., 1972, *β-Hemolytic Streptococcus as a Cancer Controller*, (H. Okamoto, ed.), Chugai Pharmaceutical Co., Japan.

OLD, L. J., AND BOYSE, E. A., 1965, Antigens of tumors and leukemias induced by viruses, *Fed. Proc.* **24**:1009.

OLD, L. J., BOYSE, E. A., CLARKE, D. A., AND CARSWELL, E. A., 1962, Antigenic properties of chemically induced tumors, *Ann. N.Y. Acad. Sci.* **101**:80.

OLD, L. J., BOYSE, E. A., AND STOCKERT, E., 1964, Typing of mouse leukemias by serological methods, *Nature (London)* **201**:777.

OLD, L. J., BOYSE, E. A., AND STOCKERT, E., 1965, The G (Gross) leukemia antigen, *Cancer Res.* **25**:813.

OLD, L. J., STOCKERT, E., BOYSE, E. A., AND KIM, J. H., 1968, Antigenic modulation, loss of TL antigen from cells exposed to TL antibody: Study of the phenomenon *in vitro*, *J. Exp. Med.* **127**:523.

OLDSTONE, M. B. A., AOKI, T., AND DIXON, F. J., 1972a, The antibody response of mice to murine leukemia virus in spontaneous infection: Absence of classical immunologic tolerance, *Proc. Natl. Acad. Sci. U.S.A.* **69**:134.

OLDSTONE, M. B. A., TISHON, A., TONIETTI, G., AND DIXON, F. J., 1972b, Immune complex disease associated with spontaneous murine leukemia: Incidence and pathogenesis of glomerulonephritis, *Clin. Immunol. Immunopathol.* **1**:6.

OROSZLAN, S., FISHER, C. L., STANLEY, T. B., AND GILDEN, R. V., 1970, Proteins of the murine C-type RNA viruses. I. Isolation of a group-specific antigen by isoelectric focusing, *J. Gen. Virol.* **8**:1.

ORTALDO, J. R., TING, C. C., AND HERBERMAN, R. B., 1974, Modulation of fetal antigen(s) in mouse leukemia cells, *Cancer Res.* **34**:1366.

ORTEZ DE LANDAZURI, M., KEDAR, E., AND FAHEY, J. L., 1974, Studies of antibody dependent cellular cytotoxicity (ADCC) to a syngeneic Gross virus-induced lymphoma, *J. Natl. Cancer Inst.* **52**:147.

PARKS, W. P., AND SCOLNICK, E. M., 1972, Radioimmunoassay of mammalian type C viral protein: Interspecies antigenic reactivities of the major internal polypeptide, *Proc. Natl. Acad. Sci. U.S.A.* **69**:1766.

PARKS, W. P., SCOLNICK, E. M., ROSS, J., TODARO, G. J., AND AARONSON, S. A., 1972, Immunological relationships of reverse transcriptases from ribonucleic acid tumor viruses, *J. Virol.* **9**:110.

PARKS, W. P., HOWK, R. S., SCOLNICK, E. K., OROSZLAN, S., AND GILDEN, R. V., 1974, Immunochemical characterization of two major polypeptides from murine mammary tumor virus, *J. Virol.* **13**:1200.

PLATA, E. J., AOKI, T., COLLINS, F., AND SIBAL, L. R., 1973, Mammary tumor virus (MTV): Soluble antigen (MSA) in the plasma of infected mice, Annual Meeting of the American Society of Microbiology, abst. 133, p. 216.

POURREAN-SCHNEIDER, N., STEPHENS, R. J., AND GARDNER, W. U., 1968, Viral inclusions and other cytoplasmic components in a Leydig cell murine tumor: An electron microscopic study, *Int. J. Cancer* **3**:155.

SALAMAN, M. H., AND WEDDERBURN, N., 1966, The immunodepressive effect of Friend virus, *Immunology* **10**:445.

SCHÄFER, W., SŹANTÓ, J., ANDERER, F. A., FRANK, H., GELDERBLOM, H., LANGE, J., AND PISTER, L., 1970, Tests for mouse leukemia viruses and isolation of some of their components, in: *Comparative Leukemia Research* (R. M. Dutcher, ed.), pp. 327–332, Karger, New York.

SHERR, C. J., LIEBER, M. M., BENVENISTE, R. E., AND TODARO, G. J., 1974, Endogenous baboon type C virus (M7): Biochemical and immunologic characterization, *Virology* **58**:492.

SILOBREIC, V., AND SUIT, H. D., 1967, Tumor specific antigen(s) in a spontaneous mammary carcinoma of C3H mice. I. Quantitative cell transplants into mammary-tumor-agent-positive and free mice, *J. Natl. Cancer Inst.* **39**:1113.

SJÖGREN, H. O., HELLSTRÖM, I., BANSAL, S. C., AND HELLSTRÖM, K. E., 1971, Suggestive evidence that the "blocking antibodies" of tumor bearing individuals may be antigen–antibody complexes, *Proc. Natl. Acad. Sci. U.S.A.* **68**:1372.

SNELL, G. D., AND STIMPFLING, J. H., 1966, Genetics of tissue transplantation, in: *The Biology of the Laboratory Mouse* (E. L. Green, ed.), pp. 457–492, McGraw-Hill, New York.

SOUTHAM, C. M., 1960, Relationships of immunology to cancer, a review, *Cancer Res.* **20**:271.

STEPHENSON, J. R., TRONICK, S. R., REYNOLDS, R. K., AND AARONSON, S. A., 1974, Isolation and characterization of C-type viral gene products of virus-negative mouse cells, *J. Exp. Med.* **139**:427.

STOCKERT, E., OLD, L. J., AND BOYSE, E. A., 1971, The G_{IX} system: A cell surface alloantigen associated with murine leukemia virus; implications regarding chromosomal integration of the viral genome, *J. Exp. Med.* **133**:1334.

STRAND, M., AND AUGUST, J. T., 1973, Structural proteins of oncogenic ribonucleic acid viruses: Interspec 11, a new interspecies antigen, *J. Biol. Chem.* **248**:5627.

STRAND, M., AND AUGUST, J. T., 1974, Structural proteins of mammalian oncogenic RNA viruses: Multiple antigenic determinants of the major internal protein and envelope glycoprotein, *J. Virol.* **13**:171.

STÜCK, B., OLD, L. J., AND BOYSE, E. A., 1964a, Occurrence of soluble antigen in the plasma of mice with virus-induced leukemia, *Proc. Natl. Acad. Sci. U.S.A.* **52**:950.

STÜCK, B., OLD, L. J., AND BOYSE, E. A., 1964b, Antigenic conversion of established leukemias by an unrelated leukemogenic virus, *Nature (London)* **202**:1016.

SUIT, H. D., AND SILOBREIC, V., 1967, Tumor specific antigen(s) in a spontaneous mammary carcinoma of C3H mice. II. Active immunization of mammary-tumor-agent-free mice, *J. Natl. Cancer Inst.* **39**:1121.

TERAMOTO, Y. A., PUENTES, M. J., YOUNG, L. J. T., AND CARDIFF, R. D., 1974, Structure of the mouse mammary tumor virus: Polypeptides and glycoproteins, *J. Virol.* **13**:411.

TING, C. C., AND HERBERMAN, R. B., 1974, Serological analysis of the immune response to Friend virus-induced leukemia, *Cancer Res.* **34**:1676.

TING, C. C., SHIU, G., RODRIGUES, D., AND HERBERMAN, R. B., 1974, Cell-mediated immunity to Friend virus-induced leukemia, *Cancer Res.* **34**:1684.

TODARO, G. J., 1972, "Spontaneous" release of type C viruses from clonal lines of "spontaneously" transformed BALB/3T3 cells, *Nature (London)* **240**:157.

TRONICK, S. R., STEPHENSON, J. R., AND AARONSON, S. A., 1973, Immunological characterization of a low molecular weight polypeptide of murine leukemia virus, *Virology* **54**:199.

TRONICK, S. R., STEPHENSON, J. R., AND AARONSON, S. A., 1974, Comparative immunological studies of RNA C-type viruses: Radioimmunoassay for a low molecular weight polypeptide of woolly monkey leukemia virus, *Virology* **57**:347.

VAAGE, J., 1968a, Non-virus-associated antigens in virus-induced mouse mammary tumors, *Cancer Res.* **28**:2477.

VAAGE, J., 1968b, Non-cross-reacting resistance to virus-induced mouse mammary tumors in virus-infected C3H mice, *Nature (London)* **218**:101.

WEDDERBURN, N., AND SALAMAN, N. H., 1968, The immunodepressive effect of Friend virus. II. Reduction of splenic hemolysin-producing cells in primary and secondary responses, *Immunology* **15:**439.

YOSHIKI, T., MELLORS, R. C., HARDY, W. D., JR., AND FLEISSNER, E., 1964, Common cell surface antigens associated with mammalian C-type RNA viruses: Cell membrane-bound *gs* antigen, *J. Exp. Med.* **139:**925.

YOSHIKI, T., MELLORS, R. C., AND HARDY, W. D., JR., 1973, Common cell-surface antigen associated with murine and feline C-type RNA leukemia viruses, *Proc. Natl. Acad. Sci. U.S.A.* **7:**1878.

183

RNA
ONCOGENIC
VIRUS-
ASSOCIATED
ANTIGENS

6

DNA Virus (SV40)
Induced Antigens

Satvir S. Tevethia and Mary J. Tevethia

1. Introduction

DNA-containing tumor viruses, in contrast to RNA tumor viruses, differ from one another in morphology, nucleic acid content, host range, mode of replication, and ability to cause neoplasia in their natural host (Green, 1970). They include viruses which cause neoplasia in the host in which they replicate (herpesviruses) and viruses that induce tumors in the experimental animals in which they undergo abortive infection (papovaviruses, adenoviruses). Great variations exist within each group of DNA tumor viruses: some members of the papovavirus group induce tumors in their natural host (papilloma viruses) and others induce tumors in a heterologous host only (SV40, human papovaviruses).

Although DNA-containing tumor viruses were shown to cause neoplasia in experimental animals over a decade ago, it is only recently that some of these viruses have been seriously considered as etiological agents in human neoplasia. A strong relationship between Epstein–Barr herpesvirus and Burkitt's lymphoma is indicated (Klein, 1971), and an association between herpes simplex virus type 2 and carcinoma of the cervix has been made (Rapp, 1974). These observations have renewed an interest in DNA tumor viruses.

Several approaches can be used in associating a DNA virus as an etiological agent of a certain tumor: (1) direct isolation or rescue of the virus by cocultivation with susceptible cells, (2) demonstration of virus DNA integrated into or associated with the host cell genome, (3) demonstration of the synthesis of messenger RNA complementary to viral DNA, and (4) synthesis of virus-induced antigens.

SATVIR S. TEVETHIA and MARY J. TEVETHIA • Department of Pathology and Cancer Research Center, Tufts University School of Medicine, Boston, Massachusetts.

186

SATVIR S.
TEVETHIA
AND
MARY J.
TEVETHIA

The detection of antigens in transformed cells has been used as an excellent tool to identify the transforming virus even when a defective viral genome is integrated into the genome of transformed cells. Virus-induced proteins that are antigenic in the autochthonous or syngeneic host can be found either in the nucleus, in the cytoplasm, or at the surface of cells. The immune response to these antigens has not only been used to associate a tumor virus with transformed cells but may also alter the progression of the neoplastic disease. This immune manipulation of these tumors is directed against cell surface antigens which are responsible for inducing cellular and humoral immune responses.

This chapter will concentrate on antigens induced by one of the DNA tumor viruses, simian papovavirus SV40, a virus which has been studied extensively and is a well-understood model DNA-containing tumor virus. The virus has limited genetic information and its nucleic acid can be isolated in an infectious form. It can be readily propagated *in vitro* and its mode of replication at the molecular level has been studied. SV40 induces tumors in hamsters and readily transforms mammalian cells *in vitro*. The transformed or tumor cells are free of infectious virus but contain virus-specific nonvirion antigens and cross-reactive embryonic antigens. Immune response to these antigens has been well characterized, and some of these antigens have been isolated and characterized (Butel *et al.*, 1972; Sambrook, 1973). Other DNA viruses will be mentioned when appropriate. Excellent reviews have been published on the role of herpesviruses in neoplasia (Klein, 1971; Rapp, 1974; Deinhardt *et al.*, 1974; Volume 2 of this series).

2. Tumor Induction and Cell Transformation by SV40

SV40 induces tumors readily at the site of virus inoculation in hamsters only when they are inoculated as newborns (Table 1). Other species are resistant to tumor induction by SV40, including monkeys, in which the virus replicates and produces

TABLE 1
Tumor Induction and Cell Transformation by SV40 and Transplantability of Transformed Cells

Host species	Tumor induction *in vivo*	Immuno-suppression used	Cell Trans-formation *in vitro*	Transplant-ability in syngeneic host	Immuno-suppression used
Monkey	No	—[a]	Yes	No	Yes
Human	No	—	Yes	No	—
Rabbit	No	—	Yes	No	—
Mice	No	—	Yes	Yes[c]	Yes
Rats	Yes	Yes	Yes	Yes[c]	Yes
Mastomys	Yes	No	Nt[b]	Nt	Nt
Hamster	Yes	No	Yes	Yes	No

[a] —, No information available.
[b] Nt, Not tested.
[c] Cells transplantable only after prolonged *in vitro* passage and in immunosuppressed animals.

latent infection. Mastomys have been shown to develop brain tumors upon SV40 inoculation; however, no evidence was provided to prove that the induced tumors contained SV40 information (Rabson *et al.*, 1962). Generally, the tumors induced by SV40 in hamsters have a long latent period (3 months to 1 year), and the tumor incidence depends on the concentration of the virus used and the age of the animals (Eddy, 1964). The resistance of young adults to SV40 oncogenesis is mediated by the immune response of the host against the antigenic tumor. The evidence for this is provided by the following observations: (1) X-irradiation of adult animals prior to virus inoculation enhances their susceptibility to tumor induction (Allison *et al.*, 1967); (2) adult hamsters when inoculated with SV40 in the cheek pouch, an immunologically privileged site, develop tumors (Allison *et al.*, 1967); (3) animals thymectomized and treated with antilymphocyte serum (ALS) are more susceptible to tumorigenesis by similar small DNA viruses than their immunocompetent littermates (Allison and Law, 1968). Recently, adult immunocompetent hamsters have been shown to be susceptible to SV40 tumorigenesis when inoculated by the intravenous route. The induced neoplasms in this case were reticulum cell sarcomas, lymphosarcomas, and lymphocytic leukemias (Diamandopoulos, 1973). Whether the development of these tumors in adult hamsters following the intravenous virus infection is due to the failure of immunosurveillance, which operates when adults are inoculated subcutaneously, is not known. The lymphoid cell tumors, however, have been shown to contain SV40-specific transplantation antigen (Tevethia, 1974).

The complete viral genome is not required for tumor induction. Both artificially produced defective viruses (irradiated and hydroxylamine-treated viruses) and naturally occurring defective viruses [T-antigen-inducing defective particles and PARA (defective SV40–adenovirus hybrid populations)] have been shown to be oncogenic in hamsters (Uchida and Watababe, 1968; Defendi and Jensen, 1967; Alstein, 1967; Rapp, 1973). The irradiated virus showed enhanced tumorigenesis over the untreated virus.

The tumor virus interaction with a cell may be either (1) productive, resulting in the synthesis of new virus and cell death, or (2) abortive, often leading to cell transformation and eventually to a malignant state. The criteria for transformation of cells by a tumor virus generally include the following: (a) loss of contact inhibition, (b) altered morphology, (c) increased growth rate, (d) increased capacity to persist in serial subcultures, (e) chromosomal abnormalities, (f) membrane changes which include changes in transport or permeability, (g) impaired intercellular communication and junction, (h) change in adhesiveness, (i) change in agglutinability by lectins, (j) change in electrophoretic mobility, and (k) biochemical changes involving glycoproteins and glycolipids. Transformation is accompanied by the synthesis of virus-induced nonvirion proteins which are antigenic in the autologous, autochthonous, or syngeneic host. The transformed cells, under certain circumstances, are also transplantable in the syngeneic host.

Even though SV40 produces tumors consistently only in hamsters, it can transform a wide variety of cells *in vitro* (Table 1). The virus can transform human, monkey, rabbit, mouse, rat, reptile, and bovine cells in addition to

188

SATVIR S.
TEVETHIA
AND
MARY J.
TEVETHIA

hamster cells. The virus can transform cells from a variety of organs and tissues. The cells from kidney, lung, liver, heart, skin, lens epithelium, brain, prostate, and pituitary can be transformed by SV40 (see Butel *et al.*, 1972). Lymphoid cells have also been demonstrated to be susceptible to transformation (Collins *et al.*, 1974; Diamandopoulos, 1973).

Since *in vitro* transformation of mammalian cells by SV40 results in the loss of contact inhibition and a gain in the ability to grow indefinitely *in vitro*, it is assumed that the transformation observed *in vitro* is analogous to tumor induction *in vivo*. This analogy seems to hold for hamster cells only, which upon transformation by SV40 are invariably transplantable in syngeneic host (Duff and Rapp, 1970). However, variation in the transplantability has been reported (Butel *et al.*, 1971). Mouse cells, which are more susceptible to transformation by SV40 *in vitro* than are hamster cells, become transplantable only after the transformed cells have been cultivated *in vitro* for prolonged periods (Tevethia and McMillan, 1974; Kit *et al.*, 1969; Takemoto *et al.*, 1968). The similar situation holds true for rat cells transformed by SV40 *in vitro*. Even then an immunosuppressed host is required. This apparent lack of transplantability of inbred mouse transformed cells in syngeneic animals raises the question of the role of the SV40 viral genome in malignancy. Studies in this laboratory (Tevethia and McMillan, 1974) have shown that freshly derived mouse embryo cells upon transformation by SV40 fail to produce tumors in immunocompetent or immunosuppressed syngeneic newborn or adult mice, thus ruling out the possibility that the lack of tumor induction by these transformed cells is due to the immune response of the host to SV40 TSTA present at the surface of SV40-transformed cells. The cells become transplantable in immunosuppressed hosts only after prolonged *in vitro* cultivation. Thus, at least in the case of mouse cells, morphological transformation (acquisition of virus antigens, integration of viral genome, and other cellular changes) can be separated from malignant transformation, and the malignant property seems to be acquired independently. What factors may be required for turning on the malignant potential of the morphologically transformed cells is not known. It has been speculated that the activation of an endogenous type C virus genome may be needed for the cells to become malignant (Todaro and Huebner, 1972). However, efforts to relate the acquisition of malignant properties by SV40-transformed BALB/c embryo cells to the activation type C gs antigen expression were not successful. Temperature-sensitive mutants defective in the initiation of DNA synthesis at nonpermissive temperature (*ts*A mutants) have been used to transform mammalian cells in order to delineate the role of this gene in cell transformation (Butel *et al.*, 1974). Cells transformed at a permissive temperature with these mutants have been established which demonstrate a normal cell phenotype at the nonpermissive temperature while exhibiting transformed cell phenotype at the permissive temperature. The criteria used for transformation were morphology, saturation density, colony formation on plastic, cell monolayers, and, in soft agar, uptake of hexose. Thus the *ts*A function appears to be required for the maintenance of morphological transformation. There is no clear evidence, however, which demonstrates that any of the above criteria can be correlated with malignant behavior of tumor cells *in vivo*.

TABLE 2

189

DNA VIRUS
(SV40)
INDUCED
ANTIGENS

Nature of Intracellular Antigens Specified by SV40[a]

Property	Antigens		
	T	U	V
Location	Nucleus, Cytoplasm	Nucleus perinuclear	Nuclear
Present in tumor cells	Yes	Yes	No
Present in transformed cells	Yes	Yes	No
Induced in cytolytic cycle	Yes	Yes	Yes
Detected by	IF, CF	IF, CF	IF, CF
Time of appearance (after virus infection)	12–24 (h)	12–24 (h)	24–40 (h)
Inhibited by araC	No	No	Yes
Inhibited by actinomycin D	Yes	?	Yes
Specific for SV40	Yes	Yes	Yes
Mol wt	70,000	?	?
Susceptibility to heat	Susceptible	Resistant	Resistant
Immune response in tumor-bearing host	Yes	Yes	+ Primary tumors − Transplanted tumors
Role in tumor rejection	None	None	None

[a] Abbreviations: T, tumor antigen; U, intra- or perinuclear antigen distinct from T antigen; V, Virion antigen; IF, immunofluorescence test; CF, complement fixation test.

3. Antigens in Tumor or Transformed Cells

The antigens induced by the members of papovavirus group in transformed cells are nonvirion in nature but are specifically induced by the transforming virus. These virus-induced nonvirion antigens can be classified into two categories based on their location within the transformed cells: (1) tumor or T and U antigens

TABLE 3

Nature of Surface Antigens Associated with SV40-Transformed Cells[a]

Property	Surface antigens			
	TSTA	S antigen	Embryonic antigens	Normal cell antigens
Specific for transforming virus	+	+	−	−
Present in transformed cells	+	+	+	+
Present in normal cells	−	−	+[b]	+
Induced in cytolytic cycle	+	?	?	?
Antigenic in syngeneic host	+	+	+	+
Detected by				
a. Transplantation rejection test	+	−	?	−
b. Serological tests	+	+	+	+
c. Cellular immunity test	+	?	?	−
Role in tumor rejection	+	−	?	−

[a] Symbols: +, present or yes; −, absent or none; ?, unknown.
[b] Repressed.

190

SATVIR S.
TEVETHIA
AND
MARY J.
TEVETHIA

located in the nucleus of transformed cells and (2) surface antigens located at the surface of transformed cells. The properties of antigens associated with SV40-transformed cells and those induced in the virus productive cycle are listed in Tables 2 and 3.

3.1. Intracellular Antigens

3.1.1. Tumor or T Antigen

The tumor or T antigen in SV40 tumor or transformed cells was first demonstrated by means of the complement fixation (CF) test by using sera from hamsters bearing SV40-induced tumors (Black *et al.*, 1963). The nuclear localization of T antigen was later demonstrated by the indirect immunofluorescence test (Pope and Rowe, 1964; Rapp *et al.*, 1964a). Demonstration of the synthesis of an antigenically similar T antigen during the productive infection by SV40 in monkey cells provided evidence for associating the virus with the virus-free transformed cells (Rapp *et al.*, 1964b). The T antigen induced by SV40 is specific for SV40, but an antigenically similar T antigen has been demonstrated in tumors induced by human papovaviruses (Walker *et al.*, 1973; Takemoto and Mullarkey, 1973). The T antigen has also been localized in the cytoplasm of cells infected with or transformed by mutants of defective SV40 populations (Butel *et al.*, 1969). The cytoplasmic localization of T antigen as detected by the indirect immunofluorescence technique did not alter its antigenic properties or the malignant behavior of the tumor cells. Kinetic studies have shown that T antigen appears 12–24 h after infection of monkey cells by SV40. The synthesis of T antigen is inhibited by actinomycin D but not by inhibitors of DNA synthesis, showing that T antigen synthesis is dependent on an early viral function and that the synthesis of viral DNA is not required for its expression (Rapp *et al.*, 1965). It is also susceptible to inhibition by interferon during the infectious cycle (Oxman and Black, 1966). T antigen is heat labile, resistant to deoxyribonuclease and ribonuclease, but susceptible to trypsin. It has a molecular weight of 70,000 (Del Villano and Defendi, 1973). The biological function of T antigen is unknown; however, the findings that T antigen binds to double-stranded DNA (Carroll *et al.*, 1974) and is not produced at normal levels by mutants which are defective in viral DNA synthesis (Tegtmeyer and Ozer, 1971) suggest that T antigen may play a role in viral DNA synthesis.

The presence of T antigen in the transformed cells has been used to follow the development of SV40-induced tumors *in vivo*. By using the indirect immunofluorescence test, Diamandopoulos (1973) was able to demonstrate the induction of SV40-induced lymphocytic leukemia, lymphosarcoma, and reticulum cell sarcomas in hamsters inoculated intravenously with SV40 as adults. The presence of T antigen was demonstrated in the nucleus of cells in imprints made from lymph nodes of animals inoculated with SV40. Even when only rare cells containing T antigen were present, they could be easily demonstrated in the tissue imprint.

Animals bearing tumors induced either by the virus or by transformed cells
develop antibody to T antigen. In hamsters, the antibody to T antigen is located in
the γ_2 fraction of 7 S immunoglobulin (Tevethia, 1967). The presence of antibody
to T antigen in the animals inoculated with the virus has generally been correlated
with the presence of a virus-induced tumor; however, it has been demonstrated
that a certain percentage of virus-inoculated hamsters develop T antibody in the
absence of neoplasia (Diamandopoulos and McLane, 1974). Also, the development of T antibody has been demonstrated in animals (rabbits and monkeys)
which support virus replication but do not develop neoplasia (Rapp *et al.*, 1967;
Tevethia, 1970). SV40 T antigen, because of its location in the nucleus of tumor
cells, does not play a role in the rejection of SV40 tumor cells by the virus-
immunized animals. This conclusion is further supported by the observation that
hamsters bearing tumors induced by one of the lines of SV40-transformed cells do
not synthesize antibodies to SV40 T antigen but are still capable of rejecting a
transplant of syngeneic SV40 tumor cells (Lausch *et al.*, 1970).

When the presence of SV40 T antigen was first demonstrated, it was thought to
be specific for SV40 virus, a unique property in light of the observations with T
antigen induced by various adenoviruses. Cross-reaction between T antigen of
human and simian adenoviruses has also been demonstrated (Riggs *et al.*, 1968).
Viruses of papovavirus morphology have been isolated from human cases of
progressive multifocal leukoencephalopathy and from the urine of patients who
had undergone renal transplantation (Padgett *et al.*, 1971; Weiner *et al.*, 1972;
Gardner *et al.*, 1971; Dougherty and Distefano, 1974). These human viruses grow
in human cells, and can transform hamster cells and induce tumors in hamsters.
The human papovaviruses, although distinct, are antigenically related to SV40.
These viruses induce T antigen in the nucleus of infected cells which is
antigenically similar to SV40 T antigen. Hamster tumors induced by the J. C. virus
develop antibodies to T antigen of J.C. and SV40 viruses (Walker *et al.*, 1973).

3.1.2. U Antigen

U antigen is specific for SV40. Several lines of evidence indicate that U may be
antigenically distinct from T antigen (Lewis and Rowe, 1971). Like the T antigen,
it is located in the nucleus of cells infected or transformed by SV40. In cells
infected by $Ad2^+ND_1$ virus, which contain a portion of SV40 DNA covalently
linked to human adenovirus 2 DNA, U antigen is located at the nuclear
membrane. The synthesis of U antigen by SV40 is not inhibited by araC, and, as
with T antigen, appears 12–24 h after virus infection. In the case of $Ad2^+ND_2$
virus, however, U antigen synthesis is diminished in the presence of araC, whereas
T antigen synthesis is unaffected. U antigen is more heat stable than T antigen and
can be distinguished from T by using temperature-sensitive mutants of SV40.
The mutant *ts B11* induces T but not U antigen at the nonpermissive temperature
(Robb *et al.*, 1974). Hamsters bearing tumors induced by SV40 develop antibodies
to U antigen as well as to T antigen. The antibody to T antigen is present in higher
titers than is the antibody to U antigen. It has been reported that U antigen cannot
be demonstrated in mouse cells transformed by SV40 (Robb *et al.*, 1974).

SATVIR S.
TEVETHIA
AND
MARY J.
TEVETHIA

3.2. Surface Antigens Associated with SV40-Transformed Cells

3.2.1. Tumor-Specific Transplantation Antigen

Cells transformed *in vitro* or *in vivo* by simian papovavirus SV40 undergo alterations in their cell membrane. Some of these changes result in the acquisition of new antigens to which the syngeneic host reacts with either a humoral or a cellular immune response or both. Perhaps the most important new antigen at the surface of virus-transformed cells is the tumor-specific transplantation antigen (TSTA). TSTA mediates the development of a cellular immune response in the host, leading to rejection of tumor cells carrying the same antigen. TSTA is specific for the transforming virus but cross-reacts from tumor to tumor and also across species lines with cells that are transformed by the same virus (see Butel *et al.*, 1972).

TSTA is not a virion antigen. Antiviral antibodies have no effect on the growth of SV40 tumor cells (Khera *et al.*, 1963), and the tumor cells themselves have been shown to be free of the infectious virus and the virion antigens.

TSTA present in cells transformed *in vitro* is identical to the antigen in tumor cells; immunization of animals with *in vitro* transformed cells can protect hamsters against a challenge of cells derived from a tumor induced by SV40 and *vice versa* (Khera *et al.*, 1963). The cross-reactivity of SV40 TSTA is not limited to tumors induced by SV40 within the same animal species. TSTA in SV40-transformed cells of one species cross-reacts with the TSTA in SV40-transformed cells from another species (Girardi, 1965). The TSTA in transformed cells remain stable during the growth of tumor cells either *in vitro* or *in vivo*. However, it has been shown that in the SV40 system the expression of TSTA at the surface of tumor cells can be altered in such a way that the immunoresistant cells escape rejection by an immunized host. The immunoresistant cells retain immunogenicity (Tevethia *et al.*, 1971).

SV40 TSTA is located at the cell surface and has been isolated in soluble form by use of 3 M KCl and by papain digestion. The activity of soluble SV40 TSTA was monitored by the *in vitro* macrophage migration inhibition test (Blasecki and Tevethia, 1973). Soluble TSTA has also been shown to be immunogenic in a syngeneic host (Drapkin *et al.*, 1974). The biochemical nature of TSTA remains unknown.

3.2.2. Surface (S) Antigens Detected by Serological Means

Tevethia *et al.* (1965) first demonstrated specific antigens at the surface of SV40-transformed hamster cells by the indirect immunofluorescence test using sera from SV40-vaccinated hamsters that had rejected a transplant of virus-free SV40 tumor cells. The reaction was specific for SV40-transformed cells since antibody against S antigen did not react either with normal hamster cells or with cells transformed by unrelated viruses. Tevethia *et al.* (1968a) later demonstrated that hamsters synthesized S antibody when immunized with SV40 virus alone, thereby ruling out the participation of isoantigens in the membrane reaction. The presence and specificity of S antigen in SV40-transformed cells were later

confirmed and extended (Kluchareva *et al.*, 1967; Girardi, 1967).

Specific antigens at the surface of SV40-transformed cells were also demonstrated *in vitro* by the mixed hemadsorption test (Hayry and Defendi, 1968; Metzgar and Oleinick, 1968), the colony inhibition test (Tevethia *et al.*, 1970), the isotopic antiglobulin test (Ting and Herberman, 1971), and the cytotoxic test using ^{51}Cr-labeled target cells (Wright and Law, 1971) and *in vivo* by inhibition of tranformed cell replication in diffusion chambers implanted in the peritoneal cavity of immune hamsters (Coggin and Ambrose, 1969). All of these studies, including our own, show beyond a doubt that antigen(s) detected at the surface of SV40-transformed cells using humoral antibodies are specific for SV40.

4. Antigens Induced in Productive Cycle

Antigens present in transformed cells have also been shown to be produced during the virus lytic cycle. T, U, and TSTA are produced during the productive cycle, and all available evidence indicates that the antigens produced in the productive cycle are identical to antigens in transformed cells. Virion antigens as well as nonvirion antigens are synthesized during the productive cycle.

SV40 virion has been shown to contain six different polypeptides ranging in molecular weight from 11,000 to 43,000. The major coat protein, which accounts for approximately 70% of the total virion protein, has a molecular weight of 43,000 daltons (Estes *et al.*, 1971). It is not clear, however, whether these polypeptides represent different antigenicities.

The virion of V antigen can be detected by the indirect immunofluorescence and complement fixation tests by using sera from animals immunized with SV40. The V antigen appears 20–40 h after infection of permissive monkey cells. The V antigen is inhibited by inhibitors of DNA synthesis (Rapp *et al.*, 1965). Transformed cells do not contain V antigen. On occasion, human and rabbit cells transformed by SV40 which release infectious virus contain V antigen in addition to T antigen. For the detection of V antigen, it is essential that the antisera to viral antigen be free from antibody to T and U antigens.

5. Genetic Origin of SV40 Induced Antigens

There is considerable argument concerning the origin of nonvirion antigens in SV40-transformed cells. Two schools of thought have developed: (1) that the antigens are derepressed host cell proteins and (2) that the antigens are coded by the virus genome.

The evidence that T antigen may be virus coded is twofold: (1) the antigenically identical T antigen is produced in all transformed and infected cells regardless of species of origin, and (2) the synthesis of SV40 T antigen in the productive cycle is

194

SATVIR S.
TEVETHIA
AND
MARY J.
TEVETHIA

inhibited by interferon (Oxman and Black, 1966), suggesting that a prereplicative SV40 gene product is required for the production of T antigen during the viral lytic cycle. Evidence has been presented that T antigen has altered sedimentation properties at nonpermissive temperature in cells infected with a temperature-sensitive mutant of SV40 which is defective in the initiation of DNA synthesis at the nonpermissive temperature (Osborne and Weber, 1973).

One difficulty in determining the genetic origin of T antigen is the lack of knowledge about its function. Therefore, the T antigen produced at nonpermissive temperature by the cells infected with a temperature-sensitive mutant of SV40 may be nonfunctional but may still be antigenic. Direct proof that SV40 T antigen is coded by the viral genome is lacking.

Similar criticisms can be raised about the genetic origin of TSTA. The evidence that the same TSTA is induced in SV40-transformed cells from different species suggests that it is coded by the viral genome. Its production during the virus infectious cycle also supports this contention. On the other hand, it is possible that SV40 TSTA may not be directly coded by the virus genome but may be produced as a result of derepression of the host cell genome triggered by the virus. The proponents of this theory argue that SV40 possesses enough DNA to code for only six to eight polypeptides and it appears that most of the DNA codes for viral structural proteins. By use of temperature-sensitive mutants, four nonoverlapping complementation groups of SV40 have been identified (Tegtmeyer and Ozer, 1971; Chou and Martin, 1974; Dubbs $et\ al.$, 1974). Mapping studies indicate that mutants in three of the groups can be localized in distinct regions of the SV40 genome, indicating that at least three of the SV40 genes have been identified (Lai and Nathans, 1974). Two of these genes appear to code for late viral proteins and are located in the late-transcribing region of the SV40 genome. None of the existing temperature-sensitive mutants of SV40 has been characterized with respect to its ability to express TSTA at the nonpermissive temperature. Efforts have been made to associate TSTA and other early SV40 antigens with a specific region of the viral genome (Lewis and Rowe, 1973). Nondefective adenovirus 2–SV40 hybrid viruses ($Ad2^+ND_1$ $Ad2^+ND_5$), which contain adenovirus type 2 DNA covalently linked to SV40 DNA, were used. These viruses, which produce only early SV40-specific RNA, were tested for their ability to induce SV40-specific transplantation immunity in hamsters. Only two of the hybrids ($Ad2^+ND_2$ and $Ad2^+ND_4$), which contain 32% and 43% of the SV40 genome, respectively, induced specific resistance to the transplantation of SV40 tumor cells. $Ad2^+ND_1$, $Ad2^+ND_3$, and $Ad2^+ND_5$ failed to induce resistance in hamsters. $Ad2^+ND_1$, which contains 18% of the SV40 DNA segment, was capable of inducing U antigen only, whereas $Ad2^+ND_5$, which contains 28% of the SV40 segment, did not induce any of the known SV40 specific antigens (U, T, TSTA, V). It should be emphasized that the $Ad2^+ND_5$ hybrid virus, which contains as much SV40 information as $Ad2^+ND_2$ virus, does not induce detectable SV40 TSTA, whereas $Ad2^+ND_2$ does. The failure of $Ad2^+ND_5$ to induce TSTA in hamsters may be due to a host-dependent block in transcription of the minus strand of the early SV40 region. Recent evidence obtained in our laboratory (Tevethia and

Lewis, unpublished) shows that one of the Ad2⁺-SV40 hybrid viruses (LEY) which
was unable to induce SV40 TSTA in hamsters induces TSTA in mouse cells,
indicating that host factors may be involved in the expression of early viral
information.

A portion of the early-transcribing region of the SV40 genome has been
identified as corresponding to the information required for synthesis of the
initiator protein for SV40 DNA replication (Tegtmeyer, 1972). Whether this
initiator protein corresponds to one of the early SV40 antigens remains in
question.

Since the TSTA and the S antigen(s) are both present at the cell surface, it has
been tempting to assume that the *in vitro* serological tests are actually measuring
TSTA. Tevethia *et al.* (1968*b*) demonstrated the lack of relationship between
TSTA and S antigen in certain hamster cell lines which became oncogenic after
exposure to SV40 (Diamandopoulos *et al.*. 1968). Some of these cell lines,
although positive for S antigen, were found to be negative for detectable TSTA.
The S^+ $TSTA^-$ cells were later shown to lack detectable amounts of both SV40
messenger RNA (Levin *et al.*, 1969) and SV40 DNA (Levine *et al.*, 1970), which
suggests that S antigen in these cells may not be coded by a persistent viral
genome.

Studies by Hayry and Defendi (1970) using the mixed hemadsorption test
suggested that S antigen may be a normal cell antigen which is specifically
unmasked during SV40 transformation. This conclusion was based on the
observation that after brief treatment with trypsin spontaneously oncogenic or
polyoma virus transformed cells reacted with SV40 S antibody.

Butel *et al.* (1974) have demonstrated that the hamster and mouse cells
transformed by temperature-sensitive mutants of SV40 which are defective in
early functions (*tsA*) show normal cell phenotype at the nonpermissive temperature and a transformed cell phenotype at the permissive temperature. Concomitant with the change of morphology to normal cell type at the restrictive
temperature, the presence of S antigen cannot be detected at the nonpermissive
temperature. These observations, although they do not prove that S antigen is the
product of the *A* cistron, indicate that the appearance of S antigen is dependent
on a virally determined function.

Serological evidence has been presented which supports the presence of fetal
antigens at the surface of SV40-transformed cells by use of either sera from
pregnant hamsters or anti-mouse-egg sera prepared in guinea pigs. Ting *et al.*
(1972) prepared antisera to fetal antigens by immunizing male C_3H mice with
X-irradiated syngeneic minced fetal tissue. These sera reacted with all the tumors
tested irrespective of the transforming agent. The antibody activity could be
adsorbed with any of the tumor types or with fetal tissues. Interestingly, the
antibody prepared against the tumor cells themselves in the syngeneic host
reacted specifically only with the tumor type used for immunization. Immunization with fetal tissue failed to provide protection against challenge by virus-
transformed cells. On the other hand, work carried out by Coggin and associates
indicates that the cross-reacting antigens present in embryonic cells may represent

SATVIR S.
TEVETHIA
AND
MARY J.
TEVETHIA

TSTA which is capable of inducing resistance to a challenge of SV40-transformed cells. These conclusions are based on the following observations: (1) immunization with fetal tissue from the midgestational period interrupts primary SV40 tumorigenesis in hamsters and also elicits a state of resistance in adult male hamsters against a challenge of SV40 tumor cells (Coggin *et al.*, 1971; Girardi *et al.*, 1973); (2) pregnant hamsters develop antibody which is cytostatic for the SV40 tumor cells and sensitized lymphocytes reactive with SV40 tumor cells (Coggin and Anderson, 1974); (3) the fetal antigen from hamster embryos capable of inducing tumor resistance is not species specific, as mouse and human embryo cells can also elicit resistance (Ambrose *et al.*, 1971*a*).

From a review of the data so far published, it now appears that during transformation of cells by SV40 the embryonic antigen appears at the cell surface. Indeed, more than one embryonic antigen may be present (Ting *et al.*, 1973). The data also suggest that the embryonic antigens under cetain circumstances induce a cellular immune response in the host which may delay the appearance of either primary or transplanted SV40 tumors. The published data strongly suggest, however, that the weakly immunogenic embryonic antigens are distinct from the virus-specific transplantation antigen (TSTA): (1) immunization of an adult host with either live virus or irradiated tumor cells results in the development of specific cellular immune responses to the TSTA specified by the particular virus (Zarling and Tevethia, 1973*a*); (2) specific immunity *in vivo* using irradiated tumor cells is stronger than the immunity induced by the fetal cells (Girardi *et al.*, 1973); (3) female hamsters do not develop detectable rejection response upon immunization with fetal cells whereas females can be immunized rather easily to TSTA by either the live virus or irradiated tumor cells (Girardi *et al.*, 1973). Additional evidence that TSTA and embryonic antigens are distinct comes from the work of Baldwin *et al.* (1974), who showed that both TSTA and cross-reactive embryonic antigens are present at the surface of chemically induced rat tumors but can be distinguished by the use of blocking antibody. Lymph node cells from multiparous female rats and from tumor-cell-immunized animals are cytotoxic to embryonic and tumor cells. The sera from multiparous females can abrogate the cytotoxicity of lymph node cells from multiparous females against both embryonic and tumor cells but not the activity of tumor-immune lymph node cells against tumor cells. Only the sera from tumor-immune animals can block the cytotoxicity of tumor-immune lymph node cells against tumor cells.

The evidence discussed above indicates that embryonic antigens as well as TSTA are present at the surface of SV40-transformed cells, as stated above. The genetic origin of TSTA is still unresolved. That finding that TSTA appears during the infectious cycle indicates that SV40 plays an active role in the production of TSTA. Several possibilities for the genetic origin of TSTA exist: (1) TSTA may be a host protein which is derepressed by an SV40 gene product; (2) an SV40 gene product may modify a normal cell protein, thereby converting it to TSTA; (3) TSTA may be a protein translated from a heterogenomic messenger RNA product of the integrated SV40 DNA containing both host and viral sequences; or (4) TSTA may itself be the product of an SV40 gene. The use of temperature-sensitive and deletion mutants of SV40 which are defective in the synthesis of TSTA may be needed to resolve the role of viral genome in the production, maintenance, and expression of TSTA in transformed cells.

6. Immune Response

6.1. Immune Response in Permissive Host

SV40 frequently produces latent subclinical infections in rhesus and African green monkeys (Ashkenazi and Melnick, 1962). These animals respond to the virus by producing viral neutralizing antibodies. The antibodies to virion antigens can also be detected by the complement fixation and immunofluorescence tests. In spite of the magnitude of the immune response to viral antigens in naturally infected animals, antibodies to T antigen, which is briefly synthesized during the virus replicative cycle, are not made to a significant degree. When T antigen was discovered as a nonvirion antigen present in the transformed cells, the presence of antibodies to T antigen was thought to be a way of predicting the progression of neoplasia. The lack of significant amounts of antibodies to T antigen in the naturally infected host was later shown to be dependent on the dose of infecting virus. Using the rabbit as a model animal in which the virus both grows and transforms cells, it was demonstrated (Tevethia, 1970) that infection of adult rabbits with a high dose of SV40 (1×10^{11} virus particles) resulted in the synthesis of antibodies to both T and V antigens. The synthesis of antibody to T antigen in rabbits or monkeys infected with the live virus in the absence of neoplasia indicated that the presence of T antibody cannot always be used as evidence for the presence of tumor in the host.

No experimental evidence is available as to if the permissive and semipermissive hosts develop either humoral or cellular immune responses to either the embryonic antigens or TSTA. Recently, viruses resembling SV40 in morphology have been isolated from human cases of progressive multifocal leukoencephalopathy and from the urine of patients who have undergone renal transplantation. Human develop antibodies to virion antigen only. These newly isolated viruses have oncogenic potential in hamsters and are antigenically related to SV40. The human papovaviruses grow in human cells but their association with human neoplasia has not been established.

6.2. Immune Response in Nonpermissive Host

Immune response to SV40-induced antigens in a nonpermissive host (hamster and mouse) has been studied only under experimental conditions. Hamsters inoculated with live virus within 24 h after birth develop tumors at the site of inoculation after a long latent period. Adults also develop tumors when inoculated with a large dose of virus intravenously. Mice have not yet been shown to develop tumors by SV40 even under immunosuppressed conditions. Hamsters inoculated as newborns with live SV40 will develop antibodies to viral antigens

198
SATVIR S.
TEVETHIA
AND
MARY J.
TEVETHIA

which can be measured by the virus neutralization, immunofluorescence, and complement fixation tests. The animals before tumor development will synthesize antibodies to SV40-specific surface antigens. These antibodies have been demonstrated in the tumor-resistant animals by the indirect immunofluorescence test (Tevethia et al., 1968a) and by an in vivo cytostasis test (Ambrose et al., 1971b). Adult animals (hamster and mice) immunized with either live SV40 or SV40-transformed cells will also develop antibodies to specific surface antigens which can be measured by the in vitro colony inhibition test (Tevethia et al., 1970), cytotoxic test (Wright and Law, 1971), and isotopic antiglobulin test (Ting and Herberman, 1971). The antibodies to S antigen cannot be demonstrated in tumor-bearing animals.

Animals bearing tumors induced either by SV40 or by virus-free SV40 tumor cells develop antibodies to intranuclear T antigen. The antibody activity to T antigen was demonstrated to be located in the γ_2 fraction of 7 S immunoglobulins (Tevethia, 1967). Animals bearing tumors invariably develop antibody to T antigen. The amount of antibody synthesized does not seem to correlate with the tumor mass. Occasionally, antibodies to T antigen cannot be demonstrated in animals bearing large tumors. In a carefully carried out study, it was demonstrated (Lausch et al., 1970) that hamsters bearing tumors induced by a particular line of SV40 tumor cells did not develop antibodies to T antigen during the entire course of tumor development. This immunological unresponsiveness to T antigen was shown to be due to the immunological tolerance to T antigen. This tolerance could be terminated by tumor resection and reimmunization with tumor homogenate with Freund's complete adjuvant. In the nonpermissive host, the presence of high levels of T antibody can be used as an indication of the growing neoplasm of SV40 etiology. However, the presence of low amounts of antibody to T antigen has also been detected in hamsters in the absence of visible tumor (Diamandopoulos and McLane, 1974).

Animals undergoing primary viral carcinogenesis or adult animals inoculated with the virus or SV40 tumor or transformed cells develop a specific cellular immune reactivity to SV40-specific transplantation antigen. Such animals are resistant to transplantation of syngeneic SV40 tumor cells (See Butel et al., 1972). Hamsters undergoing primary SV40 tumorigenesis when immunized during the latent period with irradiated cells will not develop tumors (Girardi, 1965; Tevethia et al., 1968b). Further, virus-inoculated thymectomized animals cannot be immunized during the latent period with SV40-transformed cells carrying SV40 TSTA (Girardi and Roosa, 1967). The involvement of lymphoid cells in SV40-induced tumor resistance was shown by demonstrating the ability of peritoneal exudate cells from tumor-immune mice to neutralize the tumor-forming capacity of syngeneic SV40 tumor cells (Coggin et al., 1967; Zarling and Tevethia, 1973a). Anti-hamster-thymocyte serum (ATS), a potent suppressor of cellular immunity, prevented sensitization of hamsters to SV40 TSTA when administered during the period of virus immunization (Tevethia et al., 1968c). The failure to become sensitized to TSTA was demonstrated by the fact that treated animals were unable to reject a challenge of SV40-transformed cells. The administration of ATS to hamsters which developed tumors had no effect on the synthesis of humoral antibody to SV40 T antigen. In addition, spontaneous regression of primary tumors induced by SV40 in hamsters has been observed (Tevethia *et al.*, 1968a; Deichman, 1969).

Considerable progress has been made toward understanding the nature of cellular immune response of the host to SV40 TSTA, which leads to tumor cell rejection. To meet this goal, the SV40 tumor system in inbred mice was chosen, as mouse lymphoid cells have been characterized well and the basic biology of immune response is well understood. Since SV40 does not produce tumors in mice, inbred BALB/c cells were transformed *in vitro*. These *in vitro* transformed cells possess SV40 T antigen and TSTA but are free of either the infectious virus or viral antigens and produce progressively growing tumors in adult syngeneic mice after prolonged cultivation *in vitro* (Tevethia and McMillan, 1974). These cells are both immunosensitive and immunogenic. SV40 TSTA can be isolated from the cell surface, the activity of which can be measured by the macrophage migration inhibition test (Blasecki and Tevethia, 1973). Syngeneic adult mice inoculated with one such a line of SV40 cells (Zarling and Tevethia, 1973a), before and after tumor development, will develop sensitized lymphocytes which are capable of neutralizing the tumor-producing capacity *in vivo* of both mouse and hamster cells transformed by SV40. Kinetic studies showed that the immune lymphocytes appear between 5 and 10 days after tumor cell inoculation. In animals bearing tumors induced by one such cell line (TU-5), sensitized lymphocytes can be demonstrated even when the tumor is growing progressively. The animals bearing a subcutaneous tumor will develop concomitant immunity and are able to reject specifically a transplant of SV40 tumor cells at another site. This concomitant immunity develops even before the tumor becomes palpable (Zarling and Tevethia, 1973a). The presence of sensitized lymphocytes in a tumor-bearing host, however, seems to be dependent on properties determined by the tumor cells since the sensitized lymphocytes in syngeneic BALB/c mice bearing tumors induced by another line of SV40-transformed cells (VLM) cannot be demonstrated at any stage of tumor growth. The sensitized lymphocytes can, however, be demonstrated in animals whose tumors have been removed by surgery. The lymphocytes from animals bearing tumors induced by VLM cells can be made reactive to SV40 tumor cells by either culturing them *in vitro* for 4–5 days or treating them with very low concentrations of proteolytic enzymes, suggesting that the lymphocytes from tumor-bearing animals may actually be sensitized but may be blocked, probably by soluble SV40 TSTA (Blasecki and Tevethia, unpublished results). This point was further confirmed by use of the macrophage migration inhibition test to measure the cellular immune response throughout tumorigenesis of mice inoculated with VLM cells. A specific cellular immune response can be demonstrated in mice bearing barely palpable tumors. The mice become nonreactive until the tumor is removed by surgery. Peritoneal exudate (PE) cells from tumor-bearing animals mixed in equal quantity with PE cells from immune animals will abrogate the reactivity of the latter in the migration test. This abrogation is specific in nature as the PE cells from mice bearing

200

SATVIR S.
TEVETHIA
AND
MARY J.
TEVETHIA

methylcholanthrene-induced tumors had no effect on the immune reactivity of SV40-immune PE cells in the migration inhibition test. PE cells from the tumor-bearing animals when cultured *in vitro* for 5 days not only lost their blocking activity but also responded positively in the migration test, suggesting that the lymphocytes from tumor-bearing animals are probably blocked by the soluble antigen which can be removed by culturing *in vitro* (Blasecki and Tevethia, 1974).

Lymphocytes which react with the tumor cells in the tumor cell neutralization test are thymus-derived (T) lymphocytes. T lymphocytes are also required for generation of sensitized lymphocytes capable of inhibiting SV40 tumor cells *in vivo*. This was indicated by the observation that mice lacking T-cell function (thymectomized, lethally irradiated, and bone marrow reconstituted) cannot be immunized to SV40 TSTA and the sensitized lymphocytes cannot be demonstrated in these mice. In addition, the immune reactivity of lymphocytes from animals specifically immune to SV40 TSTA can be abolished by prior treatment with anti-θ serum and complement, which selectively kills T cells. Also, lymphocyte populations depleted of B cells can still inhibit tumor development by SV40 tumor cells *in vivo* (Tevethia *et al.*, 1974).

There is now compelling evidence that T lymphocytes may not directly kill SV40 tumor cells *in vivo* but may actually recruit uncommitted bone marrow cells, probably macrophages, for killing of syngeneic SV40-transformed BALB/c tumor cells *in vivo*. This conclusion (Zarling and Tevethia, 1973b) is based on the following observations: (1) T lymphocytes in an *in vitro* microcytotoxicity assay did not cause a sufficient killing of syngeneic SV40 tumor cells to explain tumor destruction *in vivo* (Tevethia and Tevethia, unpublished data); (2) a low number of sensitized lymphocytes when mixed with syngeneic SV40 tumor cells in a 1 : 1 ratio and inoculated into young BALB/c mice prevented tumor formation by the SV40 tumor cells; (3) irradiated, sensitized lymphocytes, which were unable to replicate, inhibited tumor growth; (4) tumor growth inhibition by the immune lymphoid cells was less efficient in irradiated adult and in newborn mice; (5) bone marrow cells, after differentiation in irradiated (700 R) syngeneic hosts, provided the cells necessary for tumor cell neutralization by immune lymphoid cells; (6) tumor cell neutralization by immune lymphoid cells was diminished in animals pretreated with silica, a specific macrophage toxin.

7. Role of Antigens in Neoplasia

Cells derived from tumors induced by viruses, chemical carcinogens, and physical agents, and from human tumors of unknown etiology, synthesize macromolecules which normal adult cells do not. Only those macromolecules which are antigenic in the autochthonous host and to which the host reacts by making either a humoral or a cellular immune response take part in immunoregulation of tumor growth. Specific antigens in tumor cells, depending on their location in the cells, will determine the tumor behavior *in vivo*, depending on the nature and magnitude of immune response being elicited by the host against these antigens. Viruses differ from chemical carcinogens in that a particular virus always induces a cross-reacting antigen in tumor cells regardless of the species of animal. This virus specificity of induced antigens can be used for linking a particular virus to certain cancers.

The antigens located within the cell, such as T antigen in the nucleus of the transformed cell, do not play any role in the immunological modulation of the growth of SV40-induced tumors. TSTA by virtue of its location at the cell surface of SV40-transformed cells does play a very significant role in the progression and repression of virus-induced neoplasia. Animals receiving virus as newborns will ultimately develop tumors with a long latent period. However, inoculation of virus into weanling animals will not lead to the production of tumors at the site of inoculation.

The lack of tumor development in adult animals or tumor development in immunosuppressed adults upon virus administration indicates that an antigen (TSTA) is synthesized in the transformed cells which does play an important role in the rejection of an antigenic tumor by inducing specific cellular immune response in the host. Recently, we have obtained evidence for the appearance of TSTA *in vitro* at the surface of mouse cells abortively infected with SV40. Normal lymphocytes can be specifically sensitized *in vitro* by cultivating them on the infected monolayers. The sensitized lymphocytes will inhibit the growth of SV40-transformed cells *in vivo*, indicating that the sequence of events observed *in vitro* actually takes place *in vivo* upon virus inoculation (Tevethia and McMillan, 1973).

Why, then, do animals inoculated at birth with SV40 go on to develop tumors after a long period, in spite of a cellular immune response? The original suggestion that newborn animals inoculated with SV40 would develop immunological tolerance to SV40 TSTA, thereby allowing the emergence and eventual growth of the tumor cells, can be ruled out, since primary carcinogenesis can be aborted by immunizing the animals either with the virus or with SV40-transformed cells during the latent period (Girardi, 1965; Tevethia *et al.*, 1968b). Also, a specific cellular immune response to SV40 TSTA can be demonstrated in these hamsters prior to tumor development (Blasecki and Tevethia, 1973). Several explanations have been offered for the appearance of tumors in spite of a cellular immune response to these tumors: (1) The immune response may simply lag behind tumor development. This argument, although attractive, cannot explain the tumor induction by SV40 when a cellular immune response can be detected long before a detectable tumor is present. Newborn mice inoculated with SV40 will develop sensitized lymphocytes by 21 days of age. (2) The hypothesis of immunostimulation put forward by Prehn (1972) proposes that a weak immune response to an antigenic tumor may be stimulating whereas a strong immune response would lead to tumor rejection. Prehn (1972) demonstrated that a low number of sensitized lymphocytes when mixed with syngeneic tumor cells and inoculated into X-irradiated animals actually stimulated the growth of the tumor in comparison with the effect of normal lymphocytes. Higher numbers of sensitized lymphocytes were inhibitory to the tumor. Additionally, it

202

SATVIR S.
TEVETHIA
AND
MARY J.
TEVETHIA

has been argued that nude mice, which lack T cell function, are no less resistant to tumorigenesis by known biological and chemical carcinogens than are normal mice. However, contrary evidence has been presented which demonstrates that tumors induced by murine sarcoma virus do not regress in nude mice, but do in immunocompetent littermates (Stutman, personal communication). Nude mice have also been shown to be very susceptible to polyoma virus oncogenesis (Allison, personal communication). (3) One probable reason for the growth of tumors may be the presence of blocking factors in the sera of animals undergoing carcinogenesis. The blocking of the cellular immune response may occur either at the target cell level or at the level of T lymphocytes.

Immune response to TSTA may also affect the behavior of tumor cells *in vivo*. The tumor cells may develop immunoresistance. In this case, tumor cells, although themselves immunogenic, are not rejected by the immunized host. Cells derived from primary SV40 tumors allowed to grow for prolonged periods and the cells derived from metastasis were claimed to have lost TSTA since they were not rejected by the SV40-immunized hamsters (Deichman and Kluchareva, 1966). It was later demonstrated (Tevethia *et al.*, 1971) that such tumor cells possessed TSTA and could immunize hamsters against a challenge of immunosensitive SV40 tumor cells but could not be rejected by the immunized hamsters.

The presence of TSTA in virus-induced tumor cells offers an excellent opportunity to control the growth of antigenic tumors by manipulating the immune response to these antigens. SV40 produces tumors only in the hamster, which is a nonpermissive host. No tumors have been reported in the natural host in which the virus replicates. This apparent nononcogenity of the virus in its natural host may be due to the fact that SV40 induces TSTA in infected cells to which the host becomes sensitized. The infected cells eventually release virus progeny and die. Subsequently, each time the progeny viruses infect cells, synthesis of TSTA occurs and the cellular immune response of the host is initiated and potentiated. This initiation and potentiation of the host response to TSTA may be responsible for eliminating potentially transformed cells. The phenomenon may be applicable to DNA viruses such as herpesviruses, which are both oncogenic and permissive in the natural host. Experimental evidence does exist that monkey cells infected with SV40 synthesize SV40-specific TSTA, the activity of which can be demonstrated by both *in vivo* and *in vitro* tests (Girardi and Defendi, 1970; Tevethia and Tevethia, unpublished results), and which may explain the apparent nononcogenicity of SV40 virus in monkeys.

8. Conclusion

Virus-specified antigens have several functions in studies of viral carcinogenesis. The presence of specific intracellular antigens in tumor cells such as the intranuclear tumor or T antigen and the appearance of the identical antigen in the virus productive cycle indicate that the transformation whether *in vitro* or *in vivo* was caused by a particular oncogenic virus. The immune response to T antigen in the tumor-bearing host is also helpful in following viral oncogenesis. The synthesis of T antigen whether in permissive or nonpermissive cells has served as a marker for early viral functions.

Cells transformed by DNA tumor viruses also possess specific antigens at the cell surface. These antigen(s) can be detected by the classical transplantation rejection test *in vivo* and by *in vitro* techniques which measure cellular immune reaction. Serological tests have also been used to measure specific cell surface antigens. Among the cell surface antigens, TSTA is the most important since it mediates the development of cellular immune response in the host which leads to the rejection of developing tumors. TSTA also appears in the virus cytolytic cycle, indicating that the transformation of cells is not a prerequisite for its appearance.

Besides TSTA and other specific surface antigens, transformed cells contain cross-reacting embryonic antigens. Embryonic antigens under certain circumstances can act as weak transplantation antigens. The existence of specific transplantation antigens and embryonic antigens which induce tumor immunity offers an excellent opportunity for immunoregulation of virus-induced tumors. However, in order to exploit specific surface antigens for immunotherapeutic purposes, it is essential that we understand the nature and genetic origin of these antigens. If the antigens which induce a rejection response in the syngeneic host are found to be specified by cellular genes rather than by viral genes, then efforts may be directed toward finding means by which these antigens can be derepressed or their expression on the tumor cells increased. A combined genetic, biochemical, and immunological approach is needed to understand the biology of virus-specific antigens.

ACKNOWLEDGMENTS

This study was suported in part by research grants CA 14939 and CA 12924 from the National Cancer Institute, National Institutes of Health, Bethesda, Maryland. The authors sincerely thank Ms. Beth Gerry for excellent secretarial help.

9. *References*

ALLISON, A. C., AND LAW, L. W., 1968, Effects of antilymphocyte serum on virus oncogenesis, *Proc. Soc. Exp. Biol. Med.* **127:**207.

ALLISON, A. C., CHESTERMAN, F. C., AND BARON, S., 1967, Induction of tumors in adult hamsters with simian virus 40, *J. Natl. Cancer Inst.* **38:**567.

ALSTEIN, A. D., 1967, Oncogenic and transforming activity of hydroxylamine-inactivated SV40 virus, *Virology* **33:**746.

AMBROSE, K. R., ANDERSON, N. G., AND COGGIN, J. H., 1971*a*, Interruption of SV40 oncogenesis with human foetal cells, *Nature (London)* **233:**194.

AMBROSE, K. R., ANDERSON, N. G., AND COGGIN, J. H., 1971*b*, Cytostatic antibody and SV40 tumor immunity in hamsters, *Nature (London)* **233:**321.

204

SATVIR S.
TEVETHIA
AND
MARY J.
TEVETHIA

ASHKENAZI, A., AND MELNICK, J. L., 1962, Induced latent infection of monkeys with vaculating SV40 papovavirus in kidneys and urine, *Proc. Soc. Exp. Biol. Med.* **111**:367.

BALDWIN, R. W., EMBLETON, M. J., PRICE, M. R., AND VOSE, B. M., 1974, Embryonic antigen expression on experimental rat tumors, *Transplant. Rev.* **20**:77.

BLACK, P. H., ROWE, W. P., TURNER, H. C., AND HUEBNER, R. J., 1963, A specific complement-fixing antigen present in SV40 tumor and transformed cells, *Proc. Natl. Acad. Sci. U.S.A.* **50**:1148.

BLASECKI, J. W., AND TEVETHIA, S. S., 1973, *In vitro:* assay of cellular immunity to tumor specific antigen(s) of virus-induced tumors by macrophage migration inhibition, *J. Immunol.* **110**:590.

BLASECKI, J. W., AND TEVETHIA, S. S., 1975, Cell mediated immunity to tumors induced by SV40 transformed cells. I. *In vitro* studies on the immune response of lymphoid cells from tumor bearing mice, *J. Immunol.* **114**:244.

BUTEL, J. S., GUENTZEL, M. J., AND RAPP, F., 1969, Variants of defective simian papovavirus 40 (PARA) characterized by cytoplasmic localization of simian papovavirus 40 tumor antigen, *J. Virol.* **4**:632.

BUTEL, J. S., TEVETHIA, S. S., AND NACHTIGAL, M., 1971, Malignant transformation *in vitro* by "nononcogenic" variants of defective SV40 (PARA). *J. Immunol.* **106**:969.

BUTEL, J. S., TEVETHIA, S. S., AND MELNICK, J. L., 1972, Oncogenicity and cell transformation by papovavirus SV40: The role of viral genome, *Adv. Cancer Res.* **15**:1.

BUTEL, J. S., BRUGGE, J. S., AND NOONAN, C. A., 1974, Transformation of primate and rodent cells by temperature sensitive mutants of SV40, *Cold Spring Harbor Symp. Quant. Biol.* **39:** in press.

CARROLL, R. B., HAGER, L., AND DULBECCO, R., 1974, Simian virus 40 T antigen binds to DNA, *Proc. Natl. Acad. Sc:. U.S.A.* **71**:3754.

CHOU, J. Y., AND MARTIN, R. B., 1974, Complementation analysis of simian virus 40 mutants, *J. Virol* **13**:1101.

COGGIN, J. H., AND AMBROSE, K. R., 1969, A rapid *in vivo* assay for SV40 tumor immunity in hamsters, *Proc. Soc. Exp. Biol.* **130**:246.

COGGIN, J. H., AND ANDERSON, N. G., 1974, Cancer, differentiation and embryonic antigens: Some central problems, *Adv. Cancer Res.* **19**:105.

COGGIN, J. H., LARSON, V. M., AND HILLEMAN, M. R., 1967, Immunologic responses in hamsters to homologous tumor antigens measured *in vivo* and *in vitro, Proc. Soc. Exp. Biol. Med.* **124**:1295.

COGGIN, J. H., AMBROSE, K. R., BELLAMY, B. B., AND ANDERSON, N. G., 1971, Tumor immunity in hamsters immunized with fetal tissue, *J. Immunol.* **107**:520.

COLLINS, J. J., BLACK, P. H., STROSBERG, A. D., HABER, E., AND BLOCH, K. J., 1974, Transformation by simian virus 40 of spleen cells from a hyperimmune-rabbit: Evidence for synthesis of immunoglobulin by the transformed cells, *Proc. Natl. Acad. Sci. U.S.A.* **71**:260.

DEFENDI, V., AND JENSEN, F., 1967, Oncogenicity by DNA tumor viruses: Enhancement after ultraviolet and cobalt-60 radiations, *Science* **157**:703.

DEICHMAN, G. I., 1969, Immunological aspects of carcinogenesis by deoxyrubonucleic acid tumor viruses, *Adv. Cancer Res.* **12**:101.

DEICHMAN, G. I., AND KLUCHAREVA, T. E., 1966, Loss of transplantation antigen in primary simian virus 40 tumors and their metastasis, *J. Natl. Cancer Inst.* **36**:647.

DEINHARDT, F. W., FALK, L. A., AND WOLF, L. G., 1974, Simian herpes viruses and neoplasia, *Adv. Cancer Res.* **19**:167.

DEL VILLANO, B. C., AND DEFENDI, V., 1973, Characterization of SV40 T antigen, *Virology* **51**:34.

DIAMANDOPOULOS, G. T., 1973, Induction of lymphocytic leukemia, lymphosarcoma, reticulum cell sarcoma and osteogenic sarcoma in the Syrian golden hamster by oncogenic DNA simian virus 40, *J. Natl. Cancer Inst.* **50**:1347.

DIAMANDOPOULOS, G. T., AND MCLANE, M. F., 1974, Development of antibodies to viral and tumor antigens before tumor induction, *J. Immunol.* **13**:1450.

DIAMANDOPOULOS, G. T., TEVETHIA, S. S., RAPP, F., AND, ENDERS, J. F., 1968, Development of S and T antigens and oncogenicity in hamster embryonic cell lines exposed to SV40, *Virology* **34**:331.

DOUGHERTY, R. M., AND DISTEFANO, H. S., 1974, Isolation and characterization of a papovavirus from human urine, *Proc. Soc. Exp. Biol. Med.* **146**:481.

DRAPKIN, M. S., APPELLA, E., AND LAW, L. W., 1974, Immunogenic properties of a soluble tumor specific transplantation antigen induced by simian virus 40, *J. Natl. Cancer Inst.* **52**:259.

DUBBS, D. R., RACHMELER, M., AND KIT, S., 1974, Recombination between temperature-sensitive mutants of simian virus 40, *Virology* **57**:161.

DUFF, R., AND RAPP, F., 1970, Quantitative characteristics of the transformation of hamster cells by PARA (defective simian virus 40)-adenovirus 7, *J. Virol.* **5**:568.

EDDY, B., 1964, Simian virus 40 (SV40); an oncogenic virus, *Proc. Exp. Tumor Res.* **4**:1.

ESTES, M. K., HUANG, E. S., AND PAGANO, J. S., 1971, Structural polypeptides of simian virus 40, *J. Virol.* **7**:635.

GARDNER, S. D., FIELD, A. M., COLEMAN, D. V., AND HULME, B., 1971, New human papovavirus (B.K.) isolated from urine after renal transplantation, *Lancet* **1**:1253.

GIRARDI, A. J., 1965, Prevention of SV40 virus oncogenesis in hamsters. I. Tumor resistance induced by human cells transformed by SV40, *Proc. Natl. Acad. Sci. U.S.A.* **54**:445.

GIRARDI, A. J., 1967, Tumor resistance and tumor enahancement with SV40 virus-induced tumors, in: *Germinal Centers in Immune Responses* (H. Cottier, N. Odartchenko, R. Schindler, and C. C. Congdon, eds.), ph. 422–427, Springer, New York.

GIRARDI, A. J., AND DEFENDI, V., 1970, Induction of SV40 transplantation antigen (Tr Ag) during the lytic cycle, *Virology* **42**:688.

GIRARDI, A. J., AND ROOSA, R. A., 1967, Prevention of SV40 virus oncogenesis in hamsters. II. The effect of thymectomy on induction of tumor resistance by SV40 transformed human cells, *J. Immunol.* **99**:1217.

GIRARDI, A. J., REPPUCCI, P., DIERLAM, P., RUTALA, W., AND COGGIN, J. H., 1973, Prevention of simian virus 40 tumors by hamster fetal tissue: Influence of parity status of donor females on immunogenicity of fetal tissue and on immune cell cytotoxicity, *Proc. Natl. Acad. Sci. U.S.A.* **70**:183.

GREEN, M., 1970, Oncogenic viruses, *Ann. Rev. Biochem.* **39**:701.

HAYRY, P., AND DEFENDI, V., 1968, Use of mixed hemagglutination technique in detection of virus-induced antigen(s) on SV40 transformed cell surface, *Virology* **36**:317.

HAYRY, P., AND DEFENDI, V., 1970, Surface antigen(s) of SV40 transformed tumor cells, *Virology* **41**:22.

KHERA, K. S., ASHKENAZI, A., RAPP, F., AND MELNICK, J. L., 1963, Immunity in hamsters to cells transformed *in vitro* and *in vivo* by SV40: Tests for antigenic relationship among papovavirus, *J. Immunol.* **91**:604.

KIT, S., KURIMURA, T., AND DUBBS, D. R., 1969, Transplantable mouse tumor line induced by injection of SV40 transformed mouse kidney cells, *Int. J. Cancer* **4**:384.

KLEIN, G., 1971, Immunological aspects of Burkitts, lymphoma, *Adv. Immunol.* **14**:187.

KLUCHAREVA, T. E., SHACHANINA, K. L., BELOVA, S., CHIBISOVA, V., AND DEICHMAN, G. I., 1967, Use of immunofluorescence for detection of specific membrane antigens in simian virus 40-infected nontransformed cells, *J. Natl. Cancer Inst.* **39**:825.

LAI, C., AND NATHANS, D., 1974, Mapping temperature-sensitive mutants of simian virus 40: Rescue of mutants by fragments of viral DNA, *Virology* **60**:461.

LAUSCH, R. N., TEVETHIA, S. S., AND RAPP, F., 1970, Evidence for tolerance to SV40 tumor antigen in hamsters bearing PARA-adenovirus 12 tumor transplants, *J. Immunol.* **104**:305.

LEVIN, M. J., OXMAN, M. N., DIAMANDOPOULOS, G. T., LEVINE, A. S., HENRY, P. H., AND ENDERS, J. F., 1969, Virus-specific nucleic acids in SV40 exposed hamster embryo cell lines: Correlation with S and T antigens, *Proc. Natl. Acad. Sci. U.S.A.* **62**:589.

LEVINE, A. S., OXMAN, M. N., HENRY, P. H., LEVIN, J. J., DIAMANDOPOULOS, G. T., AND ENDERS, J. F., 1970, Virus-specific deoxyribonucleic acid in simian virus 40 exposed hamster cells: Correlation with S and T antigens, *J. Virol.* **6**:199.

LEWIS, A. M., AND ROWE, W. P., 1971, Studies on nondefective adenovirus simian virus 40 hybrid viruses. I. A newly characterized simian virus 40 antigen induced by the $Ad2^+ND_1$ virus, *J. Virol.* **7**:189.

LEWIS, A. M., AND ROWE, W. P., 1973, Studies of nondefective adenovirus 2-simian virus 40 hybrid viruses. VIII. Association of simian virus 40 transplantation antigen with a specific region of the early viral genome, *J. Virol.* **12**:836.

METZGAR, R. S., AND OLEINICK, S. R., 1968, The study of normal and malignant cell antigens by mixed agglutination, *Cancer Res.* **28**:1366.

OSBORNE, M., AND WEBER, K., 1973, Abstract, Cold Spring Harbor Tumor Virus Meeting.

OXMAN, M. N., AND BLACK, P. H., 1966, Inhibition of SV40 T antigen formation by interferon, *Proc. Natl. Acad. Sci. U.S.A.* **55**:1133.

PADGETT, B. L., WALKER, D. L., ZURHEIN, G. M., ECKROADE, R. J., AND DELSEL, B. H., 1971, Cultivation of papova-like virus from human brain with progressive multifocal leukoencephalopathy, *Lancet* **1**:1257.

POPE, J. H., AND ROWE, W. P., 1964, Detection of specific antigen in SV40 transformed cells by immunofluorescence, *J. Exp. Med.* **120**:121.

PREHN, R., 1972, The immune reaction as a stimulator of tumor growth, *Science* **176**:170.

SATVIR S. TEVETHIA AND MARY J. TEVETHIA

RABSON, A. S., O'CONNER, G. T., KIRSCHSTEIN, R. L., AND BRANIGAN, V. J., 1962, Papillary ependymomas produced in *Rattus (Mastomys) natalensis* inoculated with vacuolating virus (SV40), *J. Natl. Cancer Inst.* **29:**765.

RAPP, F., 1973, The PARA-adenoviruses, *Proc. Exp. Tumor Res.* **18:**104.

RAPH, F., 1974, Herpes viruses and cancer, *Adv. Cancer Res.* **19:**268.

RAPP, F., BUTEL, J. S., AND MELNICK, J. L., 1964a, Virus induced intranuclear antigen in cells transformed by papovavirus SV40, *Proc. Soc. Exp. Biol.* **116:**1131.

RAPP, F., KITAHARA, T., BUTEL, J. S., AND MELNICK, J. L., 1964b, Synthesis of SV40 tumor antigen during replication of simian papovavirus (SV40) *Proc. Natl. Acad. Sci. U.S.A.* **52:**1138.

RAPH, F., BUTEL, J. S., FELDMAN, L. A., KITAHARA, T., AND MELNICK, J. L., 1965, Differential effects of inhibitors on the steps leading to the formation of SV40 tumor and virus antigens, *J. Exp. Med.* **121:**935.

RAPP, F., TEVETHIA, S. S., RAWLS, W. E., AND MELNICK, J. L., 1967, Production of antibodies to papovavirus SV40 tumor antigen in African green monkeys, *Proc. Soc. Exp. Biol. Med.* **125:**794.

RIGGS, J. L., TAKEMORI, N., AND LENNETTE, E. H., 1968, Cross reactivity between T antigens of adenoviral immunotypes of proved and currently unproved oncogenic potential, *J. Immunol.* **100:**348.

ROBB, J. A., TEGTMEYER, P. ISHIKAWA, A., STARK, G. R., AND OZER, H. L., 1974, Antigenic phenotypes and complementation groups of temperature-sensitive mutants of simian virus 40, *Virology* **13:**677.

SAMBROOK, J., 1973, Transformation by polyoma virus and simian virus 40, *Adv. Cancer Res.* **16:**141.

TAKEMOTO, K. K., AND MULLARKEY, M. F., 1973, Human papovaviruses, BK strain: Biological studies including antigenic relationship to simian virus 40, *J. Virol.* **12:**625.

TAKEMOTO, K. K., TING, R. C. Y., OZER, H. L., AND FABISCH, P., 1968, Establishment of a cell line from an inbred mouse strain for viral transformation studies: Simian virus 40 transformation and tumor production, *J. Natl. Cancer Inst.* **41:**1401.

TEGTMEYER, P., 1972, Simian virus 40 deoxyribonucleic acid synthesis: The viral replicon, *J. Virol.* **10:**591.

TEGTMEYER, P., AND OZER, H. L., 1971, Temperature-sensitive mutants of simian virus 40: Infection of permissive cells, *J. Virol.* **8:**516.

TEVETHIA, S. S., 1967, Characterization of hamster antibody reacting with papovavirus SV40 tumor antigen, *J. Immunol.* **98:**1257.

TEVETHIA, S. S., 1970, Immune response of rabbits to purified papovavirus SV40, *J. Immunol.* **104:**72.

TEVETHIA, S. S., 1974, Evidence for virus-specific transplantation antigen in cells of lymphoid neoplasms induced by papovavirus SV40, *Int. J. Cancer* **13:**494.

TEVETHIA, S. S., AND MCMILLAN, V. L., 1973, *In vitro* induction of tumor specific transplantation antigen in mouse cells abortively infected with papovavirus SV40, *Proc. Am. Assoc. Cancer Res.* **13:**57.

TEVETHIA, S. S., AND MCMILLAN, V. L., 1974, Acquisition of malignant potential by SV40 transformed cells: Relationship to type C viral antigen expression, *Intervirology* (in press).

TEVETHIA, S. S., KATZ, M., AND RAPP, F., 1965, New surface antigen in cells transformed by simian papovavirus SV40, *Proc. Soc. Exp. Biol. (N.Y.)* **119:**896.

TEVETHIA, S. S., COUVILLON, L. A., AND RAPP, F., 1968a, Development in hamsters of antibodies against surface antigens present in cells transformed by papovavirus SV40, *J. Immunol.* **100:**358.

TEVETHIA, S. S., DIAMANDOPOULOS, G. T., RAPP, F., AND ENDERS, J. F., 1968b, Lack of relationship between virus-specific and transplantation antigens in hamster cells transformed by simian papovavirus SV40, *J. Immunol.* **101:**1192.

TEVETHIA, S. S., DREESMAN, G. R., LAUSCH, R. N., AND RAPP, F., 1968c, Effect of anti-hamster thymocyte serum on papovavirus DV40 induced transplantation immunity, *J. Immunol.* **101:**1105.

TEVETHIA, S. S., CROUCH, N. A., MELNICK, J. L., AND RAPP, F., 1970, Detection of specific surface antigens by colony inhibition in cells transformed by papovavirus SV40, *Int. J. Cancer* **5:**176.

TEVETHIA, S. S., MCMILLAN, V. L., KAPLAN, P. M., AND BUSHONG, S. C., 1971, Variation in immunosensitivity of SV40 transformed hamster cells, *J. Immunol.* **106:**1295.

TEVETHIA, S. S., BLASECKI, J. W., WANECK, G., AND GOLDSTEIN, A., 1974, Requirement of thymus derived θ positive lymphocytes for rejection of DNA virus (SV40) tumors in mice, *J. Immunol.* **113:**1417.

TING, C. C., AND HERBERMAN, R. B., 1971, Detection of tumor-specific antigen of simian virus 40 induced tumors by the isotopic antiglobulin technique, *Int. J. Cancer* **7:**499.

TING, C. C., LARVIN, D. H., SHIV, G., AND HERBERMAN, R. B., 1972, Expression of fetal antigens in tumor cells, *Proc. Natl. Acad. Sci. U.S.A.* **69:**1664.

TING, C. C., RODRIGUES, D., AND HERBERMAN, R. B., 1973, Expression of fetal antigens and tumor specific antigens in SV40 transformed cells. II. Tumor transplantation studies, *Int. J. Cancer* **12:**519.

TODARO, G. J., AND HUEBNER, R. J., 1972, The viral oncogene hypothesis: New evidence, *Proc. Natl. Acad. Sci. U.S.A.* **69:**1009.

UCHIDA, S., AND WATANABE, S., 1968, Tumorigenicity of the antigen-forming defective virions of simian virus 40, *Virology* **35:**166.

WALKER, D. L., PADGETT, B. L., ZU RHEIN, G. M., ALBERT, A. E., AND MARSH, R. F., 1973, Human papovavirus (JC): Induction of brain tumors in hamsters, *Science* **181:**674.

WEINER, L. P., HERNDON, R. M., NARAYAN, O., AND JOHNSON, R. T., 1972, Further studies of a simian virus 40 like virus isolated from human brain, *J. Virol.* **10:**147.

WRIGHT, P. W., AND LAW, L. W., 1971, Quantitative *in vitro* measurement of simian virus 40 tumor-specific antigens, *Proc. Natl. Acad. Sci. U.S.A.* **68:**973.

ZARLING, J. M., AND TEVETHIA, S. S., 1973a, Transplantation immunity to simian virus 40 transformed cells in tumor bearing mice. I. Development of cellular immunity to simian virus 40 tumor specific transplantation antigens during tumorigenesis by transformed cells, *J. Natl. Cancer Inst.* **50:**137.

ZARLING, J. M., AND TEVETHIA, S. S., 1973b, Transplantation immunity to simian virus 40 transformed cells in tumor bearing mice. II. Evidence for macrophage participation of the effector level of tumor cell rejection, *J. Natl. Cancer Inst.* **50:**149.

7

Immunobiology of Chemically Induced Tumors

Michael R. Price and Robert W. Baldwin

1. Introduction

A prerequisite to the analysis of cellular and humoral immune responses to neoantigens associated with chemically induced tumors is that their occurrence and specificity must be adequately defined. This has been achieved with a number of experimental tumor models, and, as indicated in a previous volume of this series, a major conclusion is that transformation by chemical carcinogens frequently results in the expression of neoantigens which function to promote tumor rejection reactions, although this is by no means a universal feature of chemical neoplasia (Baldwin and Price, Vol. 1, Chap. 12). Tumor-associated rejection antigens are, however, almost uniformly characterized by a high degree of specificity so that immunity to transplanted tumors in syngeneic hosts is directed only against cells of the immunizing tumor. There have proved to be very few exceptions to this, and individually specific neoantigens have even been demonstrated on cells transformed *in vitro* by chemical carcinogens (see Baldwin and Price, Vol. 1, Chap. 12, for further discussion of this point). One disparity recently observed has been with murine bladder tumors induced with 3-methylcholanthrene (MCA). With these, cross-reactivity was demonstrated by *in vitro* lymphocytotoxicity assays, although in tumor rejection tests individually distinct neoantigens were revealed (Taranger *et al.*, 1972; Wahl *et al.*, 1974).

Michael R. Price and Robert W. Baldwin • Cancer Research Campaign Laboratories, University of Nottingham, Nottingham, England.

210
MICHAEL R.
PRICE
AND
ROBERT W.
BALDWIN

Comparably, with carcinogen-induced and spontaneous rat mammary carcinomas, lymph node cells from tumor-bearing animals were cross-reactive in cytotoxicity tests (Baldwin and Embleton, 1974). However, tumor rejection reactions are not regularly observed with these examples, and the targets for the lymphocytotoxic reactions are viewed as being tumor-associated embryonic antigens. Embryonic antigens are widely distributed on carcinogen-induced tumors, some showing a broad cross-reactivity between tumors of different histological type while others are restricted to individual organs, e.g., rat mammary and colon carcinomas (Baldwin *et al.*, 1974*d*; Steele *et al.*, 1974). These reexpressed embryonic components have in several instances been shown to be separate products from the tumor rejection antigens, although it is not clear whether embryonic antigens can under appropriate conditions function effectively as rejection antigens. This is a major question to be resolved since embryonic antigens displaying organ-type specificity (e.g., in rat mammary and colonic carcinomas) may be analogous to the neoantigens detected on human tumors by use of comparable *in vitro* assays of lymphocytotoxic reactions (Hellström and Hellström, 1974).

2. Nature of Immune Reactions Elicited Against Tumor Antigens

A battery of immunological techniques is available for the analysis of the various facets of the immune response elicited against tumor antigens. While these have been used to define a variety of potential mechanisms for tumor cell killing, it is still a major problem to determine the relative importance of each in the control of neoplasia in the tumor-bearing individual. These difficulties will be further elaborated following discussion of the immune parameters which may contribute to tumor cell destruction.

2.1. Cell-Mediated Responses

Cell-mediated immune reactions against tumor-associated antigens are widely considered to be of prime importance in the induction of resistance against transplanted tumors (reviewed by Hellström and Hellström, 1974). In a number of studies, tumor immunity has been successfully transferred to normal syngeneic recipients with lymphoid cells taken from immune donors (adoptive transfer of immunity). Alternatively, the cytotoxic effect of lymphoid cells from immunized animals may be detected by their capacity to inhibit *in vivo* the growth of tumor following their admixture *in vitro* with the tumor cell inoculum (Winn, 1961). These cell-mediated antitumor reactions have been accomplished using cells from a variety of sources including lymph node, spleen, peritoneal cavity, peripheral blood, and thoracic duct. It is significant that the transfer of immunity may be achieved not only with lymphoid cells from animals actively immunized against transplanted tumor but also with cells from tumor-bearing hosts, emphasizing the existence of tumor rejection responses in these individuals.

Cell-mediated immune reactions have been more comprehensively evaluated using *in vitro* assays of cytotoxicity or cytostasis (Hellström and Hellström, 1974) as well as macrophage migration inhibition assays, which can be correlated with *in vivo* tests for delayed hypersensitivity (Halliday and Webb, 1969; Littman *et al.*, 1973). Lymphocyte transformation tests have been less extensively employed, but tumor-specific responses following stimulation with either tumor cells or solubilized antigen fractions have been demonstrated with diethylnitrosamine-induced guinea pig hepatomas (Littman *et al.*, 1973).

211

IMMUNO-
BIOLOGY OF
CHEMICALLY
INDUCED
TUMORS

The colony inhibition test originally introduced by Hellström (1967) for the demonstration of tumor cell killing by immune lymphoid cells has now been largely superseded by cytotoxicity assays performed with small numbers of cells cultured in the wells of microtest plates. However, the colony inhibition test offers the advantage of measuring the ability of the effector cells both to kill and to inhibit the growth of the surviving tumor cells, in this way reflecting more appropriately the *in vivo* situation (Hellström and Hellström, 1970b). In order to avoid the necessity of counting large numbers of tumor cell colonies, attempts have been made to incorporate a radiolabel into the surviving tumor cells (Jagarlamoody *et al.*, 1970). The successor to the colony inhibition assay, the microcytotoxicity test, is less consuming of reagents, although many workers still rely exclusively on visual counting to assess tumor cell killing. With this test, tumor cells are cultured in the wells of plastic microtest plates, and immune or normal preparations of lymphoid cells are added. After appropriate incubation (2–3 days), the nonadherent cells are removed by washing and the remaining surviving tumor cells are counted. Further refinements of this test using radiolabeled target cells have been introduced in order to avoid the problem of visual counting. For example, Cohen *et al.* (1971) detected cell-mediated cytotoxic reactions of spleen cells from immunized guinea pigs against two MCA-induced sarcoma cell lines, the target cells being labeled prior to the addition of lymphocytes with [^{125}I]iododeoxyuridine. In this way, the test was used to measure cell death (cytotoxic test), whereas by labeling the target cells at the end of the experiment, inhibition of growth (cytostasis) may be determined. Alternatively, Menard *et al.* (1972) have measured the release of ^{51}Cr from cells labeled with [^{51}Cr]sodium chromate to assess cell killing in a syngeneic 7,12-dimethylbenz[*a*]anthracene-induced murine sarcoma model. This method has limited application for measuring tumor-specific responses to carcinogen-induced tumors, since many solid tumors do not readily release intracellularly localized ^{51}Cr during incubation for a few hours and longer periods of incubation result in nonspecific isotope release.

Many of the proposed mechanisms for tumor cell destruction by sensitized effector cells have been elucidated in *in vitro* studies defining allogeneic immune reactions. These include direct cytotoxicity of sensitized, thymus-derived, T lymphocytes (Wagner *et al.*, 1973) and amplification by macrophages (Evans and Alexander, 1972; Lohmann–Matthes and Fisher, 1973). Nonsensitized lymphoid cells may also exert a cytotoxic effect when cultured with target cells that have been coated with anti-target cell antibody (MacLennan, 1972; Forman and Möller, 1973; Perlmann *et al.*, 1974). Arming of effector cells by specific immune

212

MICHAEL R.
PRICE
AND
ROBERT W.
BALDWIN

complexes is a further mechanism by which cytotoxicity may be demonstrated (Greenberg and Shen, 1973).

In studies on allograft rejection, the thymus-derived or T cell has been shown to mediate specific cytotoxicity against alloantigen (Cerottini *et al.*, 1972; Wagner *et al.*, 1972). Cell contact is essential for cytolysis, this being mediated by the interaction of a single effector cell with a single target cell. In tumor immunity, T-cell killing has been demonstrated with murine sarcoma virus induced tumors (Plata and Levy, 1974) with the EL-4 (C57BL) leukemia, originally induced by 7,12-dimethylbenz[*a*]anthracene (Vasudevan *et al.*, 1974) and with mineral oil induced murine plasmacytomas (Rouse *et al.*, 1972, 1973). With the latter system, θ-antigen-bearing cells were initially found to be essential for the adoptive transfer of immunity (Rouse *et al.*, 1972). Further, the abolition of the transfer of immunity with anti-θ serum and the failure to induce specific immune responses in nude mice against a murine plasmacytoma strongly indicate that T-cell killing plays a predominant role in tumor immunity (Rouse *et al.*, 1973; McCoy *et al.*, 1974).

The nature of the effector cells involved in tumor rejection reactions is still far from established, however, and the relative importance of T and non-T cells is likely to vary between different tumor systems and even with different neoantigens on one tumor. This is emphasized by *in vitro* studies with murine sarcoma virus induced tumors where effector cells involved in the ^{51}Cr release assay of cell-mediated cytotoxicity have been identified as T cells since they are inactivated by anti-θ serum and complement (Leclerc *et al.*, 1973). On the other hand, Lamon *et al.* (1973*b,c*) have reported that B cells were responsible for cytotoxicity of lymph node cells from regressor mice as assayed by the microcytotoxicity assay. In addition to these studies, there is evidence that different subclasses of lymphocytes may be involved in specific functional reactions. This is illustrated by studies on splenic T lymphocytes derived from mice immunized against an allografted tumor (mastocytoma P-815) where different subclasses of effector cells were found to be associated with cytolytic activity and the ability in the presence of stimulating antigen to cause inhibition of nonmacrophage cell populations (Tigelaar and Gorczynski, 1974).

Peritoneal exudate cells from immunized hosts are generally highly effective for adoptively transferring immunity to chemically induced tumors, including MCA-induced murine sarcomas (Old *et al.*, 1962) and aminoazo dye induced rat hepatomas (Baldwin and Barker, 1967*a*; Ishidate, 1967), suggesting a specific role *in vivo* for macrophages in tumor cell killing. This is further emphasized by tests with SV40-induced tumors, where the capacity to adoptively transfer immunity with sensitized spleen cells was diminished by pretreating recipients with silica (Zarling and Tevethia, 1973), this being a specific macrophage toxin (Allison *et al.*, 1966). Also, it has been shown that growth inhibition of tumor cells by lymphoid cells from mice bearing murine sarcoma virus induced tumors is mediated by macrophages (Senik *et al.*, 1974*a,b*). This assay, originally described by Chia and Festenstein (1973), measures inhibition of tumor growth as distinct from the cytolytic response detected by the ^{51}Cr-release assays, where, as already described, there is evidence for T-cell participation (Plata *et al.*, 1973; Plata and Levy, 1974).

The cytotoxicity of cell monolayers of sensitized macrophages for murine lymphoma cells has also been demonstrated (Evans and Alexander, 1972). As with T-cell cytotoxicity, direct cell contact between macrophage and tumor cell is required for cell killing which is not dependent on phagocytosis, although this may occur following death and fragmentation of the tumor cell. One problem with macrophage–tumor cell cocultivation experiments is associated with excluding contaminating T cells from the cultures. This may be achieved by prior irradiation of macrophage monolayers since T cells display radiosensitivity (Ritter et al., 1973) or by adequate washing of monolayer cultures (Lohmann-Matthes and Fisher, 1973), although cell separation studies have indicated that some activated T cells have adherent properties (Shortman et al., 1972). Normal macrophages may be rendered cytotoxic in vitro by contact with spleen cells from tumor-immune donors together with target cells or by their contact with specific macrophage arming factor (SMAF), this being found in supernatants from cultures of sensitized spleen cells and target cells (Evans and Alexander, 1972). Evans et al. (1973) have further proposed that "armed" macrophages after contact with the specific antigen are activated and may nonspecifically inhibit the growth of unrelated target tumor cells, although Lohmann-Matthes and Fisher (1973), using an in vitro tumor allograft model system, have indicated a greater specificity in the cytotoxic phase. For the purpose of definition, the term "armed" as opposed to "activated" denotes the ability of macrophages to destroy specifically tumor cells as compared with their ability to destroy nonspecifically a variety of tumors. For example, in one study (Krahenbuhl and Remington, 1974) armed macrophages capable of a specific cytostatic effect were produced in experiments in which C57BL mice were immunized with living L-5178YE lymphoma cells (DBA/2). However, activated macrophages were obtained from mice chronically infected with intracellular protozoan parasites and these exerted marked cytostasis on a variety of unrelated tumor target cells.

The nature of the specific macrophage arming factor is at present unknown, although one group has suggested that IgG, IgM, and immune complexes are not involved and that a possible candidate may be shed cytotoxic receptors released during the interaction of T cells with target cells (Lohmann-Matthes and Fisher, 1973).

Normal lymphoid cells may be recruited to effect tumor cell destruction in vitro when the target cells are coated with specific antibody. This cell-dependent antibody cytotoxicity is expressed only when the antibody has an intact Fc portion (MacLennan, 1972; Möller and Svehag, 1972) through which effector cell to target cell binding may occur and cytotoxicity is triggered (Perlmann et al., 1972). The present evidence suggests that the effector cell is not a T cell, and until recently it was considered that it may belong to a subpopulation of B cells (Forman and Möller, 1973). However, it has been proposed that the cytotoxic effector cell may be a "null" or "K" cell, probably of the monocyte series, which may also be capable of binding antigen–antibody complexes (Greenberg and Shen, 1973).

Hersey (1973) has suggested that cell-dependent antibody killing may account for the antitumor effects of antibody in a syngeneic rat lymphoma system. Antilymphoma antisera (prepared in allogeneic or xenogeneic donors) prolonged

213

IMMUNO-
BIOLOGY OF
CHEMICALLY
INDUCED
TUMORS

214

MICHAEL R.
PRICE
AND
ROBERT W.
BALDWIN

the survival of rats injected with lymphoma cells, and these observations correlated well with the cell-dependent antibody titers in the sera of treated animals.

Immune antisera are further capable of increasing the *in vitro* cytotoxicity of reactive lymphocytes with both experimental animal (Skurzak *et al.*, 1972) and human tumors (Hellström *et al.*, 1973). The mechanism of this so-called potentiation effect is at present unknown, although one possibility is that potentiating serum factors (antibody?) act by arming reactive lymphoid cell populations in a manner comparable to that found with cell-dependent antibody killing. This arming effect combined with the cytotoxicity of sensitized lymphocytes (as detected when no serum is present) may act synergistically to produce the high cytotoxicity observed.

2.2. Humoral Antibody

Humoral antibody directed against tumor-associated antigens capable of specific tumor cell destruction (in the presence of added complement) has been detected in several chemically induced tumor systems. By use of the colony inhibition test, complement-dependent cytotoxic antibody has been demonstrated in sera from mice immunized by surgical excision of primary MCA-induced sarcomas (Hellström *et al.*, 1968) and from rats immunized against irradiated grafts of transplanted MCA-induced sarcomas (Baldwin and Moore, 1971). With these examples, the individually distinct specificity of these tumor-immune reactions was confirmed. Complement-dependent tumor-specific cytotoxic antibody against MCA-induced sarcomas has also been detected using the microassay technique of Takasugi and Klein (1970), in this case cytotoxicity being defined by the survival capacity of treated cells (Bloom, 1970). This test has been further modified to incorporate radiolabeled target cells in order to avoid visual counting of the survivors. Le Mevel and Wells (1973) showed that serum from mice immunized against an MCA-induced sarcoma was specifically cytotoxic at high dilutions (1/64 to 1/512) for target cells of the immunizing tumor. The target cells were, in this case, labeled with [^{125}I]iododeoxyuridine 18 h after incubation with normal or test serum and complement in order to minimize the isotopic and chemical toxicity known to be associated with this label (Le Mevel *et al.*, 1973). Comparably, Cleveland *et al.* (1974) have detected antibody against tumor-associated antigens of MCA-induced murine sarcoma cells by measuring the ability of cells to incorporate [^{3}H]thymidine after exposure to immune serum and complement, this test reflecting both cytostasis as well as cytolysis.

The specificity of complement-dependent serum cytotoxic reactions has been more comprehensively analyzed in the 4-dimethylaminoazobenzene (DAB) induced rat hepatoma system using the colony inhibition test (Baldwin and Embleton, 1971a). In a series of 77 cross-tests, in no case did the serum from immunized rats react with cells other than those derived from the immunizing tumor. Comparably, Borsos *et al.* (1973) prepared xenogeneic antisera against viable cells from diethylnitrosamine-induced guinea pig hepatomas, and after appropriate absorption these exhibited complement-dependent serum cytotoxic- 215

IMMUNO-
BIOLOGY OF
CHEMICALLY
INDUCED
TUMORS
ity directed predominantly against the tumor-specific antigens associated with
these tumors. These findings were confirmed using the indirect membrane
immunofluorescence test and by complement fixation, by which it was also
estimated that each cell expressed a minimum of 10^5 specific tumor antigen sites.
As well as the individually distinct tumor-specific antigens expressed by these
tumors, cross-reacting embryonic antigens were detected on cells of the two tumor
lines, a finding not revealed by analysis of syngeneic cellular immune and
transplantation reactions (Rapp et al., 1968; Zbar et al., 1969; Meltzer et al., 1972).
Embryonic antigens have, however, been demonstrated with reagents prepared
in syngeneic hosts using the aminoazo dye induced rat hepatoma model (Baldwin
et al., 1974d) and with MCA-induced sarcomas in the rat (Baldwin et al., 1974d)
and mouse (Brawn, 1970). In these studies, cross-reacting embryonic antigens
were detected by their reaction with sera from syngeneic multiparous animals
either by indirect membrane immunofluorescence or by complement-dependent
serum cytotoxicity.

An isotopic antiglobulin assay was adopted by Burdick et al. (1973) to analyze
hyperimmune serum prepared by immunization of mice with MCA-induced
sarcomas. The predominant reaction of antibody with cell-surface-expressed
tumor antigens was directed against cells of the immunizing tumor, although
cross-reactions, ascribed to antibody against an embryonic component(s), were
observed with other MCA-induced sarcoma cell lines. These findings are somewhat at variance with those determined by membrane immunofluorescence
whereby individual, serologically defined antigens have been detected on MCA-
induced sarcomas and DAB-induced hepatomas in rats (Baldwin and Price,
Vol. 1, Chap. 12). In these examples, cross-reactivity with syngeneic antisera
produced by immunization with tumor cells was not demonstrable and the
individually specific antibody responses observed correlated with the specificity of
the tumor rejection reactions. In addition to complement-dependent antibody
mediated cytotoxicity, tumor cell killing by normal lymphoid cells in the presence
of specific antibody has been implicated in a number of systems (MacLennan,
1972; Perlmann et al., 1972, 1974).

3. Immunological Reactions Correlated with Tumor Status

3.1. Cell-Mediated Immunity

Immunological reactions in the autochthonous host to neoantigens associated
with chemically induced tumors have been well documented. These responses
were originally detected in studies showing inhibition or suppression of growth of
reimplanted biopsies of MCA-induced sarcomas following destruction of the
primary tumors by ligation of their blood supply (Takeda et al., 1966) or following
complete resection (Mikulska et al., 1966). It is interesting to note that incomplete

216

MICHAEL R.
PRICE
AND
ROBERT W.
BALDWIN

excision of subcutaneous tumors was less effective in producing tumor immunity so that whereas tumor cell challenge inocula (2×10^6 cells) were rejected by 90% of rats whose tumors were completely excised, only 30% of rats having partial tumor excision rejected equivalent challenge inocula (Mikulska et al., 1966). The failure to demonstrate tumor rejection responses in rats bearing established tumor grafts or treated by only partial excision was ascribed to the neutralization of effector lymphoid cells, and recently this concept has been re-stated in terms of humoral factors interfering with cell-mediated immunity (see Section 3.3).

The view that tumor-bearing individuals elicit substantial immunity against the primary tumor is supported by studies on "concomitant immunity" showing that tumor-bearing animals have the capacity to reject a challenge with cells of the same tumor, but not one which is immunologically different. For example, Lausch and Rapp (1969) demonstrated that hamsters bearing syngeneic transplants of a 7,12-dimethylbenz[a]anthracene-induced sarcoma rejected a second challenge of cells from this tumor but not cells from unrelated SV40-induced tumors. Comparably, concomitant immunity has been detected in mice bearing syngeneic transplants of MCA-induced sarcomas (Bard et al., 1969; Fisher et al., 1970; Deckers et al., 1971; Vaage, 1971, 1972; Belehradek et al., 1972; Chandradasa, 1973). From these studies, however, it is clear that the capacity of the tumor-bearing individual to respond against the autochthonous tumor is dependent on the extent of tumor growth. In this way, Belehradek et al. (1972) determined that mice bearing 10-day-old but not 30-day-old sarcoma grafts were able to reject a second challenge with the same tumor. This variability in the concomitant immune response has been further emphasized by Chandradasa (1973), who determined that the highest level of concomitant immunity occurred in the relatively early stages (10–14 days) of growth of an immunogenic MCA-induced murine sarcoma. Thereafter, there was a progressive decline in transplantation resistance so that by 5 wk of tumor growth tumor-bearing mice were unable to reject a fiftyfold-lower tumor cell challenge inoculum.

Adoptive transfer studies have also indicated that the tumor-bearing host produces an immune response against tumor-associated neoantigens, this response being modified by the presence of a tumor mass. Spleen cells from mice bearing grafts of MCA-induced sarcomas were found not to suppress tumor growth in recipients challenged immediately with cells of the same tumor, although resistance was observed when recipients were challenged 7 days after transfer (Old et al., 1962). These findings have subsequently been confirmed by Mikulska et al. (1966) and Bard and Pilch (1969). Sequential studies on the adoptive transfer of immunity with spleen cells from mice bearing transplanted MCA-induced sarcomas have been reported by Deckers et al. (1971). The capacity of spleen cells from tumor bearers to transfer immunity was found to develop 7–10 days after tumor implantation, although again an interval of at least 7 days between spleen cell transfer and tumor challenge was necessary for transplantation resistance to be detected. Chandradasa (1973) also demonstrated that spleen cells taken at early stages (10–14 days) of tumor growth from recipients bearing a transplanted MCA-induced murine sarcoma were effective in transferring tumor immunity. However, the transfer of spleen cells from mice bearing more well-established tumors (21- to 45-day-old tumor grafts) did not induce such a pronounced immune response. In these tests, where lymphoid cells were mixed with tumor cells and injected into compatible recipients, regional lymph node cells were much less effective in transferring tumor immunity than spleen cells from tumor-bearing mice. In most instances, concomitant immunity exhibits the individual specificity characteristic of chemically induced tumors. However, Nelson (1974) determined that, late in the development of MCA-induced murine sarcomas, resistance to a second tumor was less specific so that tumor bearers showed a degree of protection against other MCA-induced sarcomas.

There is now substantial evidence that lymphoid cells from tumor-bearing animals or cancer patients are cytotoxic *in vitro* for cultured tumor target cells (reviewed by Hellström and Hellström, 1974). To take one example, lymph node cells from rats bearing transplanted DAB-induced hepatomas are cytotoxic or inhibit the colony formation of tumor target cells (Baldwin *et al.*, 1973*d*). The specificity of these reactions again correlated with the presence of individually distinct tumor rejection antigens present on the rat hepatomas. Comparably, lymph node cells from rats bearing primary DAB-induced rat hepatomas were cytotoxic for cells prepared from biopsies of the original tumor but not from other primary hepatomas (Baldwin *et al.*, 1973*d*). These studies, demonstrating the presence of cytotoxic lymphoid cells in hepatoma-bearing rats, add to the growing body of evidence derived from experimental tumors induced by chemical carcinogens (Hellström and Hellström, 1970*b*; Taranger *et al.*, 1972; Cohen *et al.*, 1972; Baldwin and Embleton, 1974; Steele *et al.*, 1974) and oncogenic viruses (Hellström and Hellström, 1969; Datta and Vandeputte, 1971; Sjögren and Borum, 1971; Ankerst *et al.*, 1974), indicating that tumor-bearing animals have developed a tumor-specific cell-mediated immune response. The interpretation of these findings as being predictive of an active tumor rejection response should, however, be viewed with reservation, since in not all instances does the specificity of *in vitro* lymphocytotoxic reactions correlate with the results of rejection tests. This is well exemplified in the case of MCA-induced murine bladder tumors. With these, cross-reactivity between different transplanted tumors was regularly demonstrated by *in vitro* lymphocytotoxic reactions and bladder carcinogenesis could be inhibited by immunization with tumor cells (Taranger *et al.*, 1972). However, subsequent rejection tests against tumors transplanted in syngeneic mice showed that these bladder tumors exhibit individually distinct neoantigens (Wahl *et al.*, 1974). Comparably, in a recent study on spontaneously arising sarcomas and mammary carcinomas and N-2-fluorenylacetamide-induced mammary carcinomas, lymph node cells from tumor-bearing rats reacted with cells of the autochthonous tumor as well as tumors of the same histological type (Baldwin and Embleton, 1974). With these examples, tumor transplantation techniques have generally failed to reveal rejection antigens (Baldwin and Embleton, 1969*a,b*, 1971*b*), and it has been determined that the *in vitro* lymphocytotoxic reactions were directed against tumor-associated embryonic antigens since the cytotoxicity of tumor-bearer lymph node cells was "blocked" by preexposure of

217

IMMUNO-
BIOLOGY OF
CHEMICALLY
INDUCED
TUMORS

218

MICHAEL R.
PRICE
AND
ROBERT W.
BALDWIN

the plated tumor cells to multiparous rat serum (Baldwin and Embleton, 1974). Similarly, the cytotoxicity of lymph node cells from multiparous rats for embryo cells was blocked by pretreating the plated embryo cells with tumor-bearer serum (Baldwin and Embleton, 1974).

As already discussed, different lymphoid cell populations may be involved in the response to tumor-associated antigens and so the immune response in the tumor-bearing host may be highly complex. This is illustrated by studies with Moloney virus induced sarcomas in mice where T and non-T lymphocytes were found to be cytotoxic during the early phase of tumor development, this being dependent to some extent on the *in vitro* assay procedure for detecting effector cell cytotoxicity (Lamon *et al.*, 1973b,c; Plata *et al.*, 1973). In comparison, lymphocytes taken at times following spontaneous regression of tumors were found to be non-T cells (Lamon *et al.*, 1973b, 1974). Similar studies have now been carried out to characterize the dynamics of the immune response to the Gross virus induced lymphoma (C 58 NT)D in W/Fu rats. This tumor is highly immunogenic, producing transient growths which rapidly spontaneously regress unless tumor cells are implanted into immunosuppressed recipients or relatively large tumor cell inocula are injected (Shellam, 1974). Cytotoxic lymphocytes, assayed by ^{51}Cr release, were found early after tumor cell inoculation, although these gradually declined in rats bearing either progressing or regressing tumors (Oren *et al.*, 1971). However, lymphocytes taken after 40 days or more, while inactive on removal from rats, become activated following *in vitro* incubation (Ortiz de Landazuri and Herberman, 1972). The mechanism of this activation is still unresolved but similar reactivation has been observed following *in vitro* culture of peritoneal exudate cells from mice bearing SV40-induced tumors (Blasecki and Tevethia, 1975) or spleen cells from hamsters bearing PARA-7 tumors (Laux and Lausch, 1974). In the Gross lymphoma–rat system, attempts to analyze the initial steps in tumor antigen recognition using a one-way mixed lymphocyte–tumor cell interaction indicated that significant stimulation was not detectable until 14 days after tumor implantation. This response then reached a peak between days 20 and 40 and gradually decline to low levels by day 90 (Glaser *et al.*, 1974). These effects were observed only in rats where tumors regressed, although they show no concordance with comparable time-course assays of cell-mediated immunity detected using the ^{51}Cr release test. In fact, the data indicated that the mixed lymphocyte–tumor cell response, viewed as an early recognition phase of the cellular reaction, followed rather than preceded the cytotoxic response.

Time-course studies of the evolution of various facets of the cell-mediated immune response to chemically induced tumors have not so far been extensively reported. Lymph node cells taken from rats between 13 and 30 days after implantation of DAB-induced hepatomas were specifically cytotoxic for tumor cells (Baldwin *et al.*, 1973d). Also, cytotoxic lymph node cells, as well as a humoral arming factor rendering normal lymphoid cells cytotoxic, have been demonstrated in mice within 1–2 days after implantation of an MCA-induced sarcoma (Pollack and Nelson, 1974).

3.2. Humoral Antibody

219

IMMUNO-
BIOLOGY OF
CHEMICALLY
INDUCED
TUMORS

For some time, tumor-specific antibody has been considered as playing little or no role in the immunological control of carcinogen-induced tumors. This assumption is based primarily on unsuccessful attempts to passively transfer tumor immunity with tumor-immune antisera (Möller, 1964, Bubeník and Koldovsky, 1964; Bloom and Hildemann, 1970; Baldwin and Barker, 1967*b*). Furthermore, while tumor-specific antibody can be demonstrated in serum of syngeneic hosts immunized against transplanted tumor by a variety of methods (e.g., complement fixation, membrane immunofluorescence, complement-dependent cytotoxicity), similar reactivities were considered not to be present in the tumor-bearing host. For example, Harder and McKhann (1968), using an indirect ^{125}I-labeled antibody technique, observed tumor-specific antibody against MCA-induced sarcoma cells only after surgical resection of tumor grafts. Similarly, resection of transplanted DAB-induced hepatomas in rats has been shown to lead to the development of significant levels of tumor-specific antibody in serum which shows complement-dependent cytotoxicity *in vitro* for cells of the appropriate tumor (Baldwin *et al.*, 1973*d*). It should also be realized that early studies with Moloney virus induced sarcomas showing that tumor-bearer serum contained factors interfering *in vitro* with lymphocyte cytotoxicity (Hellström and Hellström, 1969) suggested a possible role *in vivo* for "blocking antibody," this being in accord with enhancement studies (Möller, 1964; Bloom and Hildemann, 1970). Blocking factors in serum of tumor-bearing hosts are now considered to be tumor-specific immune complexes (see Section 3.3). Also, while similar blocking effects can be produced by tumor-specific antibody, the donors of the antisera are often capable of rejecting tumor challenge so that in these cases blocking does not reflect the *in vivo* immune status (Baldwin *et al.*, 1973*d*).

There are several recent studies which suggest that tumor-specific antibody may play a more positive role in tumor rejection, and this possibility is currently being reevaluated. A significant feature in this respect is the finding that nonimmune lymphoid cells may be cytotoxic *in vitro* for tumor cells following interaction with specific antibody molecules bound to the tumor cell surface. This cell-dependent antibody response (reviewed by MacLennan, 1972; Perlmann *et al.*, 1972) may be much more effective than complement-mediated cytotoxicity and has been demonstrated in a number of experimental tumor systems. For example, sera taken during the early stages of growth of syngeneic transplants of an MCA-induced rat sarcoma were highly cytotoxic *in vitro* for cells of this tumor when normal spleen cells were added, but none of the sera showed complement-dependent reactivity (Basham and Currie, 1974). These observations are similar to the reported early appearance of lymphoid arming factor in sera of mice bearing primary or transplanted Moloney virus induced sarcomas or transplanted MCA-induced sarcomas (Pollack and Nelson, 1974), the sera being specifically cytotoxic for tumor cells in the presence of normal lymph node cells.

It has been suggested that cell-dependent antibody responses may play a role in the spontaneous regression of Moloney virus induced sarcomas (Lamon *et al.*,

220

MICHAEL R.
PRICE
AND
ROBERT W.
BALDWIN

1973*a*, 1974; Harada *et al.*, 1973). Comparably, cell-dependent antibody cytotoxicity has been demonstrated against a Gross virus induced lymphoma in rats (Ortiz de Landazuri *et al.*, 1974) which again usually produces transiently growing tumors that spontaneously regress. With both these tumor systems, however, complement-dependent cytotoxic antibody reactions can be detected in tumor-bearing hosts (Herberman and Oren, 1971; Herberman *et al.*, 1974; Tamerius and Hellström, 1974). In the Gross lymphoma system, for example, hosts in which tumors regressed developed a biphasic antibody response with an initial 19 S peak at 10 days and a second 7 S peak at about 30 days (Herberman and Oren, 1971). In this context, it is also relevant to note that tumor-specific antibody is demonstrable during the terminal phase of growth of a transplanted DAB-induced hepatoma D-23 so that the original concept relating humoral antibody responses to tumor burden needs to be evaluated (Bowen *et al.*, 1974).

Finally, in considering the relevance of humoral antibody to immunological control of tumor it is pertinent to note that there are circumstances where passively transferred antiserum will suppress growth of transplanted tumor cells. This has been most clearly established with murine leukemias (Old and Boyse, 1964), and in addition immune serum has been found to be effective in the treatment of Moloney virus induced sarcomas (Fefer, 1969). Again, little conclusive evidence has been presented to indicate that carcinogen-induced solid tumors are susceptible to serotherapy, but it is pertinent to note that while antibody alone was only weakly effective in preventing growth of the murine EL-4 lymphoma, this treatment enhanced the combination therapy with cyclophosphamide and chlorambucil (Davies *et al.*, 1974*a,b*).

3.3. Nature of Serum Factors Modifying Cell-Mediated Immunity

The efficacy of the cellular immune response *in vivo* may be diminished by the presence of humoral factors which specifically modify host immunity and thereby provide the tumor with an escape route from host immunological control. This concept was originally proposed and developed by the Hellströms to account for their finding that pretreatment of tumor cells with heat-inactivated serum from tumor-bearing individuals prevented them from being killed by lymphocytes specifically sensitized to the tumor (Hellström and Hellström, 1970*b*, 1974). Subsequently, the blocking reactivity of tumor-bearer serum has been demonstrated by other assays of cell-mediated immunity. For example, using the macrophage migration inhibition test, Halliday (1971) showed that serum from mice bearing either a Moloney virus induced sarcoma or an MCA-induced sarcoma had the capacity to specifically reverse the inhibition of migration of sensitized peritoneal exudate cells produced by appropriate tumor extracts. Comparably, after treatment of hamster melanoma cells with tumor-bearer serum, they were no longer able to inhibit the migration of peritoneal exudate cells from melanoma-bearing animals (Henderson *et al.*, 1973). Also serum from mice bearing MCA-induced sarcomas and cancer patients had the capacity to block the leukocyte adherence inhibition reaction by soluble tumor extracts

(Halliday *et al.*, 1974; Maluish and Halliday, 1974). With each of these tests, there is only suggestive evidence that the blocking reactions observed may be attributed to the same humoral factor(s) which protects tumor cells from *in vitro* lymphocytotoxic attack. Furthermore, in view of the complexity of effector cell interactions with tumor cells (Section 2) it is not possible to precisely define the mechanism by which humoral factors modify cell-mediated immune reactions, although in several systems correlation of serum factors with tumor status provides a model for immunoprognosis.

221

IMMUNO-
BIOLOGY OF
CHEMICALLY
INDUCED
TUMORS

The observation that serum from mice bearing progressively growing Moloney virus induced sarcomas protected tumor cells *in vitro* from attack by sensitized lymphoid cells was interpreted by the Hellströms to indicate that this effect modifying lymphocytotoxicity was mediated by antibody (termed "blocking antibody") interacting with tumor cell surface antigens (Hellström and Hellström, 1969). This conclusion was supported by experiments showing that the blocking factor in tumor-bearer serum could be neutralized by the addition of goat anti-mouse 7 S immunoglobulin and its activity in serum could be removed by adsorption with intact tumor cells. Chromatographic separation of tumor-bearer serum by Sephadex G200 gel filtration also indicated that the blocking factor eluted with the 7 S globulins (Hellström and Hellström, 1969). Comparably, fractionation of serum from rats bearing transplanted aminoazo dye induced hepatomas either by Sephadex G200 column chromatography or by sucrose density gradient centrifugation reinforced the proposal that 7 S antibody was implicated in the blocking phenomenon (Baldwin *et al.*, 1973*f*). Experiments with sera from rats immunized against hepatoma cells attenuated by γ-irradiation substantiate that blocking reactions can be induced by antibody since these sera contain tumor-specific antibody demonstrable by complement-dependent serum cytotoxicity and indirect membrane immunofluorescence reactions (Baldwin *et al.*, 1973*d*). There are also indications that only some immunoglobulins are associated with the blocking activity of tumor-bearer serum. This is supported by studies on the effects of adsorbing serum from rats bearing either virus-induced kidney sarcomas or chemically induced rat colon carcinomas, with protein-A-containing *Staphylococcus aureus*, which is known to combine specifically with some IgG subclasses (Steele *et al.*, 1974). This adsorption procedure removed the blocking activity of the serum and resulted in the appearance of complement-dependent serum cytotoxicity, suggesting to the authors that there may be competition between various antitumor antibodies and that the relative concentration of different antibodies may determine the predominating activity of the serum *in vitro* and *in vivo* (Steele *et al.*, 1974). Jose and Skvaril (1974) have further demonstrated with serum from human neuroblastoma patients that, blocking activity is associated with IgG_1 and IgG_3 and to a lesser extent IgG_4, but not IgG_2.

It is not possible in all instances to ascribe blocking reactions to antibody alone, and several findings suggest that the reactivity of tumor-bearer serum may involve tumor-specific immune complexes. Following complete surgical resection of tumor or tumor regression, the persistence of blocking activity is limited (Hellström and Hellström, 1969; Hellström *et al.*, 1970; Baldwin *et al.*, 1973*d*), and with

222

MICHAEL R.
PRICE
AND
ROBERT W.
BALDWIN

the aminoazo dye induced rat hepatoma model no detectable activity was present 3–4 days after tumor excision, although at this stage complement-dependent serum cytotoxicity became demonstrable. Nevertheless, blocking reactivity could be restored to "postexcision" serum (containing tumor-specific antibody) by the addition of papain-solubilized hepatoma-specific antigen (Baldwin *et al.*, 1972, 1973*e*). When antigen was added in excess, however, blocking activity was lost, indicative of a requirement of free antibody determinants in the immune complexes to allow interaction with the target tumor cell. Similarly, addition of papain-solubilized antigen to tumor-bearer serum (which is blocking and has been shown to contain immune complexes, Bowen *et al.*, 1974) results in a comparable loss of blocking activity (Baldwin *et al.*, 1972).

Consistent with the concept that tumor-bearer serum contains immune complexes capable of exerting blocking reactions, Sjögren *et al.* (1971, 1972) showed that the blocking factor in serum from mice bearing Moloney virus induced sarcomas or human cancer patients can be adsorbed onto intact tumor cells, eluted with low pH buffer, and separated by membrane ultrafiltration into high (more than 100,000 daltons) and low (less than 100,000 daltons) molecular weight components. Neither of these fractions alone displayed blocking activity when added to cultured tumor cells, although this was restored when the two fractions were recombined.

Although serum from individuals rendered tumor free does not block cell-mediated cytotoxicity, it has the capacity to neutralize the blocking activity of tumor-bearer serum, indicating the involvement of tumor-specific antigen in the blocking reaction. This unblocking effect was initially observed in mice with regressing Moloney virus induced sarcomas (Hellström and Hellström, 1970*a*) and has subsequently been explored using the aminoazo dye induced rat hepatoma model. In these studies, the blocking activity of serum from rats bearing transplanted hepatomas could be neutralized by addition of three types of antiserum, all of which contained antihepatoma antibody (Robins and Baldwin, 1974). These sera in increasing order of potency as assessed by indirect membrane immunofluorescence or complement-dependent cytotoxicity were postexcision serum, syngeneic immune rat serum, and rabbit antiserum produced by immunization with intact tumor cells. The capacity of these antisera to neutralize the blocking effect of tumor-bearer serum also increased in the same order, the inference being that conversion of immune complexes to a state of antibody excess prevented their participation in blocking reactions. In these studies, the specificity of the unblocking effect was equivalent to that of the individually distinct neoantigens associated with the hepatoma examined. These findings are consistent with those obtained with Moloney virus induced sarcomas in mice, where "regressor" serum neutralized the blocking activity of serum from mice bearing progressively growing tumors (Hellström and Hellström, 1970*a*).

Under the conditions of the microcytotoxicity test, it is not clear how serum factors may protect tumor cells from cell-mediated immune cytotoxicity. The mechanism of simple masking of surface antigens by bound antibody or immune complexes is unsatisfactory from several considerations. During the long incubation periods involved in the microcytotoxicity assay, release of bound reactants

223
IMMUNO-
BIOLOGY OF
CHEMICALLY
INDUCED
TUMORS

may occur as a consequence of cell membrane synthesis and regeneration, thus providing the possibility of modification of cytotoxicity at the effector cell level. It is perhaps relevant to this point that blocking reactions have been detected with sera from mice bearing murine sarcoma virus induced tumors using the long-term microcytotoxicity assay, whereas the same sera were inactive when cell-mediated immunity was determined by the short-term ^{51}Cr release test (Plata and Levy, 1974). This might imply that the blocking reaction detected was dependent on cell metabolism and surface turnover, so allowing interaction of previously bound macromolecules (immune complexes?) with sensitized effector cells. Alternatively, as suggested by Plata and Levy (1974), different subpopulations of T cells committed to tumor cell killing may be detected by the two assays. A further complication of the microcytotoxicity test is that during the relatively long incubation (up to 72 h) of effector cells with plated tumor cells, lymphocyte activation may be initiated.

Blocking reactions have, however, been detected with the ^{51}Cr release assay in analyses on the effects of hyperimmune antiserum on lymphocyte cytolysis of allogeneic murine leukemia cells (Todd *et al.*, 1973). In this study, serum blocking of lymphocytotoxicity was attributed to prevention of binding of sensitized effector cells to the tumor cells. The blocking antiserum was also shown to prevent cytolysis by displacing bound lymphocytes from tumor cells prior to irreversible tumor cell damage.

There is evidence to suggest that immune complexes may represent more efficient blocking agents than antibody alone. Previous studies have shown that serum obtained following resection of transplanted hepatomas, while exhibiting complement-dependent serum cytotoxicity, is not blocking but may be made so by the addition of solubilized tumor-specific antigen (Baldwin *et al.*, 1972). Comparably, in a recent investigation on neuroblastoma patients, maximal serum blocking was demonstrated when immune complexes were at antigen–antibody equivalence (Jose and Seshadri, 1974). This concept is consistent with experiments already described whereby antibody is effective in neutralizing the blocking activity of tumor-bearer serum. Although immune complexes may represent more effective steric blocking agents at the tumor cell surface than antibody alone (possibly modifying surface antigen redistribution), they may alternatively exert their effect through the antigen component of the bound complex which interacts with the effector cell, preventing recognition of surface antigens.

The proposal that blocking reactions may be mediated by a process in which reactants bound to tumor cell surface antigens are released and modify lymphocytotoxicity at the effector cell level suggests an alternative mechanism by which the tumor escapes immunological growth control *in vivo*. By use of the DAB-induced rat hepatoma model, it has been possible to directly demonstrate modification of cell-mediated immunity by antigen in experiments showing that the cytotoxicity of tumor-immune lymph node cells was inhibited by their pretreatment with papain-solubilized hepatoma antigen (Baldwin *et al.*, 1973g). The specificity of this effect was confirmed since the antigen preparation did not inhibit the cytotoxicity of lymph node cells sensitized against another immunologically distinct DAB-induced hepatoma. This phenomenon, involving tests where

224

MICHAEL R.
PRICE
AND
ROBERT W.
BALDWIN

the effector cells are first exposed to the reactants, has been termed "inhibition" of lymphocytotoxicity to differentiate it on an operational level from blocking reactions in which reactants are added to the target cells. Comparably, inhibitory reactions have been demonstrated with murine sarcoma virus induced sarcomas and specific inhibition of cytotoxicity was observed using autologous tumor extracts and either sensitized whole spleen cells or purified populations of spleen T cells (Plata and Levy, 1974).

With human tumors, in particular colon carcinoma and melanoma, specific inhibition of blood lymphocyte cytotoxicity has been obtained following exposure of the effector cells to papain-solubilized tumor membrane fractions (Baldwin *et al.*, 1973c, 1974c). These findings are consistent with the increased cytotoxicity observed following repeated washing of blood lymphocytes from patients with disseminated malignant melanoma, bladder carcinoma, hypernephroma, and sarcoma, and this may reflect the removal of bound tumor antigen (Currie and Basham, 1972; Currie, 1973). Analogous to these observations, Laux and Lausch (1974) determined that spleen cells from tumor-bearing hamsters were not cytotoxic for PARA-7 target cells, although after overnight incubation *in vitro* at 37°C the cells became specifically reactive. That products originating from the tumor may interfere with lymphocytotoxicity reactions has been demonstrated by Currie and Alexander (1974), who determined that specific inhibition of lymph node cell cytotoxicity directed against an MCA-induced sarcoma was produced by material shed from cultured tumor cells.

The conclusion from each of these studies is that circulating antigens or antigen-containing moieties may play a biologically important role in the tumor–host relationship by interaction with sensitized effector cells. Comparably, circulating factors in the serum of tumor-bearing hosts which are specifically inhibitory for sensitized lymphoid cells have been detected with DAB-induced rat hepatomas (Baldwin *et al.*, 1973g) as well as other experimental tumor models (Plata and Levy, 1974; Blair and Lane, 1974). Correlation of serum activity with tumor status in sequential studies with the transplanted rat hepatoma system has provided evidence for a specific role for circulating tumor antigens (Baldwin *et al.*, 1973d,f,g). Tumor-bearer serum was shown to contain factors which specifically inhibited the cytotoxicity of immune lymph node cells for plated target cells. This activity was, however, lost following surgical resection of tumor, a finding comparable to the disappearance of blocking activity after tumor excision and indicative of the rapid loss of antigen or immune complexes from the circulation. Conversely, syngeneic or heterologous antisera produced against intact hepatoma cells were lacking in inhibitory activity, although these sera displayed the capacity to specifically neutralize the inhibitory factor in tumor-bearer serum, again implying the involvement of tumor-specific antigen (Robins and Baldwin, 1974).

Cohen *et al.* (1974) have also reported experiments on the abrogation of cell-mediated immunity by antigen, antibody, and immune complexes using an allogeneic murine tumor system. As with the rat hepatoma studies, both antibody and immune complexes were blocking when added to the tumor target cells and effector cell cytotoxicity was specifically inhibited by alloantigens. Alloantibody did not, however, affect cytotoxicity when added to the effector lymphocytes.

Although the tumor rejection responses in the transplanted rat hepatoma system are directed against the individually distinct antigens and the *in vitro* blocking and inhibition reactions already discussed also show this characteristic tumor specificity, these tumors in addition express cross-reacting embryonic antigens (Baldwin and Price, Vol. 1, Chap. 12; Baldwin *et al.*, 1974*d*). These components do not, however, appear to significantly contribute to the induction of a rejection response (Baldwin *et al.*, 1974*e*), although lymphocytotoxic reactions may be modified *in vitro* by circulating serum factors. For example, the cytotoxicity of lymph node cells from multiparous or hepatoma-immune rats for 14- to 15-day embryo cells may be blocked by preexposing the target cells to multiparous rat serum, while similar treatment of tumor target cells did not prevent the cytotoxic response of tumor-immune lymph node cells (Baldwin *et al.*, 1974*f*). In comparison, tumor-immune lymph node cell reactivity was blocked only when tumor cells were pretreated with tumor-immune serum. These findings indicated that immunization against tumors results in the production of separate populations of lymphoid cells sensitized against both the tumor-specific and embryonic antigens, whereas lymph node cells of the multiparous rat are sensitized only to the embryonic component (Baldwin *et al.*, 1974*f*). In addition, exposure of multiparous rat lymph node cells to soluble hepatoma-associated embryonic antigen, which is demonstrable in the serum of tumor-bearing rats (Rees *et al.*, 1974*b*), inhibits their cytotoxicity for tumor or 14-day embryo target cells (Rees *et al.*, 1974*a*).

In accord with the now substantial evidence indicating that humoral factors may modify tumor immunity in the tumor-bearing host, it has been possible to manipulate the *in vivo* responses in a number of ways. Specific desensitization of concomitant immunity in mice bearing syngeneic transplants of MCA-induced fibrosarcomas has been achieved by injecting radiation-killed tumor cells (Vaage, 1972). It was postulated that this effect was produced by tumor antigen interacting with sensitized lymphoid cells. In this context, it is noteworthy that rapid release of tumor antigen into the serum of rats receiving syngeneic implants of MCA-induced sarcomas has been observed, this being attributed to autolysis of transplanted tumor cells (Thomson *et al.*, 1973*a*). Comparably, it has been established with a number of tumors labeled with isotopic markers that a high proportion of the isotopic label may be excreted following tumor implantation, indicating rapid lysis of injected cells (Bowen *et al.*, 1974; Pimm, unpublished findings).

Facilitation of polyoma tumor growth has been achieved by treating tumor recipients with either tumor-bearer serum or fractions eluted to pH 3 from tumor tissue (Bansal *et al.*, 1972). In these tests, enhancement was manifested by a more rapid tumor growth when compared to that in controls, and the effect was specific since extracts from normal kidney tissue or an MCA-induced sarcoma were without effect. Both the tumor-bearer serum and polyoma tumor extracts blocked polyoma tumor cells *in vitro* against the cytotoxicity of sensitized blood lymphocytes, and serum obtained following tumor cell challenge and injection of polyoma tumor eluates showed blocking activity. Fractions eluted at acid pH from MCA-induced murine sarcomas have also been reported to enhance tumor

225

IMMUNO-
BIOLOGY OF
CHEMICALLY
INDUCED
TUMORS

226

MICHAEL R.
PRICE
AND
ROBERT W.
BALDWIN

growth (Witz, 1973), but in these tests a degree of cross-reactivity was observed and the nature of the enhancing factor, containing immunoglobulin (IgG_2), has not been completely resolved. One possibility which so far has not been investigated is that the cross-reactive material enhancing tumor growth of unrelated tumors may contain embryonic antigen complexed with antibody (Rees *et al.*, 1974*b*). The nature of these serum factors and their function *in vivo* remain to be established. If, as seems likely, tumor eluates contain tumor-specific immune complexes, these may act *in vivo* either in the complexed form or following dissociation into antibody and antigen components. A specific role for immunoglobulins in tumor enhancement is well established in tumor allograft systems (Voisin, 1971). Likewise, solubilized transplantation antigens have been found to enhance tumor allografts (Rosenberg *et al.*, 1973), although there is still no conclusive proof that similar tumor antigen preparations can modify tumor growth. However, it must be recognized that treatment with isolated tumor antigen preparations may directly lead to a specific host response which acts synergistically or antagonistically to the response produced by the developing tumor. For example, plasma membrane fractions from DAB-induced hepatomas, as well as papain- or β-glucosidase-solubilized antigens, elicit specific antibody responses in syngeneic hosts, although this form of immunization does not produce immune protection against subsequent challenge with tumor cells and this treatment may even lead to a suppression of the tumor rejection response (Baldwin and Glaves, 1972; Baldwin *et al.*, 1973*b*, 1974*b*; Price and Baldwin, 1974*a,b*). In contrast, solubilized membrane fractions with some chemically induced tumors (e.g., see Baldwin and Price, Vol. 1, Chap. 12, Table 3) may be capable of eliciting an immune response which is protective against tumor challenge.

While there is still considerable uncertainty as to the role of passively transferred "blocking factors" in enhancing tumor growth, the effects of "unblocking" sera have been more clearly established. This was originally demonstrated by Bansal and Sjögren (1972), who showed that administration of various types of antisera to rats which had previously received an implant of the polyoma tumor resulted in complete rejection of the tumor. The antisera used in these experiments were produced either in syngeneic rats or in xenogeneic animals (rabbits), and correlated with the observed regression of tumors was the finding that serum of the tumor recipients no longer exhibited blocking activity. These tests were further extended to show that a combination of inoculation of unblocking antisera and splenectomy significantly inhibited the growth of primary polyoma tumors. Also, combination of treatment with unblocking sera and BCG was effective in inducing regression of polyoma tumors (Bansal and Sjögren, 1973*a,b*).

The type and degree of interference with cell-mediated immune responses by circulating serum factors will be dependent on several parameters: the immunocompetence of the host, the relative immunogenicities of the various tumor-associated neoantigens, and their capacity to undergo release or shedding from the tumor cell may each contribute to the level of circulating serum factors. Antigen release will also be dependent on cellular expression, metabolic processes, cell death, and consequent autolytic degradation. Antigens may be liberated by secretion if localized within the cell cytoplasm, or, for cell-surface-expressed antigens, membrane turnover, synthesis, and regeneration may determine release. In addition, other factors such as the ability of the host to remove antigen or immune complex from the circulation are implicated: immune complexes deposited in the kidneys may be differentially removed according to their relative quantities and/or compositions, and the kidney has different thresholds for different proteins (Anderson *et al.*, 1974). Moreover, removal of antigen via the kidneys may be variable during tumor development since in terminal cancer patients the permeability of the kidney increases and the level of urinary protein rises (Rudman *et al.*, 1969).

The nature and occurrence of circulating factors which may be involved in the modification of cell-mediated immune responses during tumor growth have been examined with several chemically induced tumor systems, notably with aminoazo dye induced rat hepatomas and murine plasmacytomas. Figure 1 summarizes the data obtained with one transplanted rat hepatoma in studies on the identification of various serum factors by membrane immunofluorescence techniques. During early tumor growth, free tumor-specific antigen became detectable in the serum and these tumor-bearer sera were weakly inhibitory against hepatoma-immune lymph node cells in assays of cell-mediated immunity, although they were not

227

IMMUNO-
BIOLOGY OF
CHEMICALLY
INDUCED
TUMORS

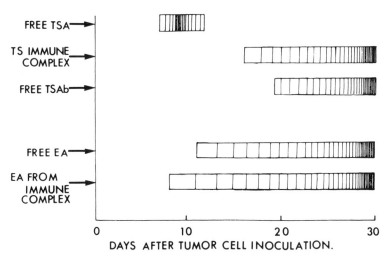

FIGURE 1. Diagrammatic representation of the serum factors detected during the subcutaneous growth of the DAB-induced rat hepatoma D23. Free circulating tumor-specific antigen (TSA) was demonstrable during the early phase of growth of hepatoma D23 (between days 7 and 11), while at later stages (from about day 16) free antibody (TSAb) was detectable. Tumor-specific (TS) immune complexes were detected before free antibody activity was evident, although both factors then persisted in the serum throughout tumor development. Immune complexes containing hepatoma-associated embryonic antigen (EA) were identified after about 1 wk following tumor cell inoculation, this being accompanied by the appearance of free circulating embryonic antigen activity shortly afterward which remained in excess during tumor growth. Data compiled from Bowen *et al.* (1974) and Rees *et al.* (1974*b*).

MICHAEL R.
PRICE
AND
ROBERT W.
BALDWIN

blocking at the level of the target cell (Bowen et al., 1974). With MCA-induced rat sarcomas, tumor-specific antigenic activity became detectable by radioimmunoassay much earlier during tumor development (within 1–2 days after implantation), but in this case the activity was attributed to autolysis of many of the injected tumor cells (Thomson et al., 1973a).

After the early release of tumor-specific antigen into the serum of hepatoma-bearing rats, the level of activity declined with tumor development, this being accompanied by the appearance of immune complexes in the serum and at later stages of tumor growth specific antibody became detectable (Baldwin et al., 1974a; Bowen et al., 1974). The appearance of tumor-specific immune complexes coincided with an increased blocking and inhibitory activity in these sera, supporting the concept that immune complexes may be more effective in the abrogation of tumor immunity than antibody alone. However, when free antibody was detectable together with immune complexes (Fig. 1), inhibitory responses directed against sensitized effector cells were no longer demonstrable, suggesting the requirement of free antigenic determinants for interaction with the immune lymph node cells.

The proposal that released tumor antigen may play a prominent role in modifying immunity in the tumor-bearing host is supported by a series of investigations with MCA-induced rat sarcomas where it was determined that antigen was rapidly released into the blood and lymph and circulating immune complexes were demonstrated (Thomson et al., 1973a,b). Tumor-bearer serum also inhibited the cytotoxicity of immune lymphoid cells for cultured sarcoma cells, although in converse to the rat hepatoma studies free antibody was demonstrable only following surgical resection of tumor (Currie and Alexander, 1974; Thomson et al., 1973b). It was further suggested that the rate of membrane turnover and antigen release could be correlated with the capacity of the tumor to metastasize and that with intense antigen shedding even small tumor foci may escape host immunological control (Currie and Alexander, 1974; Alexander, 1974).

The identification of tumor-specific antibody at later stages of growth of subcutaneous transplanted rat hepatomas (Fig. 1) is contrary to the findings obtained with murine plasmacytomas; in this case, antibody was most frequently associated with the early phase of tumor growth (Kolb et al., 1974). However, as already discussed, many factors may be operative in determining whether tumor-associated antigen, antibody, or immune complexes are present at any one time following tumor cell inoculation. In this respect, in the rat hepatoma model, when tumors are maintained in the peritoneal cavity instead of by the subcutaneous route, free circulating antigen together with immune complexes is present at terminal stages of tumor growth (Baldwin et al., 1973a). However, the growth characteristics of rat hepatomas passaged by the two routes are markedly different, the intraperitoneal tumors developing more rapidly with little necrosis, and this is most likely of significance in determining the levels of circulating factors.

It is evident that the release of factors into the circulation follows no general pattern. This is further exemplified in studies in the rat hepatoma system, in which tumor-associated embryonic antigen is demonstrable soon after tumor cell inoculation, with increasing activity during tumor development (Fig. 1). The presence of free embryonic antigen in the serum of these tumor bearers coincided with the appearance of embryonic antigen isolated from immune complexes, although this activity was also detectable at an earlier stage of growth. These findings resemble those of Kolb *et al.* (1974) showing that, with murine plasmacytomas, tumor-associated antigen was present in a free form together with immune complexes in sera from the mid and late stages of tumor growth and sera containing an excess of antigen were most frequently associated with large tumors. While it was not established whether or not this antigen functioned to promote rejection responses, its characteristics are similar to those of the rat hepatoma associated embryonic antigen in that with both components antigenic activity may be readily obtained in a soluble form following tumor cell disruption and in that isolated antigen preparations share comparable molecular weights (approximately 70,000 daltons) and α electrophoretic mobilities (Baldwin *et al.*, 1974*d*; Kolb *et al.*, 1974; Price, 1974).

229
IMMUNO-
BIOLOGY OF
CHEMICALLY
INDUCED
TUMORS

4. Conclusion

The studies discussed clearly establish that chemically induced tumors exhibit neoantigens which under appropriate conditions may elicit immune responses that have the capacity to evoke tumor rejection. These responses have been extensively demonstrated using transplanted tumor systems, and many of the cell-mediated immune reactions which are considered to be important in causing tumor rejection are demonstrable in the tumor-bearing host. Under these circumstances, however, it has been shown that circulating humoral factors may specifically interfere with cell-mediated immunity. These *in vitro* studies have defined several pathways by which tumors may escape immunological control, although more extensive analyses of *in vivo* correlates are required to assess their significance in host control of tumors.

These studies lead to the conclusion that immunological phenomena are involved in chemical carcinogenesis, but evidence supporting this hypothesis is still limited and often contradictory. To take one example, experiments designed to show increased tumor development following treatment of immunosuppressed hosts with chemical carcinogens are far from convincing (reviewed by Baldwin, 1973; Rubin, 1971). This is further exemplified by work by Stutman (1974) demonstrating that athymic-nude (*nu/nu*) mice and normal (*nu/+*) mice show no differences in either latent period or incidence of local sarcomas or lung adenomas after treatment with MCA. These results argue strongly against an active role of thymus-dependent immunity in modifying carcinogenesis. As

230

MICHAEL R.
PRICE
AND
ROBERT W.
BALDWIN

already discussed, however, the role of different effector mechanisms can now be considered as a multicomponent process. In this context, Prehn and Lappe (1971) have argued that slight immunostimulation may actually enhance rather than retard tumor growth. Clearly, each of these concepts requires further elaboration and refinement so that the relative contributions of the various immunological phenomena discussed may be restated on a more integrated basis.

ACKNOWLEDGMENTS

This work was supported by grants from the Cancer Research Campaign and the Medical Research Council.

5. References

ALEXANDER, P., 1974, Escape from immune destruction by the host through shedding of surface antigens: Is this a characteristic shared by malignant and embryonic cells? *Cancer Res.* **34**:2077.

ALLISON, A. C., HARRINGTON, J. S., AND BIRBECK, M., 1966, An explanation of the cytotoxic effects of silica on macrophages. *J. Exp. Med.* **124**:141.

ANDERSON, N. G., HOLLADAY, D. W., CATON, J. E., CANDLER, E. L., DIERLAM, P. J., EVELEIGH, J. W., BALL, F. L., HOLLEMAN, J. W., BREILLAT, J. P., AND COGGIN, J. F., 1974, Searching for human tumor antigens, *Cancer Res.* **34**:2066.

ANKERST, J., STEELE, G., AND SJÖGREN, H. O., 1974, Cross-reacting tumor-associated antigen(s) of adenovirus type 9-induced fibroadenomas and a chemically induced mammary carcinoma in rats, *Cancer Res.* **34**:1794.

BALDWIN, R. W., 1973, Immunological aspects of chemical carcinogenesis, *Adv. Cancer Res.* **18**:1.

BALDWIN, R. W., AND BARKER, C. R., 1967a, Tumor-specific antigenicity of aminoazo-dye-induced rat hepatomas, *Int. J. Cancer* **2**:355.

BALDWIN, R. W., AND BARKER, C. R., 1967b, Demonstration of tumour-specific humoral antibody against aminoazo dye-induced rat hepatomata, *Br. J. Cancer* **21**:793.

BALDWIN, R. W., AND EMBLETON, M. J., 1969a, Immunology of 2-acetylaminofluorene-induced rat mammary adenocarcinomas, *Int. J. Cancer* **4**:47.

BALDWIN, R. W., AND EMBLETON, M. J., 1969b, Immunology of spontaneously arising rat mammary adenocarcinomas, *Int. J. Cancer* **4**:430.

BALDWIN, R. W., AND EMBLETON, M. J., 1971a, Demonstration by colony inhibition methods of cellular and humoral immune reactions to tumour-specific antigens associated with aminoazo-dye-induced rat hepatomas, *Int. J. Cancer* **7**:17.

BALDWIN, R. W., AND EMBLETON, M. J., 1971b, Tumor-specific antigens in 2-acetylaminofluorene-induced rat hepatomas and related tumors, *Israel J. Med. Sci.* **7**:144.

BALDWIN, R. W., AND EMBLETON, M. J., 1974, Neoantigens on spontaneous and carcinogen-induced rat tumours defined by *in vitro* lymphocytotoxicity assays, *Int. J. Cancer* **13**:433.

BALDWIN, R. W., AND GLAVES, D., 1972, Solubilization of tumour-specific antigen from plasma membrane of an aminoazo-dye-induced rat hepatoma, *Clin. Exp. Immunol.* **11**:51.

BALDWIN, R. W., AND MOORE, M., 1971, Tumour-specific antigens and tumour-host interactions, in: *Immunological Tolerance to Tissue Antigens* (N. W. Nisbet and M. W. Elves, eds.), pp. 299–313, Orthopaedic Hospital, Oswestry, England.

BALDWIN, R. W., PRICE, M. R., AND ROBINS, R. A., 1972, Blocking of lymphocyte-mediated cytotoxicity for rat hepatoma cells by tumour-specific antigen–antibody complexes, *Nature New Biol.* **238**:185.

BALDWIN, R. W., BOWEN, J. G., AND PRICE, M. R., 1973a, Detection of circulating hepatoma D23 antigen and immune complexes in tumour bearer serum, *Brit. J. Cancer* **28**:16.

BALDWIN, R. W., EMBLETON, M. J., AND MOORE, M., 1973b, Immunogenicity of rat hepatoma membrane fractions, *Br. J. Cancer* **28**:389.

231

IMMUNO-
BIOLOGY OF
CHEMICALLY
INDUCED
TUMORS

BALDWIN, R. W., EMBLETON, M. J., AND PRICE, M. R., 1973c, Inhibition of lymphocyte cytotoxicity for human colon carcinoma by treatment with solubilized tumour membrane fractions, *Int. J. Cancer* **12**:84.

BALDWIN, R. W., EMBLETON, M. J., AND ROBINS, R. A., 1973d, Cellular and humoral immunity to rat hepatoma-specific antigens correlated with tumour status, *Int. J. Cancer* **11**:1.

BALDWIN, R. W., HARRIS, J. R., AND PRICE, M. R., 1973e, Fractionation of plasma membrane-associated tumour-specific antigen from an aminoazo dye-induced rat hepatoma, *Int. J. Cancer* **11**:385.

BALDWIN, R. W., PRICE, M. R., AND ROBINS, R. A., 1973f, Significance of serum factors modifying cellular immune responses to growing tumours, *Br. J. Cancer* **28**:37 (Suppl. I).

BALDWIN, R. W., PRICE, M. R., AND ROBINS, R. A., 1973g, Inhibition of hepatoma-immune lymph node cell cytotoxicity by tumour-bearer serum, and solubilized hepatoma antigen, *Int. J. Cancer* **11**:527.

BALDWIN, R. W., BOWEN, J. G., EMBLETON, M. J., PRICE, M. R., AND ROBINS, R. A., 1974a, Cellular and humoral immune interactions during neoplastic development, in: *Role of Immunological Factors in Viral and Oncogenic Processes* (R. F. Beers, R. C. Tilghman, and E. G. Bassett, eds.), pp. 393–407, Johns Hopkins University Press, Baltimore.

BALDWIN, R. W., BOWEN, J. G., AND PRICE, M. R., 1974b, Solubilization of membrane-associated tumour-specific antigens by β-glucosidase, *Biochim. Biophys. Acta* **367**:47.

BALDWIN, R. W., EMBLETON, M. J., PRICE, M. R., AND ROBINS, R. A., 1974c, Immunity in the tumor-bearing host and its modification by serum factors, *Cancer* **34**:1452.

BALDWIN, R. W., EMBLETON, M. J., PRICE, M. R., AND VOSE, B. M., 1974d, Embryonic antigen expression on experimental rat tumours, *Transplant. Rev.* **20**:77.

BALDWIN, R. W., GLAVES, D., AND VOSE, B. M., 1974e, Immunogenicity of embryonic antigens associated with chemically induced rat tumours, *Int. J. Cancer* **13**:135.

BALDWIN, R. W., GLAVES, D., AND VOSE, B. M., 1974f, Differentiation between the embryonic and tumour specific antigens on chemically induced rat tumours, *Br. J. Cancer* **29**:1.

BANSAL, S. C., AND SJÖGREN, H. O., 1972, Counteraction of the blocking of cell-mediated tumor immunity by inoculation of unblocking sera and splenectomy: Immunotherapeutic effects on primary polyoma tumors in rats, *Int. J. Cancer* **9**:490.

BANSAL, S. C., AND SJÖGREN, H. O., 1973a, Effects of BCG on various facets of the immune response against polyoma tumours in rats, *Int. J. Cancer* **11**:162.

BANSAL, S. C., AND SJÖGREN, H. O., 1973b, Regression of polyoma tumor metastasis by combined unblocking and BCG treatment: Correlation with induced alterations in tumor immunity status, *Int. J. Cancer* **12**:179.

BANSAL, S. C., HARGREAVES, R., AND SJÖGREN, H. O., 1972, Facilitation of polyoma tumor growth in rats by unblocking sera and tumor eluate, *Int. J. Cancer* **9**:97.

BARD, D. S., AND PILCH, Y. H., 1969, The role of the spleen in immunity to a chemically induced sarcoma in C3H mice, *Cancer Res.* **29**:1125.

BARD, D. S., HAMMOND, W. G., AND PILCH, Y. H., 1969, The role of the regional lymph nodes in the immunity to a chemically induced sarcoma in C3H mice, *Cancer Res.* **29**:1379.

BASHAM, C., AND CURRIE, G. A., 1974, Development of specific cell-dependent antibody during growth of a syngeneic rat sarcoma, *Br. J. Cancer* **29**:189.

BELEHRADEK, J., BARSKI, G., AND THONIER, M., 1972, Evolution of cell mediated antitumour immunity in mice bearing a syngeneic chemically induced tumor: Influence of tumor growth, surgical removal and treatment with irradiated tumor cells, *Int. J. Cancer* **9**:461.

BLAIR, P. B., AND LANE, M. A., 1974, Serum factors in mammary neoplasia; Enhancement and antagonism of spleen cell activity *in vitro* detected by different methods of serum factor assay, *J. Immunol.* **112**:439.

BLASECKI, J. W., AND TEVETHIA, S. S., 1975, *In vitro* studies on the cellular immune response of tumor-bearing mice to SV40-transformed cells, *J. Immunol.* **114**:244.

BLOOM, E. T., 1970, Quantitative detection of cytotoxic antibodies against tumor-specific antigens of murine sarcomas induced by 3-methylcholanthrene, *J. Natl. Cancer Inst.* **45**:443.

BLOOM, E. T., AND HILDEMANN, W. H., 1970, Mechanisms of tumor-specific enhancement versus resistance toward a methylcholanthrene-induced murine sarcoma, *Transplantation* **10**:321.

BORSOS, T., RICHARDSON, A. K., OHANIAN, S. H., AND LEONARD, E. J., 1973, Immunochemical detection of tumor-specific and embryonic antigens of diethylnitrosamine-induced guinea pig tumors, *J. Natl. Cancer Inst.* **51**:1955.

BOWEN, J. G., ROBINS, R. A., AND BALDWIN, R. W., 1974, Serum factors modifying cell mediated immunity to rat hepatoma D23 correlated with tumour status, *Int. J. Cancer* **15**:640.

232

MICHAEL R.
PRICE
AND
ROBERT W.
BALDWIN

BRAWN, R. J., 1970, Possible association of embryonal antigen(s) with several primary 3-methylcholanthrene-induced murine sarcomas, *Int. J. Cancer* **6**:245.

BUBENÍK, J., AND KOLDOVSKY, P., 1964, The mechanism of antitumour immunity studied by means of transfers of immunity, *Folia Biol. (Prague)* **10**:427.

BURDICK, J. F., COHEN, A. M., AND WELLS, S. A., 1973, A simplified isotopic antiglobulin assay: Detection of tumor cell antigens, *J. Natl. Cancer Inst.* **50**:285.

CEROTTINI, J.-C., NORDIN, A. A., AND BRUNNER, K. T., 1972, *In vitro* cytotoxic activity of thymus cells, sensitized to alloantigens, *Nature (London)* **227**:72.

CHANDRADASA, K. D., 1973, The development of specific suppression of concomitant immunity in two syngeneic tumor–host systems, *Int. J. Cancer* **11**:648.

CHIA, E., AND FESTENSTEIN, H., 1973, Specific cytostatic effect of lymph node cells from normal and T-cell deficient mice on syngeneic tumour target cells *in vitro*, and its specific abrogation by syngeneic fluid from tumour-bearing mice, *Eur. J. Immunol.* **3**:483.

CLEVELAND, P. H., McKHANN, C. F., JOHNSON, K., AND NELSON, S., 1974, A microassay for humoral cytotoxicity demonstrating sublethal effects of antibody, *Int. J. Cancer* **14**:417.

COHEN, A. M., BURDICK, J. F., AND KETCHAM, A. S., 1971, Cell-mediated cytotoxicity: An assay using ^{125}I-iododeoxyuridine-labeled target cells, *J. Immunol.* **107**:895.

COHEN, A. M., MILLAR, R. C., AND KETCHAM, A. S., 1972, Host immunity to a growing transplanted methylcholanthrene-induced guinea pig sarcoma, *Cancer Res.* **32**:2421.

COHEN, J. M., YANG, S. S., AND LAW, L. W., 1974, Abrogation of cell-mediated immunity by hyperimmune alloantiserum: Mechanisms and correlation with allograft enhancement, *Int. J. Cancer* **13**:463.

CURRIE, G. A., 1973, The role of circulating antigen as an inhibitor of tumour immunity in man, *Br. J. Cancer* **28**:153 (Suppl. I).

CURRIE, G. A., AND ALEXANDER, P., 1974, Spontaneous shedding of TSTA by viable sarcoma cells: Its possible role in facilitating metastatic spread, *Br. J. Cancer* **29**:72.

CURRIE, G. A., AND BASHAM, C., 1972, Serum-mediated inhibition of the immunological reactions of the patient to his own tumour: A possible role for circulating antigen, *Br. J. Cancer* **26**:427.

DATTA, S. K., AND VANDEPUTTE, M., 1971, Studies on cellular and humoral immunity to tumor-specific antigens in polyoma virus-induced tumors of rats, *Cancer Res.* **31**:882.

DAVIES, D. A. L., BUCKHAM, S., AND MANSTONE, A. J., 1974*a*, Protection of mice against syngeneic lymphomata. II. Collaboration between drugs and antibodies, *Br. J. Cancer* **30**:305.

DAVIES, D. A. L., MANSTONE, A. J., AND BUCKHAM, S., 1974*b*, Protection of mice against syngeneic lymphomata. I. Use of antibodies, *Br. J. Cancer* **30**:297.

DECKERS, P. J., EDGERTON, B. W., THOMAS, B. S., AND PILCH, Y. H., 1971, The adoptive transfer of concomitant immunity to murine tumor isografts with spleen cells from tumor-bearing animals, *Cancer Res.* **31**:734.

EVANS, R., AND ALEXANDER, P., 1972, Mechanism of immunologically specific killing of tumour cells by macrophages. *Nature (London)* **236**:168.

EVANS, R., COX, H., AND ALEXANDER, P., 1973, Immunologically specific activation of macrophages armed with specific macrophage arming factor, *Proc. Soc. Exp. Biol. (N.Y.)* **143**:256.

FEFER, A., 1969, Immunotherapy and chemotherapy of Moloney sarcoma virus-induced tumors in mice, *Cancer Res.* **29**:2177.

FISHER, B., SAFFER, E. A., AND FISHER, E. R., 1970, Comparison of concomitant and sineconcomitant tumor immunity, *Proc. Soc. Exp. Biol. (N.Y.)* **135**:68.

FORMAN, J., AND MÖLLER, G., 1973, The effector cell in antibody induced cell mediated immunity, *Transplant. Rev.* **17**:108.

GLASER, M., HERBERMAN, R. B., KIRCHNER, H., AND DJEU, J. Y., 1974, Study of the cellular immune response to Gross virus-induced lymphoma by the mixed lymphocyte–tumor interaction, *Cancer Res.* **34**:2165.

GREENBERG, A. H., AND SHEN, L., 1973, A class of specific cytotoxic cells demonstrated *in vitro* by arming with antigen–antibody complexes, *Nature New Biol.* **245**:282.

HALLIDAY, W. J., 1971, Blocking effect of serum from tumor-bearing animals on macrophage migration inhibition with tumor antigens, *J. Immunol.* **106**:855.

HALLIDAY, W., AND WEBB, M., 1969, Delayed hypersensitivity to chemically induced tumors in mice and correlation with an *in vitro* test, *J. Natl. Cancer Inst.* **43**:141.

HALLIDAY, W. J., MALUISH, A., AND MILLER, S., 1974, Blocking and unblocking of cell-mediated antitumor immunity in mice, as detected by the leucocyte adherence inhibition test, *Cell. Immunol.* **10**:467.

HARADA, M., PEARSON, G., PETTIGREW, H., REDMON, L., AND ORR, T., 1973, Enhancement of normal lymphocyte cytotoxicity by sera with high antibody titers against *H-2* or virus-associated antigens, *Cancer Res.* **33**:2886.

HARDER, F. H., AND MCKHANN, C. F., 1968, Demonstration of cellular antigens on sarcoma cells by an indirect ^{125}I-labeled antibody technique, *J. Natl. Cancer Inst.* **40**:231.

HELLSTRÖM, I., 1967, A colony inhibition (CI) technique for demonstration of tumor cell destruction by lymphoid cells *in vitro*, *Int. J. Cancer* **2**:65.

HELLSTROM, I., AND HELLSTRÖM, K. E., 1969, Studies on cellular immunity and its serum-medicated tumor-cell destruction by certain patient sera, *Int. J. Cancer* **12**:348.

HELLSTRÖM, I., AND HELLSTRÖM, K. E., 1970a, Colony inhibition studies on blocking and non-blocking serum effects on cellular immunity to Moloney sarcomas, *Int. J. Cancer* **5**:195.

HELLSTRÖM, I., HELLSTRÖM, K. E., AND PIERCE, G. E., 1968, *In vitro* studies of immune reactions against autochthonous and syngeneic mouse tumors induced by methylcholanthrene and plastic discs, *Int. J. Cancer* **3**:467.

HELLSTRÖM, I., HELLSTRÖM, K. E., AND SJÖGREN, H. O., 1970, Serum-mediated inhibition of cellular immunity to methylcholanthrene-induced murine sarcomas, *Cell. Immunol.* **1**:18.

HELLSTRÖM, I., HELLSTRÖM, K. E., AND WARNER, G. A., 1973, Increase of lymphocyte-mediated tumor-cell destruction by certain patient sera, *Int. J. Cancer* **12**:348.

HELLSTRÖM, K. E., AND HELLSTRÖM, I., 1970b, Immunological enhancement as studied by cell culture techniques, *Ann. Rev. Microbiol.* **24**:373.

HELLSTRÖM, K. E., AND HELLSTRÖM, I., 1974, Lymphocyte-mediated cytotoxicity and blocking serum activity to tumor antigens, *Adv. Immunol.* **18**:209.

HENDERSON, W. R., FUKUYAMA, K., EPSTEIN, W. L., AND SPITLER, L. E., 1973, Blocking of a cellular immune reaction to malignant melanoma by immunoglobulin from tumor-bearing animals, *J. Reticuloendothel. Soc.* **13**:155.

HERBERMAN, R. B., AND OREN, M. E., 1971, Immune responses to Gross virus-induced lymphoma. I. Kinetics of cytotoxic antibody response, *J. Natl. Cancer Inst.* **46**:391.

HERBERMAN, R. B., TING, C. C., KIRCHNER, H., HOLDEN, H., GLASER, M., BONNARD, G. D., AND LAVRIN, D., 1974, Effector mechanisms in tumor immunity, in: *Progress in Immunology*, Vol. II, Academic Press, New York.

HERSEY, P., 1973, New look at antiserum therapy of leukaemia, *Nature New Biol.* **244**:22.

ISHIDATE, M., 1967, Recognition of the individuality of tumour strain by peritoneal lymphoid cells, *Nature (London)* **215**:184.

JAGARLAMOODY, S., AUST, J. C., TEW, R. H., AND MCKHANN, C. F., 1970, Tumor-specific immunity assayed in vitro by cell growth inhibition, *Proc. Am. Assoc. Cancer Res.* **11**:40.

JOSE, D. G., AND SESHADRI, R., 1974, Circulating immune complexes in human neuroblastoma: Direct assay and role in blocking specific cellular immunity, *Int. J. Cancer* **13**:824.

JOSE, D. G., AND SKVARIL, F., 1974, Serum inhibitors of cellular immunity in human nephroblastoma: IgG subclass of blocking activity, *Int. J. Cancer* **13**:173.

KOLB, J. P., POUPON, M. F., AND LESPINATS, G., 1974, Tumor-associated antigen (TAA) and anti-TAA antibodies in the serum of BALB/c mice with plasmacytomas, *J. Natl. Cancer Inst.* **52**:723.

KRAHENBUHL, J. L., AND REMINGTON, J. S., 1974, The role of activated macrophages in specific and non specific cytostatis of tumor cells, *J. Immunol.* **113**:507.

LAMON, E. W., KLEIN, E., ANDERSSON, B. FENYÖ, E. M., AND SKURZAK, H. M., 1973a, The humoral antibody response to a primary viral neoplasm (MSV) through its entire course, *Int. J. Cancer* **12**:637.

LAMON, E. W., WIGZELL, H., ANDERSSON, B., AND KLEIN, E., 1973b, Anti-tumour cell activity *in vitro* dependent on immune B lymphocytes, *Nature New Biol.* **244**:209.

LAMON, E. W., WIGZELL, H., KLEIN, E., ANDERSSON, B., AND SKURZAK, H., 1973c, The lymphocyte response to primary Moloney sarcoma virus tumors in Balb/c mice: Definition of the active subpopulations at different times after infection, *J. Exp. Med.* **137**:1472.

LAMON, E. W., ANDERSSON, B., WIGZELL, H., FENYÖ, E. M., AND KLEIN, E., 1974, The immune response to primary Moloney sarcoma virus tumors in BALB/c mice: Cellular and humoral activity of long-term regressors, *Int. J. Cancer* **13**:91.

LAUSCH, R. N., AND RAPP, F., 1969, Concomitant immunity in hamsters bearing DMBA-induced tumor transplants, *Int. J. Cancer* **4**:226.

LAUX, D., AND LAUSCH, R. N., 1974, Reversal of tumor-mediated suppression of immune reactivity by in vitro incubation of spleen cells, *J. Immunol.* **112**:1900.

LECLERC, J. C., GOMARD, E., PLATA, F., AND LEVY, J. P., 1973, Cell-mediated immune reaction against tumors induced by oncornaviruses: Nature of the effector cells in tumor cell cytolysis, *Int. J. Cancer* **11**:426.

233

IMMUNO-
BIOLOGY OF
CHEMICALLY
INDUCED
TUMORS

234

MICHAEL R.
PRICE
AND
ROBERT W.
BALDWIN

LE MEVEL, B. P., AND WELLS, S. A., 1973, A microassay for the quantitation of cytotoxic antitumor antibody; Use of ^{125}I-Iododeoxyuridine as a tumor cell label, *J. Natl. Cancer Inst.* **50**:803.

LE MEVEL, B. P., OLDHAM, R. K., WELLS, S. A., AND HERBERMAN, R. B., 1973, An evaluation of ^{125}I-iododeoxyuridine as a cellular label for *in vitro* assays: kinetics of incorporation and toxicity, *J. Natl. Cancer Inst.* **51**:1551.

LITTMAN, B. H., MELTZER, M. S., CLEVELAND, R. P., ZBAR, B., AND RAPP, H. J., 1973, Tumor-specific, cell-mediated immunity in guinea pigs with tumors, *J. Natl. Cancer Inst.* **51**:1627.

LOHMANN-MATTHES, M. L., AND FISHER, H., 1973, T-cell cytotoxicity and amplification of the cytotoxic reaction by macrophages, *Transplant. Rev.* **17**:150.

MACLENNAN, I. C. M., 1972, Antibody in the induction and inhibition of lymphocyte cytotoxicity, *Transplant. Rev.* **13**:67.

MALUISH, A., AND HALLIDAY, W. J., 1974, Cell-mediated immunity and specific serum factors in human cancer: The leukocyte adherence inhibition test, *J. Natl. Cancer Inst.* **52**:1415.

MCCOY, J. L., DEAN, J. H., LAW, L. W., WILLIAMS, J., MCCOY, N. T., AND HOLIMAN, B. J., 1974, Immunogenicity, antigenicity and mechanisms of tumor rejection of mineral oil induced plasmacytomas in syngeneic BALB/c mice, *Int. J. Cancer* **14**:264.

MELTZER, M. S., OPPENHEIM, J. J., LITTMAN, B. H., LEONARD, E. J., AND RAPP, H. J., 1972, Cell-mediated tumor immunity measured *in vitro* and *in vivo* with soluble tumor-specific antigens, *J. Natl. Cancer Inst.* **49**;727.

MENARD, S., PIEROTTI, M., AND COLNAGHI, M. I., 1972, A ^{51}Cr microtest for cellular immunity, *Transplantation* **14**:155.

MIKULSKA, Z. B., SMITH, C., AND ALEXANDER, P., 1966, Evidence for an immunological reaction of the host directed against its own actively growing primary tumor, *J. Natl. Cancer Inst.* **36**:29.

MÖLLER, G., 1964, Effect on tumour growth in syngeneic recipients of antibodies against tumour-specific antigens in methylcholanthrene-induced mouse sarcomas, *Nature (London)* **204**:846.

MÖLLER, G., AND SVEHAG, S. E., 1972, Specificity of lymphocyte-mediated cytotoxicity induced by *in vitro* antibody-coated target cells, *Cell. Immunol.* **4**:1.

NELSON, D. S., 1974, Immunity to infection, allograft immunity and tumour immunity: Parallels and contrasts, *Transplant. Rev.* **19**:226.

OLD, L. J., AND BOYSE, E. A., 1964, Immunology of experimental tumors, *Ann. Rev. Med.* **15**:167.

OLD, L. J., BOYSE, E. A., CLARKE, D. A., AND CARSWELL, E. A., 1962, Antigenic properties of chemically induced tumors, *Ann. N.Y. Acad. Sci.* **101**:80.

OREN, M. E., HERBERMAN, R. B., AND CANTY, T. G., 1971, Immune response to Gross virus-induced lymphoma. II. Kinetics of the cellular immune response, *J. Natl. Cancer Inst.* **46**:621.

ORTIZ DE LANDAZURI, M. AND HERBERMAN, R. B., 1972, *In vitro* activation of cellular immune response to Gross virus-induced lymphoma, *J. Exp. Med.* **136**:969.

ORTIZ DE LANDAZURI, M., KEDAR, E., AND FAHEY, J. L., 1974, Antibody-dependent cellular cytotoxicity to a syngeneic Gross virus-induced lymphoma, *J. Natl. Cancer Inst.* **52**:147.

PERLMANN, P., PERLMANN, H., AND WIGZELL, H., 1972, Lymphocyte mediated cytotoxicity *in vitro*: Induction and inhibition by humoral antibody and nature of effector cells. *Transplant. Rev.* **13**:91.

PERLMANN, P., WIGZELL, H., GOLDSTEIN, P., LAMON, E. W., LARSSON, A., O'TOOLE, C., PERLMANN, H., AND SVEDMYR, E. A. J., 1974, Cell-mediated cytolysis *in vitro*: Analysis of active lymphocyte subpopulations in different experimental systems, *Adv. Biosci.* **12**:71.

PLATA, F., AND LEVY, J. P., 1974, Blocking of syngeneic effector T cells by soluble tumour antigens, *Nature (London)* **249**:271.

PLATA, F., GOMARD, E., LECLERC, J. C., AND LEVY, J. P., 1973, Further evidence for the involvement of thymus-processed lymphocytes in syngeneic tumor cell cytolysis, *J. Immunol.* **111**:667.

POLLACK, S., AND NELSON, K., 1974, Early appearance of lymphoid arming factor and cytotoxic lymph node cells after tumor induction, *Int. J. Cancer* **14**:522.

PREHN, R. T., AND LAPPÉ, M. A., 1971, An immunostimulation theory of tumor development, *Transplant. Rev.* **7**:26.

PRICE, M. R., 1974, Isolation of embryonic antigens from chemically induced rat hepatomas, *Biochem. Soc. Trans.* **2**:650.

PRICE, M. R., AND BALDWIN, R. W., 1974a, Preparation of aminoazo dye-induced rat hepatoma membrane fractions retaining tumour specific antigen, *Br. J. Cancer* **30**:382.

PRICE, M. R., AND BALDWIN, R. W., 1974b, Immogenic properties of rat hepatoma subcellular fractions, *Br. J. Cancer* **30**:394.

RAPP, H. J., CHURCHILL, W. H., KRONMAN, B. S., ROLLEY, R. T., HAMMOND, W. G., AND BORSOS, T., 1968, Antigenicity of a new diethylnitrosamine-induced transplantable guinea pig hepatoma: Pathology and formation of ascites variant, *J. Natl. Cancer Inst.* **41**:1.

235

IMMUNO-
BIOLOGY OF
CHEMICALLY
INDUCED
TUMORS

Rees, R. C., Price, M. R., Baldwin, R. W., and Shah, L. P., 1974a, Inhibition of rat lymph node cell cytotoxicity by hepatoma-associated embryonic antigen, *Nature (London)* **252:**751.

Rees, R. C., Price, M. R., Shah, L. P., and Baldwin, R. W., 1974b, Detection of hepatoma-associated embryonic antigen in tumour-bearer serum, *Transplantation* **19:**424.

Ritter, J., Lohmann-Matthes, M.-L., and Fisher, H., 1973, Specific inactivation of cytotoxic lymphocytes after adsorption on ^{51}Cr labeled fibroblast monolayers, *Transplantation* **16:**579.

Robins, R. A., and Baldwin, R. W., 1974, Tumour specific antibody neutralization of factors in rat hepatoma bearer serum which abrogate lymph node cell cytotoxicity, *Int. J. Cancer*, **14:**589.

Rosenberg, E. B., Hill, J., Ferarri, A., Herberman, R. B., Ting, C.-C., Mann, D. L., and Fahey, J., 1973, Prolonged survival of tumor allografts in mice pretreated with soluble transplantation antigens, *J. Natl. Cancer Inst.* **50:**1453.

Rouse, B. T., Röllonghoff, M., and Warner, N. L., 1972, Anti-θ serum-induced suppression of cellular transfer of tumour-specific immunity to a syngeneic plasma cell tumour, *Nature (London)* **238:**116.

Rouse, B. T., Röllinghoff, M., and Warner, N. L., 1973, Tumor immunity to murine plasma cell tumors. II. Essential role of T lymphocytes in immune response, *Eur. J. Immunol.* **3:**218.

Rubin, B. A., 1971, Alteration of the homograft response as a determinant of carcinogenicity, *Progr. Exp. Tumor Res.* **14:**138.

Rudman, D., Del Rio, A., Akgun, S., and Frumin, E., 1969, Novel proteins and peptides in the urine of patients with advanced neoplastic disease, *Am. J. Med.* **46:**174.

Senik, A., De Giorgi, L., Gomard, E., and Levy, J. P., 1974a, Cytostasis of lymphoma cells in suspension: Probable non-thymic origin of the cytostatic lymphoid cells in mice bearing MSV-induced tumors, *Int. J. Cancer* **14:**396.

Senik, A., De Giorgi, L., and Levy, J. P., 1974b, Cell-mediated anti-tumor immunity in oncornavirus-induced tumors: Specific cytostasis of tumor cells by spleen and lymph node cells, *Int. J. Cancer* **14:**386.

Shellam, G. R., 1974, Studies on a Gross-virus-induced lymphoma in the rat. I. The cell-mediated immune response, *Int. J. Cancer* **14:**65.

Shortman, K., Byrd, W., Williams, N., Brunner, K. T., and Cerottini, J.-C., 1972, Separation of different cell classes from lymphoid organs, *Aust. J. Exp. Biol. Med. Sci.* **50:**323.

Sjögren, H. O., and Borum, K., 1971, Tumor-specific immunity in the course of primary polyoma and Rous tumor development in intact and immunosuppressed rats, *Cancer Res.* **31:**890.

Sjögren, H. O., Hellström, I., Bansal, S. C., and Hellström, K. E., 1971, Suggestive evidence that the "blocking antibodies" of tumor bearing individuals may be antigen–antibody complexes, *Proc. Natl. Acad. Sci.* **68:**1372.

Sjögren, H. O., Hellström, I., Bansal, S. C., Warner, G. A., and Hellström, K. E., 1972, Elution of "blocking antibodies" from human tumors, capable of abrogating tumor cell destruction by specifically immune lymphocytes, *Int. J. Cancer* **9:**274.

Skurzak, H. M., Klein, E., Yoshida, T. O., and Lamon, E. W., 1972, Synergistic or antagonistic effect of different antibody concentrations on *in vitro* lymphocyte cytotoxicity in the Moloney sarcoma virus system, *J. Exp. Med.* **135:**997.

Steele, G., Ankerst, J., and Sjögren, H. O., 1974, Alteration of *in vitro* antitumor activity of tumor bearer serum by absorption with *Staphylococcus aureus*, Cowan I, *Int. J. Cancer* **14:**83.

Stutman, O., 1974, Tumor development after 3-methylcholanthrene in immunologically deficient athymic-nude mice, *Science* **183:**534.

Takasugi, M., and Klein, E., 1970, A microassay for cell-mediated immunity, *Transplantation* **9:**219.

Takeda, K., Aizawa, M., Kituchi, Y., Yamawaki, S., and Nakamura, K., 1966, Tumour autoimmunity against methylcholanthrene-induced sarcomas of the rat, *Gann* **57:**221.

Tamerius, J. D., and Hellström, I., 1974, *In vitro* demonstration of complement-dependent cytotoxic antibodies to Moloney sarcoma cells, *J. Immunol.* **112:**1987.

Taranger, L. A., Chapman, W. H., Hellström, I., and Hellström, K. E., 1972, Immunological studies on urinary bladder tumors of rats and mice, *Science* **176:**1337.

Thomson, D. M. P., Eccles, S., and Alexander, P., 1973a, Antibodies and soluble tumour-specific antigens in blood and lymph of rats with chemically induced sarcomata, *Br. J. Cancer* **28:**6.

Thomson, D. M. P., Sellens, V., Eccles, S., and Alexander, P., 1973b, Radioimmunoassay of tumor-specific transplantation antigen of a chemically-induced rat sarcoma: Circulating soluble tumour antigen in tumour bearers, *Brit. J. Cancer* **28:**377.

Tigelaar, R. E., and Gorczynski, R. M., 1974, Separable populations of activated thymus-derived identified in two assays for cell-mediated immunity to murine tumor allografts, *J. Exp. Med.* **140:**267.

236

MICHAEL R.
PRICE
AND
ROBERT W.
BALDWIN

TODD, R. F., STULTING, R. D., AND BERKE, G., 1973, Mechanism of blocking by hyperimmune serum of lymphocyte-mediated cytolysis of allogeneic tumor cells, *Cancer Res.* **33**:3203.

VAAGE, J., 1971, Concomitant immunity and specific depression of immunity by residual or reinjected syngeneic tumor tissue, *Cancer Res.* **31**:1655.

VAAGE, J., 1972, Specific desensitization of resistance against a syngeneic methylcholanthrene-induced sarcoma in C3Hf mice, *Cancer Res.* **32**:193.

VASUDEVAN, D. M., BRUNNER, K. T., AND CEROTTINI, J.-C., 1974, Detection of cytotoxic T lymphocytes in the EL4 mouse leukemia system: Increased activity of immune spleen and peritoneal cells following preincubation and cell fractionation procedures, *Int. J. Cancer* **14**:301.

VOISIN, G. A., 1971, Immunological facilitation, a broadening of the concept of the enhancement phenomenon, in: *Progress in Allergy,* Vol. 15 (P. Kallós, B. H. Waksman, and A. de Weck, eds.), pp. 328–485, Karger, Basel.

WAGNER, H., HARRIS, A. W., AND FELDMANN, H., 1972, Cell-mediated immune response *in vitro.* II. The role of thymus and thymus-derived lymphocytes, *Cell. Immunol.* **4**:39.

WAGNER, H., RÖLLINGHOFF, M., AND NOSSAL, G. J. V., 1973, T-cell-mediated immune responses induced *in vitro*: A probe for allograft and tumor immunity, *Transplant. Rev.* **17**:3.

WAHL, D. V., CHAPMAN, I., HELLSTRÖM, I., AND HELLSTRÖM, K. E., 1974, Transplantation immunity to individually unique antigens of chemically induced bladder tumors in mice, *Int. J. Cancer* **14**:114.

WINN, H. J., 1961, Immune mechanisms in homotransplantation. II. Quantitative assay of the immunologic activity of lymphoid cells stimulated by tumor homografts, *J. Immunol.* **86**:228.

WITZ, I., 1973, The biological significance of tumor-bound immunoglobulins, in: *Current Topics in Microbiology and Immunology,* Vol. 61 (W. Arber, R. Haas, W. Henle, P. H. Hofschneider, N. K. Jerne, P. Koldovsky, H. Koprowski, O. Maaløe, R. Rott, H. G. Schweiger, M. Sela, L. Syrucek, P. K. Vogt and E. Wecker, eds.), pp. 151–171, Springer, Berlin.

ZARLING, J., AND TEVETHIA, S. S., 1973, Transplantation immunity to simian virus 40-transformed cells in tumor-bearing mice. II. Evidence for macrophage participation at the effector level of tumor cell rejection, *J. Natl. Cancer Inst.* **50**:149.

ZBAR, B., WEPSIC, H. T., RAPP, H. J., BORSOS, T., KRONMAN, B. S., AND CHURCHILL, W. H., 1969, Antigenic specificity of hepatomas induced in strain-2 guinea pigs by diethylnitrosamine, *J. Natl. Cancer Inst.* **43**:833.

8

Immunological Surveillance Against Tumor Cells

A. C. ALLISON

1. Introduction

Many tumor cells have antigens distinct from those of adult host cells, including virus-specific antigens, embryonic antigens, and others of unknown origin. These antigens can stimulate a variety of immune responses which are demonstrable by serological methods, rejection of tumor transplants *in vivo*, and cell-mediated cytotoxicity *in vitro*. One important question is the effectiveness of such immune responses in limiting tumor formation in normal humans and experimental animals. Ehrlich (1906), who anticipated many concepts of contemporary immunology, suggested that immunity might be directed not only against microbial and parasitic pathogens but also against malignant cells arising within the body. Such surveillance against malignant cells has been postulated more recently by Thomas (1959) and the concept has been elaborated by Burnet (1971) and others. Burnet suggests that immunity directed against autonomous cell variants may have arisen early in the evolution of multicellular organisms and may have been of importance comparable with that of protection against pathogenic organisms from outside the body.

Doubts about the effectiveness of immunological surveillance have arisen from reports that mice treated for long periods with antilymphocytic serum (Nehlsen, 1971) and nude mice (Rygaard and Poulsen, 1974) do not show a greatly increased incidence of spontaneously occurring tumors. However, there is no doubt that

A. C. ALLISON • Clinical Research Centre, Harrow, Middlesex, England.

when such animals are exposed to oncogenic viruses the incidence of tumors is much higher than in controls (Allison, 1974, and below). There is an interesting interaction of inherited factors affecting susceptibility to virus oncogenesis which are exerted through the immune system and those which affect the probability of transformation of target cells by the viruses.

During the past 5 years, it has become clear that there is an increased incidence of tumors in humans with immunodeficiency syndromes and in immunosuppressed recipients of organ grafts. The interpretation of the latter observation has been complicated by the presence of the graft, a relatively large mass of antigenic material; this has raised the possibility that prolonged antigenic stimulation may contribute to neoplasia, especially of the lymphoreticular system. In experimental animals, continued antigenic stimulation, especially in chronic graft-vs.-host reactions, is associated with lymphoreticular malignancy. However, data now being accumulated suggest that humans immunosuppressed for reasons other than organ grafting have an increased risk of developing malignant disease.

Studies of immunosuppressed animals also provide information about which mechanisms of antitumor immunity are effective *in vivo*. Four major *in vitro* reactions against tumor cells have been described:

1. Lysis of tumor cells in the presence of antibody and complement.
2. Lysis of tumor cells by activated T lymphocytes.
3. Lysis of tumor cells with bound antibody by nonspecific effector lymphoid cells (K cells).
4. Tumor cell lytic or cytostatic effects of macrophages.

However, the importance of each of these mechanisms in preventing tumor development is difficult to evaluate. The most informative approach is to compare the incidence of tumor in normal animals and in animals with one or more of these immune reactions suppressed. Thymectomy followed by administration of antilymphocytic serum, for example, suppresses reactions mediated by T lymphocytes. This includes not only cell-mediated immunity but also helper effects in the formation of thymus-dependent antibodies. Treatment of animals with cyclophosphamide or other drugs or X-irradiation strongly suppresses formation of IgG antibody, but also inhibits cell-mediated immunity and produces at least temporary depletion of circulating K cells, monocytes, and granulocytes. To obtain information about which immune reaction is most important in any particular situation, it is therefore necessary to restore selectively immune responses by transfer of serum containing antibody, in the presence or absence of effector cells from nonimmune donors, or by transfer of sensitized lymphocytes from immune donors. In this chapter, for reasons of space, only a single example will be given in detail of each type of investigation in experimental animals, together with a short list of other comparable situations and a brief description of the incidence of malignant disease in immunosuppressed human subjects. Since immunosuppressive treatments would not be expected to increase the incidence of tumors if there were tolerance of tumor-specific antigens, evidence bearing on this question is also mentioned.

Another prediction of the surveillance hypothesis is that the probability of escape of tumor cells from immunological control is low. Hence the likelihood of two or more clones of tumor cells emerging at the same time is small, and tests with genetic markers will show that most tumors in fact arise from single cells. Evidence has also accumulated in support of this view.

2. Polyoma Virus in Mice

It has been suggested that surveillance against polyoma virus and other oncogenic viruses is a laboratory artifact that has no relevance under natural conditions. This view is inconsistent with the natural history of polyoma virus infections, which are common in wild as well as laboratory colonies of mice (Huebner, 1963).

Polyoma virus is a small DNA virus about 45 nm in diameter which when injected into newborn mice of susceptible strains induces tumors in a high proportion of recipients (salivary and mammary adenocarcinomas, osteosarcomas, and others) (see Chap. 9 in Volume 2 of this series). Normal adult mice are resistant to polyoma oncogenesis even though the virus multiplies extensively in host organs. Unlike the indigenous leukemogenic viruses and the mammary tumor agent, polyoma virus is not vertically transmitted from mothers to offspring. Indeed, a mother which has been infected passes antibodies to her offspring, which are then protected for some weeks against infection by the virus. Only when passive protection has waned do the young mice become horizontally infected by polyoma virus from other mice in the colony. The lateness of the infection probably explains why tumors hardly ever arise.

A basic question which can be asked is, therefore, why newborn animals are susceptible to polyoma virus oncogenesis (and also that by many other viruses) whereas adult animals are resistant. Two main explanations can be considered. There might be some feature of differentiation by which adult cells are relatively resistant to polyoma virus transformation. Alternatively, there might be an efficient immune response in the adult against the virus-specific antigens demonstrable by transplantation tests on the surface of the transformed cells, thereby preventing them from growing into a tumor, whereas the immune response is absent, weak, or delayed in newborn animals.

These alternatives can be tested by the use of immunosuppression of adult mice infected by contact or inoculated with polyoma virus. The most efficient immunosuppressive procedure has been thymectomy (3 days or 6 wk after birth) followed by repeated injections of antilymphocytic globulin (ALG). As shown in Table 1, all mice so treated develop polyoma tumors after infection as adults. The tumors are antigenic and the importance of cell-mediated immunity in the prevention of tumor growth is emphasized by the results of restoration experiments. Immune serum from infected mice confers some protection when given 24 h after the virus—apparently because it limits the dissemination of the infection—but when given 7 days after virus it has no protective effect. Likewise,

TABLE 1

Development of Tumors in CBA Mice Infected as Adults with Polyoma Virus

Preliminary treatment	Restoration at 7 wk	Number of animals	Percent with tumors
Normal rabbit globulin	None	24	0
Thymectomy and anti-lymphocyte globulin	None	14	100
	Normal lymphoid cells	10	90
	Sensitized lymphoid cells	11	0
	Sensitized lymphoid cells	10	0
Thymectomy and anti-lymphocyte globulin	Sensitized lymphoid cells treated with anti-θ serum and complement	6	83
Thymectomy and anti-lymphocyte globulin	Antibody at 24 h	12	17
	Antibody at 7 days	10	90
Thymectomy	None	20	0

[a] From Allison (1974).

normal syngeneic lymphoid cells given after the cessation of the ALG treatment provide no protection. In contrast, transfer of lymphoid cells from syngeneic donors immunized with a polyoma tumor protects the animals very efficiently. Transfer of lymphocytes from donors immunized with a tumor induced in the same strain by an unrelated virus (adenovirus type 12) provides no protection. Treatment of the specifically sensitized lymphoid cells by anti-θ serum and complement, to destroy thymus-dependent (T) lymphocytes, abolishes the protective effect (see Gaugas *et al.*, 1973; Allison, 1974).

The importance of T lymphocytes in control of polyoma virus oncogenesis has been emphasized by recent observations in my laboratory (Allison *et al.*, 1974) and that of Professor M. Vandeputte in Louvain that congenitally athymic (*nu/nu*) mice infected with the virus at the age of 6–8 wk develop multiple tumors whereas their *nu/+* littermates with an intact T-lymphocyte system do not. Three months after infection, all the nudes have multiple skin tumors including carcinomas of the hair follicles and sebaceous glands (Figs. 1 and 2), and many have osteosarcomas, and tumors of the salivary gland, kidney, and other sites as well.

Thus the main reason why older mice contracting polyoma virus infections do not develop tumors is that they mount an effective cell-mediated immune response against the tumor cells. This response is mediated by T lymphocytes, but whether these lymphocytes are themselves responsible for killing polyoma tumor cells is not known. However, there is substantial evidence that T cells transformed in the presence of antigen can kill target cells (see Cerottini and Brunner, 1974), so it is reasonable to suppose that this can happen with polyoma tumor cells.

There are at least two explanations for the susceptibility of newborn animals to virus oncogenesis. The traditional explanation is that early exposure to the tumor antigens induces immunological tolerance. An alternative interpretation is that in the adult animal a cell-mediated immune response is mounted rapidly whereas in the newborn animal the response develops only slowly. These possibilities can be distinguished by transferring spleen cells from mice inoculated as newborns with

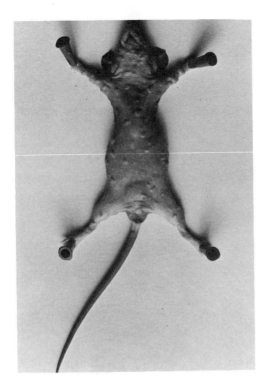

FIGURE 1. Congenitally hypothymic (*nu/nu*) mouse
8 wk after inoculation with polyoma virus, showing
multiple skin tumors.

polyoma virus into immunosuppressed recipients. The results show that both in
mice (Allison, 1970) and in rats (Vandeputte and Datta, 1972) inoculation of
newborns results in efficient cell-mediated immunity, but only after several weeks.
Hence there is no tolerance to the polyoma-specific transplantation antigen, but a
delay in mounting cell-mediated immunity allows the virus-transformed cells to
grow into masses too large for control by the developing immune response.

Genetic differences between mouse strains in susceptibility to tumor induction
by polyoma virus are also explicable in terms of the efficiency of their immune
responses. If genetically resistant strains such as the C57Bl are immunosuppressed with ALG, they all develop tumors (Allison and Law, 1968). This
contrasts with the strong inherited resistance against leukemogenic viruses which
is manifested by all cells of resistant animals and does not depend on the reactions
of immunocompetent cells (see Rowe, 1973).

Immune responses to other DNA oncogenic viruses are also strong and
surveillance mechanisms against tumor formation in adult animals are efficient.
Thus the incidence of adenovirus-induced tumors in mice, especially genetically
resistant strains, is increased by ALG administration (Allison *et al.*, 1967*a*).
Newborn hamsters inoculated with vacuolating virus (SV40) all develop tumors in
about 100 days, whereas only about one-fifth of adult animals develop
tumors—after a very long interval representing the greater part of the life span of

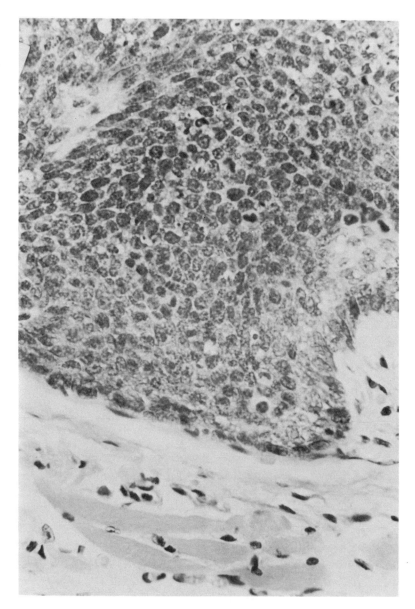

FIGURE 2. Skin carcinoma in a congenitally hypothymic (*nu/nu*) mouse inoculated with polyoma virus, × 670.

the animals. Antigenic markers show that such tumors are indeed induced by the virus. The incidence of tumors is increased and the latent period is reduced if the adults are irradiated (Allison *et al.*, 1967*b*).

Another interesting situation is the rapid induction by fibroma virus in rabbits and Yaba virus in monkeys (both poxviruses) of tumors that regress after 1–3 months. The importance of the immune system in the regression is illustrated by the much greater size and delayed regression of the tumors in animals treated with methotrexate, as well as spread to distant sites (Allison and Friedman, 1970). In these cases, the role of immunological reactions in eliminating neoplastic growths is evident. In newborn rabbits, the immunological reactions are again inefficient and fibromas grow to massive size and kill the hosts (Allison, 1970).

3. Leukemogenic Viruses in Mice

Effects of immunosuppression on leukemias and lymphomas of mice are of special interest in view of the raised incidence of lymphoreticular malignancy in immunosuppressed human patients. There are several groups of leukemogenic viruses in mice. One consists of indigenous leukemogenic viruses related to Gross virus that are vertically transmitted in most—if not all—strains of mice. These variants of Gross virus share major antigens but differ in certain properties, e.g., host-range specificity. In addition, there are several varieties of laboratory-passaged murine leukemogenic viruses that share major transplantation and other antigens (Friend, Moloney, and Rauscher viruses). Host-range differences are due to segregation of major genetic factors that affect the susceptibility of host cells to infection by leukemogenic viruses (see Rowe, 1973). In addition genes at another locus, $Rgv-1$, affecting susceptibility to Gross virus, are closely linked to the K end of the H-2 complex (Lilly and Pincus, 1973), and may influence effectiveness of the immune response against leukemic cells.

It has long been known that early thymectomy greatly decreases the incidence of leukemia in mice inoculated with Gross or Moloney viruses. The most plausible explanation is that the target cells transformed by the virus are T lymphocytes, which are depleted after thymectomy, and the presence of thymus-specific antigens on tumor cells supports this interpretation. Hence thymectomy cannot be used as an immunosuppressive procedure with these viruses. However, ALG was shown by Allison and Law (1968) to increase greatly the leukemogenic effect of Moloney virus in BALB/c mice. Leukemia could be delayed or prevented by transferring normal syngeneic lymphoid cells to the mice after the cessation of ALG treatment (see Law, 1972). These results support the view that the immunosuppressive effect of ALG was responsible for the increased susceptibility observed, rather than other effects such as ALG-induced proliferation of lymphoid cells.

Again, the question of tolerance arises. If mice were fully tolerant to antigens of vertically transmitted leukemogenic viruses, they should show no antibody and no cell-mediated immunity against these antigens. Mice of the BALB/c strain with vertically transmitted Moloney virus were found to have complexes of viral antigen and antibody in the circulation and especially in the renal glomeruli (Hirsch et al., 1969). Similar results have been obtained with Gross virus antigens in the high leukemic AKR strain of mice (Oldstone et al., 1972). Thus these mice are certainly capable of producing some antibody against leukemogenic virus antigens. Doré et al. (1969) reported that in AKR mice immunization with a syngenic Gross tumor (K-36) produces antibodies cytotoxic for Gross leukemia cells. Two investigations indicate that—contrary to earlier suggestions—these mice are also able to mount a cell-mediated response against leukemic cells with virus-specific antigens. Wahren and Metcalf (1971) reported that lymphoid cells from preleukemic AKR mice can exert a cytotoxic effect on target cells bearing Gross virus specific antigens. Haran-Ghera (1971) has found that C57BL mice can, by appropriate manipulations, be immunized with the strain of Gross virus which they themselves carry (radiation leukemia virus) and are then resistant to transplantation of syngenic Gross tumor cells. Thus they are not tolerant, an important question when the effects of immunosuppression are considered. In fully tolerant animals, immunosuppression would not be expected to increase the incidence of malignancy. In several of these mouse strains, aging animals spontaneously develop leukemias, sometimes (as in the AKR strain) when they are still relatively young. Presumably, immune responses help to delay the onset of leukemia until the animals have had an opportunity to reproduce. Under these circumstances, it would be expected that the incidence of leukemia or lymphoma would be increased by immunosuppression. Casey (1968) showed that in NZB mice treatment with azathioprine increased the incidence of lymphoreticular malignancies, and C57BL mice treated with 6-mercaptopurine show a higher proportion with leukemia than untreated mice (Doell *et al.*, 1967). Repeated administration of ALG to AKR mice under the appropriate conditions accelerates the onset of leukemia (Allison, 1970). However, this result is not always observed, apparently because some batches of ALG are cytotoxic for Gross leukemia cells. Administration of ALG also accelerates the onset of lymphoreticular malignancy in the SJL/J strain in mice, which is not known to be related to a virus (Burstein and Allison, 1970). One of the effects of radiation when eliciting leukemia in strains such as the C57BL is immunosuppression (Haran-Ghera, 1971).

4. Murine Sarcoma Virus

The different strains of murine sarcoma virus (MSV) are antigenically related to Moloney leukemogenic virus. All appear to be defective, in the sense that for sarcoma virus to be liberated from cells they must be concomitantly infected with MLV (see Harvey and East, 1971). When inoculated intramuscularly or subcutaneously into young mice or rats, progressively growing tumors soon develop at the sites of inoculation; there is usually also splenomegaly. In mice a few weeks old, injections of MSV give rise to local tumors which in some animals continue to grow until they kill the animal (progressors) while in other animals they regress (regressors). The regression of palpable tumors is a striking phenomenon, and suggests that immune reactions against tumor cells are strong. This is confirmed by the immunity against transplantation of syngenic tumor cells bearing virus-specific antigens (MSV or MLV).

Adult mice are again relatively resistant to tumor induction with MSV, but they become susceptible after thymectomy or ALG administration or both (Law *et al.*,

1968), or after treatment with cortisone or X-irradiation (Fefer, 1970). In contrast to the situation with polyoma virus, injections of serum from regressor or hyperimmune animals, even when made several days after virus inoculation, protect the animals against sarcoma development, but not against later onset of leukaemia (Law, 1972). The protective effect of sera is not correlated with the levels of antiviral antibody; and serum confers protection against transplants of tumor cells bearing Moloney-specific antigens. Hence the effect is exerted against the tumor cells rather than the virus itself. Preliminary results suggest that the regressor serum becomes attached to the target cells and collaborates with nonspecific effector cells (K cells) in the host to destroy the target cells in a manner analogous to that described by Perlmann and Holm (1969). Serum from animals immune to MSV can increase the cytotoxicity of immune lymphoid cells and can sensitize target cells for killing by normal lymphoid cells (Hellström and Hellström, 1969; Skurzak et al., 1972).

Collaboration between antibody and effector cells in immunity against tumors in vivo can be shown by experiments of the type described by Shin et al. (1972). Specific antibody mixed with tumor cells suppresses growth of the cells as a graft in normal syngenic recipients but not in X-irradiated (500 rads) recipients. Inoculation of peritoneal cells and antibody into irradiated recipients prevented tumor growth. These results suggest that antibody is unable by itself to prevent multiplication of tumor cells but that a cell in the recipient, production of which is radiosensitive, collaborates with antibody to protect recipients. Whether the radiosensitive cell is a K cell, macrophage, or some other cell type has not yet been established.

5. Effects of Immunosuppression on Other Tumors in Experimental Animals

Numerous reports have appeared on the effects of neonatal thymectomy or administration of ALS on chemical carcinogenesis (see Balner, 1970; Penn, 1970). Some striking results have been described, for example, an increase of late-developing, apparently nonviral mammary tumors in neonatally thymectomized mice (Burstein and Law, 1971), the appearance of nephroblastomas in rats given oral 7,12-dimethylbenzanthracene only when they were also given ALS (Bourgoin et al., 1972), and the finding of bladder tumors in rats after intravenous administration of nitrosomethylurea only when they were given ALS, although neurogenic tumors were induced both in the presence of ALS and in controls given normal horse serum (Denlinger et al., 1973). Some decrease in the latent period for induction of skin tumors by hydrocarbons has been noted when ALS is administered (Balner, 1970), but in general the effects of immunosuppression are less striking with carcinogenesis by chemicals than by viruses (Allison and Taylor, 1967; Penn, 1970; Wagner and Haughton, 1971).

Facilitation by ALS of the spread of a hamster lymphoma (Gershon and Carter, 1970) and rat tumors (Fisher et al., 1970) has been reported.

A. C. ALLISON

The increasing use over the past decade of powerful immunosuppressive drugs has had obvious clinical benefits, of which the most notable has been making kidney transplantation possible in human patients. However, the use of long-term immunosuppression in transplantation has had complications, including severe infections with viruses that are normally controlled by cell-mediated immune responses, such as cytomegalovirus (Craighead, 1969) and herpes simplex virus (Montgomerie *et al.*, 1969).

Spencer and Anderson (1970) have reported that in a group of Danish renal transplant recipients under immunosuppression for more than 1 year the incidence of common warts was 42%—significantly higher than in control populations. A similar figure is given by Penn (1974), who states that in some patients the skin is covered with warts.

Six years ago, reports from widely separated centers in the United States, New Zealand, and Scotland of reticulum-cell sarcomas in patients on immunosuppressive therapy after renal transplantation drew attention to an even more serious problem. The occurrence of several cases of so rare a disease in a relatively small group of transplant recipients was unlikely to be due to chance. Informal registries of malignant neoplasis in organ transplant recipients have been kept by I. Penn and T. Starzl in Denver, Colorado, and L. Kinlen and W. R. S. Doll in Oxford, England. Penn and Starzl (1972) have reported that of a group of 7581 renal and 179 cardiac homograft recipients on immunosuppressive therapy until the end of 1971, 31 had mesenchymal tumors. The striking fact is that, of these, 28 had lymphoreticular malignancies, 20 being reticulum-cell sarcomas, while four were other lymphomas (three unclassified and one lymphosarcoma). Since lymphoreticular tumors within the central nervous system are uncommon (the incidence being 0.04–1.5% in the large series of Richmond *et al.*, 1962, and Rosenberg *et al.*, 1961), it is also of interest that the brain and spinal cord were involved in 11 of the lymphoreticular tumors in transplant patients. By May 1963, 49 cases of solid lymphomas had been recorded in transplant recipients (Penn, 1974), with the central nervous system involved in 23 (47%). The increased incidence of reticulum-cell sarcomas in immunosuppressed transplant recipients is statistically highly significant and is conservatively estimated to be at least 100 times the incidence expected in an untreated populations of comparable age.

Several explanations for the lymphoreticular malignancies can be considered. The first is that a surveillance mechanism is normally operating in man against leukemogenic viruses or lymphoma cells and that this mechanism is inhibited by immunosuppression. However, it is also possible that lymphoreticular malignancies in transplant recipients may be due to carcinogenic effects on lymphoreticular cells of the azathioprine or steroids used in nearly all cases. The possible role of the grafted tissue itself has to be borne in mind. In mice, graft-vs.-host reactions and prolonged antigenic stimulation have been associated with lymphoreticular malignancy (see below). For this and other reasons it would be important to know whether patients receiving immunosuppressive therapy for reasons other than transplantation also develop malignancies. This question is discussed in the next section.

Whether there is an increased risk of developing other neoplasms in transplant recipients is another important question. Penn (1974) states that in the Denver tumor registry there are records of *de novo* cancers in 170 organ homograft recipients; the risk of development of *de novo* cancer between 6 months and 10 years after transplantation being 5–6%. Skin cancers (51 cases, 45%) were the most common of the epithelial lesions. The skin tumors were often multiple, and in some cases extensive areas of skin were either frankly malignant or showed evidence of intraepithelial cancer (Bowen's disease). Skin cancers have also attracted the attention of transplant surgeons in Australia, where the strong solar radiation and genetic constitution of the population combine to make this tumor relatively common. Walder *et al.* (1971) reported the observation of malignant tumors of the skin in seven out of 51 kidney allograft recipients (14%). They conclude that under the influence of immunosuppression cutaneous hyperkeratoses more rapidly evolve into squamous-cell carcinoma, skin cancers tend to be multiple, and keratoacanthoma is not only frequent but also prone to early recurrence. This poses a semantic problem since recurrence is regarded by many pathologists as diagnostic of carcinoma rather than keratoacanthoma. Marshall (1973) reports that skin cancer was the commonest type of malignancy in the registry of transplants in Australia and New Zealand. Of a personal series of 151 patients, eight had skin carcinomas (5.3%), five had keratoacanthomas, and 13 had hyperkeratoses. Multiple primary carcinomas of the skin sometimes heal spontaneously (Currie and Ferguson-Smith, 1952), possibly because of immunological reactions, and it is conceivable that in the transplant recipients such rejection mechanisms are less effective than in normal persons.

The Denver Tumor Registry in May 1963 had records of tumors in 170 organ transplant recipients, including 119 epithelial malignancies and 58 mesenchymal malignancies. The excess of lymphoreticular and skin cancers over U.S. whites of the same age group (Doll *et al.*, 1970) is unlikely to be due to chance. Whether the transplant recipients are especially prone to develop other tumors is more difficult to evaluate because carefully matched control figures are not yet available.

7. Malignancy in Other Immunosuppressed Patients

Penn and Starzl (1972) listed 30 patients with a variety of non malignant diseases who were treated with immunosuppressive agents without organ transplantation and developed cancer. Among the 30 were patients with the nephrotic syndrome, systemic lupus erythematosus, ulcerative colitis, psoriasis, cryoglobulinemia, and rheumatoid arthritis. More recent reports have been published of a cerebral lymphoma in a patient with systemic lupus erythematosus treated with azathioprine (Lipsemeyer, 1972), and of reticulum-cell sarcoma in an unusual site (the vulva) in a 34-year-old woman with dermatomyositis treated with prednisolone and azathioprine (Sneddon and Wishart, 1972).

Such individual case reports are difficult to evaluate, and comparisons of groups of patients treated with immunosuppressive drugs with other patients not so treated and matched control normal subjects are required. Parsons *et al.* (1974) found that eight of 28 patients (29%) dying with rheumatoid arthritis treated with cytotoxic drugs had neoplasias, in contrast to only 6% of patients in the classical manner. More remarkable is that fact that seven of the eight patients had lymphoproliferative neoplasia, a figure significantly in excess of expectation in comparable local and national populations. Penn (1974) states that more than 20 psoriasis patients treated with methotrexate have developed lymphomas, but the total number of patients treated and the precise incidence of this complication are not yet known.

There are thus indications that patients treated with immunosuppressive drugs such as cyclophosphamide and methotrexate have an increased risk of developing lymphomas. Since this is an important clinical point, careful comparisons should be made of subjects so treated and suitable controls in order that the risk can be assessed accurately. The cases treated with immunosuppressive drugs should not have been selected because of severe disease or any other special reasons. Even if such a risk is proved, it could imply that the immunosuppressive drugs are carcinogens for lymphoreticular cells rather than neoplasia being an effect of impaired surveillance. However, the results would be consistent with the latter interpretation.

8. Malignant Disease in Children with Immunodeficiency

Now that children with immunodeficiency are given replacement therapy and antibiotic treatment, they are surviving to adolescence, and it is becoming apparent that they are unusually prone to malignant disease (Table 2). The highest incidence has been in ataxia-telangiectasia, in which a defect of cell-mediated immunity is accompanied by low levels of Iga and IgE. Comparison between the number of cases with malignancy and the total number of known cases (about 500) suggests that more than 10% of patients develop malignant disease. The true incidence may be even higher, since about 35% of patients coming to autopsy have shown evidence of cancer (Good, 1974). Much the most common type of malignancy has been that of the lymphoreticular system, but tumors of other sites, including epithelia, are also unusually frequent. A similar incidence and organ distribution of malignant disease are seen in patients with the Wiskott–Aldrich syndrome, in which defective T-lymphocyte-mediated immune responses are accompanied by low circulating IgM.

Selective deficiency of circulating IgM is likewise associated with lymphoreticular neoplasia. Another syndrome has been termed the "common variable form of primary immunodeficiency." In this condition, immunoglobulin levels in the circulation are markedly depressed, sometimes with variable manifestations in a

TABLE 2

Incidence of Malignant Disease in Children with Immunodeficiency

Disease	Number of cases	Estimated risk[a] (%)	Lympho-reticular malignancy[b] (%)	Leukemia[b] (%)
Congenital X-linked immunodeficiency	6	6	12	83
Severe combined system immunodeficiency	9	2	67	33
IgM deficiency	6	8	83	0
Wiskott–Aldrich syndrome	24	8	79	4
Ataxia-telangiectasia	52	10	62	2
Common variable immunodeficiency	41	8	56	2
All children under 15	—	0.19[c]	8[d]	48[d]

[a] Estimated from the approximate number of cases of the syndrome (Good, 1974).
[b] Proportion of all malignancies (Good, 1974).
[c] Cumulative incidence in United States (Doll *et al.*, 1970).
[d] Death certificates of 29,457 U.S. children (Miller, 1969).

single family (e.g., one child with low IgG, a second with low IgA and IgM but normal IgG, and a third with selective deficiency of IgG and IgM). In addition, T-cell functions may be depressed. Again, far more malignancies of the lymphoreticular system (lymphomas and reticulum-cell sarcomas) have been seen than in normal children. Moreover, carcinomas of the gastrointestinal tract have been commoner than expected, and achlorhydria and pernicious anemia have been described in some children (Twomey *et al.*, 1971). Why achlorhydria and pernicious anaemia should be associated with an immunodeficiency syndrome involving a failure of terminal differentiation of B lymphocytes is not yet understood. In patients with X-linked infantile agammaglobulinemia, the incidence of neoplasms is less raised, but leukemias appear to be far more common than in controls.

In general, the incidence of neoplasia (some 7% of cases) is much higher in children with immunodeficiency involving T-lymphocyte function than in controls. The excess of lymphoreticular malignancy is of the order of 1000 times that seen in children with intact immune systems. Although the association is established, the interpretation is uncertain. If simple lack of surveillance were involved, an increase of tumors of all sites would be expected, whereas the increase is obviously selective, involving mainly lymphoreticular organs. It is still possible that in normal humans these organs are especially prone to malignancy, because of virus infections or for some other reason, but that the tumors are highly antigenic and immunological surveillance is normally very efficient. Alternatively, antigenic stimulation from chronic infection, or the disorder in the lymphoid system itself, may predispose the patients to malignancy. The relatively high incidence of epithelial tumors, especially in the gastrointestinal tract, of six patients with ataxia-telagiectasia and 12 with the common variable form of immunodeficiency, is remarkable in patients of the age group under 15 and may be attributable to lack of surveillance.

Since cancer cells bear major histocompatibility antigens, they would be expected to provoke strong homograft reactions when inoculated into normal recipients. This is usually the case: Southam (1969) reported that cancer cell homotransplants into normal human recipients produce subcutaneous nodules that usually reach maximum size by 14 days, regress rapidly during the third or fourth week, and have completely disappeared 6 wk after inoculation. However, such experiments have been discontinued because of some unfortunate results. Thus, in the hope of stimulating the production of sensitized lymphocytes, melanoma cells were transplanted from a mother to her healthy daughter; the melanoma grew in the daughter and killed her (Schwartz, 1974). In patients with advanced cancer, the rejection of tumor cell homotransplants is also slower than in normal recipients (Southam, 1964).

Penn (1974) reviewed observations on transplanted cancers in 16 of 42 patients who received grafts of organs, usually kidneys, from donors with cancer. All recipients received prednisone and azathioprine, and some received other immunosuppressives as well. In ten of the recipients, cancer had spread from the transplanted organ to distant sizes. After cessation of immunosuppression in three patients, the cancers apparently underwent rejection. This type of experience has convinced most transplant surgeons of the inadvisability of using organs from cadaver donors who died of cancer. They also suggest that immunological mechanisms are usually able to reject tumor cell homotransplants in normal humans even when they have grown to visible tumors, but that in patients with advanced cancer or immunosuppressed for organ transplants the rejection mechanism may be impaired.

Human tumor xenografts grow in immunodeficient *nu/nu* mice (Poulson *et al.*, 1973) and in mice effectively immunosuppressed with ALS (Franks *et al.*, 1973).

10. *Immunological Stimulation and Malignancy*

Metcalf (1963) observed a high incidence of lymphomas in mice undergoing repeated antigenic stimulation. Observations in the laboratory of R. S. Schwartz showed that transfer of lymphocytes from parental inbred mice to young adult hybrid offspring results in graft-vs.-host reactions of varying severity and with various consequences. One of these was the development of lymphomas in recipients of some strains (Armstrong *et al.*, 1970). It has been found by Hirsch (1974) that leukemogenic viruses are activated in the spleens of mice undergoing graft-vs.-host reactions. The activated virus could be seen budding from the cells by electron microscopic examination, produced cytopathic effects in XC mixed cultures, and induced reticulum-cell sarcomas in newborn hybrid mice. Mixed lymphocyte cultures from the same strains of mice also show activation, whereas this was not seen in lymphocytes transformed by mitogens. In mice bearing skin allografts treated with ALS, activation of leukemogenic virus was seen in lymph nodes and spleen.

The results of these studies suggest that immunostimulation and immunosuppression may be complementary mechanisms leading to virus activation and replication in a carefully balanced system. Graft-vs.-host reactions are themselves immunosuppressive, and the relative importance of activation of leukemogenic viruses, immunosuppression, and other factors in the genesis of reticulum-cell sarcomas of experimental animals is not yet known. Whether these observations shed light on the development of reticulum-cell sarcomas in human organ transplant recipients is also uncertain.

11. Infectious Mononucleosis and Burkitt's Lymphoma

Retrospective (Niederman et al., 1968) and prospective (Evans and Niederman, 1972) studies have established beyond reasonable doubt that infectious mononucleosis is caused by EB virus. The prospective study showed that no cases of infectious mononucleosis occurred in a group of more than 1100 seropositive college students during observation periods of several months to several years. In the corresponding seronegative group of more than 900 students, infectious mononucleosis occurred in about 10%, accompanied by regular seroconversion.

In the presence of EB virus, lymphocytes from cord blood or seronegative donors are regularly transformed into lymphoblastoid cell lines. The reaction can be used in microwells to titrate EB virus (Moss and Pope, 1972). In the absence of the virus, lymphoblastoid cell lines capable of unlimited growth are seldom obtained from lymphocytes of seronegative persons (see Klein, 1974). Herpesviruses inducing lymphoproliferative malignancy include the agent of Marek's disease in chickens and *Herpesvirus saimiri* and *H. ateles* in marmosets and owl monkeys (Biggs *et al.*, 1972). EB virus can induce lymphomalike lesions in marmosets (Shope *et al.*, 1973). The combination of the peripheral blood picture and mononuclear infiltration of internal organs during acute infectious mononucleosis (Carter, 1972) has led to the view that the disease is a form of lymphoproliferative neoplasia which is self-limited because of an effective immune response. The characteristics of the cells in the peripheral blood and the nature of the immune response in infectious mononucleosis are therefore of interest. The cells in the peripheral blood might be lymphoid cells stimulated to proliferate by EB virus. In that case, they would probably be of the B-lymphocyte lineage, since most of the lymphoblastic cell lines obtained *in vitro* from patients with infectious mononucleosis synthesize readily detectable amounts of immunoglobulin and have other B-cell markers (Steel and Ling, 1973). Alternatively, the cells in the peripheral blood might be derived from T lymphocytes reacting against virus-infected cells.

Mixed lymphocyte reactions have been demonstrated between blood lymphocytes obtained after recovery from infectious mononucleosis and autochthonous lymphoblastoid cell lines initiated at the height of the disease or with atypical cells obtained at this time and preserved with cryoprotective agents (Junge *et al.*, 1971; Steel and Ling, 1973). Steel and Ling (1973) also described cytotoxic reactions of convalescent lymphocytes against autochthonous lymphoblastoid cells lines. Denman and Pelton (1974) have separated the blood mononuclear cells from 46 patients with infectious mononucleosis into populations of normal and atypical cells by velocity sedimentation. The atypical cells showed both T- and B-cell markers, and the authors concluded that the atypical cells consist of two populations, a major one which is part of the host reaction to EB virus infected cells and a minor one which is the target for immunological responses and may represent cells transformed by the virus.

The relationship of EB virus to Burkitt's lymphoma is also well known. Antibody against virus and virus-associated antigens is consistently found in lymphoma-bearing patients and the virus genome is incorporated into the host cell genome even in "virus-free" lines of Burkitt cells (zur Hausen and Szhulte-Holthausen, 1970). The much higher frequency of Burkitt's lymphoma in some populations living in tropical environments than elsewhere has suggested that chronic malarial infection may play a role in the pathogenesis of the disease (Burkitt, 1969). Malaria could provide a powerful and continuing antigenic stimulus which might favor lymphoma induction (see above); it can be immunosuppressive or by antigenic competition diminish the effectiveness of immune responses against unrelated antigens (see Pross and Eidinger, 1974). Acute malarial infections are immunosuppressive and increase lymphoprolifera-tive neoplasia in experimental animals (Wedderburn, 1974). The coincidence of repeated malarial infection and EB virus infection might allow occasional clones of cells transformed by the virus to escape from immunological surveillance and grow into lymphomas. Once these attain reasonable size, antigen shed from the tumor cells could inhibit immune responses directly or through the formation of blocking immune complexes.

On this hypothesis, Burkitt lymphomas would be expected to originate from single clones or small numbers of clones. The uniclonality of Burkitt's lymphoma has been demonstrated by use of glucose-6-phosphate dehydrogenase and immunoglobulins as markers (Fialkow *et al.*, 1970, 1973). As a rule, multiple tumors of the same patient are due to proliferation of the same clone. Recurrences are usually of the same clonal type as the original tumor, although occasional exceptions have been observed in patients after chemotherapy (Fialkow *et al.*, 1972, 1973). Since the EB virus infection is always present, new clones of cells could arise continuously, and the chemotherapy itself is immunosuppressive and might allow the clones to grow into tumors. Evidence suggestive of continued transformation is the observation that tumors can be contaminated *in vivo* by foreign lymphocytes, presumably derived from transfusions, and that the contaminant cells may themselves contribute to tumor growth (Fialkow *et al.*, 1971; Manolov *et al.*, 1970). This may be analogous to the "trans-formation" of transplanted bone marrow cells in a leukemic patient (Thomas *et al.*, 1972).

Another group of viruses that produce well-controlled infections in normal persons but overt infections in patients with immunodeficiency or those undergoing immunosuppressive therapy has recently been defined. Progressive multifocal leukoencephalopathy is a rare demyelinating disease of man occurring in patients with Hodgkin's disease, sarcoidosis, and other conditions in which cell-mediated immunity is often defective. The suggestion that this disease is the result of a viral infection was strengthened when electron microscopic studies revealed papovavirus-like particles in nuclei of oligodendrocytes in demyelinated areas of brain. Padgett *et al.* (1971) isolated a papovavirus from the brain of a patient with progressive multifocal leukoencephalopathy complicating Hodgkin's disease. Primary cultures of fetal glial cells were inoculated with extracts of brain made at necropsy. The virus (J.C.) isolated was similar in size and shape to the polyoma–SV40 group of viruses. The J.C. virus did not produce a cytopathic effect in African green monkey kidney cells and infected cells did not show immunofluorescence with antibody against SV40. Other viruses isolated from patients with progressive multifocal leukoencephalopathy (Weiner *et al.*, 1971) are antigenically closely related to SV40.

A third virus of the same group was isolated from the urine of an immunosuppressed renal transplant recipient by Gardner *et al.* (1971). The patient had a fibrotic obstruction of the donor ureter, which was excised, and many virus particles were seen in nuclei of epithelial cells bordering the lumen. The virus (B.K. virus) again resembled polyoma virus and SV40 in size and shape but was distinct from SV40 in that it agglutinated human erythrocytes and showed antigenic differences as well as some common reactions with SV40. Four similar isolates have been made from immunosuppressed transplant recipients, and B.K. virus has been found to induce tumors after inoculation into newborn hamsters (Gardner, 1974).

The B.K. and J.C. viruses are smaller than human papilloma virus and serologically unrelated to it. The morphological similarity and partial serological relationship to SV40 suggest that these viruses are representatives of a group of human papovaviruses that commonly produce latent infections in humans, as SV40 does in rhesus monkeys. The high incidence of antibodies in normal humans suggests that the infection is frequent. It seems reasonable to conclude that normally the virus infection is controlled by an immune response, although prolonged latent infections can occur, and that only in subjects with secondary immunodeficiency (as in Hodgkin's disease) or immunosuppressed subjects (renal transplant recipients) do infections become overt, with virus demonstrable by electron microscopy in the tissues and available for isolation. Whether these viruses are oncogenic in humans is another problem of interest that requires further investigation. There is no evidence that SV40 induces tumors in the natural host, the rhesus monkey, but the B.K./J.C. group of viruses might produce tumors in some humans. Studies on immunosuppressed monkeys would be of interest.

A. C. ALLISON

In this chapter, evidence has been reviewed in support of the view that immunological surveillance in adult animals operates efficiently against virus-induced tumors and some chemically induced tumors but not others. Several explanations can be offered for this difference. The virus-related tumor antigens are strong, in the sense that they induce immunity against transplants of many more tumor cells than are required to establish tumors in unimmunized animals; in contrast, the antigens associated with chemically induced and spontaneously occurring tumors are often weak or difficult to demonstrate at all (see Baldwin, 1973). Moreover, chemical carcinogens themselves have immunosuppressive effects, which may facilitate the carcinogenic process when tumors are antigenic.

Most of the nude mice have been studied for relatively short periods (7 months) under artificial (pathogen-free) conditions (Rygaard and Poulsen, 1974). They have a markedly depleted population of T- lymphocytes, which are the target of endogenous leukemogenic virus transformation. Moreover, although they lack an efficient T-lymphocyte-mediated immune system, they have antibody-dependent cytotoxic (K cells) and the possible existence of a surveillance system independent of or minimally dependent on T lymphocytes must be borne in mind. The great sensitivity of nude mice to virus oncogenesis (Allison *et al.*, 1974) has already been mentioned.

Reports that mice treated chronically with antilymphocytic serum do not show an increased incidence of spontaneously occurring tumors (Nehlsen, 1971) do not carry much weight since this procedure is now known to inhibit only partially T-cell-mediated immunity. In the case of polyoma virus oncogenesis, ALS treatment is much less effective than this procedure following thymectomy. Moreover, the ALS used was not tested for capacity to neutralize leukemogenic viruses or lyse leukemic or lymphoma cells; most samples of ALS have these effects. Also, very few strains of mice have been treated with ALS, for less than a normal life span. Genetic variations apart from those affecting immune responses may well influence susceptibility to oncogenesis, as known for the leukemogenic viruses.

With regard to humans, the evidence for immunological surveillance is best for lymphoreticular neoplasms, as shown by their increased incidence in children with immunodeficiency and in immunosuppressed patients. However, the immunosuppression has been much less powerful than that used in experimental animals, and it is likely that some surveillance mechanisms (mediated, for example, by antibody and K cells) may escape.

Hence only limited tests of the surveillance hypothesis have been possible. They have strongly supported the hypothesis in the case of virus-induced tumors in experimental animals. These are uniform antigenically and induce relatively strong immune responses, as exemplified by polyoma virus in mice. Natural selection may well have operated to retain immune response genes efficiently limiting oncogenesis by polyoma virus, which is common in colonies of mice. Likewise, the induction of lymphoreticular neoplasms by endogenous leukemogenic viruses is delayed by immune responses (again under genetic control) until the animals have bred. In contrast, the antigens induced by chemically induced tumors are diverse, so that in this artificial situation there would be no selection pressure favoring genes allowing efficient responses to most of them. Hence antigens in chemically induced and spontaneous tumors are usually "weak," and surveillance is not readily demonstrable. Similar arguments may account for the efficiency of immune responses against lymphoreticular neoplasms in man.

14. References

ALLISON, A. C., 1966, Immune responses to Shope fibroma virus in adult and newborn rabbits, *J. Natl. Cancer Inst.* **36:**389.

ALLISON, A. C., 1970, On the absence of tolerance in virus oncogenesis, *in:* Proceedings of the IV Quad, *International Conference on Cancer,* (L. Severi, ed.), p. 653.

ALLISON, A. C., 1974, Interactions of antibodies, complement components and various cell types in immunity against viruses and pyogenic bacteria, *Transplant. Rev.* **19:**3.

ALLISON, A. C., AND FRIEDMAN, R. M., 1970, Effects of immunosuppressive agents on Shope rabbit fibroma, *J. Natl. Cancer Inst.* **36:**869.

ALLISON, A. C., AND LAW, L. W., 1968, Effects of antilymphocyte serum on virus oncogenesis, *Proc. Soc. Exp. Biol. Med.* **127:**707.

ALLISON, A. C., AND TAYLOR, R. B., 1967, Observations on thymectomy and carcinogenesis, *Cancer Res.* **207:**703.

ALLISON, A. C., BERMAN, L. D., AND LEVEY, R. H., 1967a, Increased tumour induction by adenovirus type 12 in thymectomized mice and mice treated with antilymphocytic serum, *Nature* (London) **215:**185.

ALLISON, A. C., CHESTERMAN, F. C., AND BARON, S., 1967b, Induction of tumors in adult hamsters with simian virus 40, *J. Natl. Cancer Inst.* **38:**567.

ALLISON, A. C., MONGA, J. N., AND HAMMOND, V., 1974, Increased susceptibility to virus oncogenesis of congenitally thymus-deprived nude mice, *Nature* (London) **252:**746.

ARMSTRONG, M. Y. K., GLEICHMANN, E., GLEICHMANN, H., BELDOTTI, L., ANDRÉ-SCHWARTZ, J., AND SCHWARTZ, R. S., 1970, Chronic allogeneic disease. II. Development of lymphomas, *J. Exp. Med.* **137:**417.

BALDWIN, R. W., (1973), Immunological aspects of chemical carcinogenesis, *Adv. Cancer Res.* **18:**1.

BALNER, H., 1970, Immunosuppression and neoplasia, *Rev. Eur. Etud. Clin. Biol.* **15:**199.

BIGGS, P. M., DE THÉ, G., AND PAYNE, L. N., eds., 1972, *Oncogenesis and Herpes Viruses,* IARC, Lyon.

BOURGOIN, J. J., CUEFF, J., BAILLY, C., AND DARGENT, M., 1972, Incidence de néphroblastomas chez le rat Sprague–Dawley immunodeprine soumis au D.M.B., *Bull. Cancer (Paris)* **59:**429.

BURKITT, D., 1969, Etiology of Burkitt's lymphoma—An alternative hypothesis to a vectored virus, *J. Natl. Cancer Inst.* **42:**19.

BURNET, F. M., 1971, Immunological surveillance in neoplasia, *Transplant. Rev.* **7:**3.

BURSTEIN, N. A., AND ALLISON, A. C., 1970, Effect of antilymphocyte serum on the appearance of reticular neoplasma in SJL/J mice, *Nature (London)* **225:**1139.

BURSTEIN, N. A., AND LAW, L. W., 1971, Neonatal thymectomy and non-viral mammary tumours in mice, *Nature (London)* **231:**450.

CARTER, R. L., 1972, The pathology of infectious mononucleosis—A review, in: *Oncogenesis and Herpes Viruses* (P. M. Biggs, G. de Thé, and L. N. Payne, eds.), p. 230, IARC, Lyon.

CASEY, T. P., 1968, Azathioprine (Imuran) administration and the development of malignant lymphomas in NZB mice, *Clin. Exp. Immunol.* **3:**305.

CEROTTINI, J. C., AND BRUNNER, K. T., 1974, Cell-mediated cytotoxicity, allograft rejection, and tumour immunity, *Adv. Immunol.* **18:**67.

CRAIGHEAD, J. E., 1969, Immunologic response to cytomegalovirus infection in renal allograft recipients, *Am. J. Epidemiol.* **90:**506.

CURRIE, A. R., AND FERGUSON-SMITH, J., 1952, Multiple primary spontaneous-healing squamous carcinomata of the skin, *J. Pathol. Bacteriol.* **64**:827.

DENLINGER, R. H., SWENBERG, J. A., KOESTNER, A., AND WECHSLER, W., 1973, Differential effect of immunosuppression on the induction of nervous system and bladder tumours by *N*-methyl, *N*-nitroserurea, *J. Natl. Cancer Inst.* **50**:87.

DENMAN, A. M., AND PELTON, B. K., 1974, Control mechanisms in infectious mononucleosis, *Clin. Exp. Immunol.* **18**:13.

DOELL, R. G., DE VAUX ST. CYR, C., AND GROBER, P., 1967, Immune reactivity prior to development of thymic lymphoma in C57Bl mice, *Int. J. Cancer* **2**:103.

DOLL, R., MUIR, C., AND WATERHOUSE, J., 1970, *Cancer Incidence in Five Continents*, Springer, Berlin.

DORÉ, J. F., SCHNEIDER, M., AND MATHE, G., 1969, Reactions immunitaires chez les souris AKR leucémiques ou preleucémiques, *Rev. Fr. Etud. Clin. Biol.* **14**:1003.

EHRLICH, P., (1906), Collected studies on immunity, London, Macmillan.

EVANS, A. S., AND NIEDERMAN, J. C., 1972, Epidemiology of infectious mononucleosis: A review. in: Oncogenesis and Herpes Viruses (P. M. Biggs, G. de Thé, and L. N. Payne, eds.), p. 230, IARC, Lyon.

FEFER, A., 1970, Immunotherapy of primary Moloney sarcoma virus-induced tumours, *Int. J. Cancer* **5**:327.

FIALKOW, P. J., 1972, Use of genetic markers to study cellular origin and development of tumours in human females, *Adv. Cancer Res.* **15**:191.

FIALKOW, P. J., KLEIN, G., GARTLER, S. M., AND CLIFFORD, P., 1971*a*, Clonal origin for individual Burkitt's tumours, *Lancet* **2**:384.

FIALKOW, P. J., KLEIN, G., AND GIBLETT, F. R., GOTHOSKAR, G., AND CLIFFORD, P., 1971*b*, Foreign cell contamination in Burkitt tumours, *Lancet* **1**:883.

FIALKOW, P. J., KLEIN, F., KLEIN, G., AND CLIFFORD, P., 1972, Second malignant clone underlying a Burkitt's tumour exacerbation, *Lancet* **2**:69.

FIALKOW, P. J., KLEIN, G., CLIFFORD, P., AND SINGH, S., 1973, Immunoglobulin and G6PD as markers of cellular origin in Burkitt lymphoma, *J. Exp. Med.* **138**:89.

FISHER, B., SOLIMAN, O., AND FISHER, E. R., 1970, Further observations concerning effects of anti-lymphocyte serum on tumour growth, with special reference to allogeneic inhibition, *Cancer Res.* **20**:2035.

FRANKS, C. R., CURTIS, K., AND PERKINS, F. T., 1973, Long-term survival of Hela tumours in mice treated with antilymphocyte serum, *Br. J. Cancer* **27**:390.

GARDNER, S. D., 1974, personal communication.

GARDNER, S. D., FIELD, A. M., COLEMAN, D. V., AND HULME, B., 1971, New human papovavirus (B.K.) isolated from urine after renal transplantation, *Lancet* **1**:1253.

GAUGAS, J. M., ALLISON, A. C., CHESTERMAN, F. C., REES, R. J. W., AND HIRSCH, M. S., 1973, Immunological control of polyoma virus oncogenesis in mice, *Br. J. Cancer* **27**:10.

GERSHON, R. K., AND CARTER, R. L., 1970, Facilitation of melostatic growth by antilymphocyte serum, *Nature (London)* **226**:328.

GOOD, R. A., 1974, The lymphoid system, immunodeficiency and malignancy, *Adv. Biosci.* **12**:123.

HARAN-GHERA, N., 1971, The influence of host factors on leukaemogenesis by the radiation leukaemia virus, *Israel J. Med. Sci.* **7**:17.

HARVEY, J. J., AND EAST, J., 1971, The murine sarcoma virus (MSV), *Int. Rev. Exp. Pathol.* **10**:266.

HELLSTRÖM, I., AND HELLSTRÖM, K. E., 1969, Studies in cellular immunity and its serum-mediated inhibition in Moloney virus induced mouse sarcomas, *Int. J. Cancer* **4**:587.

HIRSCH, M. S., 1974, Immunological activation of oncogenesis viruses: Inter-relationship of immunostimulation and immunosuppression, *Johns Hopkins Med. J. Suppl.* **3**:177.

HIRSCH, M. S., ALLISON, A. C., AND HARVEY, J. J., 1969, Immune complexes in mice infected with Moloney leukaemogenic and murine sarcoma viruses, *Nature (London)* **223**:739.

HUEBNER, R. J., 1963, Tumor virus study system, *Ann. N.Y. Acad. Sci.* **108**:1129.

JUNGE, U., HOEKSTRA, J., AND DEINHARDT, F., 1971, Stimulation of peripheral lymphocytes by allogeneic and autochthonous mononucleosis cell lines, *J. Immunol.* **106**:1306.

KLEIN, G., 1974, Herpes viruses and oncogenesis, *Johns Hopkins Med. J. Suppl.* **3**:15.

LAW, L. W., 1972, Influence of immune suppression on the induction of neoplasms by the leukaemogenic virus MLV and the variant MSV, in: *The Nature of Leukaemia* (P. D. Vincent, U. C. N. Blight, eds.), p. 23, University Press, Sydney, Australia.

LAW, L. W., TING, R. C., AND ALLISON, A. C., 1968, Effects of antilymphocyte serum on tumour and leukaemia induction by murine sarcoma virus (MSV), *Nature (London)* **220**:611.

LILLY, F., AND PINCUS, T., 1973, Genetic control of resistance to murine leukemia viruses, *Adv. Cancer Res.* **17**:231.

LIPSEMEYER, E. A., 1972, Development of malignant lymphoma in a patient with systemic lupus erythematosus treated with immunosuppression, *Arthritis Rheum.* **15**:183.

MANOLOV, G., LEVAN, A., NADKARNI, J. S., NADKARNI, J. J., AND CLIFFORD, P., 1970, Burkitt's lymphoma with female karyotype in an African male child, *Hereditas* **66**:79.

MARSHALL, V. D., 1973, Skin tumours in immunosuppressed patients, *Aust. N.Z. J. Surg.* **43**:214.

METCALF, D., 1963, Induction of reticular tumours in mice by repeated antigenic stimulation, *Acta Unio Int. Contra Cancrum* **19**:657.

MILLER, R. W., 1969, Fifty-two forms of childhood cancer: United States mortality experience 1960–1966, *J. Pediatn.* **75**:685.

MONTGOMERIE, J. Z., BECROFT, D. M. O., CROXSON, M. C., DOAK, P. B., AND NORTH, J. D. K., 1969, Herpes-simplex-virus infection afterr renal transplantation, *Lancet* **22**:867.

MOSS, D. J. AND POPE, J. H., (1972), Assay of the infectivity of Epstein–Barr virus by transformation of human leukocytes *in vitro*, *J. Gen. Virol.* **17**:233.

NEHLSEN, S. J., 1971, Prolonged administration of antithymocyte serum in mice, *Clin. Exp. Immunol.* **9**:63.

NIEDERMAN, J. C., MCCOLLUM, R. W., HENLE, G., AND HENLE, W., 1968, Infectious mononucleosis, *J. Am. Med. Assoc.* **203**:205.

OLDSTONE, M. B. A., AOKI, T., AND DIXON, F. J., 1972, The antibody response of mice to murine leukemia virus in spontaneous infection: Absence of classical immunological tolerance, *Proc. Natl. Acad. Sci. U.S.A.* **69**:134.

PADGETT, B. L., ZU RHEIN, G. M., WALKER, D. L., ECKRODE, R. J., AND DESSEL, B. H., 1971, Cultivation of papova-like virus from human brain with progressive multifocal leucoencephalopathy, *Lancet* **1**:1257.

PARSONS, J. L., SERANG, J. S., AND FORSDICK, W. M., 1974, The causes of death in patients with rheumatoid arthritis treated with cytotoxic agents, *J. Rheumatol. Suppl.* **1**:135.

PENN, I., 1970, *Malignant Tumours in Organ Transplant Recipients* Springer, New York.

PENN, I., 1974, Malignancies in recipients of organ transplants, *Johns Hopkins Med. J. Suppl.* **3**:211.

PENN, I., AND STARZL, T., 1972, Malignant tumours arising *de novo* in immunosuppressed organ transplant recipients, *Transplantation* **14**:407.

PERLMANN, P., AND HOLM, G., 1969, Cytotoxic effects of lymphoid cells *in vitro*, *Adv. Immunol.* **11**:117.

POULSON, C. O., FIALKOW, P. J., KLEIN, E., RYGAARD, J., AND WEINER, F., 1973, Growth and antigenic properties of a biopsy-derived Burkitt's lymphoma in thymus-less (nude) mice, *Int. J. Cancer* **11**:30.

PROSS, H. F., AND EIDINGER, D., 1974, Antigenic competition: A review of non-specific antigen-induced suppression, *Adv. Immunol.* **18**:133.

RICHMOND, J., SHERMAN, R. S., DIAMOND, H. D., AND CRAVER, L. E., 1962, Renal lesions associated with malignant melanomas, *Am. J. Med.* **32**:184.

ROSENBERG, S. A., DIAMOND, H. D., JASLOWITZ, B., AND CRAVER, L. F., 1961, Lymphosarcoma: 1269 cases, *Medicine* **40**:31.

ROWE, W. P., 1973, Genetic factors in the natural history of murine leukemia virus infection: G.H.A. Clowes memorial lecture, *Cancer Res.* **33**:3061.

RYGAARD, J., AND POULSEN, C. O., 1974, A dissociation between cell-mediated immunity and immunological surveillance? Observations in the mouse, in: *Workshop on Nude Mice*, Munksgaard, Copenhagen.

SCHWARTZ, R. S., 1974, Discussion, *Johns Hopkins Med. J. Suppl.* **3**:234.

SHARPSTONE, P., OGG, C. S., AND CAMERON, J. S., 1969, Nephrotic syndrome due to primary renal disease in adults. II. A controlled trial of prednisolone and azapriothine, *Br. Med. J.* **2**:535.

SHIN, H. S., KALISS, N., BORENSTEIN, D., AND GATELY, M. K., 1972, Antibody-mediated suppression of grafted lymphoma cells. II. Participation of macrophages, *J. Exp. Med.* **136**:375.

SHOPE, T., DECHAIW, D., AND MILLER, G., 1973, Malignant lymphoma in cottontop marmosets after inoculation with Epstein–Barr virus, *Proc. Natl. Acad. Sci. U.S.A.* **70**:2487.

SKURZAK, H. M., KLEIN, E., YOSHIDA, T. O., AND LAMON, E. W., 1972, Synergistic or antagonistic effect of different antibody concentrations on *in vitro* lymphocyte cytotoxicity in the Moloney sarcoma virus system, *J. Exp. Med.* **135**:997.

SNEDDON, I., AND WISHART, J. M., 1972, Immunosuppression and malignancy, *Br. Med. J.* **4**:235.

SOUTHAM, C. M., 1969, Host defence mechanisms and human cancer, *Ann. Inst. Pasteur*, **107**:585.

SPENCER, E. S., AND ANDERSON, H. K., 1970, Clinically evident, nonterminal infections with herpes viruses and the wart virus in immunosuppressed renal allograft recipients, *Br. Med. J.* **3**:251.

STEEL, C. M., AND LING, N. R., 1973, Immunopathology of infectious mononucleosis, *Lancet* **2**:861.

THOMAS, E. D., BRYANT, J. L., BUCKNER, C. D., CLIFT, R. A., FEFER, A., JOHNSON, F. L., NEIMAN, P., RAMBERG, R. E., AND STORB, R., 1972, Leukaemic transformation of engrafted human marrow cells *in vivo*, *Lancet* **1**:1310.

THOMAS, L., 1959, Reactions to homologous tissue antigens, in: Cellular and Humoral Aspects of the Hypersensitive States (H. S. Lawrence, ed.), p. 529, Cassell, London.

TWOMEY, J. J., LAUGHTON, A. H., VIHLANUEVA, N. D., KAV, Y. S., LIDSBY, M. D., AND JORDAN, P. H., 1971, Gastric secretary and serologic studies on patients with neoplastic and immunologic disorders, *Arch. Intern. Med.* **128**:746.

VANDEPUTTE, M., AND DATTA, S. K., 1972, Cell-mediated immunity in polyoma oncogenesis, *Eur. J. Cancer* **8**:1.

WAGNER, J. L., AND HAUGHTON, G., 1971, Immunosuppression by antilymphocyte serum and its effect on tumours induced by 3-methylcholanthrene in mice, *J. Natl. Cancer Inst.* **46**:1.

WAHREN, B., AND METCALF, D. L., 1971, Cytotoxicity *in vitro* of preleukaemic lymphoid cells on syngeneic monolayers of embryo or thymus cells, *Clin. Exp. Immunol.* **7**:373.

WALDER, B. K., ROBERTSON, M. R., AND JEREMY, D., 1971, Skin cancer and immunosuppression, *Lancet* **2**:1282.

WEDDERBURN, N., 1974 , Immunodepression produced by malarial infection in mice, in: Parasites in the immunized host—Mechanisms of survival, Ciba Foundation Symposium No. 25 Associated Scientific Publishers, Amsterdam, p. 123.

WEINER, L. P., HERDON, R. M., NARAYAN, O., JOHNSON, R. T., SHAH, K., RUBJNSTEIN, L. J., PREZIOSI, T. J., AND CONLEY, F. K., 1971, Isolation of virus related to SV40 from patients with progressive multifocal leukoencephalopathy, *New Engl. J. Med.* **286**:385.

ZUR HAUSEN, H., AND SZHULTE-HOLTHAUSEN, H., 1970, Presence of EB virus nucleic acid homology in a "virus-free" line of Burkitt's tumour cells, *Nature (London)* **227**:245.

9

Host Immune Response to Human Tumor Antigens

SIDNEY H. GOLUB

> *Some of what follows is true . . .*
> (Opening credits in the film "Butch Cassidy and the Sundance Kid")

1. Introduction

This chapter assumes that human tumor-associated antigens exist, and that the tumor-bearing host makes an immune response to these antigens. The weight of experimental evidence supports this assumption. However, tumor immunology is a relatively young science that is burdened with inexact and often cumbersome techniques and is working from a base of knowledge of the fundamentals of immunology and tumor biology that is only now beginning to make sense. Thus there can be no dogma of tumor immunology. The literature of this field must be approached critically and with a healthy dose of skepticism. The one prediction that can be made with confidence is that there will be many surprises in tumor immunology in the near future.

Any review of this type must begin with a series of disclaimers, as it is impossible to adequately examine all aspects of this field. Therefore, it is the intention of the author to provide a basis for critically reading the literature for the individual unfamiliar with the problems of tumor immunology. This necessitates an emphasis on the problems, pitfalls, and potentials of the various techniques employed in studying human tumor immunology, rather than an extensive discussion of the theoretical implications of the findings. For the reader who wishes to obtain a more comprehensive view of human tumor immunology, there

SIDNEY H. GOLUB • Division of Oncology, Department of Surgery, and Department of Microbiology and Immunology, University of California at Los Angeles, School of Medicine, Los Angeles, California.

have been a number of relatively recent reviews (Klein, 1971; McKhann and Jagarlamoody, 1971; Fisher, 1971; Cinader, 1972; Feldman, 1972; Hellström and Hellström, 1974; Pilch *et al.*, 1975*a,b*).

This chapter will be confined to discussion of host-generated immune responses specific for tumor-associated antigens. This will omit large areas of considerable interest and importance, including such aspects as the identification of tumor-specific antigens with xenogeneic antisera, manipulation of the response by nonspecific means, or induction of responses with transfer factor or "immune RNA." These approaches may contribute significantly to our understanding of the immunology of tumors, but do not bear directly on the nature of the response elicited in the tumor-bearing host.

One area of direct importance to the host response to tumor antigens is the question of immunocompetence. Space limitations do not allow for a detailed evaluation of the influence of the efficiency of immune function on the response to the tumor, and some of these aspects are discussed by Allison in Chapter 8 of this volume. Obviously, if the immune system is impaired by the presence of a growing neoplasm, this will greatly alter the type and effectiveness of the immune response to the tumor antigens. As Eilber and Morton (1970*a*) originally described, patients with impaired immunological function, as measured by the cutaneous hypersensitivity response to a contact allergen, have a poorer prognosis.

There is a wealth of data in the literature dealing with various aspects of immunological function in cancer patients. Immunocompetence has been evaluated by determinations of serum immunoglobulin levels, antibody responses to a new antigen, lymphocyte proliferation after stimulation with mitogens, mixed lymphocyte culture reactivity, delayed cutaneous hypersensitivity reactions to common recall antigens or to a primary exposure to a contact allergen or skin-sensitizing agent, peripheral blood lymphocyte counts, enumeration of lymphocyte subpopulations, ability to manifest an inflammatory response, and reticuloendothelial system function. All of these approaches can be useful in evaluating the status of the immune system, but none of them measures a specific response for tumor-associated antigens. Interpretation of such experiments is also complicated by the finding that the frequency with which defects in immune function are found will depend on both the population studied and the assays employed (Golub *et al.*, 1974). Thus the rest of this discussion will focus on tumor-associated antigens and the responses they elicit. It must be kept in mind that the determination of immunocompetence in cancer patients is a closely related field, and may prove to be extremely useful as a guide to the extent of disease, prognosis, and the choice of an immunotherapeutic modality.

2. Methodology of Human Tumor Immunology

Unfortunately, there are almost as many techniques for studying tumor-specific reactions as there are tumor immunologists. This is not because tumor immomologists are extraordinarily creative scientists, but because no one technique can answer all the appropriate questions. Thus, by carefully examining the methodology of human tumor immunology, we can discern what questions can be asked and what type of answers obtained.

261

HOST
IMMUNE
RESPONSE TO
HUMAN
TUMOR
ANTIGENS

2.1. Methods for the Assessment of Cell-Mediated Immunity

Most of the attention of tumor immunologists has focused on the *in vitro* measurement of cellular aspects of tumor immunity, and this is an appropriate place to begin a discussion of methodology. A recent symposium examined many of the problems of cell-mediated immunity to human tumor antigens, and the proceedings of that symposium (*National Cancer Institute Monograph* No. 37, 1973) will provide an extensive bibliography for those particularly interested in this field.

2.1.1. Lymphocyte-Mediated Cytotoxicity

By far the most common, and controversial, technique used for the study of cell-mediated reactions against tumor-associated antigens is the cytotoxicity assay. This test is based on the ability of lymphocytes to lyse target tumor cells. A variation of this approach is to assess inhibition of growth of the target tumor cells rather than cytolysis. In either case, the purpose is to determine whether putatively immune lymphocytes will damage the tumor cells. Assessment of the damage can be accomplished either by visual observation or by the use of a radioactive isotope to label the target cell. The former, visual observation, was the original approach in this area (Hellström *et al.*, 1968a; Takasugi and Klein, 1970), and is still widely used. This was based on the observation that sensitized lymphocytes could lyse appropriate target cells (Rosenau and Moon, 1961) or could inhibit the outgrowth of target cells into colonies (Hellström, 1967). However, colony inhibition is a time-consuming assay in that the target cells must be allowed to grow out into colonies, and the criteria used for designation of a colony may be difficult to establish. Thus most laboratories have abandoned colony inhibition in favor of one of the various microcytotoxicity assays. If the results of this assay are read visually, this is also a tedious and time-consuming procedure. One alternative approach is to read the results of microcytotoxicity tests electronically (Takasugi *et al.*, 1973a), but this technology is not available to most laboratories.

Many laboratories have turned to isotopic labels to permit the automated enumeration of target cell survival. Much of the work on the cell-mediated cytotoxic reaction against antigens of the histocompatability systems has been accomplished using the release of ^{51}Cr from labeled target cells as a marker of cytolysis (Brunner *et al.*, 1968; Canty and Wunderlich, 1970). Unfortunately, this potentially very useful assay has been difficult to adapt to human target cells. The test requires a target cell which will readily bind the isotope, will not release it spontaneously in appreciable amounts, and will promptly release sufficient

quantities of the label upon cytolysis by immune lymphocytes. These requirements are well fulfilled by many murine tumors, especially ascites tumors, but are
marginally, if at all, fulfilled by cells from human solid tumors. Thus the
^{51}Cr-release assay has been exploited effectively only in studies of responses
against human leukemia cells (Rosenberg *et al.*, 1972).

The problems associated with the chromium-release assay have led to attempts
to utilize other isotopic markers for human tumor target cells. One relatively new
approach that will probably see application to human studies is the label
technitium-99*m* (Barth and Gillespie, 1974). Among the more promising labels
now in use are [^{125}I]iododeoyxuridine (^{125}IdUrd) (Cohen *et al.*, 1971) and the
tritiated compounds [^{3}H]thymidine, [^{3}H]uridine, and [^{3}H]proline (MacPherson
and Pilch, 1972; Jagarlamoody *et al.*, 1971; Bean *et al.*, 1973). In all these assays,
the usual procedure is to prelabel the target cells with the isotope, add the effector
cells, and count the isotope remaining in the target cells as a function of the
number of surviving cells. This often requires a rather long labeling period,
especially for slowly growing target cells, and is not often useable for early
subcultures of the tumor targets that have not been adapted to growth *in vitro*.
Alternative procedures involve the measurement of inhibition of target cell
growth as assessed by incorporation of [^{3}H]thymidine (Ming *et al.*, 1966) or of
^{125}IdUrd (Seeger and Owen, 1973) or by the release of ^{125}IdUrd from labeled
target cells (Oldham and Herberman, 1973). The ^{125}IdUrd assays have the
advantage of simplicity of counting, as that isotope, being a γ-emitter, can be
counted more readily than the tritiated labels, which require liquid scintillation
counting. However, IdUrd is toxic to target cells, whereas the tritiated labels are
innocuous. It is possible that the cell damage induced by the IdUrd may enhance
the sensitivity of the assay by making partially damaged cells more susceptible to
lymphoid-mediated cell destruction. In any case, there do not appear to be any
fundamental differences between these assays, and researchers continue to use
the assay with which they feel most comfortable.

2.1.2. The Problem of Specificity and the Question of Controls

Since cytotoxicity is probably the most widely used assay for cell-mediated
reactions against human tumor cells, it is not surprising that considerable
controversy about the technical aspects of the test has emerged. Since the original
finding by the Hellströms that neuroblastoma patients had lymphocytes that
damaged neuroblastoma cells *in vitro* (Hellström *et al.*, 1968b), there have been
innumerable reports that lymphocytes from cancer patients can kill target tumor
cells of the same histological type as the patients' disease, while lymphocytes from
normal donors or cancer patients with histologically different diseases would not
kill the target cells. Among the many reports of this type are studies showing
"specific" cytotoxicity against breast carcinomas (Fossati *et al.*, 1972), brain tumors
(Levy *et al.*, 1972; Kumar *et al.*, 1973), bladder carcinoma (Bubenik *et al.*, 1970;
O'Toole *et al.*, 1973b), melanoma (Fossati *et al.*, 1971; Currie and Basham, 1972;
DeVries *et al.*, 1972; Hellström *et al.*, 1973c; Heppner *et al.*, 1973), and sarcomas

263

HOST
IMMUNE
RESPONSE TO
HUMAN
TUMOR
ANTIGENS

(Sinkovics *et al.*, 1972; Cohen *et al.*, 1973). With this wealth of data available, only one conclusion would seem possible: cancer patients have circulating lymphoid cells that are specifically cytotoxic for tumor cells of the appropriate histological type.

But this conclusion has been seriously challenged. Many laboratories, including those that have reported "specific" cytotoxicity, have also found situations where "non-specific" reactions occur. For example, the Discussion section of the Conference and Workshop on Cellular Immune Reactions to Human Tumor-Associated Antigens (*National Cancer Institute Monograph* No. 37, 1973) details many observations of reactivities that are not specific for the appropriate target tumor cells. These reactions can be grouped into two types: cytotoxicity by inappropriate effector cells (cytotoxicity by lymphoid cells from normal individuals or cancer patients with a different type of cancer than the target cell) and cytotoxicity against inappropriate target cells. For some time, these "nonspecific" aspects were simply dismissed as technical errors and were not critically examined. Now it is apparent that such responses are commonly found, and must be explained. In a study of extraordinary proportions, Takasugi *et al.* (1973*b*) described cell-mediated cytotoxicity from normal donor lymphocytes as being equivalent or greater against target tumor cells than the cytotoxicity obtained by lymphocytes from patients with tumors of the appropriate histological type. In these experiments, involving over 2000 separate assays, no evidence for "specific" cytotoxicity was found. Similarly, Rosenberg *et al.* (1974) found that all normal donors tested were cytotoxic in a ^{51}Cr-release assay against certain human lymphoblastoid target cells.

Sometimes both specific and nonspecific cytotoxicity can be detected. For example, Bloom *et al.* (1974) confirmed the finding of O'Toole *et al.* (1973*b*) that the degree of cytotoxicity of lymphocytes from bladder carcinoma patients correlated with the stage of the disease, and that lymphocyte cytotoxicity against bladder carcinoma cells was greater for those of the patients than for those obtained from normal donors. However, Bloom *et al.* also found increased cytotoxicity from effector cells of patients with nonmalignant genitourinary disorders. Similarly, Skurzak *et al.* (1973) found patients with gliomas to possess cytotoxic lymphocytes when tested against glioma target cells, but patients with subarachnoid hemorrhages also possessed such effector cells. Takasugi *et al.* (1973*b*) documented what had long been suspected—that laboratory personnel are more cytotoxic than are other normal donors. The most intriguing finding of unexpected cytotoxicity is the report of Hellström *et al.* (1973*a*) that healthy black individuals have lymphocytes specifically cytotoxic to melanoma cells. This finding has interesting implications for the epidemiology and biology of that malignancy. Thus the choice of a control population can greatly influence the specificity of the results.

Similar problems are posed by the choice of target cells. For example, Wahlström *et al.* (1973) demonstrated cytotoxicity against glioma cells with lymphocytes from patients with this disease, but were also able to show cytotoxicity against normal and fetal glial cells. These results suggest a "tissue-specific" antigenicity (Taranger *et al.*, 1972) rather than a truly tumor-specific response.

Allogeneic tumor cells of a different histological type are the most commonly used controls, but reactivity against such cells might be encountered due to histocompatibility differences or the presence of fetal antigens. Autochthonous fibroblasts are also often used, but are generally considered to be rather resistant to cytolysis. However, fibroblast lines can be found that are sensitive to cell-mediated cytotoxicity (Golub *et al.*, 1975) and can serve as control target cells. Even so, lymphocytes both from melanoma patients and from normal donors were more cytotoxic against the tumor-derived target cells than the fibroblasts of known sensitivity (H. Sulit and S. Golub, unpublished data). Several laboratories have detailed the greater sensitivity of tumor cell lines as compared to short-term tumor cell cultures (Takasugi *et al.*, 1973*b*; DeVries *et al.*, 1974). Cell line sensitivity to cytolysis can also be influenced by the serum used to grow the target cells, with fetal calf serum grown cells being more sensitive than human serum grown cells (Sulit *et al.*, 1975) and the growth phase of the target cell (Leneva and Svet-Moldavsky, 1974).

Some of the aspects of "nonspecific" cytotoxicity are probably due to differences in the method of preparation of the effector cells. This is not an appropriate place for the detailed examination of all the technical aspects of the various cytotoxicity assays. However, DeVries *et al.* (1975) have carefully examined the two most widely used methods for preparation of effector lymphocytes (Plasmagel sedimentation and nylon-wool columns vs. Ficoll–Hypaque discontinuous gradients) and found that although the former technique resulted in less cytotoxicity from normal donors, both techniques resulted in considerable "nonspecific" cytotoxicity.

In summary, the main pillar on which many conclusions about cellular immunity to human tumor antigens rests, the cytotoxicity assay, has come into serious question. It is extremely unlikely the conflicting data of different groups of skilled researchers are due to simple technical differences or that only one point of view can discern the truth. The reactivity of lymphoid cells from cancer patients is undoubtably real. The reactivity of lymphoid cells from normal donors is also very probably a real phenomenon, and warrants much closer examination. All of us are under continual bombardment by potentially oncogenic stimuli. It would not be surprising if this were reflected in a sensitive assay for immunity to tumor-associated antigens. Characterization of the nature of the *in vitro* response and identification of the antigens involved in the cytolysis of tumor cells by lymphoid cells from donors without cancer may prove to be a particularly important advance in our comprehension of the neoplastic process.

The technical problems associated with the cytotoxicity assay, and the question of specificity, have consumed much of the discussion about their use. This has tended to obscure a more fundamental question. Does *in vitro* cytotoxicity reflect a phenomenon which is pertinent to tumor immunity *in vivo*? There is an obvious appeal to the conceptual correlation of tumor rejection and the ability of a lymphoid cell to kill a tumor cell *in vitro*. However, hard evidence that the cell that mediates cytolysis *in vitro* is identical to the cell that mediates tumor rejection *in vivo* is difficult, if not impossible, to obtain. It is hard to imagine that the presence

265

HOST
IMMUNE
RESPONSE TO
HUMAN
TUMOR
ANTIGENS

within an organism of lymphoid cells that have the ability to kill tumor cells can be anything but beneficial. However, even this simple logic has been challenged by the work of Prehn (1972), who has suggested that a weak immune response that is insufficient to destroy the tumor may actually promote tumor growth.

In human solid tumors, as discussed above, the nearly universal finding has been that lymphoid cells from cancer patients evince cytotoxic activity against tumor cells of the same histological type. Since almost all patients with that type of cancer appear to produce cytotoxic lymphocytes, much research has centered on the interaction of cytotoxic cells with serum factors. This has tended to obscure the very real possibility that quantitative differences in numbers or efficiency of cytotoxic lymphocytes may greatly influence, or reflect, the progress of the disease. To a large extent, this difficulty is due to the inability to accurately quantitate lymphocyte-mediated cytotoxicity, and most work has tended to classify lymphocytes simply as cytotoxic or noncytotoxic. However, there are data that in bladder carcinoma (O'Toole *et al.*, 1972*a,b*) and in melanoma (Hellström *et al.*, 1973*c*) the magnitude of the *in vitro* response does indeed correlate with the stage or clinical course of the disease. If this is the case, then it provides indirect evidence that cytotoxic lymphocytes are not simply an *in vitro* phenomenon but do play an important role in the host–tumor relationship. At the very minimum, it indicates that cytotoxicity may be a useful monitor of the clinical status of the patient.

2.1.3. Blastogenesis Assays

Cytotoxicity reflects the final event in a series of cellular reactions. The earlier phases of the initiation of immune reactivity to a tumor antigen, i.e., the events whereby immune lymphoid cells are triggered to some reaction by tumor antigen, may be of even greater importance. The most convenient test of triggering of lymphoid cells by tumor antigens is the blastogenesis assay. In this test, lymphocytes (termed "responder cells") are cultivated in the presence of tumor antigens, either in the form of intact tumor cells (termed "stimulator cells") or as extracts of tumor cells, and DNA synthesis or some other aspect of lymphocyte proliferation is quantitated. Authochthonous tumor cells must be employed to avoid reactions due to histocompatibility antigens. The major conceptual difficulty with blastogenesis assays is the question of what the blastogenic response represents. Does it indicate prior sensitization to tumor antigens, or does it simply indicate an antigenic disparity between the responding lymphocyte and that antigen? The evidence is conflicting and not at all conclusive. It has been known for some time that soluble antigens such as PPD (purified protein derivative) require presensitization of the individual in order to elicit a blastogenic response (Schrek, 1963). This is in contrast to nonspecific mitogens or allogeneic lymphocytes, which elicit responses without apparent presensitization. Thus it might be expected that blastogenic responses to tumor antigens by human lymphocytes would also require presensitization. Unfortunately, this cannot be tested, since lymphocytes cannot be obtained from human donors prior to tumor development. However,

Kanner *et al.* (1970) demonstrated blastogenic responses to tumor-associated antigens on syngeneic tumors in the mouse in the MLTR (mixed lymphocyte–tumor reaction) without immunizing the donor of the responder lymphocytes. Thus it is clear that lymphocyte proliferative responses can be used to demonstrate a neoantigen on a tumor cell. But whether these responses also reflect cell-mediated immunity is uncertain at present.

The blastogenesis assay has been employed most extensively in studies of cellular responses to antigens on transformed lymphoid cells. Leukemia cells have been shown to stimulate DNA synthesis in lymphocytes of the identical twin of the patient (Bach *et al.*, 1969) or the autochthonous donor (Fridman and Kourilsky, 1969; Viza *et al.*, 1969). Autochthonous stimulation has also been reported when responder lymphocytes are stimulated with mitomycin-treated or irradiated cultured lymphoblastoid cell lines derived from mononucleosis patients, leukemia patients, or normal donors (Green and Sell, 1970; Steel and Hardy, 1970; Han *et al.*, 1971; Junge *et al.*, 1971; Knight *et al.*, 1971). The most remarkable feature of these results is the magnitude of the blastogenic response. In all these cases, stimulation with autochthonous cultured lymphoblasts resulted in responses in the range of mitogen-induced stimulation rather than the usually minimal responses seen in solid tumors. This suggests some type of altered antigenicity during the adaptation of the cells to *in vitro* growth.

This last example points out one of the major drawbacks of the blastogenesis assay. It is very difficult to use this assay to distinguish between tumor-associated antigens and other neoantigens on the stimulator cell. Furthermore, the test can be complicated by the production of various soluble blastogenic factors. One approach to identification of the antigens on tumor cells that result in blast transformation of autochthonous lymphocytes is to recover the lymphocytes and test them for cytotoxic activity against a variety of target cells. This was done for Burkitt's lymphoma cells by Golub *et al.* (1972). In these experiments, lymphocytes from patients with Burkitt's lymphoma were cocultivated with mitomycin-treated autochthonous cultured lymphoblastoid cell line cells derived from the tumor. This procedure, comparable to the leukemia and infectious mononucleosis systems, resulted in a high degree of blastogenesis. The lymphocytes sensitized in this fashion showed cytotoxic activity against autochthonous and allogeneic Burkitt tumor derived lines but not against lymphoblastoid lines derived from normal donors. The original conclusion was that sensitization was specific for tumor-associated Epstein–Barr virus defined antigens. However, subsequent experimentation in this system has shown that the types of target cells affected by such *in vitro* sensitized cells include several nonvirally transformed lines (Svedmyr *et al.*, 1974a). Thus it appears more likely that *in vitro* sensitization against cultured autochthonous lymphoblasts is directed against some unknown, perhaps fetal, neoantigen. This points out the strength of this type of approach in identification of the relevant antigens.

Lymphocyte blastogenic responses can also be obtained with fresh autochthonous lymphoid tumor cells, although these responses are not usually as dramatically strong as with the cultured tumor cells. This has been shown with occasional biopsies of Burkitt's lymphomas (Stjernsward *et al.*, 1970) but has been best exploited with the leukemias. In these diseases, the usual experimental procedure is to store the acute-phase leukemia cells in viable condition by freezing in liquid nitrogen and then use them as stimulator cells. Responder lymphocytes are drawn after remission has been induced in the patient by chemotherapy. A positive blastogenic response has been shown to be correlated with a general state of stronger immunocompetence and appeared to be a good prognostic sign (Gutterman *et al.*, 1972*a*). However, interpretation of blastogenesis responses in leukemia patients is almost invariably complicated by the intensive chemotherapy administered to the patients. Hersh *et al.* (1971) studied the effect of chemotherapy and observed a "rebound" phenomenon whereby blastogenic responses to nonspecific mitogens were elevated past pretherapy levels following recovery from the immunosuppressive effects of the drugs. This may have contributed to the elevated lymphocyte blastogenic responses to autochthonous tumor cells observed in leukemia patients following immunization with leukemia cell vaccines (Powles *et al.*, 1971). In a similar immunotherapy program, Gutterman *et al.* (1974*b*) also found that autoimmunized patients gave greater blastogenic responses to autochthonous leukemia cells, but that during the early period after immunization both specific responses to the tumor antigens and nonspecific responses showed a "rebound," while several weeks after immunization only the increase in blastogenic response to leukemia cells persisted. Thus alterations in the level of blastogenesis must be cautiously evaluated. Furthermore, the blastogenesis assay is subject to much experimental variation, and altogether too little work has been done on the kinetics and dose requirements of the assay in each tumor system. Schweitzer *et al.* (1973) have questioned whether specific responses can be detected in acute lymphocytic leukemia, and point out the variability of DNA synthesis of the responder lymphocytes. Even with these problems, the blastogenesis assay remains a valuable research tool. Perhaps the most exciting potential use is the immunodiagnosis of residual disease, which has been described by Gutterman *et al.* (1974*a*) for the detection of leukemic cells in the bone marrow of patients in remission.

In solid tumor systems, the blastogenesis assay has been even more difficult to manage successfully. Positive blastogenic responses have been reported to autochthonous malignant melanoma cells (Nagel *et al.*, 1971) and sarcomas (Taylor *et al.*, 1971; Vanky *et al.*, 1971*b*). Positive responses have also been obtained with soluble extracts of tumors in a number of neoplasms (Savel, 1969; Gutterman *et al.*, 1972*b*; Mavligit *et al.*, 1973; Vanky *et al.*, 1974). In all these systems, a positive response is a relatively small increase in DNA synthesis and little information is available as to the kinetics of the response. A slight modification of this approach is the measurement of increases in protein synthesis rather than DNA synthesis, and preliminary findings suggest that this response may be useful in monitoring immunotherapy (Roth *et al.*, 1975).

The problem of specificity remains in all such systems. One approach ,to dissecting apart the antigen from nonspecific blastogenic factors has been to look for interactions with serum components. Blocking of blastogenesis has been reported for autochthonous sera from leukemia patients (Gutterman *et al.*, 1973*b*) and for sarcomas with both autochthonous and allogeneic sarcoma sera (Vanky *et al.*, 1971*a*). Perhaps the most intriguing study of this type was the report of Hattler and Soehnlen (1974) that tumor-induced blastogenesis could be blocked by the addition of a factor eluted from the responder leukocytes. This factor was thought to be antigen–antibody complexes. These interactions will be discussed again in the section on cell–serum interactions, but are mentioned here as among the few examples where any preliminary findings relevant to determining the specificity of the reaction are available. Finally, the sensitization technique can be used to study the specificities involved in the blastogenic reaction against autochthonous tumor cells. Golub and Morton (1974) reported that lymphoid cells from melanoma patients could be sensitized on autochthonous melanoma monolayers. The recovered lymphocytes displayed slightly increased DNA synthesis and augmented cytotoxic activity for autochthonous or allogeneic melanoma target cells but not for skin fibroblasts or allogeneic tumor cells of different histological type. These results suggest that the antigens involved in the sensitization procedure, although not necessarily identical to the antigens promoting the blastogenic response, are tumor associated.

2.1.4. The Detection of Lymphokines

A number of soluble substances have been identified that are elaborated by specifically sensitized lymphocytes upon contact with antigen. These substances are collectively termed "lymphokines." Only one of these many substances has been exploited thus far for the detection of responses to human tumor antigens. This lymphokine is termed "migration inhibition factor" (MIF) and is a protein that can prevent the migratory movement of macrophages. The inhibition of macrophage migration by the products of sensitized lymphocytes has been one the best-studied *in vitro* correlates of delayed hypersensitivity. In the usual MIF assay, antigen and sensitized lymphocytes are interacted and the supernatant containing MIF is tested on normal macrophages (often guinea pig peritoneal exudate cells) for the inhibition of migration. There have been a number of reports in animal model systems (e.g., Kronman *et al.*, 1969; Vaage *et al.*, 1972) of tumor-specific immunity being detected by the generation of MIF from sensitized lymphocytes in the presence of tumor cells.

With this background of positive results in animal models, and the good correlation known to exist between MIF production and delayed cutaneous hypersensitivity, it was obvious that this assay had considerable potential for the study of tumor immunity in man. This is especially true with the advent of skin testing for tumor-associated antigens in humans. However, with few exceptions (Wolberg and Goelzer, 1971; Hilberg *et al.*, 1973) attempts to use the usual "indirect" type of MIF assay described above for the detection of human tumor-associated antigens have been unsuccessful. Most of the success in this field has been obtained using a "direct" assay, in which leukocytes from cancer patients are tested for their migration in the presence or absence of tumor cell extracts.

Whether the lymphokine responsible for this migration inhibition is identical to MIF us still unclear, but the principle remains the same.

269

HOST
IMMUNE
RESPONSE TO
HUMAN
TUMOR
ANTIGENS

This leukocyte inhibition of migration (LIM) assay has been used by Andersen *et al.* (1970) in studies of immune response to human breast carcinoma antigens. The response of breast carcinoma patients to extracts of breast carcinomas in the LIM assay has been confirmed by Cochran *et al.* (1974), who also showed that extracts of nonmalignant breast pathological tissues did not inhibit the migration of carcinoma patient leukocytes. The most intriguing observation in this study was that extracts of histologically noninvolved areas of cancerous breasts also inhibited in the LIM assay of carcinoma leukocytes. This strongly suggests the antigenic modification of apparently normal cells and is in keeping with the known multifocal nature of the disease.

The LIM assay has also been studied in patients with malignant melanoma (Cochran *et al.*, 1973) and shows a good correlation to the extent of disease, with patients having widely disseminated disease not exhibiting inhibition of migration. Presumably, this indicates that patients with large tumor burdens circulate lymphoid cells that are no longer capable of elaborating the appropriate lymphokine. Furthermore, the LIM response is depressed in patients in the immediate postoperative period (Cochran *et al.*, 1972). This finding, along with the observation of depression of responses to several nonspecific mitogens in the postoperative period (Roth *et al.*, 1974), should serve as a warning to investigators to avoid sampling during this transient period of immunosuppression.

The migration inhibition assays have several notable advantages. The first is speed. These assays can be completed within a day, contrasting favorably with the several days to a week required for cytotoxicity or blastogenesis. The equipment required is minimal and either tumor cells or antigenic extracts can be employed. Quantitation is still imprecise, but is only slightly worse than in other cellular assays. Most of all, the migration assays can be used without the culturing of tumor cells *in vitro* with all the artifacts that may ensue. This allows for the study of tumors that are not easily adapted to growth *in vitro*, such as breast carcinoma, as previously discussed, and more recently lung carcinomas (Boddie *et al.*, 1974).

Unfortunately, little is known of the relationship between migration inhibition and other assays of cellular immunity to tumors, making comparisons of data difficult. It is clear that the migration assays, along with blastogenesis, are already very useful for monitoring the purification of tumor antigens. Whether they will be as useful as cytotoxicity for the analysis of interactions between immune lymphocytes and serum factors remains to be determined. The only major drawback to the LIM assay is a theoretical one: since the assay requires two cell types, a lymphocyte to generate the lymphokine and a migratory cell to respond to it, a defective migratory response does not identify the site of the defect. The migration assays seem to have avoided the controversies about specificity swirling about the other assays, and will probably see much more widespread use in the future.

There are several other assays of lymphokines that can be used for the detection of responses to tumor-associated antigens. However, these assays have yet to be fully investigated on human systems, and will be only briefly summarized here. One is the assessment of cytotoxic products of specifically immune lymphocytes—the lymphotoxin assay. Although there are many reports of lymphotoxins that are cytotoxic to tumor cells, this assay has yet to be explored for the detection of cells immune to human tumor antigens. Similarly, the leukocyte adherence inhibition assay, which is presumably mediated by a lymphokine, has been studied as a cellular assay in mice but not man. Since this assay can be used to detect "blocking factors" (Halliday *et al.*, 1974), it will probably receive increased attention. Finally, the macrophage electrophoretic migration test of Field and Caspary (1970), which depends on a lymphokine that retards the electrophoretic migration of macrophages, is an assay closely akin to the other migration assays. As frustration with the cytotoxicity and blastogenesis assays increases, the use of lymphokine assays will also undoubtedly increase, and will undoubtedly reveal new pitfalls.

2.1.5. In Vivo Assays

Ethical and legal factors greatly restrict the types of experiments that can be performed on cancer patients. Thus experiments utilizing tumor transplantation techniques, which have been of extraordinary value in animal studies, cannot be easily performed in patients. Among the few studies of this type that have been done are the important experiments of Southam *et al.* (1966). These experiments indicated that patients with progressively growing neoplasms have concomitant immunity, in that they resist implantation of small numbers of their own tumor cells at new sites. This resistance can be overcome with larger doses of cells. The admixture of a patient's own leukocytes, or less often his own plasma, inhibited the growth of the implanted tumor cells. These experiments remain as among the most convincing evidence that there is immune resistance to human tumors in the patient with cancer.

It is unlikely that much more experimentation of the type described above will be done, and other approaches must be found to examine the immune reactions against tumors *in situ*. Cancer is not a disease of the petri dish, and our current preoccupation with *in vitro* assays must not obscure the need for observations that take into account the architecture and physiology of the growing tumor. One approach is to attempt to imitate human tumor growth in experimental models, and introduce human immune components to study the ensuing interactions. Richmond and Morton (1974) observed that the growth of human melanoma cells in the cheek pouch of immunosuppressed hamsters can be inhibited by the admixture of lymphoid cells from melanoma patients. Whether this type of xenogeneic *in vivo* assay will be more useful than standard *in vitro* techniques remains to be determined.

One technique that has often been neglected is the simple observation of events. Richters and Sherwin (1974) have used sophisticated microscopic techniques to observe the interactions of lymphoid cells and tumor cells in fresh surgical explants. Their results suggest the existence of several types of effector lympho-

271

HOST
IMMUNE
RESPONSE TO
HUMAN
TUMOR
ANTIGENS

cytes as well as the relative scarcity of multiple lymphocytes interacting with a target tumor cell in tumor-containing lymph nodes. As the technology of microscopy continues to improve, it can be expected that more subtle distinctive features of the interactions of lymphoid and tumor cells will be distinguished by observational techniques. The observation of "purposeful" lymphocyte activity in fresh tumor explants (Richters *et al.*, 1971) provides a challenge to find *in vitro* assays that correlate with the events observed. This is a largely unexplored area, and may prove to be particularly fruitful.

Finally, the most commonly used *in vivo* assay is the delayed cutaneous hypersensitivity reaction. The great simplicity, ease of quantitation, speed, and safety of skin testing have resulted in more extensive study of cutaneous hypersensitivity reactions in cancer patients than any other immunological aspect. Much of this work concerns the response to common "recall" antigens of microbial origin or the responses to organic chemical haptens that do not exist naturally. The former can be used to study the function of the "memory" component of the immune response, while the latter can be used to determine whether the individual is sufficiently immunocompetent to generate a primary immune response.

More relevant to this chapter is the use of cutaneous hypersensitivity reactions to extracts of human tumor cells. Two types of tumor cell extracts have been used to elicit delayed cutaneous hypersensitivity reactions. The first is tumor cell membrane fractions (Oren and Herberman, 1971). This type of fractionation, with various modifications, has been used successfully in patients with colon carcinoma (Hollinshead *et al.*, 1970), breast carcinoma (Alford *et al.*, 1973), melanoma (Fass *et al.*, 1970*b*), Burkitt's lymphoma (Fass *et al.*, 1970*a*), cervical carcinoma (Wells *et al.*, 1973), lung carcinoma (Hollinshead *et al.*, 1974), and leukemia (Char *et al.*, 1973). The other type of antigenic preparation of wide usage is the 3 M potassium chloride extract. This procedure has the advantage of being useful simultaneously in the cutaneous hypersensitivity and blastogenesis assays (Mavligit *et al.*, 1973; Vanky *et al.*, 1974). It must be pointed out that both types of extraction procedures have been widely used for preparing histocompatibility antigens, and cannot be expected to yield highly purified tumor-specific antigens without further purification. This may account for the widely reported "nonspecific" reactivities of such preparations when tested at high dose levels. When low doses are employed, or extracts are further purified, the reaction appears to be relatively specific, although occasional individuals do react to similar extracts of normal tissues or extracts of allogeneic tumors of different histological types. In most cases, reactions to autochthonous tumor extracts appear to be strongest, although this varies with the tumor studied. For example, Char *et al.* (1973) found that acute myelogenous leukemia patients reacted to both autochthonous and allogeneic extracts. One final type of antigenic preparation should be mentioned—intact tumor cells. These appear to be relatively poor antigens for skin testing, as neither viable leukemia cells (Gutterman *et al.*, 1973*a*) nor mitomycin-treated leukemia cells (Santos *et al.*, 1973) elicit strong cutaneous reactions.

The significance of skin test reactivity remains unclear. There have been several reports that correlated cutaneous hypersensitivity reactions with clinical parameters. Fass *et al.* (1970a), in studies of Burkitt's lymphoma patients, found reactions to be much more common in remission periods than during relapse of the disease. Bluming *et al.* (1971) reported longer remission durations for Burkitt's lymphoma patients with positive reactions to autochthonous tumor extracts. In contrast, Stewart and Orizaga (1971) found breast cancer patients with positive cutaneous reactions to have poorer survival duration and Hughes and Lytton (1964) could find no correlation between cutaneous response to a crude tumor extract and any clinical parameter.

Skin testing with tumor extracts has yet to prove itself as a diagnostic test or to have an unequivocal correlation with clinical status. At best, it can be used to distinguish remission and relapse patients in the lymphoproliferative malignancies and to identify a state of anergy. However, one hardly needs an immunological test to identify a leukemic recurrence, and anergy can be shown with nontumor antigens. Thus the predominant use of cutaneous hypersensitivity reactions to tumor antigens remains in the immunochemistry of tumors. Skin testing is a useful means of monitoring the purification of tumor antigens, and has also proved of value in distinguishing common antigenicities within tumor types. For the study of the nature of the immune response to tumor antigens of man, we must continue to rely on *in vitro* assays.

2.2. Human Tumor Serology

2.2.1. The Problem of Specificity

Any serological method can be adapted for the detection of antibodies to tumor-associated antigens. The most commonly used techniques are the standard methods of immunology such as immunoprecipitation, complement fixation, complement-dependent cytolysis, and immunofluorescence. More sophisticated methods, such as radioimmunoassays and immunoelectron microscopy, are now coming into wider usage. The most important problem associated with any immunological assay is proving that the reaction is detecting an antigen that is truly tumor associated. This is particularly true when the tumor antigen is presented on a tissue culture cell. In this case, a number of artifacts have been identified that can be misinterpreted for tumor-associated antigens.

The most common problem with tissue culture tumor cells is mycoplasma contamination. There are numerous reports, mostly informal in nature, that indicate that many sera contain antibodies to these organisms, and that these antibodies will react against contaminated cell lines. One of the most definite studies of this type was performed by Bloom (1973), who showed marked increases in cytotoxic antibody activity against mycoplasma-infected cell lines as compared to noncontaminated lines. Since cancer patients are subject to more infections than healthy donors, it can be expected that the use of contaminated cell lines would result in more "false positive" reactions with patient sera than with control sera, thus compounding the error. Unfortunately, few serological studies have also included control sera from hospitalized noncancer patients, who might be expected to have higher antimycoplasma titers than healthy donors. The problem can be solved, of course, by using noncontaminated cell lines or by not using cultured cells at all. The latter solution is foolproof, but the advantages of reproducibility and convenience argue strongly for the continued use of cell cultures. Thus extreme care must be taken to avoid contamination of cell lines. Improved "biohazard"-type culture facilities should limit this problem in the future.

273

HOST
IMMUNE
RESPONSE TO
HUMAN
TUMOR
ANTIGENS

A cultured tumor cell is not a pure source of tumor antigens—it presents a wide array of antigenic specificities, most of which are irrelevant to the tumor immunologist. However, these nontumor antigens can be detected on the cultured tumor cell and can be confused with antigens unique for the tumor cell. Among such nontumor antigens are the histocompatibility antigens, which are certainly well expressed on cultured tumor cells. Since many cancer patients have received transfusions, they can be expected to have antibodies reactive with antigens of the HL-A complex. This can be easily controlled by testing, or adsorption with, normal cells bearing the same HL-A antigens.

A similar, but less often recognized problem is the expression of blood-group-like antigens on tumor cells. Bloom *et al.* (1973) demonstrated that many sera from cancer patients of blood group B or O phenotypes reacted with a variety of tumor cells. Confirming immunological tests indicated the presence of blood group A, or a cross-reacting substance, on the membrane of many cultured tumor cells. Blood group antigens could obviously distort seroepidemiological studies using cultured tumor cells.

Perhaps the most pervasive problem with cultured cells is the incorporation of exogenous antigens from the culture media. This is particularly a problem as most cells are cultured in media containing fetal calf serum (FCS), which has been shown to be incorporated into the cell membranes of cultured cells as antigenically detectable moieties (Hamburger *et al.*, 1963). The most distressing aspect about the incorporation of FCS antigens into cultured cells is that many human sera appear to have natural antibodies to FCS related antigens, which Irie *et al.* (1974b) termed "HM," for heterologous membrane antigen. The HM antigen appears to be best expressed on the cultured cells that have been most often used in human tumor immunology (sarcomas, melanomas, and lymphoblastoid cells) and less well expressed on carcinoma and normal cells in culture.

There seems to be little doubt that many studies of presumptive tumor antigens were actually studies of HM antigen. This is possibly true for the "nonspecific" cytotoxic antibodies detected against lymphoblastoid cells (Herberman, 1969), and is almost certainly true for the sarcoma antigen S-1 (Giraldo *et al.*, 1971), which was thought to be a sarcoma-associated antigen to which many healthy individuals had been exposed. However, the seroepidemiology of the S-1 antigen (Hirshault *et al.*, 1974) is identical to that of the HM antigen (Irie, 1974) and the conclusion is inescapable that this "sarcoma" antigen is a fetal calf serum substance. The seroepidemiology of HM (or S-1) antigen is interesting in that antibody levels are highest in early years of life and decline with age. Titers are also high in patients with certain malignancies besides sarcoma. This pattern emphasizes the necessity for using age-matched control donors for serological studies, as studies of osteosarcoma patients (who are young and would normally have high anti-HM titers) compared to blood bank donors (who are older and would have low levels of anti-HM) would result in an apparent tumor specificity.

The studies on HM antigen point out the great care that must be employed in serological studies utilizing cultured cells. Many studies are now going to have to be reinterpreted in light of the peculiar seroepidemiology of the natural antibody to this antigen. For example, the meningioma-associated antigen detected on cultured meningioma cells by Catalono *et al.* (1972) probably represents two antigenic specificities: HM antigen, which would explain its cross-reactivity with sarcoma sera, and a truly meningioma-associated antigen. The existence of the latter is evidenced by the reactivity of meningioma patient sera with extracts of fresh tumor (Rich and Winters, 1974). Using tumor cells or extracts rather than cultured cells is the most effective means of ruling out the participation of HM antigen. Caution should be used whenever an antigen can be detected only on tumor cells in culture. If the same antigen cannot be detected on noncultured tumor cells or on cells cultured in human serum, it is most likely HM antigen.

A final word must be said about the use of cultured cells in the special case of Burkitt's lymphoma. The fact that the membrane antigen (MA) is poorly expressed on biopsy cells of this malignancy and strongly expressed on cultured cells might lead one to suspect HM antigen. However, the MA of Burkitt's lymphoma cells in culture has been clearly shown to be a product of the infection of the cell with Epstein–Barr virus (EBV) (Klein *et al.*, 1968). The studies on Burkitt's lymphoma have generated several new approaches to seroepidemiology that deserve mention. The use of a carefully screened positive antiserum as a reference serum, for which all other sera are tested in a blocking assay, can avoid many of the problems mentioned above (Klein *et al.*, 1967). Also, the studies of Yata and Klein (1969) indicate the effects of culture conditions on the expression of MA on cultured lymphoblastoid cells. This is a particularly important point and indicates the absolute necessity for establishing standard culture conditions for serological studies. Otherwise, the fluctuations of antigenicity in culture will prevent obtaining comparable data from any two assays not performed simultaneously.

2.2.2. A Case Study: Malignant Melanoma

It is a temptation in a chapter of this type to include a complete listing of all serological reactions against human tumor-associated antigens. Suffice it to say that for nearly every thoroughly studied human tumor there is evidence for antibodies formed in the tumor-bearing host against tumor-associated antigens. The significance of such antibodies remains unknown in most cases. Therefore, this section will discuss a single human neoplastic disease, malignant melanoma, and attempt to present the different methodologies used and the areas of agreement and difference among the laboratories studying this disease. It is hoped that this will be of use as a model in the interpretation of data on any human malignancies. By necessity, some of the data will be more applicable to the next section on the nature of the host response, but methodology and interpretation cannot be readily dissociated.

275
HOST
IMMUNE
RESPONSE TO
HUMAN
TUMOR
ANTIGENS

Malignant melanoma has received a disproportionate share of interest from tumor immunologists, as it is a relatively rare disease representing only 2–3% of malignancies in the United States. However, the unpredictable natural history of the disease and the abnormally high share of "spontaneous regressions" among melanomas (Everson and Cole, 1966) recommend this disease as one human tumor likely to be influenced by the immune system.

The first finding of antibodies to malignant melanoma cell antigens was by Morton *et al.* (1968) using indirect immunofluorescence. Antibodies were detected in sera of melanoma patients against both autochthonous and allogeneic biopsy cells. The antibodies revealed antigens both on the cell membrane and intracellularly. The presence of antibodies detectable by membrane immunofluorescence was confirmed by Romsdahl and Cox (1970), Nairn *et al.* (1972), and Fossatti *et al.* (1971). The cytoplasmic antigen detectable on fixed melanoma cells by immunofluorescence was proven to be melanoma specific and not common to other pigmented cells by Muna *et al.* (1969) and Elliott *et al.* (1973).

Other methods have been used to demonstrate antibodies to melanoma-associated antigens. Siegler *et al.* (1972) used mixed hemagglutination in addition to cytolysis and immunofluorescence to demonstrate antimelanoma antibodies. Lewis *et al.* (1969) used immunofluorescence, complement-dependent cytotoxicity, and complement-dependent inhibition of tumor cell RNA synthesis to measure reactivity against freshly explanted tumor cells. In this latter study, and in subsequent studies on the specificity of the immunofluorescent reaction (Lewis and Phillips, 1972), Lewis and colleagues maintained that there were two types of melanoma antigen: a cross-reactive cytoplasmic antigen and an individually specific membrane antigen. Bodurtha *et al.* (1975) also found individual specificity for the membrane antigen. However, the other previously mentioned studies using either biopsy cells or cultured tumor cells seemed to indicate the presence of a cross-reactive melanoma-associated membrane antigen. The most convincing evidence for a cross-reactive melanoma antigen on tumor cell membranes is that of Gupta and Morton (1975) indicating that tumor-reactive antibodies can be eluted from the membrane of tumor cells obtained at surgery, and that such eluted antibodies show reactivity in complement fixation tests with membrane extracts of both the autochthonous tumor and allogeneic melanomas but not with extracts of normal tissues or other tumors.

One interesting aspect of the serology of melanoma is the agreement that disseminated disease is associated with lower levels of antibodies. This is true for antibodies detectable by immunofluorescence (Morton *et al.*, 1971; Wood and Barth, 1974) and antibodies detectable by several techniques for reactivity to membrane antigens (Lewis *et al.*, 1969; Bodurtha *et al.*, 1975). This could well be due to adsorption of the antibodies to the tumor mass, or to a decreased immunocompetence in the patients with disseminated disease. However, since such patients can respond with cytotoxic antibodies following immunization with irradiated tumor cells (Ikonopisov *et al.*, 1970), these explanations are unlikely to be the sole reason for the low levels of antibodies in patients with disseminated disease. Another factor may be the increased circulation of soluble tumor antigens which occupy all antibody combining sites. Carrel and Theilkaes (1973) presented evidence for excreted melanoma antigens, and it seems likely from data on cellular reactivities (to be discussed in Section 3.3) that circulating antigens may have a crucial role in modulating the immune response in the disease. Lewis *et al.* (1971) considered another explanation for the loss of detectable antibodies in patients with disseminated malignant melanoma. These investigators presented evidence for anti-idiotype antibodies, i.e., antibodies reactive against the antimelanoma antibodies, in such patients. This is an area that certainly warrants further investigation, as it is the only report to date of anti-idiotype antibodies having an immunoregulatory role in human malignancy.

In summary, the serology of human malignant melanoma has utilized a wide variety of techniques—immunofluorescence (membrane and intracellular), cytotoxicity, complement fixation, precipitation, mixed agglutination, and inhibition of RNA synthesis. These techniques have revealed large areas of agreement, such as the existence of antimelanoma antibodies and the difficulty in detecting such antibodies in patients with disseminated disease. Some areas of divergence remain, such as the specificity of antimembrane antibodies, and the biological effects of such antibodies remain to be elucidated.

3. The Nature of the Host Response

3.1. Humoral Immunity

One fact must influence any consideration of the role of humoral immunity in limiting tumor growth or development: antibodies can be detected against tumors, yet tumor cells continue to proliferate and kill the host. Does this indicate that the humoral response to tumor antigens is insufficient, inefficient, or irrelevant? In this section, only those situations where a humoral immune response is correlated with some prognostic or clinical feature will be considered. Tumor immunology has now progressed beyond the point where the identification of an antibody reactive with the tumor cell is a noteworthy event.

As previously mentioned, antimelanoma antibodies appear to be present only when the disease is anatomically restricted and are difficult to detect when the disease has disseminated. Similarly, complement fixing antisarcoma antibody titers have been shown to decrease at times of recurrence of disease (Morton *et al.*, 1970, 1971). Unfortunately, the HM antigen has clouded the entire sarcoma picture, and the specificities of such antibodies remain in doubt. The antigen detected by complement fixation (Eilber and Morton, 1970*b*) appears to have a different distribution as compared to HM antigen and is suggestive of an infectious agent associated with sarcomas. Another solid tumor in which antibody levels have been correlated with clinical features is breast cancer. Hudson *et al.* (1974) reported a correlation between the presence of anti-breast-carcinoma antibodies and the degree of sinus histiocytosis of the tumor, which is thought to be a favorable prognostic sign (Black *et al.*, 1956).

One category of malignant diseases in which the humoral immune response is likely to have an important role in the host defense mechanism is the lympho-proliferative malignancies. Leukemia in experimental animals is a notoriously difficult disease to enhance immunologically. In human leukemia, Gutterman *et al.* (1973*b*) found a correlation between the presence of antibodies against leukemic cells detectable by immunofluorescence or by blocking of blastogenesis and longer periods of chemotherapy-induced remission. Yoshida and Imai (1970) found increased incidence of antileukemic antibodies detectable with the sensitive immune adherence assay in patients in remission. Thus in leukemia, as in the solid tumors, the weight of evidence so far available tends to indicate that antibodies are most often detectable when tumor burden is low. However, insufficient data are available correlating clinical factors with antibody responses to be able to visualize the role of the humoral response in the host defense against the tumor.

The question still remains as to the significance of *in vitro* detectable antibodies. Indirect evidence for an *in vivo* role for antibodies can be discerned from the observation of antibodies bound to the tumor cell growing in the host. Phillips and Lewis (1971) were able to elute antibodies from the membranes of surgical samples of Hodgkin's disease cells and detect the specific antibody by immunofluorescence. Gupta and Morton (1975) used complement fixation to detect antibodies eluted from melanoma cells. When an even more sensitive assay system was employed, immune adherence, Irie *et al.* (1974*a*) demonstrated antitumor antibodies and complement components on the membranes of tumor cells of various histologic types. Specificity was indicated by the lack of such antibodies on the normal tissues of the same patient. These studies do not indicate the function of such antibodies. Tumor-bound antibodies may be initiating mediated cytolysis of the cell, or interacting with cellular components of the immune system, or even augmenting the growth of the tumor cell (Shearer *et al.*, 1973). Thus the presence of antibodies on a tumor cell *in vivo* cannot necessarily be interpreted as a function that benefits the host.

One final area of the humoral response warrants mention. In a very few systems it is possible to discuss the humoral response against specific viral antigens in human tumor systems. One viral antigen where the humoral response appears to be of key importance is the common benign tumor known as warts. Matthews and Shirodaria (1973) showed that the presence of anti-wart-virus antibodies in the serum was closely correlated with the regression of the lesions. Whereas a very high proportion of those individuals with regressing warts had anti-wart-virus antibodies of IgM, IgG, and IgA classes in their serum, individuals with nonre-gressing warts had a much lower incidence of antibodies. Regressing wart lesions often contained the viral antigens, while nonregressing warts did not have detectable viral antigens. Neither type of lesion showed significant lymphoid cell infiltration. The implication is clear that when the wart virus antigens are expressed the humoral response mediates regression of the infected cells. The other case when antiviral antibodies have prognostic significance is in Burkitt's lymphoma. Antibodies to the cytoplasmic nonvirion early antigen (EA) of EBV-infected cells tend to higher titers in tumor-bearing patients. In patients in remission, high anti-EA titers have been correlated with higher incidence of recurrence (Henle *et al.*, 1971). Conversely, anti-MA antibodies tend to decline prior to recurrence (Klein *et al.*, 1969). Thus the antiviral antibodies in Burkitt's lymphoma may have prognostic significance as well as providing clues as to the tumor cell–virus interactions.

3.2. Cellular Response

3.2.1. Lymphocytes

For some time, the working assumption of tumor immunology was that tumor immunity was simply a variation of transplantation immunity and must be mediated by the same mechanisms as allograft rejection. The only fundamental difference was thought to be the nature of the target cell. If that were the case, one would expect tumor-specific immunity to be mediated primarily by thymus-derived lymphocytes, since the T lymphocyte has been unequivocally shown to be the cytotoxic effector cell in alloimmune systems (Cerottini *et al.*, 1970). It can even be shown that T cells are autonomous in their cytotoxic activity and do not require the participation of any other cell type in order to deliver a cytotoxic effect to an allogeneic target cell (Golstein *et al.*, 1972). However, the situation does not appear to be so well defined in tumor-specific cell-mediated immunity.

The most direct method to study the cell population responsible for antitumor cytotoxicity is to use purified cell populations in the various *in vitro* assays. This approach is complicated by the findings that the various microcytotoxicity assays appear to measure the various lymphocyte subpopulations with different efficiencies (Plata *et al.*, 1974). Thus the ^{51}Cr-release test is probably a more efficient assay for T-cell cytotoxicity and the microcytotoxicity test appears to measure both T-cell and non-T-cell cytotoxic effects. Studies on the activity of purified cell populations must take into account the assay system, as different assays may detect one population in a preferential fashion.

There are surprisingly few reports of T-cell-mediated cytotoxic effects specific for tumor antigens. Wybran *et al.* (1974) found most of the cytotoxic activity in the microcytotoxicity assay with human lymphocytes from cancer patients to be in a T-cell-rich fraction of the peripheral blood lymphocytes. In these tests, lymphocytes from cancer patients, predominantly melanoma patients, were separated into a T-cell fraction by the ability of T cells to form spontaneous rosettes with sheep erythrocytes, and tested against appropriate tumor cell targets. DeVries *et al.* (1974) used similar techniques for melanoma patients and found some cytotoxic activity in the T-cell fraction but found considerably more cytotoxic activity in the non-T-cell (nonrosetting) fraction. The explanation for the discrepancy between these two studies remains unknown.

The report of Wybran *et al.* remains the sole evidence for T-cell cytotoxicity against a human solid tumor, although there are other indications of T-cell activity in animal studies. Leclerc *et al.* (1973) demonstrated T-cell-mediated cytotoxicity against Moloney sarcoma virus induced tumor antigens, but this activity was measured only after a short period following immunization. Rouse *et al.* (1972) observed that most of the lymphocytes in Marek's disease lesions in chickens bear surface markers indicative of thymic origin.

279

HOST
IMMUNE
RESPONSE TO
HUMAN
TUMOR
ANTIGENS

One area where T-cell cytotoxic activity is better documented is the lymphoproliferative malignancies. Rouse *et al.* (1972) demonstrated that the cells capable of passively transferring immunity to syngeneic murine plasma cell tumors are sensitive to treatment with anti-θ serum and complement, indicating the T-cell dependence of this immunity. The fact that cytotoxic reactions, albeit weak ones, can be detected against autochthonous human leukemia cells in the ^{51}Cr-release assay (Rosenberg *et al.*, 1972; Herberman *et al.*, 1974) is suggestive of T-cell activity, given the preferential detection of T-cell reactions by this assay. It also appears that the reactive morphologically atypical cell in the nonmalignant lymphoproliferative disease infectious mononucleosis is a T cell and the cell with neoantigens induced by the Epstein–Barr virus is a B cell (Sheldon *et al.*, 1973; Pattengale *et al.*, 1974). Mononucleosis may be a very appropriate model for malignant lymphoid tumors, and this evidence is strongly suggestive of a T-cell mechanism beneficial to the host. With the morphological evidence for T-cell reactivity against EBV-infected cells in infectious mononucleosis, one would predict that *in vitro* T-cell-mediated reactions would be detectable against EBV-transformed cells in EBV-associated diseases such as Burkitt's lymphoma and infectious mononucleosis. However, Hewetson *et al.* (1972) could not detect cells in the peripheral blood of Burkitt's lymphoma patients that would inhibit colony formation of EBV-transformed tissue culture target cells. These lymphocytes could be sensitized *in vitro* with the autochthonous tumor-derived tissue culture cells (Golub *et al.*, 1972) and a small sampling of lymph node cells displayed effector cell activity against EBV-transformed target cells (Hewetson *et al.*, 1972; Golub *et al.*, 1973). On the other hand, Rosenberg *et al.* (1974) could find only nonspecific cytotoxic activity against tissue culture lymphoblastoid target cells *in vitro*. It may be that nonspecific reactions mask the specific T-cell cytotoxicity, and preliminary evidence (Svedmyr and Jondal, personal communication) suggests that if the non-T cells are removed, specific T-cell cytotoxicity can be detected in the peripheral blood of infectious mononucleosis patients.

One reaction which is certainly dependent on T cells is the *in vitro* sensitization of lymphocytes against tumor-associated antigens. This has been shown to be a T-cell reaction in the sensitization of mouse lymphocytes against syngeneic plasmacytomas (Wagner and Röllinghoff, 1973) and for the sensitization of human lymphocytes against autochthonous lymphoblastoid cells (Svedmyr *et al.*, 1974*b*). This is consistent with the T-cell dependence of the stimulation of lymphocytes by tumor antigens in blastogenesis assays (Gorczynski, 1974).

There is substantial evidence for non-T-cell-mediated cytotoxic effects against tumor-associated antigens. The mechanism of non-T-cell cytotoxicity in many of these cases is likely to be the "arming" of so-called K (for killer) cells in the process known as antibody-dependent cellular cytotoxicity. This process, and the nature of the K cell, will be discussed in greater detail in Section 3.3. In this section, only the evidence indicating the reactivity of non-T cells against tumor cells will be discussed.

Borum and Jonsson (1972) found that neonatally thymectomized rats were still able to produce cytotoxic lymphocytes, as measured by the colony inhibition assay, against Rous sarcoma antigens. The Moloney sarcoma tumor system in mice has been studied extensively by Lamon *et al.* (1973*a,b*). At time periods shortly after infection with the virus when the tumor was developing or regressing, T-cell cytotoxicity was detected in the lymph node and splenic lymphocytes. The T-cell-mediated cytotoxicity diminished at later time periods, but non-T-cell cytotoxicity was apparent throughout the period of T-cell activity and through much of the time of tumor progression. Neither T-cell nor non-T-cell cytotoxicity, as measured by the microcytotoxicity assay, was detectable when the tumor burden was very large.

The results in the Moloney sarcoma system are paralleled by similar findings in human bladder carcinoma. O'Toole *et al.* (1973*a*, 1974) found that all cytotoxic activity in the microcytotoxicity assay was obtained in the non-T-cell fraction of peripheral blood lymphocytes. As was the case with the Moloney sarcoma studies, the active cell was not removed by procedures that remove phagocytic cells. Non-T-cell cytotoxicity could be detected only in individuals bearing bladder carcinomas, but was diminished in those with widespread metastatic disease. DeVries *et al.* (1974) also found the active population in microcytotoxicity tests against human melanoma targets to be predominantly non-T-cell in nature.

Thus the original assumption that tumor immunity is mediated exclusively via a thymus-derived lymphocyte is probably not accurate. T cells can mediate specific cytotoxic effects against tumor target cells, and from the available evidence are probably quite important in the initial immune response to the neoplasm. However, non-T lymphocytes (not necessarily B cells) have also been detected in assays of cell-mediated immunity to tumor antigens. This population of effector cells can be detected at times when T-cell activity is low, such as during the period of maximal tumor growth. By extrapolation from the animal models, it seems likely that most human tumor studies, which by necessity are conducted after tumor development, will reflect non-T-cell activity. What remains to be determined is the biological importance of these two types of lymphocyte effector cells. The fact remains that in the animal models T-cell activity is detected at times crucial to the subsequent development of the tumor, while non-T-cell cytotoxicity is detected both at the early phases of development and after the progressive course of the disease has been determined. It is tempting to speculate that T cells may be the determinant of the progression or regression of the disease, while non-T-cell activity reflects only the antigenic disparity between the tumor and the host. This is an area of critical importance, and merits intensive investigation.

In the foregoing, lymphocyte populations were distinguished by criteria used to determine thymic or nonthymic derivation. There are other functional characteristics that can be used to identify various subpopulations of lymphocytes. For example, Grant *et al.* (1973) were able to identify several effector cell populations based on differential sensitivity to radiation of the effector cells. These experiments suggest the existence of several types of effector cells, one population of which requires the presence of antigen to proliferate and mediate a cytotoxic reaction and one or more types of effector cells able to mediate a cytotoxic reaction without an activational event. Similarly, Senik *et al.* (1973) studied lymphocytes reactive in the blastogenesis assay with syngeneic Moloney sarcoma virus induced tumors. These cells appeared in infected animals prior to the development of tumor and prior to cells specifically cytotoxic in the ^{51}Cr-release test. Wright *et al.* (1973) found that the lymphocytes that were nonreactive in the ^{51}Cr-release assay but were active in microcytotoxicity tests could be "reactivated" *in vitro* to cytotoxic activity in the ^{51}Cr assay by a simple incubation procedure. Thus there is evidence for various functional subpopulations based on the kinetics of the assay system, the presence of the sensitizing antigen, and the culture conditions. These various populations may coincide with the T-cell, B-cell, K-cell, and macrophage classifications, or they may represent memory cells of various types, or cells in different stages of maturation and differentiation. The key point is that it is becoming increasingly clear that the effector cells mediating tumor-specific immunity are a remarkably heterogeneous population. There does not appear to be a single identifiable cell type which is the sole autonomous antitumor entity in all circumstances. The immune system has apparently developed a battery of effector cells usable in its combat with the tumor cell.

3.2.2. Macrophages

Thus far, almost all *in vitro* studies of cell-mediated immunity in cancer patients have been studies of peripheral blood lymphocytes. Unfortunately, it is not nearly so easy to obtain spleen or lymph node samples from patients as it is to obtain peripheral blood. Only in breast carcinoma has any concerted and sustained effort been made to study the regional lymph nodes of patients, and such studies have concentrated on morphological features and nonspecific measurements of immunocompetence (Humphrey *et al.*, 1971; Fisher *et al.*, 1972, 1974). However, several investigators have observed interactions of lymph node cells and mammary carcinoma cells indicative of a local cellular response (Deodhar *et al.*, 1972; Richters and Sherwin, 1974). The role of regional lymphatics is an aspect of human tumor immunology that is just beginning to develop, and it is much too early to generalize about the comparative functions of regional and distant lymphoid organs. The neglect of the extravascular component of the immune system has had a pronounced effect on the present definition of cell-mediated immunity. In human tumor immunology, cell mediated is taken to mean lymphocyte mediated. However, extensive studies in animals on the role of macrophages in tumor immunity have prompted a redefinition of cell-mediated immunity to include cells of the macrophage/monocyte class. This is still an unexplored area in human studies, but the animal models have provided some valuable insights into the antitumor effects of these nonlymphocytic cells. The macrophage was first proposed as a key element in tumor immunity by Gorer (1956), but only in recent years has any progress been made on the mechanisms involved. There appear to be at least two classes of tumoricidal macrophages—the nonspecifically "activated" macrophage and the specifically "armed" macrophage. The "activated" macrophage was described by Hibbs *et al.* (1972*a*) as a nonspecifically cytotoxic cell from animals infected with parasitic organisms. Any number of microbes and microbial products have been shown to "activate" macrophages. Although these cells are nonspecifically activated, the cytotoxic activity has been most efficiently detected on transformed target cells. Target cells transformed by oncogenic viruses—spontaneously, or grown under conditions that diminish contact inhibition—were the most sensitive to this nonphagocytic macrophage-mediated cytolysis (Hibbs *et al.*, 1972*b*; Hibbs, 1973). Keller (1973) described a cytostatic effect of activated macrophages against a syngeneic rat tumor, thus indicating that activated macrophages can recognize syngeneic tumor cells.

The "armed" macrophage has been the subject of considerable investigation, and the mechanisms involved in generating a specific macrophage effector cell have not yet been entirely elucidated. Granger and Weiser (1966) found that alloimmunized animals possessed cytotoxic macrophages specific for the histocompatibility antigens of the immunizing cell, and that the specificity was determined by a cell-bound receptor structure with the characteristics of immunoglobulin. Evans and Alexander (1970) found immunologically specific cooperation between lymphocytes and macrophages. Evidence from this research group has indicated that a product of immune T lymphocytes specifically arms the macrophage (Evans and Alexander, 1972; Grant *et al.*, 1972). This product has been termed "specific macrophage arming factor" (SMAF), and these investigators consider it to be a lymphokine produced by a process similar to the other known lymphokines. Whether this SMAF is related to the rather controversial tumor-specific immunoglobulin product from the surface of sensitized T cells (Röllinghoff *et al.*, 1973) is not known at present. The major differences between activated and armed macrophages are the methods of generation and the specificity of the cytotoxic event (Krahenbuhl and Remington, 1974). Presumably the cytotoxic event itself is mediated by similar cellular events, no matter how the macrophage is activated.

The question remains as to the *in vivo* role of macrophages. The finding that the passive administration of activated macrophages can prolong survival in tumor-inoculated hosts (van Loveren and den Otter, 1974) supports the concept of the macrophage as a key element in the host defense against tumors. Furthermore, the recruitment of macrophages at a tumor site by preparations containing the injection migration inhibition factor has been shown to induce tumor rejection (Bernstein *et al.*, 1971), although other immunologically active materials besides MIF may have contributed to the tumor regression. The most impressive recent evidence of the role of the macrophage is the excellent correlation among the metastatic potential, immunogenicity, and macrophage content of rat tumors (Eccles and Alexander, 1974). Tumors with low content of macrophages were poorly immunogenic and highly metastatic, while tumors with a high proportion of macrophages at the primary tumor site were of greater immunogenicity and formed fewer metastases. Other work has linked activated or armed macrophages with the prevention of the metastatic spread of tumors (Proctor *et al.*, 1973; Fidler, 1974). Additionally, macrophages may remove tumor cell debris, thus decreasing the amount of tumor antigen able to enter the circulation and affect the function of the lymphocytes. Although macrophages can be observed in human tumors, and reactive histiocytes are seen in lymph nodes draining tumor sites, the techniques of cell-mediated immunity have yet to be thoroughly applied to the human macrophage. Of relevance is the observation that macrophage/monocyte types of cells, as well as lymphocytes, can be seen clustering around tumor cells in the pleural and ascites effusions of cancer patients (Sulitzeanu *et al.*, 1974). In summary, the macrophage has been conclusively shown to be an integral portion of the immune response to tumor antigens in animal model systems, and may have a key function in the inhibition of metastatic spread of the tumor. Similar observations are not yet available in human studies; however, it seems likely that many of the nonspecific modes of immunotherapy such as the administration of reticuloendothelial stimulants like BCG or *Corynebacterium parvum* owe some of their effectiveness to the activation of macrophages.

283

HOST
IMMUNE
RESPONSE TO
HUMAN
TUMOR
ANTIGENS

3.2.3. Cell–Cell Interactions

It is now recognized that different subpopulations of immunologically competent cells can act in synergistic or antagonistic fashions when present together. The study of any single population of cells may yield a result that is not comparable to the *in vivo* situation because it ignores the interactions of cell populations. For example, different populations of thymus-derived lymphocytes, obtained from different anatomical locations, can act synergistically in generating a graft-vs.-host reaction (Cantor and Asofsky, 1972) and the cooperation of T cells with B cells to produce a humoral response is well known. Little has been done to date on identifying interactions relevant to the response against tumors, and nothing is known about such interactions in the cancer patient. What interactions have been observed in animal studies in tumor systems have been primarily lymphocyte–macrophage interactions. Gershon *et al.* (1974) observed that T lymphocytes were necessary for tumor cells and isoantibody to suppress the appearance of macrophages able to bind tumor cells. Products of stimulated macrophages have been found to suppress the proliferative activity of lymphocytes (Nelson, 1973) and adherent cells from tumor-bearing animals can also suppress the response of lymphocytes to mitogens (Kirchner *et al.*, 1974).

On the other hand, the arming of macrophages by the products of T cells has already been discussed. The "reactivation" of lymphocytes immune to virally determined tumor antigens but unable to mediate a cytotoxic response was shown to depend on incubation *in vitro* in the presence of an adherent cell (Ortiz de Landazuri and Herberman, 1972). Thus both synergistic and antagonistic macrophage–lymphocyte interactions have been described in animal model systems. Presumably, many more such interactions among lymphocyte subpopulations, macrophage populations, and perhaps among nonlymphoid cells such as granulocytes will be discovered. It is impossible at present to discern which ones of these many possible interactions are relevant to the response against tumors, especially in humans.

3.3. Cell Interactions with Serum Factors

3.3.1. Blocking and Inhibition

No aspect of human tumor immunology has received so much attention as the interactions between serum factors and the cells mediating tumor-specific cytotoxicity. This is primarily due to the pioneering efforts of the Hellströms. The extensive literature on the blocking of cell-mediated immunity by serum factors has been reviewed in detail by them (Hellström and Hellström, 1974) and only the key features will be discussed here.

Their work has indicated that most cancer patients have lymphocytes that are cytotoxic for tumor cells of the same histopathological type as the tumor of the patient. The presence of cytotoxic lymphocytes seemed to be a relatively constant finding in a high proportion of patients except for those with extremely advanced disease, and, with that exception, was unrelated to the clinical status of the patient (Hellström et al., 1971a; Baldwin et al., 1973a). However, a strong correlation was found between the presence of "blocking factors" in the serum of patients and the clinical course. Patients who had progressive disease had a much higher incidence of serum factors that would abrogate cell-mediated cytotoxicity than did patients who were tumor free at the time of testing (Hellström et al., 1971a). The blocking activity could be removed by adsorption with tumor cells and was clearly a portion of the immunoglobulin fraction of the serum, and could thus be interpreted to represent tumor-specific antibody. However, the mechanism of blocking was not immediately apparent. Although it was possible that the tumor-specific antibodies were "masking" the antigenic determinants on the tumor cell and thereby protecting the target cell from recognition and destruction by the immune lymphoid cell, this did not explain the rapid disappearance of blocking activity in the serum of patients following resection of the tumor. It seemed nearly impossible that antibody production would cease following extirpation of a tumor.

Later findings by Sjögren et al. (1971, 1972) have suggested that blocking is due to antigen–antibody complexes rather than antibody alone. Baldwin et al. (1972) also demonstrated that the serum blocking factors are complexes and emphasized the importance of the ratio of antigen to antibody in the complexes. Since the reactive complexes can be removed by adsorption with tumor cells, the critical ratio is likely to be one of slight antibody excess. However, Thomson et al. (1973) found that rats with growing sarcomas circulated complexes with antigen in excess of antibody. Whether blocking complexes work by reacting with the lymphocyte receptor or by some masking event at the target cell level is difficult to determine, although the former seems to be more likely. At present, there is little or no evidence for blocking due to antibody alone.

A different form of blocking, termed "inhibition," has been described in which antibody apparently plays no part. This type of blocking is due to circulating tumor antigen, perhaps shed from the tumor cell membrane by metabolic turnover, which can interact with antigen-specific receptors on the membrane of the immune lymphocyte and render the cell noncytotoxic. This can be visualized as a form of cellular "desensitization" where the interaction of antigen and effector cell takes place at a site distant from the target tumor cell and the tumor cell is unaffected by the process. This form of blocking was first suggested experimentally by Brawn (1971) in allograft immunity. Solubilized antigen has been shown to inhibit cytotoxicity in the microcytotoxicity assay in rat hepatomas (Baldwin *et al.*, 1973*c*). In the previously discussed experiments of Sjögren and coworkers, inhibition could also be achieved with the low molecular weight (nonimmunoglobulin) fraction of the antigen–antibody complexes if that fraction was used to pretreat the effector cells. Plata and Levy (1974) were able to inhibit T-cell-mediated cytotoxicity against a syngeneic mouse tumor with soluble tumor antigens in the microcytotoxicity assay, although the same preparations did not inhibit cytotoxicity in the ^{51}Cr-release assay. However, conditions can be found that allow for the inhibition of alloimmune cytotoxicity by target cell membrane antigens in that assay (Bonavida, 1974) and discrepancies with that assay may be due to technical differences. Most relevant to the clinical situation is the finding by Currie and Basham (1972) of lymphocyte-bound tumor-associated antigens in cancer patients. When factors (presumably tumor antigen) were eluted from the surface of the lymphocytes, the effector cells displayed augmented cytotoxic activity against appropriate target cells. The augmented cytotoxicity could be abrogated by pretreating the lymphoid cells with tumor-bearing patient serum. These results are consistent with the hypothesis that circulating tumor antigens can inhibit the cytotoxic effects of immune effector cells. This concept has been cogently summarized by Alexander (1974).

At present, two modes of serum inhibition of specific antitumor immunity have been defined in man—blocking by antigen–antibody complexes and inhibition by tumor antigens. These are not the only means by which serum factors can inhibit cellular immunity. There is some evidence in animal models of "central inhibition" whereby the generation of effector cells is inhibited by antibody (Mitchell, 1972; Ortiz de Landazuri and Herberman, 1972). Antibody may also alter the membrane characteristics of the target cell, and thereby alter its reactivity with effector cells (Faanes *et al.*, 1973). Many other possibilities exist, including the immunoregulatory role of antibodies. Anti-idiotype antibodies and antilymphocyte receptor antibodies could modulate the activity of immune system in its interactions with tumor antigens. Rowley *et al.* (1973) have reviewed the implications of specific immunosuppression and regulation.

One final interaction with serum factors merits mention, although it is not a tumor-specific event. A host of studies have shown that serum from certain cancer patients can inhibit the response of normal lymphocytes to mitogens (e.g., Silk, 1967; Sample *et al.*, 1971; Brooks *et al.*, 1972). The factors responsible for such inhibition have not been completely characterized, but several possibilities exist. One is that some necessary nutrient has been exhausted from the serum by the tumor cells. Alternatively, some regulatory material, such as α-globulin, may be

285

HOST
IMMUNE
RESPONSE TO
HUMAN
TUMOR
ANTIGENS

elevated in cancer patients (Copperband *et al.*, 1968; Hsu and LoGerfo, 1972). Finally, some product of the tumor cell, such as tumor antigens or antigen–antibody complexes, may nonspecifically inhibit lymphocyte function. Preliminary evidence in melanoma patients has shown a good correlation between the presence of melanoma antigens in the serum and the degree of inhibition of mitogen-induced blastogenesis (Rangel, Gupta, Golub, and Morton, unpublished data). Although all these mechanisms are immunologically nonspecific, the end result would be identical to the specific inhibition of the efferent arm of the immune response. Both specific and nonspecific inhibitors may have important roles in preventing effector cells from functioning efficiently in combating tumor growth.

3.3.2. Serum Factors That Promote Cytotoxicity

Two types of serum effects that promote the cytotoxic activity of lymphoid effector cells have been described in humans. Hellström *et al.* (1971*b*) found that serum from patients who were disease free or ostensibly "cured" of their cancers seldom demonstrated blocking activity *in vitro*. Moreover, when serum samples from these tumor-free individuals were mixed with serum from patients with progressive disease that manifested blocking activity, the blocking of lymphocyte-mediated cytotoxicity was abrogated. This phenomenon was termed "unblocking." Bansal and Sjögren (1972) found that "unblocking" sera, when administered to mice with growing tumors, had an immunotherapeutic effect.

A number of possible mechanisms for unblocking can be envisioned, although definitive evidence on the mechanism is lacking. Since unblocking is clearly due to antibodies reactive with tumor-associated antigens, it may simply represent complement-dependent cytotoxic antibody. This is unlikely, although not impossible, in that the demonstration of unblocking does not require the addition of complement. A more likely mechanism, favored by the discoverers of the phenomenon, is that unblocking serum is antitumor antibodies that are not complexed with antigen. Such antibodies could saturate the available antigenic determinants in antigen–antibody complexes, and thus the complex would have no antigen exposed and reactive with the tumor-antigen-specific receptor on the immune lymphocyte. If this is the case, it would argue strongly against any significant blocking role for free (noncomplexed) antibody by masking antigenic sites on the tumor, as unblocking antibody should be able to mask even more efficiently than blocking complexes. The final hypothesis on mechanisms of unblocking is that it represents the antibody able to induce the reaction known as antibody-dependent cellular cytotoxicity, to be discussed below.

The second form of serum-promoted cytotoxicity has been termed "antibody-dependent cellular cytotoxicity" (ADCC). This phenomenon has also been described as "lymphocyte-dependent antibody" (LDA), "arming," "potentiation," "synergistic cytotoxicity," "B-cell cytotoxicity," and "K-cell cytotoxicity." The excessive nomenclature is characteristic of a new, exciting, and incompletely understood phenomenon. Much of our knowledge of ADCC is based on work in the laboratories of Perlmann and MacLennan, and both have written reviews 287

HOST
IMMUNE
RESPONSE TO
HUMAN
TUMOR
ANTIGENS
(MacLennan, 1972; Perlmann et al., 1972). Additional information is available
from the excellent review on the mechanisms of cytotoxicity by Cerottini and
Brunner (1974). Briefly summarized, the phenomenon consists of a cytotoxic
event mediated by a nonimmune effector cell in the presence of antibodies specific
for the target cell. Nonimmune cell-mediated cytotoxicity was first observed by
Möller (1965), but only in the last few years has the mechanism been at all
characterized. Antibody able to induce ADCC is of the IgG class, and must be
specific for the target cell (Larsson and Perlmann, 1972). The cell able to mediate
ADCC (the K or killer cell) has been difficult to identify with certainty, although
several characteristics are known. The K cell is not a thymus-derived lymphocyte
(van Boxel et al., 1972) and must have a receptor for the Fc portion of
immunoglobulin. The cytotoxic event is not complement dependent and not
phagocytic, although monocytes can mediate ADCC. It appears that there may be
several populations of K cells (Zighelboim et al., 1973), which is not surprising as
many non-T lymphoid cells have Fc receptors. It is not certain whether mature B
cells can mediate ADCC, and it has been suggested that the K cells are the "null"
cells lacking both T- and B-cell characteristics (Greenberg et al., 1973). It seems
probable that various types of K cells will be identified in different species.

The relevant point for tumor immunology is that there exists a population, or
populations, of cells that can mediate a cytotoxic event once armed by specific
antibody against the target cells. This K-cell population appears to be an
important effector cell in human tumor studies (see Section 3.2.1). Of particular
relevance is the finding of antibody and complement component C'3 complexed
to human tumor cells in vivo (Irie et al., 1974a), as K cells have been shown to bear
receptors for activated C'3 (Perlmann et al., 1969, 1972).

The search for the natural occurrence of antibodies able to mediate ADCC
specific for tumor cells has begun, and Pollack et al. (1972) found a small
proportion of immune sera to promote cytotoxicity in a syngeneic Moloney
sarcoma system. Parenteral administration of such sera resulted in the detection
of cytotoxic lymph node cells in treated mice (Pollack, 1973). ADCC may have
been responsible for the immunoprophylactic effectiveness of xenoantibodies
directed against a mouse leukemia (Zighelboim et al., 1974).

A few examples of ADCC have been described in human tumor systems.
Hellström et al. (1973b) found some sera that would promote cytotoxicity of
noncytotoxic normal lymphocytes ("arming") and cancer patient sera that would
augment the cytotoxicity of already reactive cancer patient lymphocytes ("potentiation"). No correlation between the appearance of antibodies that induce ADCC
and any clinical parameter was seen. Similarly, in the best-characterized ADCC
system in human tumors to date, the transitional cell carcinomas of the urinary
tract (Hakala and Lange, 1974; Hakala et al., 1974), the presence of antibody
capable of inducing ADCC was not correlated with prognosis. Actually, this may
not be surprising as the antibodies capable of promoting ADCC could be attached
to the K cells, and only in relatively rare circumstances would they be in an
appropriate concentration to be detected in the serum. Since the Fc receptor on

lymphoid cells is a relatively weak receptor, it is likely that many of the reactive K cells *in vivo* are charged with antigen–antibody complexes rather than free antibody. Complexes have been shown to induce ADCC (Greenberg and Shen, 1973) and the sera reactive against bladder carcinomas induce ADCC only when complexed with the target (Hakala *et al.*, 1974). Thus antigen–antibody complexes can mediate both blocking and ADCC—two events with entirely opposite results. Whether ADCC or blocking results from such complexes has been shown to be dependent on the immune serum concentration tested (Skurzak *et al.*, 1972). The immunotherapeutic use of sera able to induce ADCC can easily be visualized, but the potential of such sera to also induce tumor enhancement makes these antibodies a double-edged sword.

Thus ADCC helps draw together a number of observations from various experimental systems. For example, in carcinoma of the bladder in humans, much of the available data can be explained on the basis of ADCC. The greater efficiency of the microcytotoxicity assay in detecting non-T-cell-mediated reactions (Plata *et al.*, 1974) correlates with the non-T-cell characteristics of the effector cells found in this disease (O'Toole *et al.*, 1973*a*). The finding that only patients with known disease have cytotoxic lymphoid cells (O'Toole *et al.*, 1972*a*) can be interpreted as meaning that only patients circulating tumor antigen–antibody complexes can arm their lymphocytes with the appropriate complex, and such complexes can be shown *in vitro* to induce cytotoxicity (Hakala *et al.*, 1974). What remains to be determined is whether ADCC is truly responsible for tumor rejection *in vivo*.

4. Conclusions and Speculations

Figure 1 depicts ten of the various components of the immune response to tumor antigens that have been discussed. Each component has many subgroups (e.g., the different classes of immunoglobulins, the various ratios in immune complexes, all the different lymphokines). Therefore, the number of possible interactions of components of the immune response to tumor antigens is astronomical. Yet all the available evidence points to interactions of these components as crucial events in the host response. We cannot identify any single component as autonomous and preeminent in the control of neoplastic cells, and only a few of the many possible interactions have even been investigated. No single experimental approach, no single laboratory, and no single review can hope to discern more than a small portion of this extraordinarily complex series of events.

Much has been learned in human tumor immunology in the past several years, but important conflicts await resolution and vast areas remain unexplored. However, one problem stands out and should influence all studies done on the immunological relationship between the cancer patient and the disease: do any of the experimental findings have real relevance to the *in vivo* mechanisms, or are they epiphenomena? As one tumor immunologist phrased it, "Are we following armies or just flags?" Which assays are a mirror reflective of immunological events

289

HOST
IMMUNE
RESPONSE TO
HUMAN
TUMOR
ANTIGENS

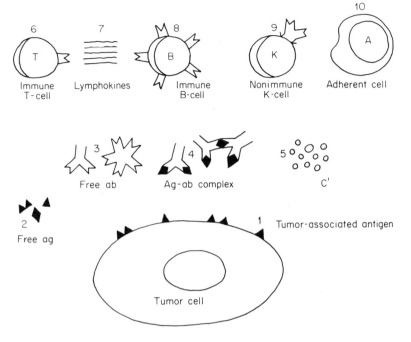

FIGURE 1. Ten of the different components of the immunological relationship of tumor and host.

in the host and which are coincidental? Such questions are extremely difficult to answer, but they emphasize the caution required in making the transition from observation of a phenomenon to understanding of a mechanism.

The wealth of available experimental data invites speculation, and a logical, if vastly oversimplified, sequence of events can be envisioned. Human tumors are immunogenic, and they elicit an immune response in the tumor-bearing host. This response can limit, and possibly terminate, the growth of a neoplasm. The most critical time is obviously early in the growth of the neoplasm, for if the tumor is not rejected then, it will become increasingly difficult for the immune system to cope with it. Early in the development of the tumor, the T-cell response is probably a key factor in determining the ultimate fate of the malignancy. A vigorous response by the thymus-derived lymphocytes will result in the elimination of the threat, while an insufficient response will allow for its continued development and perhaps even promote its growth. The macrophage response will augment the T-cell reaction, and limit the ability of the cancer to metastasize. In addition, the cytotoxic actions of specific antibodies are probably of greatest importance in the early phase of the growth of the tumor. Specific immune antibodies probably have an even more pronounced and longer-lasting role in the leukemias than in the solid tumors. This conclusion is based on the greater accessibility of the leukemic cells to humoral immunity, and the resistance of experimental leukemias to immunological enhancement.

Once a tumor has survived this onslaught of immune factors and is established and growing, a series of events takes place due to the progressive increase of circulating tumor antigen. Antigen, complexed with antibody, arms the K cells and provides a new line of defense. As more antigen enters the circulation, the proportion of antigen in the complexes increases. This results in less arming of K cells and increased inhibition of effector cells of various types. It is in this phase that most of the testing is done in cancer patients.

Finally, antigen circulating freely and not complexed with antibody results in all immunological defenses being severely impaired. The effector cells are "desensitized," antibodies are rendered ineffective, and the generation of new effector cells and antibodies diminishes. Concurrent with this specific immunosuppression is a general deterioration of the immune function. The tumor, now having escaped all immunological control, grows progressively until the host succumbs.

The relative importance of each of the components of the response and the times at which they are most critical can be expected to vary with each tumor–host system. The immunological characteristics of the tumor, such as its immunogenicity and its susceptibility to cell- or antibody-mediated lysis, will influence this sequence greatly. Nonimmunological characteristics of the tumor can also profoundly affect its relationship to the immune system. A tumor is not a static target for the immune system; it is a dynamic, growing entity. The growth rate of the tumor, its metastatic potential, its anatomical location, its invasiveness, the cohesiveness of the tumor cells, the fibrous tissue reaction surrounding the tumor, and many other factors will influence the course of the disease and the interaction of the tumor with the immune system.

The fact that immune reactions can be detected against tumors in hosts destined to die of the malignancy has been taken as evidence by some that the immune response is irrelevant to tumor growth. However, it must be remembered that the rejection of a neoplasm is not at all comparable to the rejection of an organ graft. With an allografted organ, rejection of enough of the vascular endothelium to cause ischemia will result in complete rejection. On the other hand, the immune system must reject every individual tumor cell in order to cure a cancer. Any cells that escape the immune defenses are an almost certain death sentence for the patient. We can assume that even the best therapeutic modalities seldom eliminate every tumor cell, yet a significant proportion of cancer patients are cured. With all the means of evasion of the immune system that the tumor has available, it is much more surprising that cancer is ever cured than it is surprising that it is a lethal disease.

As this chapter opened with a quotation from a rather light-hearted film, it is appropriate to close with a more serious cinema analogy. In Kurosawa's film classic "Rashomon," all the protagonists recall an event differently; the truth remains uncertain but must encompass all of their experiences. Human tumor immunology is in a similar state. Many different viewpoints are being used to study tumor immunology, and areas of conflict will necessarily arise. These will be resolved through the elucidation of basic mechanisms that can accommodate all of the varied and divergent evidence.

ACKNOWLEDGMENTS

291
HOST
IMMUNE
RESPONSE TO
HUMAN
TUMOR
ANTIGENS

The author is the recipient of a National Institutes of Health Career Development Award. Work performed in his laboratory was supported by USPHS Grants CA12582 and CA05252. The author thanks his colleagues in the UCLA Division of Oncology, Department of Surgery, for the many useful discussions and Ms. Susan Ponedel for assistance in preparation of the manuscript.

5. References

ALEXANDER, P., 1974, Escape from immune destruction by the host through shedding of surface antigens: Is this a characteristic shared by malignant and embryonic cells? *Cancer Res.* **34**:2077.

ALFORD, C., HOLLINSHEAD, A. C., AND HERBERMAN, R. B., 1973, Delayed cutaneous hypersensitivity reactions to extracts of malignant and normal breast cells, *Ann. Surg.* **178**:20.

ANDERSEN, V., BJERRUM, O., BENDIXEN, G., SCHIODT, T., AND DISSING, I., 1970, Effect of autologous mammary tumor extracts on human leukocyte migration *in vitro*, *Int. J. Cancer* **5**:357.

BACH, M. L., BACH, F. S., AND JOO, P., 1969, Leukemia-associated antigens in the mixed leukocyte culture test, *Science* **166**:1520.

BALDWIN, R. W., PRICE, M. R., AND ROBINS, R. A., 1972, Blocking of lymphocyte-mediated cytotoxicity for rat hepatoma cells by tumour specific antigen–antibody complexes, *Nature New Biol.* **238**:185.

BALDWIN, R. W., EMBLETON, M. J., JONES, J. S. P., AND LANGMAN, M. J. S., 1973a, Cell-mediated and humoral immune reactions to human tumors, *Int. J. Cancer* **12**:73.

BALDWIN, R. W., EMBLETON, M. J., AND PRICE, M. R., 1973b, Inhibition of lymphocyte cytotoxicity for human colon carcinoma by treatment with solubilized tumour membrane fractions, *Int. J. Cancer* **12**:84.

BALDWIN, R. W., PRICE, M. R., AND ROBINS, R. A., 1973c, Inhibition of hepatoma-immune lymph-node cells by tumor-bearer serum and solubilized hepatoma antigen, *Int. J. Cancer* **11**:527.

BANSAL, S. C., AND SJÖGREN, H. O., 1972, Counteraction of the blocking of cell-mediated tumor immunity by inoculation of unblocking sera and splenectomy: Immunotherapeutic effects on primary polyoma tumors in rats, *Int. J. Cancer* **9**:490.

BARTH, R. F., AND GILLESPIE, G. Y., 1974, The use of technetium-99m as a radioisotopic label to assess cell-mediated immunity *in vitro*, *Cell. Immunol.* **10**:38.

BEAN, M. A., PEES, H., ROSEN, G., AND OETGGEN, H. F., 1973, Prelabeling target cells with ^{3}H-proline as a method for studying lymphocyte cytotoxicity, *Natl. Cancer Inst. Monogr.* **37**:41.

BERNSTEIN, I. D., THOR, D. E., ZBAR, B., AND RAPP, H. J., 1971, Tumor immunity: Tumor suppression *in vivo* initiated by soluble products of specifically sensitized lymphocytes, *Science* **172**:729.

BLACK, M. M., SPEER, F. D., AND OPLER, S. R., 1956, Structural representations of tumor–host relationships in mammary carcinoma: Biologic and prognostic significance, *Am. J. Clin. Pathol.* **26**:250.

BLOOM, E. T., 1973, Microcytotoxicity tests on human cells in cultures: Effect of contamination with mycoplasma, *Proc. Soc. Exp. Biol. Med.* **143**:244.

BLOOM, E. T., FAHEY, J. L., PETERSON, I. A., GEERING, G., BERNHARD, M., AND TREMPE, G., 1973, Anti-tumor activity in human serum: Antibodies detecting blood-group-A-like antigen on the surface of tumor cells in culture, *Int. J. Cancer* **12**:21.

BLOOM, E. T., OSSORIO, R. C., AND BROSMAN, S. A., 1974, Cell-mediated cytotoxicity against human bladder cancer, *Int. J. Cancer* **14**:326.

BLUMING, A. Z., ZIEGLER, J. L., FASS, L., AND HERBERMAN, R. B., 1971, Delayed cutaneous sensitivity reactions to autologous Burkitt lymphoma protein extracts: Results of a prospective two and a half year study, *Clin. Exp. Immunol.* **9**:713.

BODDIE, A. W., JR., HOLMES, E. C., ROTH, J. A., AND MORTON, D. L., 1974, Inhibition of human leukocyte migration in agarose by KCl extracts of carcinoma of the lung, *Int. J. Cancer* **15**:823–829.

BODURTHA, A., CHEE, D., LAUCIUS, J. F., MASTRANGELO, M., AND PREHN, M., 1975, Clinical and immunological significance of human melanoma cytotoxic antibody, *Cancer Res.* **35**:189.

BONAVIDA, B., 1974, Studies on the induction and expression of T cell-mediated immunity. I. Blocking of cell-mediated cytolysis by membrane antigens, *J. Immunol.* **112**:926.

BORUM, K., AND JONSSON, N., 1972, Influence of neonatal thymectomy upon the cell-mediated tumor-specific immunity in Rous sarcoma virus tumorigenesis in rats, *Cell Immunol.* **3**:22.

BRAWN, R. J., 1971, *In vitro* desensitization of sensitized murine lymphocytes by a serum factor (soluble antigen?), *Proc. Natl. Acad. Sci. U.S.A.* **68**:1634.

BROOKS, W. H., NETSKY, M. G., NORMANSELL, D. E., AND HORWITZ, D. A., 1972, Depressed cell-mediated immunity in patients with primary intracranial tumors: Characterization of a humoral immunosuppressive factor, *J. Exp. Med.* **136**:1631.

BRUNNER, K. T., MAUEL, J., CERROTTINI, J. C., AND CHAPUIS, B., 1968, Quantitative assay of the lytic action of lymphoid cells on ^{51}Cr-labeled allogeneic target cells *in vitro*; inhibition by isoantibody and by drugs, *Immunology* **14**:181.

BUBENIK, J., PERLMANN, P., HELMSTEIN, K., AND MOBERGER, G., 1970, Cellular and humoral immune responses to human urinary bladder carcinomas, *Int. J. Cancer* **5**:310.

CANTOR, H., AND ASOFSKY, R., 1972, Synergy among lymphoid cells mediating the graft vs. host response. III. Evidence for interaction between two types of thymus-derived cells, *J. Exp. Med.* **135**:764.

CANTY, T. G., AND WUNDERLICH, J. R., 1970, Quantitative *in vitro* assay of cytotoxic cellular immunity, *J. Natl. Cancer Inst.* **45**:761.

CARREL, S., AND THEILKAES, L., 1973, Evidence for a tumor-associated antigen in human malignant melanoma, *Nature (London)* **242**:609.

CATALONO, L. W., HARTER, D. H., AND HSU, K. C., 1972, Common antigen in meningioma-derived cell cultures, *Science* **175**:180.

CEROTTINI, J. C., AND BRUNNER, K. T., 1974, Cell-mediated cytotoxicity, allograft rejection, and tumor immunity, *Adv. Immunol.* **18**:67.

CEROTTINI, J. C., NORDIN, A. A., AND BRUNNER, K. T., 1970, Specific *in vitro* cytotoxicity of thymus derived lymphocytes sensitized to allo-antigens, *Nature (London)* **228**:1308.

CHAR, D. H., LEPOURHIET, A., LEVENTHAL, B. G., AND HERBERMAN, R. B., 1973, Cutaneous delayed hypersensitivity responses to tumor-associated and other antigens in acute leukemia, *Int. J. Cancer* **12**:409.

CINADER, B., 1972, The future of tumor immunology, *Med. Clin. N. Am.* **56**:801.

COCHRAN, A. J., SPILG, W. G. S., MACKIE, R. M., AND THOMAS, C. E., 1972, Postoperative depression of tumour directed cell-mediated immunity in patients with malignant disease, *Br. Med. J.* **4**:67.

COCHRAN, A. J., MACKIE, R. M., THOMAS, C. E., GRANT, R. M., CAMERON-MOWAT, D. E., AND SPILG, W. G. S., 1973, Cellular immunity to breast carcinoma and malignant melanoma, *Br. J. Cancer* **28**:77.

COCHRAN, A. J., GRANT, R. M., SPILG, W. G., MACKIE, R. M., ROSS, C. E., HOYLE, D. E., AND RUSSELL, J. M., 1974, Sensitization to tumor-associated antigens in human breast carcinoma, *Int. J. Cancer* **14**:19.

COHEN, A. M., BURDICK, J. F., AND KETCHAM, A. S., 1971, Cell-mediated cytotoxicity: An assay using ^{125}I-iododeoxyuridine-labeled target cells, *J. Immunol.* **107**:895.

COHEN, A. M., KETCHAM, A. S., AND MORTON, D. L., 1973, Tumor-specific cellular cytotoxicity to human sarcomas: Evidence for a cell-mediated host immune response to a common sarcoma cell-surface antigen, *J. Natl. Cancer Inst.* **50**:585.

COOPERBAND, S. R., BONDEVIK, H., SCHMID, K., AND MANNIK, J. A., 1968, Transformation of human lymphocytes: Inhibition by homologous alpha globulin, *Science* **159**:1243.

CURRIE, G., AND BASHAM, C., 1972, Serum mediated inhibition of the immunological reactions of the patient to his own tumor: A possible role for circulating antigen. *Br. Med. J.* **26**:427.

DEODHAR, S. D., CRILE, G., AND ESSELSTYN, C. B., 1972, Study of the tumor cell–lymphocyte interaction in patients with breast cancer, *Cancer* **29**:1321.

DEVRIES, J. E., RÜMKE, P., AND BERNHEIM, J. L., 1972, Cytotoxic lymphocytes in melanoma patients, *Int. J. Cancer* **9**:567.

DEVRIES, J. E., CORNAIN, S., AND RÜMKE, P., 1974, Cytotoxicity of non-T versus T-lymphocytes from melanoma patients and healthy donors on short- and long-term cultured melanoma cells, *int. J. Cancer* **14**:427.

DEVRIES, J. E., MEYERLING, M., VAN DONGEN, A., AND RÜMKE, P., 1975, The effects of different isolation procedures and the use of target cells from melanoma cell lines and short term cultures on the non-specific cytotoxic effects of lymphocytes from healthy donors, submitted for publication.

ECCLES, S. A., AND ALEXANDER, P., 1974, Macrophage content of tumours in relation to metastatic spread and host immune reaction, *Nature (London)* **250**:667.

293

HOST
IMMUNE
RESPONSE TO
HUMAN
TUMOR
ANTIGENS

EILBER, F. R., AND MORTON, D. L., 1970a, Impaired immunologic reactivity and recurrence following cancer surgery, *Cancer* **25**:362.

EILBER, F. R., AND MORTON, D. L., 1970b, Sarcoma-specific antigens: Detection by complement fixation with serum from sarcoma patients, *J. Natl. Cancer Inst.* **44**:651.

ELLIOTT, P. C., THURLOW, B., NEEDHAM, P. R. G., AND LEWIS, M. G., 1973, The specificity of the cytoplasmic antigen in human malignant melanoma, *Eur. J. Cancer* **9**:607.

EVANS, R., AND ALEXANDER, P., 1970, Cooperation of immune lymphoid cells with macrophages in tumour immunity, *Nature (London)* **228**:620.

EVANS, R., AND ALEXANDER, P., 1972, Mechanism of immunologically specific killing of tumour cells by macrophages, *Nature (London)* **236**:168.

EVERSON, T. C., AND COLE, W. H., 1966, *Spontaneous Regression of Cancer*, Saunders, Philadelphia.

FAANES, R. B., CHOI, Y. S., AND GOOD, R. A., 1973, Escape from isoantiserum inhibition of lymphocyte-mediated cytotoxicity, *J. Exp. Med.* **137**:171.

FASS, L., HERBERMAN, R. B., AND ZIEGLER, J., 1970a, Delayed cutaneous hypersensitivity reactions to autologous Burkitt-lymphoma cells, *New Engl. J. Med.* **282**:776.

FASS, L., ZIEGLER, J. L., HERBERMAN, R. B., AND KIRYABWIRE, I. W. M., 1970b, Cutaneous hypersensitivity reactions to autologous extracts of malignant melanoma cells, *Lancet* **1**:116.

FELDMAN, J., 1972, Immunological enhancement: A study of blocking antibodies, *Adv. Immunol.* **15**:167.

FIDLER, I. J., 1974, Inhibition of pulmonary metastasis by intravenous injection of specifically activated macrophages, *Cancer Res.* **34**:1074.

FIELD, E. J., AND CASPARY, E. A., 1970, Lymphocyte sensitization: An *in vitro* test for cancer? *Lancet* **2**:1337.

FISHER, B., 1971, The present status of tumor immunology, *Adv. Surg.* **5**:189.

FISHER, B., SAFFER, E. A., AND FISHER, E. R., 1972, Studies concerning the regional lymph node in cancer. III. Response of regional lymph node cells from breast and colon cancer patients to PHA stimulation, *Cancer* **30**:1202.

FISHER, B., SAFFER, E. A., AND FISHER, E. R., 1974, Studies concerning the regional lymph node in cancer. VII. Thymidine uptake by cells from nodes of breast cancer patients relative to axillary location and histopathologic discriminants, *Cancer* **33**:271.

FOSSATI, G., COLNAGHI, M. I., DELLA PORTA, G., CASCINELLI, N., AND VERONESI, U., 1971, Cellular and humoral immunity against human malignant melanoma, *Int. J. Cancer* **8**:344.

FOSSATI, G., CANEVARI, S., DELLA PORTA, G., BALZARINI, G. P., AND VERONESI, U., 1972, Cellular immunity to human breast carcinoma, *Int. J. Cancer* **10**:391.

FRIDMAN, W. H., AND KOURILSKY, F. M., 1969, Stimulation of lymphocytes by autologous leukaemia cells in acute leukaemia, *Nature (London)* **224**:277.

GERSHON, R. K., MOKYR, M. B., AND MITCHELL, M. S., 1974, Activation of suppressor T cells by tumour cells and specific antibody, *Nature (London)* **250**:594.

GIRALDO, G., BETH, E., HIRSHAULT, Y., AOKI, T., OLD, L. J., BOYSE, E. A., AND CHOPRA, H. C., 1971, Human sarcomas in culture, *J. Exp. Med.* **133**:454.

GOLSTEIN, P., WIGZELL, H., BLOMGREN, H., AND SVEDMYR, E., 1972, Cells mediating specific *in vitro* cytotoxity. II. Probable autonomy of thymus-processed lymphocytes (T cells) for the killing of allogeneic target cells, *J. Exp. Med.* **135**:890.

GOLUB, S. H., AND MORTON, D. L., 1974, Sensitization of lymphocytes *in vitro* against human melanoma-associated antigens, *Nature (London)* **251**:161.

GOLUB, S. H., SVEDMYR, E. A. J., HEWETSON, J. F., KLEIN, G., AND SINGH, S., 1972, Cellular reactions against Burkitt lymphoma cells. III. Effector cell activity of leukocytes stimulated *in vitro* with autochthonous cultured lymphoma cells, *Int. J. Cancer* **10**:157.

GOLUB, S. H., HEWETSON, J. F., SVEDMYR, E. A. J., KLEIN, G., AND SINGH, S., 1973, Stimulation of lymphocytes *in vitro* to reactions against cultured Burkitt's lymphoma cells, *Natl. Cancer Inst. Monogr.* **37**:25.

GOLUB, S. H., O'CONNELL, T. X., AND MORTON, D. L., 1974, Correlation of *in vivo* and *in vitro* assays of immunocompetence in cancer patients, *Cancer Res.* **34**:1833.

GOLUB, S. H., HANSON, D. C., MORTON, D. L., PELLEGRINO, M., AND FERRONE, S., 1975, Comparison of histocompatability antigens on cultured human tumor cells and fibroblasts by sensitivity to cell-mediated cytotoxicity and quantitative antibody absorption, in press. *J. Natl. Cancer Inst.*, 1975.

GORCZYNSKI, R. M., 1974, Immunity to murine sarcoma virus-induced tumors. I. Specific T lymphocytes active in macrophage migration inhibition and lymphocyte transformation, *J. Immunol.* **112**:1815.

GORER, P. A., 1956, Some recent work on tumor immunity, *Adv. Cancer Res.* **4:**149.

GRANGER, G. A., AND WEISER, R. S., 1966, Homograft target cells: Contact destruction *in vitro* by immune macrophages, *Science* **151:**97.

GRANT, C. K., CURRIE, G. A., AND ALEXANDER, P., 1972, Thymocytes from mice immunized against an allograft render bone-marrow cells specifically cytotoxic, *J. Exp. Med.* **135:**150.

GRANT, C. K., EVANS, R., AND ALEXANDER, P., 1973, Multiple effector roles of lymphocytes in allograft immunity, *Cell. Immunol.* **8:**136.

GREEN, S. S., AND SELL, K. W., 1970, Mixed leukocyte stimulation of normal peripheral leukocytes by autologous lymphoblastoid cells, *Science* **170:**989.

GREENBERG, A. H., AND SHEN, L., 1973, A class of specific cytotoxic cells demonstrated *in vitro* by arming with antigen–antibody complexes, *Nature New Biol.* **245:**282.

GREENBERG, A. H., HUDSON, L., SHEN, L., AND ROITT, I. M., 1973, Antibody-dependent cell-mediated cytotoxicity due to a "null" lymphoid cell, *Nature New Biol.* **242:**111.

GUPTA, R. K., AND MORTON, D. L., 1975, Suggestive evidence for *in vivo* binding of specific antitumor antibodies of human melanoma, *Cancer Res.* **35:**58.

GUTTERMAN, J. U., HERSH, E. M., MCCREDIE, K. B., BODEY, G. P., RODRIQUEZ, V., AND FREIREICH, E. J., 1972*a*, Lymphocyte blastogenesis to human leukemia cells and their relationship to serum factors, immunocompetence and prognosis, *Cancer Res.* **32:**2524.

GUTTERMAN, J. U., MAVLIGIT, G., MCCREDIE, K. B., BODEY, G. P., FREIREICH, E. J., AND HERSH, E. M., 1972*b*, Antigen solubilized from human leukemia: Lymphocyte stimulation, *Science* **177:**1114.

GUTTERMAN, J. U., HERSH, E. M., FREIREICH, E. J., ROSSEN, R. D., BUTLER, W. T., MCCREDIE, K. B., BODEY, G. P., RODRIQUEZ, V., AND MAVLIGIT, G. U., 1973*a*, Cell-mediated and humoral immune response to acute leukemia cells and soluble leukemia antigen—Relationship to immunocompetence and prognosis, *Natl. Cancer Inst. Mongr.* **37:**153.

GUTTERMAN, J. U., ROSSEN, R. D., BUTLER, W. T., MCCREDIE, K. B., BODEY, G. P., FREIREICH, E. J., AND HERSH, E. M., 1973*b*, Immunoglobulin on tumor cells and tumor-induced lymphocyte blastogenesis in human acute leukemia, *New Engl. J. Med.* **288:**169.

GUTTERMAN, J. U., MAVLIGIT, G., BURGESS, M. A., MCCREDIE, K. B., HUNTER, C., FREIREICH, E. J., AND HERSH, E. M., 1974*a*, Immunodiagnosis of acute leukemia: Detection of residual disease, *J. Natl. Cancer Inst.* **53:**389.

GUTTERMAN, J. U., MAVLIGIT, G., MCCREDIE, K. B., FREIREICH, E. J., AND HERSH, E. M., 1974*b*, Auto-immunization with acute leukemia cells: Demonstration of increased lymphocyte responsiveness, *Int. J. Cancer* **11:**521.

HAKALA, T. R., AND LANGE, P. H., 1974, Serum induced lymphoid cell mediated cytotoxicity to human transitional cell carcinomas of the genitourinary tract, *Science* **184:**795.

HAKALA, T. R., LANGE, P. H., CASTRO, A. E., ELLIOTT, A. Y., AND FRALEY, E. E., 1974, Antibody induction of lymphocyte-mediated cytotoxicity against human transitional-cell carcinomas of the urinary tract, *New Engl. J. Med.* **291:**637.

HALLIDAY, W. J., MALUISH, A., AND MILLER, S., 1974, Blocking and unblocking of cell-mediated anti-tumor immunity in mice, as detected by the leukocyte adherence inhibition test, *Cell. Immunol.* **10:**467.

HAMBURGER, R. N., PIOUS, D. A., AND MILLES, S. E., 1963, Antigenic specificities acquired from the growth medium by cells in tissue culture, *Immunology* **6:**439.

HAN, T., MOORE, G. E., AND SOKAL, J. E., 1971, *In vitro* lymphocyte response to autologous cultured lymphoid cells, *Proc. Soc. Exp. Biol. Med.* **36:**976.

HATTLER, B. G., AND SOEHNLEN, B., 1974, Inhibition of tumor-induced lymphocyte blastogenesis by a factor or factors associated with peripheral lymphocytes, *Science* **184:**1374.

HELLSTRÖM, I., 1967, A colony inhibition (CI) technique for demonstration of tumor cell destruction by lymphoid cells *in vitro*, *Int. J. Cancer* **2:**65.

HELLSTRÖM, I., HELLSTRÖM, K. E., AND PIERCE, G. E., 1968*a*, Cellular and humoral immunity to different types of human neoplasms, *Nature (London)* **220:**1352.

HELLSTRÖM, I. E., HELLSTRÖM, K. E., PIERCE, G. E., AND BILL, A. H., 1968*b*, Demonstration of cell-bound and humoral immunity against neuroblastoma cells, *Proc. Natl. Acad. Sci. U.S.A.* **60:**1231.

HELLSTRÖM, I., HELLSTRÖM, K. E., SJÖGREN, H. O., AND WARNER, G. A., 1971*a*, Demonstration of cell-mediated immunity to human neoplasms of various histological types, *Int. J. Cancer* **7:**1.

HELLSTRÖM, I., HELLSTRÖM, K. E., SJÖGREN, H. O., AND WARNER, G. A., 1971*b*, Serum factors in tumor-free patients cancelling the blocking of cell-mediated tumor immunity, *Int. J. Cancer* **8:**185.

HELLSTRÖM, I., SJÖGREN, H. O., WARNER, G. A., AND HELLSTRÖM, K. E., 1971*c*, Blocking of cell-mediated tumor immunity by sera from patients with growing neoplasms, *Int. J. Cancer* **7:**226.

HELLSTRÖM, I., HELLSTRÖM, K. E., SJÖGREN, H. O., AND WARNER, G. A., 1973a, Destruction of cultivated melanoma cells by lymphocytes from healthy Black (North American Negro) donors, *Int. J. Cancer* **11**:116.

HELLSTRÖM, I., HELLSTRÖM, K. E., AND WARNER, G. A., 1973b, Increase of lymphocyte-mediated tumor-cell destruction by certain patient sera, *Int. J. Cancer* **12**:348.

HELLSTRÖM, I., WARNER, G. A., HELLSTRÖM, K. E., AND SJÖGREN, H. O., 1973c, Sequential studies on cell-mediated tumor immunity and blocking serum activity in ten patients with malignant melanoma, *Int. J. Cancer* **11**:280.

HELLSTRÖM, K. E., AND HELLSTRÖM, I., 1974, Lymphocyte-mediated cytotoxicity and blocking serum activity to tumor antigens, *Adv. Immunol.* **18**:209.

HENLE, G., HENLE, W., KLEIN, G., GUNVEN, P., CLIFFORD, P., MORROW, P. H., AND ZIEGLER, J. L., 1971, Antibodies to early EBV-induced antigens in Burkitt's lymphoma, *J. Natl. Cancer Inst.* **46**:861.

HEPPNER, G. H., STOLBACH, L., BYRNE, M., CUMMINGS, F. J., MCDONOUGH, E., AND CALABRESI, E., 1973, Cell-mediated reactivity to tumor antigens in patients with malignant melanoma, *Int. J. Cancer* **11**:245.

HERBERMAN, R. B., 1969, Studies on the specificity of human cytotoxic antibody reactive with cultures of lymphoid cells, *J. Natl. Cancer Inst.* **42**:69.

HERBERMAN, R. B., MCCOY, J. L., AND LEVINE, P. H., 1974, Immunological reactions to tumor-associated antigens in Burkitt's lymphoma and other lymphomas, *Cancer Res.* **34**:1222.

HERSH, E. M., WHITECAR, J. P., MCCREDIE, K. B., BODEY, G. P., AND FREIREICH, E. J., 1971, Chemotherapy, immunocompetence, immunosuppression, and prognosis in acute leukemia, *New Engl. J. Med.* **285**:1211.

HEWETSON, J. F., GOLUB, S. H., KLEIN, G., AND SINGH, S., 1972, Cellular reactions against Burkitt lymphoma cells. I. Colony inhibition with effector cells from patients with Burkitt's lymphoma, *Int. J. Cancer* **10**:142.

HIBBS, J. B., 1973, Macrophage nonimmunological recognition: Target cell factors related to contact inhibition, *Science* **180**:868.

HIBBS, J. B., LAMBERT, L. H., AND REMINGTON, J. S., 1972a, Control of carcinogenesis: A possible role for the activated macrophage, *Science* **177**:998.

HIBBS, J. B., LAMBERT, L. H., AND REMINGTON, J. S., 1972b, Possible role of macrophage mediated nonspecific cytotoxicity in tumour resistance, *Nature New Biol.* **235**:48.

HILBERG, R. W., BALCERZAK, S. P., AND LoBUGLIO, A. F., 1973, A migration inhibition factor assay for tumor immunity in man, *Cell. Immunol.* **7**:152.

HIRSHAULT, Y., PEI, D. T., MARCOVE, R. C., MUKHERJI, B., SPIELVOGEL, A. R., AND ESSNER, E., 1974, Seroepidemiology of human sarcoma antigen (S1), *New Engl. J. Med.* **291**:1103.

HOLLINSHEAD, A., GLEW, D., BUNNAG, B., GOLD, P., AND HERBERMAN, R., 1970, Skin reactive soluble antigen from intestinal cancer cell membranes and relationship to carcinoembryonic antigens, *Lancet* **1**:1191.

HOLLINSHEAD, A. C., STEWART, T. H. M., AND HERBERMAN, R. B., 1974, Delayed-hypersensitivity reactions to soluble membrane extracts of human malignant lung cells, *J. Natl. Cancer Inst.* **52**:327.

HSU, C. C., AND LoGERFO, P., 1972, Correlation between serum alpha-globulin and plasma inhibitory effect of PHA-stimulated lymphocytes in colon carcinoma patients, *Proc. Soc. Exp. Biol. Med.* **139**:575.

HUDSON, M. J. K., HUMPHREY, L. J., MANTZ, F. A., AND MORSE, P. A., 1974, Correlation of circulating serum antibody to the histologic findings in breast cancer, *Am. J. Surg.* **128**:756.

HUGHES, L. E., AND LYTTON, B., 1964, Antigenic properties of human tumors: Delayed cutaneous hypersensitivity reactions, *Br. Med. J.* **1**:209.

HUMPHREY, L. J., BARKER, C., BOKESCH, C., FETTER, D., AMERSON, J. R., AND BOEHM, O. R., 1971, Immunologic competence of regional lymph nodes in patients with mammary cancer, *Ann. Surg.* **174**:383.

IKONOPISOV, R. L., LEWIS, M. G., HUNTER-CRAIG, I. D., BODENHAM, D. C., PHILLIPS, T. M., COOLING, C. I., PROCTOR, J., FAIRLEY, G. H., AND ALEXANDER, P., 1970, Autoimmunization with irradiated tumour cells in human malignant melanoma, *Br. Med. J.* **2**:752.

IRIE, K., IRIE, R. F., AND MORTON, D. L., 1974a, Evidence for *in vivo* reaction of antibody and complement to surface antigens of human cancer cells, *Science* **186**:454.

IRIE, R. F., 1974, Exclusion of heterologous membrane antigen in immunologic studies of cultured human cancer cells, *Proc. Am. Assoc. Cancer Res.*, p. 87.

IRIE, R. F., IRIE, K., AND MORTON, D. L., 1974b, Natural antibody in human serum to a neoantigen in human cultured cells grown in fetal bovine serum, *J. Natl. Cancer Inst.* **52**:1051.

295

HOST
IMMUNE
RESPONSE TO
HUMAN
TUMOR
ANTIGENS

JAGARLAMOODY, S. M., AUST, J. C., TEW, R. H., AND MCKHANN, C. F., 1971, *In vitro* detection of cytotoxic cellular immunity against tumor-specific antigens by a radioisotopic technique, *Proc. Natl. Acad. Sci. U.S.A.* **68**:1346.

JUNGE, U., HOEKSTRA, J., AND DEINHARDT, F., 1971, Stimulation of peripheral lymphocytes by allogeneic and autochthonous mononucleosis cell lines, *J. Immunol.* **106**:1306.

KANNER, S. P., MARDINEY, M. R., JR., AND MANGI, R. J., 1970, Experience with a mixed lymphocyte–tumor reaction as a method of detecting antigenic differences between normal and neoplastic cells, *J. Immunol.* **106**:1052.

KELLER, R., 1973, Cytostatic elimination of syngeneic rat tumor cells *in vitro* by nonspecifically activated macrophages, *J. Exp. Med.* **138**:625.

KIRCHNER, H., CHUSED, T. M., HERBERMAN, R. B., HOLDEN, H. T., AND LAVRIN, D. H., 1974, Evidence of suppressor cell activity in spleens of mice bearing primary tumors induced by Moloney sarcoma virus, *J. Exp. Med.* **138**:1473.

KLEIN, G., 1971, Immunological aspects of Burkitt's lymphoma, *Adv. Immunol.* **14**:187.

KLEIN, G., CLIFFORD, P., KLEIN, E., SMITH, R. T., MINOWADA, J., KOURILSKY, F., AND BURCHENAL, J., 1967, Membrane immunofluorescence reactions of Burkitt lymphoma cells from biopsy specimens and tissue cultures, *J. Natl. Cancer Inst.* **39**:1027.

KLEIN, G., PEARSON, G., NADKARNI, J. S., NADKARNI, J. J., KLEIN, E., HENLE, G., HENLE, W., AND CLIFFORD, P., 1968, Relation between Epstein–Barr viral and cell membrane immunofluorescence of Burkitt tumor cells. I. Dependence of cell membrane immunofluorescence on presence of EB virus, *J. Exp. Med.* **128**:1011.

KLEIN, G., CLIFFORD, P., HENLE, G., HENLE, W., OLD, L. J., AND GEERING, G., 1969, EBV-associated serological patterns in a Burkitt lymphoma patient during regression and recurrence, *Int. J. Cancer* **4**:416.

KNIGHT, S. C., MOORE, G. E., AND CLARKSON, B. D., 1971, Stimulation of autochthonous lymphocytes by cells from normal and leukaemia lines, *Nature New Biol.* **229**:185.

KRAHENBUHL, J. L., AND REMINGTON, J. S., 1974, The role of activated macrophages in specific and nonspecific cytostasis of tumor cells, *J. Immunol.* **113**:507.

KRONMAN, B. S., WEPSIC, H. T., CHURCHILL, W. H., ZBAR, B., BORSOS, T., AND RAPP, H. J., 1969, Tumor-specific antigens detected by inhibition of macrophage migration *Science* **165**:296.

KUMAR, S., TAYLOR, G., STEWARD, J. K., WAGHE, M. A., AND MORRIS-JONES, P., 1973, Cell-mediated immunity and blocking factors in patients with tumors of the central nervous system, *Int. J. Cancer* **12**:194.

LAMON, E. W., WIGZELL, H., ANDERSON, B., AND KLEIN, E., 1973*a*, Anti-tumour activity *in vitro* dependent on immune B lymphocytes, *Nature New Biol.* **224**:209.

LAMON, E. W., WIGZELL, H., KLEIN, E., ANDERSSON, B., AND SKURZAK, H. M., 1973*b*, The lymphocyte response to primary Moloney sarcoma virus tumors in BALB/c mice: Definition of the active subpopulations at different times after infection, *J. Exp. Med.* **137**:1472.

LARSSON, A., AND PERLMANN, P., 1972, Study of Fab and F(ab')2 from rabbit IgG for capacity to induce lymphocyte mediated target cell destruction *in vitro*, *Int. Arch. Allergy* **43**:80.

LECLERC, J. C., GOMARD, E., PLATA, F., AND LEVY, J. P., 1973, Cell-mediated immune reaction against tumors induced by oncornaviruses. II. Nature of the effector cells in tumor cell cytolysis, *Int. J. Cancer* **11**:426.

LENEVA, N. V., AND SVET-MOLDAVSKY, G. J., 1974, Susceptibility of tumor cells in different phases of the mitotic cycle to the effect of immune lymphocytes, *J. Natl. Cancer Inst.* **52**:699.

LEVY, N. L., MAHALEY, M. S., AND DAY, E. D., 1972, *In vitro* demonstration of cell-mediated immunity to human brain tumors, *Cancer Res.* **32**:477.

LEWIS, M. G., AND PHILLIPS, T. M., 1972, The specificity of surface membrane immunofluorescence in human malignant melanoma, *Int. J. Cancer* **10**:105.

LEWIS, M. G., IKONOPISOV, R. L., NAIRN, R. C., PHILLIPS, T. M., FAIRLEY, G. H., BODENHAM, D. C., AND ALEXANDER, P., 1969, Tumour-specific antibodies in human malignant melanoma and their relationship to the extent of disease, *Br. Med. J.* **3**:547.

LEWIS, M. G., PHILLIPS, T. M., COOK, K. B., AND BLAKE, J., 1971, Possible explanation for loss of detectable antibody in patients with disseminated malignant melanoma, *Nature (London)* **232**:52.

MACLENNAN, I. C. M., 1972, Antibody in the induction and inhibition of lymphocyte cytotoxicity, *Transplant. Rev.* **13**:67.

MACPHERSON, B. R., AND PILCH, Y. P., 1972, Cellular cytolysis *in vitro*: Mechanisms underlying a quantitative assay for cellular immunity, *J. Natl. Cancer Inst.* **48**:1619.

MATTHEWS, R. S., AND SHIRODARIA, P. V., 1973, Study of regressing warts by immunofluorescence, *Lancet* **1:**689.

MAVLIGIT, G. M., AMBUS, U., GUTTERMAN, J. U., HERSH, E. M., AND MCBRIDE, C. M., 1973, Antigen solubilized from human solid tumors: Lymphocyte stimulation and cutaneous delayed hypersensitivity, *Nature New Biol.* **243:**188.

MCKHANN, C. F., AND JAGARLAMOODY, S. M., 1971, Immune reactivity against neoplasms, *Transplant. Rev.* **7:**55.

MING, S. C., KLEIN, E., AND KLEIN, G., 1966, Inhibitory effect of lymphocytes on DNA synthesis of target cells *in vitro*, *Ann. Med. Exp. Fenn.* **44:**191.

MITCHELL, M., 1972, Central inhibitions of cellular immunity to leukemia L1210 by isoantibody, *Cancer Res.* **32:**825.

MÖLLER, E., 1965, Contact induced cytotoxicity by lymphoid cells containing foreign isoantigens, *Science* **147:**873.

MORTON, D. L., MALMGREN, R. A., HOLMES, E. C., AND KETCHAM, A. S., 1968, Demonstration of antibodies against human malignant melanoma by immunofluorescence, *Surgery* **64:**233.

MORTON, D. L., EILBER, F. R., JOSEPH, W. L., WOOD, W. C., TRAHAN, E., AND KETCHAM, A. S., 1970, Immunological factors in human sarcoma and melanomas: A rational basis for immunotherapy, *Ann. Surg.* **172:**740.

MORTON, D. L., EILBER, F. R., AND MALMGREN, R. A., 1971, Immune factors in human cancer: Malignant melanomas, skeletal and soft tissue sarcomas, *Prog. Exp. Tumor Res.* **14:**25.

MUNA, W. M., MARCUS, S., AND SMART, C., 1969, Detection by immunofluorescence of antibodies specific for human malignant melanoma cells, *Cancer* **23:**88.

NAGEL, G. A., PIESSENS, W. F., STILMONT, M. M., AND LEJEUNE, F., 1971, Evidence for tumor specific immunity in human malignant melanoma, *Eur. J. Cancer* **7:**41.

NAIRN, R. C., NIND, A. P., GULI, E. P., DAVIES, D. J., LITTLE, J. H., DAVIS, N. C., AND WHITEHEAD, R. H., 1972, Anti-tumor immunoreactivity in patients with malignant melanoma, *Med. J. Aust.* **1:**397.

NELSON, D. S., 1973, Production by stimulated macrophages of factors depressing lymphocyte transformation, *Nature (London)* **246:**306.

OLDHAM, R. K., AND HERBERMAN, R. B., 1973, Evaluation of cell-mediated cytotoxic reactivity against tumor associated antigens with ^{125}I-iododeoxyuridine labeled target cells, *J. Immunol.* **111:**1862.

OREN, R. K., AND HERBERMAN, R. B., 1971, Delayed cutaneous hypersensitivity reactions to membrane extracts of human tumor cells, *Clin. Exp. Immunol.* **9:**45.

ORTIZ DE LANDAZURI, M., AND HERBERMAN, R. B., 1972, *In vitro* activation of cellular immune response to Gross virus-induced lymphoma, *J. Exp. Med.* **136:**969.

O'TOOLE, C., PERLMANN, P., UNSGAARD, B., MOBERGER, G., AND EDSMYR, F., 1972a, Cellular immunity to human urinary bladder carcinoma. I. Correlation to clinical stage and radiotherapy, *Int. J. Cancer* **10:**77.

O'TOOLE, C., PERLMAN, P., UNSGAARD, B., ALMGARD, L. E., JOHANSSON, B., MOBERGER, G., AND EDSMYR, F., 1972b, Cellular immunity to human urinary bladder carcinoma. II. Effect of surgery and preoperative irradiation, *Int. J. Cancer* **10:**92.

O'TOOLE, C., PERLMANN, P., WIGZELL, H., UNSGAARD, B., AND ZETTERLUND, C. G., 1973a, Lymphocyte cytotoxicity in bladder carcinoma: No requirement for thymus derived effector cells, *Lancet* **1:**1085.

O'TOOLE, C., UNSGAARD, B., ALMGARD, L. E., AND JOHANSSON, B., 1973b, The cellular immune response to carcinoma of the urinary bladder: Correlation to clinical stage and treatment, *Br. J. Cancer* **28:**266.

O'TOOLE, C., STEJSKAL, V., PERLMANN, P., AND KARLSSON, M., 1974, Lymphoid cells mediating tumor–specific cytotoxicity to carcinoma of the urinary bladder: Separation of the effector population using a surface marker, *J. Exp. Med.* **139:**437.

PATTENGALE, P. K., SMITH, R. W., AND PERLIN, E., 1974, Atypical lymphocytes in acute infectious mononucleosis: Identification by multiple T and B lymphocyte markers, *New Engl. J. Med.* **291:**1145.

PERLMANN, P., PERLMANN, H., MÜLLER-EBERHARD, H. J., AND MANNI, J. A., 1969, Cytotoxic effects of leukocytes triggered by complement bound to target cells, *Science* **163:**937.

PERLMANN, P., PERLMANN, H., AND WIGZELL, H., 1972, Lymphocyte mediated cytotoxicity *in vitro*: Induction and inhibition by humoral antibody and nature of effector cells, *Transplant. Rev.* **13:**91.

PHILLIPS, T. M., AND LEWIS, M. G., 1971, A method for elution of immunoglobulin from the surface of living cells, *Rev. Eur. Etud. Clin. Biol.* **16:**1051.

297

HOST
IMMUNE
RESPONSE TO
HUMAN
TUMOR
ANTIGENS

PILCH, Y. H., MYERS, G. H., SPARKS, F. S., AND GOLUB, S. H., 1975a, Prospects for the immunotherapy of cancer. I. Basic concepts of tumor immunology, *Curr. Prob. Surg.*, **1975**:1–46.

PILCH, Y. H., MYERS, G. H., SPARKS, F. S., AND GOLUB, S. H., 1975b, Prospects for the immunotherapy of cancer. II. Current status of immunotherapy, *Curr. Prob. Surg.*, **1975**:1–61.

PLATA, F., AND LEVY, J. P., 1974, Blocking of syngeneic effector T cells by soluble tumour antigens, *Nature (London)* **249**:271.

PLATA, F., GOMARD, E., LECLERC, J. C., AND LEVY, J. P., 1974, Comparative *in vitro* studies on effector cell diversity in the cellular immune response to murine sarcoma virus (MSV)- induced tumors in mice, *J. Immunol.* **112**:1477.

POLLACK, S., 1973, Specific "arming" of normal lymph-node cells by sera from tumor-bearing mice, *Int. J. Cancer* **11**:138.

POLLACK, S., HEPPNER, G., BRAWN, R. J., AND NELSON, K., 1972, Specific killing of tumor cells *in vitro* in the presence of normal lymphoid cells and sera from hosts immune to the tumor antigens, *Int. J. Cancer* **9**:316.

POWLES, R. L., BALCHIN, L. A., FAIRLEY, G. H., AND ALEXANDER, P., 1971, Recognition of leukemic cells as foreign before and after auto-immunization, *Br. Med. J.* **1**:486.

PREHN, R. T., 1972, The immune reaction as a stimulator of tumor growth, *Science* **176**:170.

PROCTOR, J. W., RUDENSTAM, C. M., AND ALEXANDER, P., 1973, A factor preventing the development of lung metastases in rats with sarcomas, *Nature (London)* **242**:29.

RICH, J. R., AND WINTERS, W. D., 1974, Tumor-associated antigen in human meningioma, *New Engl. J. Med.* **290**:164.

RICHMOND, R. E., AND MORTON, D. L., 1974, A hamster cheek pouch assay of human cell-mediated immunity to human melanoma xenografts, *J. Reticuloendothel. Soc.* **16**:8a.

RICHTERS, A., AND SHERWIN, R. P., 1974, Human breast cancer and the autochthonous lymph node cell responses: A tissue culture and ultrastructural study, *Cancer* **34**:328.

RICHTERS, A., SHERWIN, R. P., AND RICHTERS, V., 1971, The lymphocyte and human lung cancers, *Cancer Res.* **31**:214.

RÖLLINGHOFF, M., WAGNER, H., CONE, R. E., MARCHALONIS, J. J., 1973, Release of antigen-specific immunoglobulin from cytotoxic effector cells and syngeneic tumour immunity *in vitro*, *Nature New Biol.* **243**:21.

ROMSDAHL, M. M., AND COX, I. S., 1970, Human malignant melanoma antibodies demonstrated by immunofluorescence, *Arch. Surg.* **100**:491.

ROSENAU, W., AND MOON, H. D., 1961, Lysis of homologous cells by sensitized lymphocytes in tissue culture, *J. Natl. Cancer Inst.* **27**:471.

ROSENBERG, E. B., HERBERMAN, R. B., LEVINE, P. H., HALTERMAN, R. H., MCCOY, J. L., AND WUNDERLICH, J. R., 1972, Lymphocyte cytotoxicity reactions to leukemia associated antigens in identical twins, *Int. J. Cancer* **9**:648.

ROSENBERG, E. B., MCCOY, J. L., GREEN, S. S., DONNELLY, F. C., SIWARSKI, D. F., LEVINE, P. H., AND HERBERMAN, R. B., 1974, Destruction of human lymphoid tissue-culture cell lines by human peripheral blood lymphocytes in ^{51}Cr-release cellular cytotoxicity assays, *J. Natl. Cancer Inst.* **52**:345.

ROTH, J. A., GOLUB, S. H., GRIMM, E. A., EILBER, F. R., AND MORTON, D. L., 1974, Effect of surgery on *in vitro* lymphocyte function, *Surg. Forum* **25**:102.

ROTH, J. A., GOLUB, S. H., HOLMES, E. C., AND MORTON, D. L., 1975, Effect of BCG on the stimulation of lymphocyte protein synthesis by melanoma antigens, *Surgery* (in press).

ROUSE, B. T., RÖLLINGHOFF, M., AND WARNER, N. L., 1972, Anti-θ serum induced suppression of the cellular transfer of tumour specific immunity to a syngeneic plasma cell tumour, *Nature New Biol.* **238**:116.

ROWLEY, D. A., FITCH, F. W., STUART, F. P., KOHLER, H., AND COSENZA, H., 1973, Specific suppression of immune responses, *Science* **181**:1133.

SAMPLE, W. F., GERTNER, H. R., AND CHRETIEN, P. B., 1971, Inhibition of phytohemagglutinin-induced *in vitro* lymphocyte transformation by serum from patients with carcinoma, *J. Natl. Cancer Inst.* **46**:1291.

SANTOS, G. W., MULLINS, G. S., BIAS, W. B., ANDERSON, P. N., GRAZZIANO, K. D., KLEIN, D. L., AND BURKE, P. J., 1973, Immunologic studies in acute leukemia, *Natl. Cancer Inst. Monogr.* **37**:69.

SAVEL, H., 1969, Effect of autologous tumor extracts on cultured human peripheral blood lymphocytes, *Cancer* **24**:56.

SCHREK, R., 1963, Cell transformations and mitoses produced *in vitro* by tuberculin purified protein derivative in human blood cells, *Am. Rev. Resp. Dis.* **87**:734.

Schweitzer, M., Melief, C. M. J., and Eijsvoogel, V. P., 1973, Failure to demonstrate immunity to leukemia associated antigens by lymphocyte transformation *in vitro*, *Int. J. Cancer* **11**:11.

Seeger, R. C., and Owen, J. J. T., 1973, Measurement of tumor immunity *in vitro* with ^{125}I-iododeoxyuridine-labeled target cells, *Transplantation* **15**:404.

Senik, A., Gomard, E., Plata, F., and Levy, J. P., 1973, Cell-mediated immune reaction against tumors induced by oncornaviruses. III. Studies by mixed lymphocyte–tumor reaction, *Int. J. Cancer* **12**:233.

Shearer, W. T., Philpott, G. W., and Parker, C. W., 1973, Stimulation of cells by antibody, *Science* **182**:1357.

Sheldon, P. J., Hemsted, E. H., Papamichail, M., and Holborow, E. W., 1973, Thymic origin of atypical lymphoid cells in infectious mononucleosis, *Lancet* **1**:1153.

Siegler, H. F., Shingleton, W. W., Metzgar, R. S., Buckley, C. E., Bergoc, P. M., Miller, D. S., Fetter, B. F., and Phaup, M. B., 1972, Non-specific and specific immunotherapy in patients with melanoma, *Surgery* **72**:162.

Silk, M., 1967, Effect of plasma from patients with carcinoma on *in vitro* lymphocyte transformation, *Cancer* **20**:2088.

Sinkovics, J. G., Cabiness, J. R., and Shullenberger, C. C., 1972, Disappearance after chemotherapy of blocking serum factors as measured *in vitro* with lymphocytes cytotoxic to tumor cells, *Cancer* **30**:1428.

Sjögren, H. O., Hellström, I., Bansal, S. C., and Hellström, K. E., 1971, Suggestive evidence that the "blocking antibodies" of tumor-bearing individuals may be antigen–antibody complexes, *Proc. Natl. Acad. Sci. U.S.A.* **68**:1372.

Sjögren, H. O., Hellström, I., Bansal, S. C., Warner, G. A., and Hellström, K. E., 1972, Elution of "blocking factors" from human tumors, capable of abrogating tumor-cell destruction by specifically immune lymphocytes, *Int. J. Cancer* **9**:274.

Skurzak, H. M., Klein, E., Yoshida, T. O., and Lamon, E. W., 1972, Synergistic or antagonistic effect of different antibody concentrations on *in vitro* lymphocyte cytotoxicity in the Moloney sarcoma virus system, *J. Exp. Med.* **135**:997.

Skurzak, H., Steiner, L., Klein, E., and Lamon, E., 1973, Cytotoxicity of human peripheral lymphocytes for glioma, osteosarcoma, and glia cell lines, *Natl. Cancer Inst. Monogr.* **37**:93.

Southam, C. M., Brunswig, A., Levin, A. G., and Dizon, Q. S., 1966, Effect of leukocytes on transplantability of human cancer, *Cancer* **19**:1743.

Steel, C. M., and Hardy, D. A., 1970, Evidence of altered antigenicity in cultured lymphoid cells from patients with infectious mononucleosis, *Lancet* **1**:1322.

Stewart, T. H. M., and Orizaga, M., 1971, The presence of delayed hypersensitivity reactions in patients toward cellular extracts of their malignant tumors: The frequency, duration, and cross-reactivity of this phenomenon in patients with breast cancer and its correlation with survival, *Cancer* **28**:1472.

Stjernsward, J., Clifford, P., and Svedmyr, E., 1970, General and tumor-distinctive cellular immunological reactivity, in: *Burkitt's Lymphoma* (D. P. Burkitt and D. N. Wright, eds.), pp. 164–171, Livingstone, Edinburgh.

Sulit, H. S., Golub, S. H., Irie, R., Gupta, R., Grooms, G. A., and Morton, D. L., 1975, Fetal calf serum and human serum grown tumor cells: Influence on tests for lymphocyte cytotoxicity, serum blocking, and serum arming effects, submitted for publication.

Sulitzeanu, D., Gorsky, Y., Paglin, S., and Weiss, D., 1974, Morphologic evidence suggestive of host-tumor cell interactions *in vivo* in human cancer patients. *J. Natl. Cancer Inst.* **52**:603.

Svedmyr, E. A., Deinhardt, F., and Klein, G., 1974a, Sensitivity of different target cells to the killing action of peripheral lymphocytes stimulated by autologous lymphoblastoid cell lines, *Int. J. Cancer* **13**:891.

Svedmyr, E., Wigzell, H., and Jondal, M., 1974b, Sensitization of human lymphocytes against autologous or allogeneic lymphoblastoid cell lines: Characterization of the reactive cells, *Scand. J. Immunol.* **3**:499.

Takasugi, M., and Klein, E., 1970, A microassay for cell-mediated immunity, *Tranplantation* **9**:219.

Takasugi, M., Mickey, M. R., and Terasaki, P., 1973a, Quantitation of the microassay for cell-mediated immunity through electronic image analysis, *Natl. Cancer Inst. Monogr.*, **37**:77.

Takasugi, M., Mickey, M. R., and Terasaki, P. I., 1973b, Reactivity of lymphocytes from normal persons on cultured tumor cells, *Cancer Res.* **33**:2898.

Taranger, L. A., Chapman, W. H., Hellström, I., and Hellström, K. E., 1972, Immunological studies on urinary bladder tumors of rats and mice, *Science* **176**:1337.

299

HOST
IMMUNE
RESPONSE TO
HUMAN
TUMOR
ANTIGENS

TAYLOR, J. F., JUNGE, U., WOLFE, L., DEINHARDT, F., AND KYALWAZI, S. K., 1971, Lymphocyte transformation in patients with Kaposi's sarcoma, *Int. J. Cancer* **8**:468.

THOMSON, D. M. P., STEELE, K., AND ALEXANDER, P., 1973, The presence of tumour-specific membrane antigen in the serum of rats with chemically induced sarcomata, *Br. J. Cancer* **27**:27.

VAAGE, J., JONES, R. D., AND BROWN, B. W., 1972, Tumor-specific resistance in mice detected by inhibition of macrophage migration, *Cancer Res.* **32**:680.

VAN BOXEL, J. A., STOBO, J. D., PAUL, W. E., AND GREEN, I., 1972, Antibody-dependent lymphoid cell-mediated cytoxicity: No requirement for thymus-derived lymphocytes, *Science* **175**:194.

VANKY, F., STJERNSWARD, J., KLEIN, G., AND NILSONNE, U., 1971a, Serum-mediated inhibition of lymphocyte stimulation by autochthonous human tumors, *J. Natl. Cancer Inst.* **47**:95.

VANKY, F., STJERNSWARD, J., AND NILSONNE, U., 1971b, Cellular immunity to human sarcoma, *J. Natl. Cancer Inst.* **46**:1145.

VANKY, F., KLEIN, E., STJERNSWARD, J., AND NILSONNE, U., 1974, Cellular immunity against tumor-associated antigens in humans: Lymphocyte stimulation and skin reaction, *Int. J. Cancer* **14**:333.

VAN LOVEREN, H., AND DEN OTTER, W., 1974, *In vitro* activation of armed macrophages and the therapeutic application in mice, *J. Natl. Cancer Inst.* **52**:1917.

VIZA, D. C., BERNARD-DEGANI, O., BERNARD, C., AND HARRIS, R., 1969, Leukemia antigens, *Lancet* **2**:493.

WAGNER, H., AND RÖLLINGHOFF, M., 1973, *In vitro* induction of tumor-specific immunity. I. Parameters of activation and cytotoxic reactivity of mouse lymphoid cells immunized *in vitro* against syngeneic and allogeneic plasma cell tumors, *J. Exp. Med.* **138**:1.

WAHLSTRÖM, T., SAKSELA, E., AND TROUPP, H., 1973, Cell-bound antiglial immunity in patients with malignant tumors of the brain, *Cell. Immunol.* **6**:161.

WELLS, S. A., MELEWICZ, F. C., CHRISTIANSEN, C., AND KETCHAM, A. S., 1973. Delayed cutaneous hypersensitivity reactions to membrane extracts of carcinomatous cells of the cervix uteri, *Surg. Gynecol. Obstet.* **136**:717.

WOLBERG, W. H., AND GOELZER, M. L., 1971, *In vitro* assay of cell-mediated immunity in human cancer: Definition of a leukocyte migration inhibition factor, *Nature (London)* **229**:632.

WOOD, G. W., AND BARTH, R. F., 1974, Immunofluorescent studies of the serologic reactivity of patients with malignant melanoma against tumor-associated cytoplasmic antigens, *J. Natl. Cancer Inst.* **53**:309.

WRIGHT, P. W., ORTIZ, DE LANDAZURI, M., AND HERBERMAN, R. B., 1973, Immune response to Gross virus-induced lymphoma: Comparison of two *in vitro* assays of cell-mediated immunity, *J. Natl. Cancer Inst.* **50**:947.

WYBRAN, J., HELLSTRÖM, I., HELLSTRÖM, K. E., AND FUDENBERG, H. H., 1974, Cytotoxicity of human rosette-forming blood lymphocytes on cultivated human tumor cells, *Int. J. Cancer* **13**:515.

YATA, J., AND KLEIN, G., 1969, Some factors affecting membrane immunofluorescence reactivity of Burkitt lymphoma tissue culture cell lines, *Int. J. Cancer* **4**:767.

YOSHIDA, T. O., AND IMAI, K., 1970, Auto-antibody to human leukemic cell membrane as detected by immune adherence, *Rev. Eur. Etud. Clin. Biol.* **15**:61.

ZIGHELBOIM, J., BONAVIDA, B., AND FAHEY, J. L., 1973, Evidence for several cell populations active in antibody dependent cellular cytoxicity, *J. Immunol.* **111**:1737.

ZIGHELBOIM, J., BONAVIDA, B., AND FAHEY, J. L., 1974, Antibody-mediated *in vivo* suppression of EL4 leukemia in a syngeneic host, *J. Natl. Cancer Inst.* **52**:879.

Comparative Pathology

10

Comparative Aspects of Certain Cancers

Harold L. Stewart

1. Introduction

Descriptions of the relative frequency, age distribution, site, histological appearance, and spread of tumors of man and lower animals are numerous. Many of the sources of information detail wide differences among species. To collect all the specific details of this information in one publication would amount to an encyclopedic task. I have therefore selected a few examples of common human neoplasms of specific sites and compared them with neoplasms of similar sites in other species. These are tumors of the lung, liver, mammary gland, and soft tissues, and, because of their recent appearance in employees of the plastics industry, malignant hemangioendotheliomas induced by exposure to vinyl chloride. While there are some similarities, there are many differences among species. A point of view that many writers on comparative oncology have adopted is to overemphasize the resemblance between neoplasms of lower animals, particularly rodents, and those of man. A stated aim of these authors has been to adopt, whenever possible, the classification and terminology proposed by the WHO International Reference Centers for the histological classification of human tumors. To stress the resemblances without pointing up the differences in structural appearances and known behavior is likely to mislead investigators to believe that many animal tumors are suitable models for the human tumors. What are needed are a series of workshops and studies by collaborative committees. These would bring together pathologists with their slides and their clinical, biological, and behavioral data in order to confer and to work out acceptable definitions of cancer types in different species of lower animals.

HAROLD L. STEWART • Registry of Experimental Cancers, National Cancer Institute, National Institutes of Health, Bethesda, Maryland.

HAROLD L.
STEWART

The study of comparative oncology may be said to have begun with a query circulated in 1802 by the Medical Committee of the Edinburgh Society for Investigating the Nature and Cure of Cancer (Baillie *et al.*, 1806). This Committee was evidently the forerunner of the many cancer societies subsequently organized. The Committee's aim was "the acquisition of knowledge on a subject on which, it may be said, we are even at this time [1802] totally ignorant." The Committee's report continues: "In order to form a basis of inquiry, in which the nature and cure of cancer, it is presumed, may be pursued with all the advantages of reason and experience, the Medical Committee very early drew out and distributed queries, for the consideration not only of the corresponding members, but of all medical men to whom opportunities of answering them might, by study or by accident, occur."

All 13 of these queries are as canny as might be expected from Scots of the early nineteenth century. Query No. 10 is pertinent to the subject of comparative oncology, so I reproduce it here along with a more lengthy explanation of its aims and purposes as stated by the Medical Committee:

> Query 10th—Are brute creatures subject to any disease resembling cancer in the human body?
>
> It is not at present known whether brute creatures are subject to cancer, though some of their diseases have a very suspicious appearance. When this question is decided, we may inquire what class of animals is chiefly subject to cancer; the wild or the domesticated; the carnivorous or the graminivorus; those which do, or those which do not, chew the cud. This investigation may lead to much philosophical amusement and useful information; particularly it may teach us how far the prevalence or frequency of cancer may depend upon the manners and habits of life. As establishments are now formed for the reception of several kinds of animals, and as the treatment of their diseases has at length fallen under the care of scientific men, it is hoped that the information here required may be readily obtained. If animals which live only on herbs, and never drink any other liquid than water, prove to be the least, or not at all, subject to cancer; such proof may, in many cases, become a guide in practice.

Answers came slowly to this old, yet up-to-date, query about cancer in "brute creatures." It was 50 odd years later that Leblanc (1858, 1859) in France reviewed and appraised case reports of tumors in the horse, mule, donkey, cow, dog, cat, and pig. He emphasized the importance of histological examination in diagnosis and stated that the cellular composition of tumors of domestic animals was comparable to that of human tumors as first described some 20 years earlier by Müller (1838). Nearly 40 years elapsed before McFadyean (1891), a Scot living in London, and Sticker (1902), from Germany, published extensive data on tumors of domestic animals. About this time—that is, around the turn of the century—Bashford and Murray (1904), of the Imperial Cancer Research Fund of London, began their investigation of the distribution of neoplasms throughout the animal kingdom. It was in 1904 that they published the now historic survey entitled "The ... Zoological Distribution ... of Cancer," which formed a solid foundation for comparative oncology. They stated with certainty that cancer occurs in wild as well as in domestic animals, and they predicted that many forms of cancer would be found throughout the subphylum Vertebrata. It was also around the turn of the century that the transplantation of rodent tumors got well under way, although as early as 1876 Nowinsky in Moscow had passed the venereal tumor from one dog to another. In succeeding years, as a result of the systematic charting of the growth of transplanted tumors, it became evident that mice in which transplanted tumors had regressed were immune to subsequent transplants of the same and sometimes of other tumors as well. This basic discovery of an immunological factor associated with cancer in mice was, according to the late Dr. Clowes (personal communication), principally responsible for the expansion of cancer research laboratories in the early years of this century. Studies of cancer immunity have depended heavily on comparative pathology, of rodents in particular, and lately of other species lower on the phylogenetic tree. Comparative studies of cancer in primitive species have revealed a critical problem centering about the evolutionary development of the thymic system of cellular immunity. Bearing on this point is the recent demonstration of the induction of sarcomas in athymic nude mice by the subcutaneous injection of 3-methylcholanthrene.

Interest in comparative pathology received a new impetus in 1908 and 1910 by the respective demonstrations of the viral transmission of chicken leukemia by Ellerman and Bang (1908) and of chicken sarcoma No. 1 by Rous (1910). This was followed in the 1930s by the work of Shope (1932), Bittner (1936), Korteweg (1936), and others on viral cancers and related conditions in laboratory and wild animals. Even with these epochal discoveries of virus tumors in animals and on up through the 1930s, no university thought it worthwhile to establish a chair of virology in any medical school in this country, showing how far education lags behind research. The later work on virus-induced neoplasms and in particular on virus-induced hematopoietic and salivary gland neoplasms, initiated by the discoveries of Gross (1951, 1955), Stewart (1955), and others, has led to studies on mechanisms and pathogenesis of viral carcinogenesis that have revealed biological processess never before suspected. The World Health Organization (WHO, 1974) has encouraged research in leukemic diseases of felines and bovines. In cats, investigations on the molecular structure of the virus that causes feline leukemia and on the pathogenesis of the disease have revealed that virus injected into kittens may cause either lymphocytic or myelogenous leukemia. Failing this, the virus may destroy the thymus and T lymphocytes and thus produce an immunodeficiency disease. Recently developed immunological techniques detect leukemia virus in cats, and this has led to the possibility of developing a vaccine. The significance for human cancer is obvious. The extensive investigations of bovine leukemia with much encouragment from WHO have not led to the promising results that the feline leukemia studies have, principally because the transmission studies in bovines have been negative or doubtful. Today, support for investigations of cancer viruses runs into hundreds of millions of dollars, nearly all of it for support of comparative oncology studies, because to date viruses have not been shown to cause cancer in man. Nearly all the known agents that do cause cancer in man, be they biological, physical, or chemical, were discovered from studies in man. So studies in man are important, also. Nevertheless, for the elucidation of knowledge about carcinogenesis, and for carcinogenicity testing, recourse must be had to the lower animals, or the "brute creatures," as that very modern-thinking Committee of Scots of 1802 designated them. The mouse was the model employed by the London School for carcinogenicity testing that led to the identification and subsequent isolation of carcinogenic aromatic polycyclic hydrocarbons from the crude tar starting material through the more refined distillates.

3. Registries and Publications

Gradually, over the years, the establishment of registries for the accession and study of cancer in lower animals and the publication of monographs and nomenclatures have resulted in a better understanding of comparative oncology. The International Agency for Research on Cancer at Lyon, France, has now begun the preparation of atlases of spontaneous and induced cancers of laboratory animals starting with the rat, mouse, and hamster. These atlases will serve as training and reference guides for experimental pathologists working with laboratory rodents.

The National Cancer Institute has established the Registry of Experimental Cancers, which consists of accessions drawn from a collection of half a million necropsies, mostly of rodents with spontaneous or induced cancers, that have accumulated since 1937. At the Armed Forces Institute of Pathology, the Registry of Comparative Pathology has been expanding its accumulation of cancers chiefly from domestic animals. The European Late Effects Group is circulating among its members and finally storing at Munich, Germany, pathological material and descriptions of animal cancers from each semiannual symposium held there. These specimens are available for comparison with cancers presently induced by irradiation. Antedating by many years these collections is the priceless collection of necropsy protocols and histological slides of cancers and other diseases of captive wild animals and birds at the Philadelphia Zoo dating back to the early 1900s.

The study of naturally occurring diseases of domestic animals in which pathological processes are more easily investigated than they are in man (if proper efforts are made) has led to many important advances in human medicine. Until comparatively recently, however, neoplastic diseases, because they are of little economic importance in domestic animals, have received a low priority in veterinary medicine. Nowadays, research on these diseases is being stimulated because of the potential contribution to our knowledge of cancer in man. New epidemiological and diagnostic data are being provided by the California-based Alemeda–Contra Costa Animal Neoplasm Registry. The World Health Organization (WHO, 1974) has established an international reference center and collaborating laboratories to participate in a program of studies in comparative oncology. These groups have been collecting tumors of ten major body sites from six species of domestic animals—the horse, ox, sheep, pig, dog, and cat. They have

been working on definitions of tumor types and designing histological classifications that follow, as nearly as possible, the classification of human tumors. As they
are published, these projects will enlarge the basis for research in comparative
oncology, particularly for epidemiological studies and therapeutic trials in animal
models of human cancers.[1]

Of the cancers that occur in animals, the prevalence of different histological
types and sites of tumor differs from species to species, from breed to breed, and
from region to region. One registry supported by WHO has 3000 accessions of
canine and feline tumors with follow-up data from biopsy to necropsy. The bovine
has been important in studies of bladder cancer, which, in areas of Turkey and
Southern Africa, is endemic and which has been shown to result from the
ingestion of plants, bracken fern in the former area and a species of cycad plant in
the latter area. A substance carcinogenic for rats has been extracted from bracken
fern, and this substance has been isolated from the milk of cows eating the plant.
Whatever its significance, it has been noted that in two regions of the world where
bracken fern is prevalent there is an unusually high incidence of gastric cancer in
man. The use of transplantable tumors in rodents has, over the more than 100
years that they have been available for study by cancer investigators, proven to be
of the utmost value (Stewart *et al.*, 1959). The WHO reports that one of its
collaborators has developed techniques for the successful transplantation of
several different histological types of canine tumors which have the possibility to
make available to investigators a group of dogs bearing a similar tumor.

The Registry of Tumors in Lower Animals, at the Smithsonian Institution of
Washington, is collecting examples of cancers, and lesions confused with cancers,
from poikilothermic and invertebrate animals. A few years ago, the International
Union Against Cancer established within its framework a ten-man Committee on
Comparative Oncology, to function as a field and laboratory task force to survey
and collect naturally occurring neoplasms in aquatic animals, chiefly bottom-
feeding fish and filter-feeding mollusks. These two groups were selected because
of the now known epizootics of neoplasms among them. Moreover, their
environment and habits place them in a position of exposure to particulate and
soluble pathogens. Chlorinated hydrocarbon pesticides adsorb readily to suspended particulates in water and these particulates filter out and concentrate in
the bodies of filter-feeding mollusks. In turn, the bottom feeders eat the mollusks,
and also bottom sediment on which organochlorine pesticides may be concentrated. Apart from these practical considerations, such surveys may generate
information of value to the fundamental biological concepts of the relationships

[1] As this chapter went to press, a copy of the WHO International Histological Classification of Tumors
of Domestic Animals (*Bulletin of the World Health Organization 50*:1–142, 1974) arrived on my desk.
The contents consist of definitions, brief descriptions, abundant and elegant illustrations, and a
nomenclature of and for tumors and tumorlike lesions of ten body sites of six species. This pioneer
publication now enables pathologists to use comparable standards for reports that emanate from
different laboratories within countries and internationally. This, as the Chinese would say, is a great
leap forward.

between neoplasia and evolutionary events. This could require a reappraisal of a commonly held concept that evolutionary development of the thymic system of cellular immunity came about as a compensatory response to an increased predisposition to neoplasia in vertebrates. All of these efforts are contributing answers, albeit tardily, to the 1802 query about cancer in "brute creatures."

4. Criteria for Diagnosis of Cancer

None know better than the experimental pathologists the difficulties encountered by those who work in comparative oncology. The switch from hospital practice is a difficult transition. There are no fixed and immutable criteria for the diagnosis of cancer in all species. Some cancers of lower animals may be similar and others dissimilar to those of man. Some cancers arise in organs of laboratory animals not possessed by man. The nomenclature of animal tumors, which in the past was based largely on the nomenclature of human tumors, is confusing and contradictory. The troubles that beset a pathologist in his studies of cancer of domestic, laboratory, and captive wild animals and birds pale, however, by comparison when he extends his studies to pathological material of invertebrate and poikilothermic animals. Examination of the pathological material in the registry at the Smithsonian Institution and a perusal of the papers in the proceedings of the symposium held there a few years ago convince one how really complex are cancers and abnormalities of growth and form in the simpler systems of animal species (*National Cancer Institute Monograph*, 1969).

Over the years, the zoologists have applied massive efforts to the understanding of the normal anatomy and biology of primitive creatures, while they consistently ignored or discarded diseased and otherwise abnormal specimens. The pathologists from their side largely neglected the primitive creatures. This is now a diminishing problem. It is now known that neoplasms of primitive animals do not exhibit differentiation characteristics of tissues not yet evolved phylogenetically. Thus osteomas occur in bony fish and above but never at lower levels of organization where bone does not exist. There are no chondromas before the evolution of the cartilaginous fishes. Like comparable neoplasms of warm-blooded vertebrates, some neoplasms of fish depend on genetic variables and alteration of the environment and some can be induced by carcinogenic chemicals and viruses. In animals below the fishes, the precise identification and classification of neoplasms are not easy, and not even always possible. The question "What is cancer?" constantly confronts the experimental pathologist. Processes that had previously been classified as cancers, such as the melanotic lesions of *Drosophila* and the lesions that ensue upon nerve severance in cockroaches, are nowadays not considered neoplasms. Serial transplantability of tumors of rodents, long considered to be irrefutable proof of malignancy for lower forms, now must be evaluated in the light of transplantable insect cells. Some lines of transplantable insect cells, when subjected to appropriate hormonal influences, still retain the capacity to differentiate, like completely normal embryonic cells. Are there, moreover, at the premetazoan level of evolution, clonal phenomena analogous to neoplasia? Ever since Bashford (Bashford and Murray, 1904) pondered the possible relationship of clonal phenomena to neoplasia at the very lowest level of organization there has been much speculation about what some have termed neoplastic "equivalents." Years ago, Virchow wrote: "I do not think that a living human being can be found that even under torture could actually say what tumors really are" (Ackerknecht, 1953). Today, also, there exists no accurate definition of cancer. Working definitions do abound in textbooks, but none is accurate. Some feel that such definitions are too pragmatic and do damage by discouraging new concepts and are thus a real impediment to research. If, as we hope, the enigma of cancer will one day disappear and a proper understanding of it emerge, then the knowledge of comparative oncology will necessarily need to have been expanded.

5. Hyperplasia and Benign and Malignant

"Hyperplasia," "benign," and "malignant" are terms whose meaning every experimental pathologist should clearly define to convey to the reader the concept that he intends. To decide that a given lesion is a hyperplastic process or a benign or malignant neoplasm carries a legal implication in the area of carcinogenicity testing. If cancer develops from the administration of a potential food additive the agent is banned in this country, whereas if the lesion so induced is diagnosed as hyperplasia or simply as a nodule the agent is permitted. *Stedman's Medical Dictionary* (1961) defines hyperplasia as "an increase in number of the individual tissue elements, excluding tumor formation, whereby the bulk of the part or organ is increased." Many publications dealing with spontaneous and induced tumors at various stages during their development are full of specious arguments about their hyperplastic or benign nature. There are a number of examples. One is the common pulmonary tumor of the mouse that arises from the alveolar type II cell. At different stages of its development within the lung, it has been variously classified as alveolar cell hyperplasia, adenoma, and glandular, cystic, papillary, and solid carcinoma; after it has spread and metastasized it has been classified as undifferentiated-cell carcinoma, mixed carcinosarcoma, and sarcoma. The pulmonary tumor of the mouse grows readily when transplanted to syngeneic mice, exhibiting in the host animals autonomy, invasion, and metastasis, all characteristics of cancer. The various histological appearances simply denote different stages in the malignant progression of this cancer. The application of the term "hyperplasia" to any stage of this process is a misuse of the word as defined.

The common uterine tumor of the rabbit is another example. Beginning as an innocent-looking polypoid adenomatous formation, it enlarges and infiltrates the wall of the uterus as it progresses and finally metastasizes widely, during these events having taken on the histological appearance of a less-differentiated carcinoma or a sarcoma (Stewart, 1953b). Following treatment with chemical carcinogens, I have followed, by serial killings of the experimental animals and serial sections of the lesion, the evolution of the early innocent-looking cellular proliferations as they progressed by stages into highly malignant neoplasms of the skin, subcutaneous tissues, forestomach, glandular stomach, intestine, and liver. On this material, one would be justified to render an opinion of benign hyperplasia from the examination of a single histological section at an early point in time during the beginning histogenesis of the neoplasm.

The common hepatic tumor of the mouse arises as a small nodule composed of alternating cords of hepatic cells and blood sinusoids. Even as it enlarges, its close resemblance to the structure of liver may make distinction difficult and without any change in histological pattern it may enlarge, metastasize, and grow when transplanted to syngeneic mice. So, despite its innocent-looking appearance, it is a cancer *de novo*.

Some experimental pathologists have forgotten, while others never learned, that the field of human oncology has many examples of cancers, some that arise as innocent-looking lesions, others that pursue an indolent course over a long period of years and metastasize infrequently late in the disease, and still others so well differentiated that when sections of their metastases are placed side by side with a section of the organ of origin the two may not be distinguishable. Cancer of the urinary bladder arises in man as an innocent-looking papillary structure which, if left untreated, grows into the lumen and into the wall of the bladder and metastasizes widely, the metastases taking on the appearance of a highly malignant transitional-cell or undifferentiated-cell carcinoma. A classic example of a human tumor that may metastasize while still retaining the appearance of the organ of origin is thyroid gland cancer, formerly miscalled benign metastasizing goiter. There are additional examples of cancers in human medicine that never metastasize, such as the gliomas and basal cell carcinomas. Examples of those that persist at the site of origin for a long period of time and metastasize late in the disease and then only in a fraction of the cases, but are nevertheless malignant and lethal, are certain fibrosarcomas, leiomyosarcomas, and salivary gland tumors. It is often difficult for the clinical pathologist to distinguish between those salivary gland tumors classified as papillary cystadenoma and papillary cystadenocarcinoma, since tumors with a relatively benign histological appearance may metastasize after a long period of slow growth. Similarly, a mixed tumor of the salivary glands may after a long static period undergo rapid growth and metastasize widely. The late Dr. Joseph McFarland (1943) used to refer to this phenomenon as a ripening process of the mixed salivary gland tumor. There are thus no immutable criteria by which one can, with certainty, diagnose all cancers during all stages of their progression from their early inception to their terminal metastasis. One needs to understand very well the tumor with which he is dealing, its histological appearances, and its biological behavior at different stages of its growth. The phenomenon of tumor progression is inadequately understood in comparative pathology.

The concept of tumor progression, as formulated by Foulds (1969), is fundamental to cancer biology, deserving attention of clinician and experimentalist alike. The observations that led to Foulds' (1969) concept of progression were of a series of subcutaneous masses which developed in the mammary pads of a group of hybrid mice (RIII × C57BL) during periods of pregnancy and which regressed or became quiescent with the termination of pregnancy. Eventually, many of the growths became independent of the hormonal state of the host and grew progressively after pregnancy had ended. This set of circumstances illustrates progression, by which tumors advance from an early responsive stage to unresponsive and independent growth. The complexities of histological structure and biological behavior of new growths can be explained as expressions of numerous and diverse unit characters that make up neoplasms. One of these, unrestricted capacity for growth, while harmful to the host, is only one of many alterations in a cancer cell. The unit characters in a tumor can combine together in a variety of ways and yet be independently variable and subject to independent progression. It has been emphasized that this concept of Foulds (1969) is one of the most valuable stimuli to creative thought and research currently available to students of oncology.

On the other side of the coin, there are hyperplasias in man and animals that never behave like cancer. In man, there are the common warts, juvenile papillomatosis of the larynx, and pseudoepitheliomatous hyperplasia associated with insect bites and blastomycosis of the skin; in cattle and mules, there are the viral warts of the skin; in dogs, the viral papillomatosis of the lips and gingiva. In monkeys, there are the polypoid adenomatous lesions of the stomach caused by a parasite and the adenomatous proliferations of the mucosa of the large bowel that are induced by inhalation of aerosols of lubricating oils. Originally both of these alimentary tract lesions of monkeys were mistakenly diagnosed as cancer. Also misdiagnosed for years as adenocarcinoma was the nonneoplastic lesion of adenomatous proliferative hyperplasia of the glandular stomach of strain NHO mice. A comparable lesion occurs in strain I mice. These gastric lesions not only never progress to cancer spontaneously but also resist cancer induction even when 3-methylcholanthrene is injected into the wall of the glandular stomach. This treatment induces gastric cancer in mice of other strains which do not exhibit the spontaneous adenomatous hyperplasia. Strain DBA mice spontaneously develop benign adenomatous intestinal plaques that do not progress to cancer. The pulmonary adenomatosis and squamous metaplasia of mice, rats, and captive wild animals quartered in zoos need to be distinguished as hyperplastic processes that do not eventuate in cancer. In rats and mice, adenofibrosis of the liver, often previously misdiagnosed as cancer, heals by fibrosis. The nonneoplastic lesions of acanthosis, hyperkeratosis, and papillomatosis that develop in the forestomach of malnourished rodents have been misdiagnosed as cancers (Fibiger, 1919). Despite the atypical histological appearance of these various lesions, they do not infiltrate the adjacent tissues or metastasize or transplant to syngeneic animals of species in which it is feasable to test for transplantability. There are thus examples of human and animal lesions that are hyperplasias which never progress to cancer, and examples of cancers whose first manifestations are heralded by the appearance of innocent-looking cellular proliferations. The pathologists should not use the term "hyperplasia" for those lesions that are neoplastic from the beginning, but apply the term only to those lesions that represent a nonneoplastic overgrowth of normal cells.

6. Tumors of the Lung

When a comparative pathologist attempts to classify the pulmonary tumors of animals, he naturally turns to current classifications of pulmonary tumors in man for standards for comparison. More work, by far, has gone into the development of classifications of pulmonary tumors in man than in those of all other species combined. The WHO International Histological Classification of (Human) Lung Tumors (Kreyberg, 1967) adopted definitions for most tumor types that are generally logical and reasonable. The typing was based primarily on cytological and histological criteria, with consideration given to histogenesis, particularly in the subtyping of the adenocarcinomas. Nevertheless, the WHO nomenclature contains some loose categories which create difficulties, in particular with the classification of adenocarcinomas and oat cell carcinomas. The oat cell carcinomas, under which heading pathologists of this country classify a not inconsiderable number of pulmonary cancers, appears in the WHO nomenclature in parentheses in "II.3. *Lymphocyte-like ("oat-cell") carcinomas.*" Many pathologists have not thought that the cells of the oat cell tumor look like a lymphocyte, hence those neoplasms of the oat cell type that are composed of fusiform cells (perhaps the majority) would be classified under "II.1. *Fusiform cell carcinomas.*" The oat cell tumors are thus split two ways and there are no instructions as to where to code those that have both round cells and fusiform cells. There are also different categories for the classification of mucus-producing carcinomas which many pathologists would classify as a single entity under adenocarcinomas, irrespective of the presence of demonstrable acinar of tubular structures, or minor differences in pattern in the sections of tumor examined. One category is "III. *Adenocarcinomas,*" composed of tubules and glandlike structures with or without mucin, and often with solid masses of undifferentiated cells. Certain of these, according to the instruction, may be distinguished with difficulty from large cell carcinomas such as "IV.1. *Solid tumors with mucin-like* substances," "IV.2. *Solid tumors without mucin-like* substances," and "IV.3. *Giant cell carcinoma.*" Here then are examples of large categories of pulmonary cancers of man, the oat cell carcinoma and the adenocarcinoma, one of which is split into two and the other into four ill-defined categories. Facing these dilemmas, the comparative pathologist naturally feels frustrated when he attempts to correlate the typing of animal tumors with those of man.

In lower animals, the large group of epithelial-type tumors of the lung have been roughly classified as adenocarcinoma, squamous cell carcinoma, and undifferentiated or anaplastic carcinoma without further histological refinement

and with few attempts at the assessment of the cell of origin, the lobes or the areas
of the lung involved, the gross characteristics, the manner of spread, and the
frequency of and the sites involved by secondary deposits, and even in some
instances without a clear distinction from metastatic tumors. An exception is the
alveologenic carcinoma of the mouse. This neoplasm has been subjected to the
most intense etiological, histological, histogenetic, genetic, and biological studies
of any pulmonary tumor in the lower animals, with positive results in all of these
areas of investigation. This same type of tumor may also be seen in the rat,
mastomys, guinea pig, skunk, and perhaps dog and cat, but it has no counterpart
in man. On the other hand, some of the commonly recognized pulmonary tumors
of man have not been described in lower animals. This is true of the entire classes
of carcinoid tumors, with two possible exceptions (see 319): the mucus gland type
tumors and the cylindromas with hyaline differentiation or with mucus production, and also perhaps the mucoepidermoid tumors. Students of the morphology
of pulmonary neoplasms have taken too few advantages of the opportunities for
studies of the histogenesis of pulmonary neoplasms in laboratory animals. It is
certainly possible, with appropriate experimental designs, to determine the
histogenesis of experimentally induced tumors in animals with an accuracy not
possible for tumors in man.

6.1. Rodents

The common pulmonary tumor of the mouse, the alveologenic carcinoma, has
been the object of many studies since first identified around the turn of the
century. A large literature dealing with it has accumulated (Stewart *et al.*, 1975). As
its name implies, this neoplasm develops in the pulmonary alveoli from the type II
alveolar cell. One to four tumors may be counted in the lungs of untreated mice of
a susceptible strain and this number may increase to 100 or more per lung in such
mice treated with any of a great variety of potent carcinogenic agents. The tumors
grow expansively but are not encapsulated. Microscopically, they are composed of
columns of cuboidal and columnar cells arranged in the form of glands and often
exhibit papillary formations. Ordinarily less than 2% metastasize, but when the
tumor does extend through the lung, spread to the pleura, and metastasize the
adenomatous pattern of the primary neoplasm frequently converts to a less-
differentiated epithelial tumor pattern or to sarcoma. The same phenomenon is
seen in serial transplants carried in syngeneic hosts.

The only other histological type of spontaneous pulmonary neoplasm commonly encountered in some strains of mice is the malignant hemangioen-
dothelioma. A variety of carcinogenic regimens may induce the hemangioen-
dothelioma in a number of different strains of mice (Stewart *et al.*, 1975).
Squamous cell carcinoma is exceedingly rare in untreated mice but can be induced
by the intratracheal injection of the carcinogenic polycyclic aromatic hydrocarbons (Nettesheim and Hammons, 1971). A commonly encountered nonneoplastic
lesion of the mouse, squamous metaplasia, has frequently been mistakenly

diagnosed as squamous cell carcinoma in the past. By microscopic examination alone, the two lesions may be distinguished with difficulty or not at all. Therefore, any one claiming to induce squamous cell carcinoma in the lungs of the mouse is well advised to produce convincing evidence in the form of invasion of blood vessels or lymph vessels, metastasis of the lesion, or its successful transplantation to syngeneic mice.

Rats, unlike mice, rarely develop spontaneous tumors of the lung except for the so-called lymphoreticular neoplasms that may occur rather frequently in some stocks of rats (Pour *et al.*, 1975). Care must be taken to distinguish lymphoreticular tumors from the sequela of chronic murine pneumonitis. Also, in contrast to mice, in which the alveologenic carcinoma is the most common histological type of spontaneous tumor of the lung encountered, the rat may develop a wide range of different histological types of spontaneous pulmonary tumors even though they are rare (Stewart 1966*a,b*). In fact almost no other species has developed so wide a variety and range of different histological types of spontaneous pulmonary tumor as the rat. Moreover, the more different histological types have been encountered in untreated rats than in rats exposed to carcinogens for the purpose of inducing pulmonary tumors. Except for the bronchial polyps in Snell's material (1965) and the fibroma reported by Guèrin (1954), all the other reported tumor types are of the malignant variety.

Pour *et al.* (1975) have written a full account of, and elegantly illustrated, the different types of spontaneous and induced lung tumors of rats, the methods for their induction, and their comparative aspects. They reviewed the results obtained by the ingenious technique devised by Stanton *et al.* (1969) whereby inert beeswax is used as the vehicle for the incorporation of potential or suspected pulmonary carcinogens, such as asbestos, for screening purposes. The beeswax mixture is then warmed to a liquid state and injected into the tissues of the lung through an open thoracotomy. Beeswax pellets containing 3-methylcholanthrene induced changes that could be categorized in a progressive series as keratinizing squamous cell metaplasia, keratinizing squamous cell dysplasia with localized extension, overt squamous cell carcinoma, and undifferentiated neoplasms (Hirano *et al.*, 1974). The neoplastic response was dose related. Although pulmonary cancers have never been induced by exposure of laboratory animals to inhalation of cigarette smoke, the incorporation of cigarette smoke condensate into intrapulmonary implants of beeswax pellets yielded high incidences of pulmonary carcinomas at the site of remarkably small amounts of injected condensate (Stanton *et al.*, 1972).

Urethan induces the alveologenic type of pulmonary tumor in rats, as do a number of other classes of pulmonary carcinogens including fluorenylamines, nitrosamines, quinolines, radioactive materials, and beryllium, but some of these induce a variety of other types of pulmonary cancers as well. The prolonged feeding of *N,N'*-2,7-fluorenylenebisacetamide has induced mucoepidermoid carcinoma, adenocarcinoma arising from the bronchial glands, and hemangioendothelioma (Stewart *et al.*, 1965). Chronic murine pneumonitis may significantly enhance the development of pulmonary cancers induced by *N*-nitrosoheptamethyleneimine (Schreiber *et al.*, 1972). Squamous cell carcinomas arise at deposit sites of 3-methylcholanthrene in areas of pulmonary infarction (Stanton and Blackwell, 1964) but not in healthy lung tissue. Thus preliminary tissue damage is important in the enhancement of the effects of chemical carcinogens in the lungs of rats. The same relationship has been observed in man; there is a higher frequency of pulmonary cancer in persons with pulmonary asbestosis who smoke cigarettes than in those who don't smoke.

Radioactive compounds are among the most potent and widely used pulmonary carcinogens (Pour *et al.*, 1975), among which are radionuclide gases, vapors, and particulates that may be administered by inhalation, instillation, or implantation; these agents may emit α-, β-, or γ-radiation (*AEC Monograph No. 29*, 1973). Their use has yielded valuable information on the histological types of cancers induced, their histogenesis, and dose–response relationships, despite which the determination of a threshold carcinogenic dose has not been determined. Laskin *et al.* (1970) summarize the results of their experiments on the induction of cancer of the lung in rats by the intratracheal insertion of a radioactive substance and by combination of inhalation of benzo[*a*]pyrene and exposure to sulfur dioxide by stating that these regimens induced both squamous cell carcinomas and adenocarcinomas which metastasized to kidney.

Spontaneous primary pulmonary tumors of guinea pigs are rare. Those that I (Stewart, 1966*a*) have examined have occurred singly and were classifiable as alveologenic-type tumor, similar in all respects to this neoplasm as seen in the mouse. The same histological type of pulmonary tumor arose in large numbers (up to 27 per animal) in 30% of guinea pigs receiving carcinogenic polycyclic hydrocarbons intravenously (Heston and Deringer, 1952*b*). Smaller numbers of tumors arose in fewer animals subjected to whole body γ-radiation (Lorenz *et al.*, 1954). I have not observed any of the alveologenic tumors of the guinea pig to have spread through the lung, metastasize, or convert to an undifferentiated neoplasm or sarcoma as does the alveologenic pulmonary tumor of the mouse. In their comprehensive review of the literature, Hoch-Ligeti and Argus (1970) confirmed the rare occurrence of spontaneous pulmonary tumors in guinea pigs and described the different types of neoplasms and proliferative lesions that oral administration of diethylnitrosamine and dioxane induced in this species, maintained in their laboratories. In addition to the alveologenic types of tumor, they observed large intrabronchial papillomas. They carefully distinguished these neoplasms from areas of adenomatous hyperplasia composed of mucus-secreting cells and commented on the resemblance of this latter lesion to the lesion of pulmonary adenomatosis in mice and to jaagsiekte in sheep.

In the Syrian hamster, the histological types of bronchial papilloma, squamous cell carcinoma, adenocarcinoma, and undifferentiated carcinoma may arise in the lung when animals are treated with carcinogenic polycyclic hydrocarbons given intratracheally. Montesano *et al.* (1974) have shown that combined treatment of Syrian hamsters with a low-effect dose schedule of benzo[*a*]pyrene plus ferric oxide, given intratracheally and followed by a low dose of diethylnitrosamine given systemically, resulted in a synergistic tumor response that induced many squamous cell carcinomas of the tracheobronchial tract. Each carcinogen administered singly did not at that dose induce squamous cell tumors, suggesting that low-level exposure to a variety of carcinogens may produce a synergistic tumor response. The implication for man is obvious. I have examined a number of sections of hamster lung showing the lesion of pulmonary adenomatosis, some florid, which had been initially misdiagnosed as mucinous adenocarcinoma.

The wild European hamster, it has been suggested, may serve as a model for human squamous cell carcinoma of the lung. This neoplasm develops spontaneously and can be induced by treatment with N-diethylnitrosamine (Mohr *et al.*, 1972).

The primary pulmonary tumors that I have examined in our colony of mastomys have all been alveologenic carcinoma. They occur in less than 10% of animals.

Rabbits are exceedingly resistant to the development of spontaneous pulmonary tumors, but these can be readily induced by chemical carcinogens (Fumio *et al.*, 1972).

6.2. Domestic Animals

Stünzi (1973) observed primary lung carcinomas in 99 or approximately 1% of 8650 dogs and in 58 or approximately 0·8% of 6960 cats which he necropsied. The corresponding age distribution was more or less the same in the dog and cat as has been reported for man, but the prevalence of the histological types of tumor differed. In the lower animals, in contrast to man, adenocarcinomas predominated, while squamous cell carcinomas were rare and the undifferentiated small-cell and large-cell types were exceedingly rare in dogs. The adenocarcinomas occurred at the age of $11\frac{1}{2}$ yr in the dog and 13 yr in the cat and there was no predilection based on sex. Stünzi (1973) classified more than 90% of the tumors in cats as adenocarcinomas and more than 80% of those in the dog as being of this histological type.

In the dog, Nielsen (1966, 1970) described more than 80% of the papillary glandular tumors of the lung he observed or others reported in the literature as being composed of two distinguishable types. One he described as composed of low cuboidal cells resembling those of the epithelium lining the terminal bronchiole. This tumor, he believes, pursues a benign biological course and so may be mislabeled when classified with the carcinomas. The other tumor type he describes as composed of tall cylindrical cells. This tumor pursues a malignant course and may invade lung tissue and metastasize. Most of the lung tumors induced in dogs by the inhalation of radionuclides or by whole-body radiation have been multicentric, peripherally located bronchoalveolar-type neoplasms, although other types including well-differentiated and anaplastic mucinous carcinomas, squamous cell carcinomas, and small-cell carcinomas have occurred (Park *et al.*, 1966; Andersen and Guttman, 1966; Howard, 1970).

6.3. Cattle

In a review of the literature several years ago, Dahme (1966) collected 123 case reports of lung tumors of cattle. The majority were epithelial types, and in descending order of frequency were typed as adenocarcinoma, squamous cell carcinoma, scirrhous carcinoma, microcellular carcinoma, and adenoma. Many experienced veterinary pathologists, including Nielsen (1970), have expressed skepticism about the validity of case reports of primary cancer of the lung from abattoir material, because of the likelihood that primary cancers of other sites that may have metastasized to lung were overlooked. Two rather common tumors of cattle, adenocarcinoma of the uterus and squamous cell carcinoma of the eye, may yield pulmonary metastasis. Nielsen (1970) categorized the relatively few, well-documented, malignant pulmonary tumors as adenocarcinoma and undifferentiated medullary carcinoma, both of which types spread throughout the lung tissue and metastasize to lymph nodes. A benign neoplasm of young animals that some have categorized as hamartoma consists of multifocal adenomas composed of mucin-secreting columnar cells that possibly originate from bronchial mucous glands. Migaki *et al.* (1974) described and illustrated this lesion as observed in eight cattle aged 1–2 yr. Cattle rather frequently develop diffuse alveolar cell hyperplasia or adenomatosis (Seaton, 1958), as a reaction to inflammation due to parasites, ingestion of poisonous plants, or inhalation of noxious gases or fungal spores. As with somewhat similar lesions of other species, this lesion of alveolar epithelialization may be mistakenly diagnosed as cancer.

Primary pulmonary cancers are rare in sheep, goats, and horses, while in swine Nielsen (1970) was unable to find a single acceptable description in the literature. Some of the cases reported in sheep in the past have been rejected as being inadequately differentiated from pulmonary adenomatosis or from proliferative changes in lung tissue in the vicinity of parasites. The sheep is unique in developing two different hyperplastic proliferative diseases of the lung caused by infectious agents with long incubation periods, from 1 to 3 yr. One, jaagsiekte or adenomatosis, is a multifocal papillary tumorlike lesion which progresses slowly and which eventually kills by suffocation. Electron microscopic studies of the cells of pulmonary adenomatosis of Awassi sheep showed that they are derived from type B alveolar cells (Perk *et al.*, 1971). Some claim that the process may metastasize (Nobel *et al.*, 1969; Cuba-Caparo *et al.*, 1961). The etiology has not been clarified as yet but a herpesvirus is suspected as the cause. The second ovine pulmonary disease, maedi, falls within the category of slow latent infections; a myxovirus has been isolated from the lesions. The disease is characterized by progressive interstitial infiltration of lymphoreticular cells that eventually kill the animal, also by suffocation. Both jaagsiekte and maedi are contagious to other sheep but not to man or other species and each exhibits a specific geographic distribution.

The horse develops a comparable hyperplastic proliferative process of the alveolar and bronchiolar cells described as equine jaagsiekte that may progress to fibrosis and lead to emphysema. In Australia, the cause of the disease has been attributed to the effects of the alkaloids of ingested *Crotalaria crispa*, which alkaloids, when injected into rabbits, induced pulmonary adenomatosis (Gardiner *et al.*, 1965).

6.4. Zoo Animals

From 1901 to 1963, more than 19,000 captive wild animals and birds came to necropsy at the Philadelphia Zoo. Originally cancer of the lung was diagnosed in 36 animals, and of these I was able to examine histological preparations from 31 (Stewart, 1966*a*). The diseases in these 31 animals were 14 adenocarcinomas in 11 birds of the family Anatidae, a silver pheasant, a red jungle fowl, and a coypu; one squamous cell carcinoma in a North American otter; one undifferentiated small-cell carcinoma in a Java sparrow; one alveologenic carcinoma in a striped skunk; two pleural mesotheliomas in a Cape hunting dog and a clouded leopard; ten adenomatosis or squamous metaplasia or both in a red fox, puma, North American otter (also had squamous cell carcinoma of lung), squirrel monkey, peafowl, African eared vulture, Chinese myna, two toucan barbets, and a rabbit-eared bandicoot; one tuberculosis in a civet; one pneumonia in a kangaroo; and one metastatic renal carcinoma of the lung in a red wolf. Thus 11 or more than one-half of the pulmonary cancers in this group occurred in birds of the family Anatidae. Six were either shoveler ducks or redhead ducks. The majority of the birds had been on exhibit at the Philadelphia Zoo for relatively long periods of time so that one may safely assume that their exposure to hypothetical carcinogens could have taken place while they were in captivity. The birds of the family Anatidae merit careful study to determine whether they have a genetic susceptibility to pulmonary cancer, whether special circumstances at the Philadelphia Zoo contributed to the induction of this neoplasm, or whether both of these factors played a role.

There is a pronounced contrast between the adenocarcinomas, with their relatively uniform structural pattern, that developed in the wild ducks of the Philadelphia Zoo and the diversified histological types of tumors that Rigdon (1966) induced in the domestic white Pekin duck. Rigdon classified the pulmonary tumors in the 29 of 66 ducks that received intratracheal instillations of 3-methylcholanthrene in Tween 80 as ganglioneuroma, neurofibroma, hemangioendothelioma, osteofibroma, fibrosarcoma, adenoosteoma, adenocarcinoma, adenoacanthoma, carcinosarcoma, and embryonal carcinoma. There is no record, that I know of, of such a wide range of histological types of pulmonary neoplasm having been induced in any species of animal other than the duck by the instillation of a carcinogen into the trachea or by any other single experimental procedure designed to induce lung tumors. The large variety of different histological types of lung cancer that develop in ducks following the intratracheal instillation of a carcinogen, by comparison with the few types that this treatment induces in mammals, is dependent in large part on the differences in the anatomy of the respiratory tract in these two contrasting classes of animals. The duck possesses nine air sacs, which may hold insufflated fluids, the lungs attach directly to the thoracic cage, and a muscular diaphragm is absent; there are thus direct communications between the respiratory tract and the skeleton. Hence in the duck insufflated carcinogen has the opportunity to come in contact with many more varieties of tissues than in mammals.

It would be highly desirable from a practical point of view to have available laboratory models of the different histological types of human lung cancers for tests of suspected pulmonary carcinogens and for other purposes, because lung cancers are among the most important neoplasms developing in man. During the past several decades, the reported incidence of respiratory cancer has increased at an alarming rate and a variety of environmental pollutants are suspected as causative factors. But, with the possible exception of the spontaneous squamous cell carcinoma of the wild European hamster, no spontaneous lung cancers in animals exactly replicate the histological types and clinical courses of the different types of pulmonary cancers of man. There are many differences. In lower animals, spontaneous lung cancers are likely to be multiple, multicentric, and peripherally located. They generally originate from alveoli, bronchioles, and small bronchi, and they grow more by expansion than by infiltration. An adenomatous pattern prevails in the lung tumors of lower animals, but generally the glandular cells do not secrete mucus. Squamous cell carcinomas are infrequent in all lower animals except the wild European hamster. Only once did I diagnose an oat cell carcinoma and that was in the lungs of a Java sparrow from the Philadelphia Zoo. We are, of course, ignorant of the origin and histopathogenesis of the oat cell carcinoma of man. Pulmonary carcinoids, with the exception of those reported by Schiller (1970) in four dogs and in one cat, have not been reported in animals, nor have other so-called bronchial adenomas.

In lower animals with lung tumors the sex ratio is more nearly equal. The disease progresses more slowly than in man; mice, in particular, may live a long time and in apparent good health even with their lungs riddled with multiple tumors. Generally fewer lower animals than human beings develop lung tumors, the incidence being negligible in rats, hamsters, guinea pigs, large domestic animals, rabbits, and the domestic fowl. Yet nearly 100% of mice of some inbred strains spontaneously develop alveologenic carcinoma in old age and close to 1% of necropsied old dogs and old cats may exhibit primary pulmonary cancer. By the use of various carcinogens and different experimental methods it has been possible to induce squamous cell carcinomas, mucus-producing adenocarcinomas, hemangioendotheliomas, and undifferentiated- and mixed-cell types of cancers in several species of animals, but these fall far short of duplicating the biological characteristics and clinical course of lung cancers in man. In the cat, the pulmonary tumors that have been carefully studied are nearly all adenocarcinomas. In the dog, the glandular type of tumor also prevails and outranks by a wide margin squamous cell carcinoma, adenocanthoma, and undifferentiated-cell carcinoma. Most of the spontaneous and induced pulmonary tumors of the dog are peripherally located in the lung and are classified as alveolar or bronchioalveolar in origin and a large proportion pursue a benign course. Among the 31 initially diagnosed primary cancers of the lung of captive wild mammals and birds from Philadelphia Zoo, I could confirm the diagnosis in only 19 of these, showing how frequently mistakes are made in this field of comparative pathology. The nonneoplastic proliferative lesions of the zoo animals, initially and mistakenly diagnosed as cancer, were pulmonary adenomatosis and squamous metaplasia of alveoli and bronchi and they occurred in a wide range of wild species. Comparable nonneoplastic proliferative lesions may become widespread and destructive of lung tissue in most domestic and laboratory animals and these lesions need to be distinguished with care from genuine cancers.

7. Tumors of the Liver

7.1. Mouse

7.1.1. Common Spontaneous Hepatic Tumor

Evidence attesting to the malignant neoplastic nature of the common spontaneous hepatic tumor of the mouse was first presented nearly 60 years ago (Murray, 1908); this was followed 7 years later by a report of its metastasis (Slye *et al.*, 1915) and 20 years later by a report of its transplantability to other mice (Strong and Smith, 1936). Subsequent studies have continued to confirm these acceptable criteria of a malignant neoplasm in properly executed experiments. More than 30 years ago, Edwards *et al.* (1942) adduced additional evidence from elegant cytological studies that the spontaneous hepatic lesion of the mouse is a genuine neoplasm and advanced cogent arguments that contradicted those advanced by others who contended that the lesion is a hyperplastic nodule of regenerated tissue or a developmental anomaly. Among the arguments advanced then and now to imply the nonneoplastic nature of the hepatic growth is the high degree of differentiation of the cells, together with their definite tendency to form liverlike cords alternating with endothelial-lined sinuses and the capacity for storing fat and glycogen. That the lesion is regenerative in character is difficult to reconcile with the absence of any demonstrable damage in liver tissue away from the hepatoma. The fact that the lesion is seen in mice consistently after middle age contradicts the idea of a congenital anomaly. Moreover, the fact that the cells may be well-differentiated does not rule out neoplasm, since the metastasis of spontaneous hepatic cell carcinomas of man, the cow, and other species, and of certain of the induced liver carcinomas of the rat, may closely resemble normal hepatic cells.

Although the cells of the hepatic tumor of the mouse may closely resemble normal hepatic cells in sections stained with hematoxylin and eosin, special stains reveal that both the golgi apparatus and the mitochondria are profoundly unlike those respective subcellular constituents of the cells of normal liver or regenerating liver following hepatectomy or chemical injury. Indeed, the golgi apparatus of the cells of the mouse tumor is virtually indistinguishable from that of cells of induced hepatic carcinomas of the rat. Functionally, fat and glycogen are natural products of mouse hepatic cells and the retention of these functions by neoplastic hepatic cells is not surprising. Cells of other tissues may function similarly when they convert to cancer, as, for example, production mucus of by intestinal tumors, keratin by cutaneous tumors, and hormones by endocrine tumors. Thus the evidence adduced by these early studies clearly supports the view that the spontaneous hepatic tumor of the mouse is a genuine cancer, although it has not laid to rest the temptation to revive the arguments against this conception.

The gross appearance of hepatic tumors is rather uniform. They are generally visible on the surface and exhibit a rounded, elevated, lumpy, and bumpy growth, the larger ones often exhibiting a central umbilicate depression. They are covered by the original capsule of the liver, so that ordinarily they are not adherent to the surrounding viscera. They are softer and more homogeneous than the normal liver tissue but rarely cystic. Those of any considerable size may be pedunculated. Small tumors are the precursors of the large ones and the smallest appear simply as nodules within the liver substance first revealed on section of the organ. The cut surface may show fusion of adjacent nodules. The nodules are frequently solitary, or number two or three per mouse, but may be multiple, amounting to as many as a dozen in the same liver. They may vary in size from a few millimeters to as large as 20 or 30 mm in greatest diameter; they may thus become larger than the original liver, distending the abdomen and being easily palpable through the abdominal wall. Commonly they are lighter colored than the normal liver—brownish, yellow, straw-colored, pinkish, or whitish. When richly vascularized, they appear mostly red or hemorrhagic.

Microscopically the spontaneous hepatic tumor consists essentially of a circumscribed area or nodular growth or tumor mass of liver cells, differing from normal tissue by the variability in size and staining reactions of the cells, the irregularity in the arrangement of the cords of liver cells, the absence of regular relation to central veins, the lack of lobule formation, and especially the absence of bile ducts or other evidences of portal systems within the lesion (Lippincott *et al.*, 1942). They are never encapsulated by connective tissue but are often marked off by a surrounding zone of compressed and atrophied liver cells in which the normal reticulum fibres may be condensed. The expansive character of the lesions is usually marked. Occasionally, the tumor cells appear to be continuous with apparently normal hepatic cords at the periphery of the growth, a condition which human liver cell tumors may duplicate. Frequently and in particular with the smaller ones, the tumor is so well differentiated and reproduces so closely the cordlike pattern of normal liver tissue that at first glance the lesion may be overlooked. A conspicuous feature of most of the growths, however, is the formation of extremely large liver cells, sometimes multinuclear but more often with a single giant nucleus. The sinusoids present the same relation to the tumor cells as they do in the normal liver, although often they are much wider and irregular in size and shape, forming large blood spaces. Mitotic figures are infrequent in the better-differentiated growths. Fatty change, glycogen deposition, or intracellular vacuoles of an unidentified nature may, when present, differ in quantity and distribution from those of the surrounding liver. The amount of connective tissue in the tumors is usually minimal. Other tumors vary from the well-differentiated tumors in the degree of deviation from normal hepatic cells and liver structure. In these, the cords of tumor cells are more often multinuclear, with enlarged and nucleoli eosinophilic inclusions. They are more irregular in arrangement, often in sheet formation, and more subject to retrogressive change and hemorrhage; atypical nuclear forms are common. They may show areas of papilliform and adenoid formation of tumor cells. Some of the hepatic cancers induced in mice by heavy doses of powerful carcinogens may exhibit all the cytological and structural abnormalities with much necrosis that characterize the more malignant hepatic cancers of rats similarly treated. Although spontaneous hepatomas of the mouse do not metastasize within the liver, those induced by diethylnitrosamine may invade the portal vessels (Kyriazis *et al.*, 1974). In none of the livers of mice bearing spontaneous tumors is there ever any cirrhosis or other evidence of any particular inflammatory or other pathological condition acting as a predisposing cause of the tumor. Indeed, in untreated mice of any age cirrhosis is so exceedingly rare as to be virtually nonexistent. The situation is different in man, in whom liver cancer is frequently associated with cirrhosis, especially in the peoples living in sub-Saharan Africa.

Andervont and Dunn (1952) noted that many spontaneous hepatic tumors of the mouse are composed, especially at the margins, of cells having smaller nuclei and a small amount of cytoplasm that is considerably more basophilic than that of the normal cells. Nests of larger cells are frequently found within a hepatoma which compress the surrounding hepatoma cells, much as a hepatoma compresses normal liver tissue. This is referred to as a tumor within a tumor. Focal areas made up entirely of small cells are usual, rather than a haphazard intermingling of cells of different shapes. Miyaji (1952) found that the volume of the nuclei of hepatoma cells showed roughly the same proportionate variation in size—i.e., in a 1 : 2 : 4 : 8 ratio—as do normal liver cell nuclei, and the differences in size are not haphazard. The cytoplasm of the hepatoma cells may contain hyaline inclusion bodies (waxy bodies), and intranuclear inclusion bodies occasionally occur. The nuclear inclusions are invaginations of the nuclear membrane by histologically demonstrable cytoplasmic components (Edwards *et al.*, 1942; Edwards and Dalton, 1942; Leduc and Wilson, 1959*a,c*; Liebelt *et al.*, 1971). Study of these objects by electron microscopy and histochemistry has indicated that the cytoplasmic inclusion bodies are intracisternal proteins with relatively little polysaccharide and varying amounts of phospholipid but with no detectable neutral fat or nucleic acids. As stated in the foregoing, although the neoplastic cells may closely resemble normal hepatic cells in sections stained with hematoxylin and eosin, special stains reveal that both the golgi apparatus and the mitochondria are profoundly dissimilar to those respective subcellular constituents of the cells of normal liver or of regenerating liver following hepatectomy or chemical injury (Edwards *et al.*, 1942).

The ability of the spontaneous hepatoma to metastasize (Slye *et al.*, 1915) has been confirmed by many, although the frequency of metastasis is usually low,

often in the range of 1–2%, even in animals allowed to live out their full life span.
Gorer (1940) observed one pulmonary metastasis among 17 male and female
untreated CBA mice aged 11 months, and Turusov *et al.* (1973*a*) found one
metastasis among 97 untreated CF-1 male mice shown to have hepatomas at
necropsy at the average age of 114 wk. In the DDT-treated males that developed
hepatomas and that lived on an average of 84–104 wk, 1.4% had metastasis
(Tomatis *et al.*, 1972; Turusov *et al.*, 1973*a*). In a study by Thorpe and Walker
(1973) in which noninbred mice of both sexes ingested a diet containing 10 ppm of
dieldrin, they found pulmonary metastasis in three of 24 males (12+%) and in 17
of 28 females (60+%). In a study by Geliatly (1975) in which inbred C57BL male
and female mice ingested, for 47 wk, a diet containing butter yellow in the amount
of 0.06% dietary level, he reported pulmonary metastasis in three of 23 animals
(13%), A study of the metastatic rate of liver tumors induced in mice by
diethylnitrosamine revealed that upon detailed histological examination of the
lungs 22% had metastasis (Kyriazis *et al.*, 1974). The tumors metastasized mainly
by the hematogenous route, but the pulmonary deposits were not always confined
within blood vessels.

Over the years, variable results have attended the transplantation of the
common hepatic tumor of the mouse, although now more than 38 years have
passed since Strong and Smith (1936) first demonstrated this possibility. Various
factors have accounted for subsequent failures: the number of recipient mice into
which the primary tumor was transplanted was too small; noninbred or hybrid,
instead of inbred, strains of mice were used; the receipients were not held long
enough for the transplants to grow to palpable size; different sites for the
transplants were used; and insufficient attention was given to sex, for it is well
known that male grafts of a variety of tissues to female hosts may be rejected.
Hence, one can understand why, with the failures encountered and the successes
achieved, investigators were surprised and puzzled that lesions they had classified
histologically as highly malignant hepatic carcinomas failed to transplant, while
others that looked more innocent did transplant.

In their definitive studies of the transplantation of spontaneous and induced
hepatic tumors of the mouse, Andervont and Dunn (1952, 1955) used inbred
mouse strains C3H and BALB/c and succeeded in transplanting nine of ten
spontaneous tumors, 28 of 30 tumors induced with carbon tetrachloride, and all
of six tumors induced with *o*-aminoazotoluene. They carried in serial passage
many of the transplants for more than six transplant generations. The latent
period, before the first generation transplant grew to palpable size, varied from 2
months to 1 yr or more. The slow growth of some transplantable tumors is
consistent with the appearance of the primary tumor late in life and its
relatively slow rate of evolution in older mice. During serial passage, most
transplanted tumors studied by Andervont and Dunn (1952, 1955) exhibited
increased growth rates and shorter latent periods; a number of them transformed
in part or entirely into neoplasms they classified as adenocarcinoma, anaplastic
carcinoma, carcinosarcoma, fibrosarcoma, and osteogenic sarcoma. Some transformed to completely undifferentiated neoplasms that these investigators could

not further classify histologically. These switches in histological pattern evolved on transplantation, irrespective of the histological appearance of the primary neoplasm. Moreover, their histological study of the primary hepatic neoplasms revealed no consistent differences in pattern between those that transplanted successfully and those that failed to grow. Hence they concluded, as others have in comparative studies of morphology and biological behavior of tumors of other sites, that malignant growth is not necessarily associated with dedifferentiation, that retention of virtually complete differentiation is compatible with the malignant neoplastic state and is no certain indication of benignancy. The thoroughness of the transplantation studies of Andervont and Dunn (1952, 1955) has not been matched by any subsequent studies, although segments of their results have been confirmed.

Thus Leduc and Wilson (1959*b*), like Andervont and Dunn (1952, 1955), could not distinguish histologically between those CCL_4-induced hepatic tumors that transplanted and those that did not. They observed in addition that the longer the mice lived following the initiating doses of CCL_4 and the greater the size of the tumor, the more likely it was to transplant. This result is consistent with, as stated above, the appearance of the spontaneous primary tumors late in life and their relatively slow rate of evolution in older animals. In man, also, time plays a decisive role in the progression of many cancers, as discussed in the foregoing.

The study of Reuber (1971) is vitiated by his use of hybrid mice, both as the source for the spontaneous primary tumors and as recipients for transplantation. He used C3H × Y hybrid mice to transplant autologously and isologously. He reported that only the primary tumors that he had classified histologically as hepatocellular carcinomas grew on transplantation. Those that did not grow he classified as areas of hyperplasia or nodules of hyperplasia. Cancer investigators have known since the development of strains of inbred mice earlier in this century by Little and Strong (1924) that valid results of tumor transplantation from one animal to another must be based on the use of syngeneic animals. Moreover, when one attempts autologous transplantation he must be aware of Leduc and Wilson's observation that hepatic tumors require a certain period of time in their natural habitat, the liver, before neoplastic progression has reached the point at which these tumors will always continue to grow when disturbed by removal to another site. Hence Reuber's (1971) attempt to discredit the findings of Andervont and Dunn (1952, 1955) must be weighed against the quality of the two experiments: the use of inbred mice by the latter and the use of hybrid mice by the former.

Thorpe and Walker (1973) used the results of transplantation to devise a histological classification scheme of the common hepatic tumor of the mouse as hyperplastic foci, type (a) growth, a simple nodular growth of parenchymal cells, and type (b) growth, with areas of papilliform and adenoid formations of tumor cells. Within a liver containing multiple confluent nodules they found it difficult to sort out these different histological patterns because hyperplastic foci and type (a) growths might be present in the same or other lobes where type (b) tumors were also found. They were able to transplant successfully only those lesions they had classified as the type (b) growth and not the others, and so concluded that the

others were simply hyperplastic lesions and not genuine neoplasms. However,
their results, like those of Reuber (1971), must be weighed against the fact that,
like him, they based their results of transplantation on the use of random-bred
mice and not syngeneic animals.

Geliatly (1975) classified the common liver tumors of the mouse into three
categories: type I, well-differentiated foci of hypertrophy and nodular hyperplasia; type II, a heterogeneous mixed group that evolved from type I; and type
III, which he considered to be cancer. In a transplantation experiment involving
11 untreated donor animals and 64 recipient animals carried out in his laboratory
over a 1-yr period with inbred C57BL mice, four type I and two type II lesions
failed to grow, while three type II and two type III lesions did grow when the
donor tissue was inserted beneath the capsule of the kidney of the syngeneic
C57BL mice. A similar short-term transplantation study was carried on for
6-10 wk. Obvious deficiencies in these studies are that too few tumors were put to
test and the experiment conducted was too limited in time. Moreover, the renal
subcapsular site has been too infrequently employed for the transplantation of
tumors to permit comparisons with the results obtained by using other conventional sites such as the subcutaneous and intramuscular tissues in the host animal
as employed by Andervont and Dunn (1952, 1955). It was, however, on the basis
of this histological scheme that Geliatly (1975) classified the lesions arising in mice
that had ingested the food additives Flavour G and Flavour F. Compared to
controls, the number of mice with nodules and the number of nodules per mouse
were both greater in the test animals, but since most of them were type I nodules
Geliatly concluded that the agents tested were not carcinogenic!

Akamatsu and associates (for references, see Akamatsu et al., 1969) have had
considerable experience in the transplantation of spontaneous and induced
hepatic cell tumors of mice. Biochemical studies of one such tumor revealed
enzymatic activities similar to those of normal liver parenchymal cells, and these
activities persisted after 4 yr of transplantation through 15 transplant generations
(Akamatsu et al., 1969).

There are therefore two views that have been expressed about this subject. One
is that the tumors—or lesions as some prefer to designate them—that are rather
well-differentiated histologically remain static, while other lesions that are less
differentiated may also arise. The other view is that with time the well-
differentiated lesions progress through stages to biologically less-differentiated
lesions, and this view has support from the transplant data of Andervont et al.
(1952, 1955) and Leduc and Wilson (1959b).

A number of factors influence the induction, retardation, and incidence of
hepatic tumors. These include strain and sex of the mouse, diet, obesity,
overfeeding, underfeeding, and ablation of endocrine organs. Hypophysectomy
decreases the tumor frequency. The frequency of tumors increase with longevity
and longevity is based in part on the quality of the diet and proper hygienic care of
the animals, and the control of infections and infestation with ectoparasites. The
tumor is more frequent in males than females, in obese and overfed mice than in
those that are underfed. Different diets affect the incidence in different directions.

A number of carcinogens induce the tumors and decrease the latent period, among which are carbon tetrachloride, chloroform, aldrin, dieldrin, DDT, and urethan, as well as some of the azo dyes and nitroso compounds. Most investigators who have studied CCL_4-induced tumors have classified them histologically as well differentiated. This treatment induces severe cirrhosis in the remainder of the liver in which Leduc and Wilson (1959b) grossly identified foci that they classified as nodular hyperplastic lesions, and that regressed and disappeared upon cessation of the carcinogenic regimen, while the hepatomas persisted and enlarged. The feeding of butter yellow and other hepatic carcinogens, in addition to inducing multiple, large, invasive, undifferentiated-appearing hepatic tumors, may induce lesions of adenofibrosis (Kimbrough and Linder, 1974), as well as bile retention and degeneration resulting in anemia, ascites, and early death.

As has so frequently happened with so many spontaneous tumors of the mouse, the first indication of a genetic influence on hepatic tumors was reported by Slye *et al.* (1915). Since then others have studied genetic influences in more refined genetic material and in great depth. The tumor occurs in a varying, though usually low, incidence in a number of inbred strains of mice (Smith *et al.*, 1973); Geliatly, 1975). Strain C57BL has a low tumor incidence, while strains CBA and C3H are high tumor strains (Andervont, 1950a). Andervont and Dunn (1962) found hepatomas in 4.9% of wild house mice raised in captivity. Deringer (1959) was the first to report an exceedingly high incidence: 91% tumors in males and 58% in virgin females in C3HeB mice, derived by transferring ova from strain C3H to strain C57BL females to remove the mammary tumor virus (MTV), thus allowing the mice to live out their life span. Genetic studies continued by Heston and Vlahakis (1961) showed that the lethal yellow gene, A^y, increased susceptibility to the point that all male A^yA F_1 hybrid mice surviving for 16 months developed hepatomas. In a further study with the viable yellow mutation (A^{vy}), which like the lethal yellow (A^y) mutation increases the body weight considerably and induces a yellow coat color, Heston and Vlahakis (1968) developed the substrain (C3H-A^{vy}fB), which they had freed of the mammary tumor virus by a combination of caesarean section and foster-nursing: they found that 98.8% of the males of the parent strain C3H-A^{vy} developed hepatomas by 12 months of age and 96.9% of the females of the substrain C3H-A^{vy}fB freed of the MTV developed tumors by 16 months of age. In a group of C3HfB mice used as controls for another experiment, Heston *et al.* (1973) found hepatomas in 75% of females just under 2 yr of age. Mice of strain C3H-A^{vy} and substrain C3H-A^{vy}fB developed far fewer liver tumors when bred and maintained in Australia, suggesting possible dietary or other influences (Sabine *et al.*, 1973). For further discussion of this observation, see p. 348. Rowlatt *et al.* (1973) demonstrated that simple dietary restriction can reduce or abolish the development of hepatomas in strain C3H-A^{vy} mice.

It is evident from the foregoing that for years following Murray's 1908 report of the first observation of the common hepatic tumor of the mouse, this small neoplasm was the object of serious scientific study by those interested in the pursuit of knowledge for its own sake. Their studies resulted in the accumulation

of a large body of facts dealing with the morphology of the spontaneous and
induced tumors, the metastases and transplants, the characteristics of the subcellular constituents, the incidence in different inbred strains of mice, and the
influence of genetics, age, sex, diet, castration, and hormones. These scientific
studies proved this lesion to be cancer. Then suddenly all this changed. This small
tumor, often not as large as the tip of a man's finger, began to engage the attention
of wealthy and powerful industrial concerns, the chemical and pharmaceutical
companies in particular, whose products including drugs, chemicals, food additives, and pesticides, when subjected to carcinogenicity testing in the mouse,
might induce this tumor. Examples are aldrin, dieldrin, and DDT. Two questions
were asked: Is the common liver tumor of the mouse a genuine malignant
neoplasm? Should a chemical compound that induces the common liver tumor of
the mouse but tumors at no other site in this species, and no tumors at any site in
other species of laboratory animal, be banned from the human environment
because the agent under test poses a carcinogenic hazard for man? There are
those who have said yes and those who have said no to one or the other or both of
these questions.

Train (1974), in prohibiting the environmental use of aldrin and dieldrin
(except for three minor uses), based his decision on the testimony of expert
witnesses who are recognized authorities on carcinogenesis and carcinogenicity
testing. A crucial piece of testimony given by one of the experts, Dr. U. Saffiotti of
the National Cancer Institute, was that the proposition is unacceptable, that the
induction of liver tumors in mice is a tissue response that is not representative of
carcinogenic effects such as are seen in other organs and other species. Moreover, Train (1974) held that there is no distinction between the induction of so-
called benign or malignant tumors in determining the carcinogenicity of a
compound. Butler (1971) agreed that the ability of the hepatoma to transplant
suggests that the lesion is neoplastic but not necessarily carcinomatous, since
according to him transplantation *per se* cannot be considered an absolute indication of malignancy. Roe (1968) in a paper entitled "Carcinogenesis and Sanity"
argued that evidence for carcinogenicity must be sought in more than one
biological system since an increase of a type of tumor that arises commonly in a test
species is suggestive of a cocarcinogenic rather than a carcinogenic effect. This
opinion was later expressed by Roe and Grant (1970) and by Grasso and
Crampton (1972). Fouts (1970) argued that the mouse is an unsatisfactory test
animal because hepatic microsomal enzyme inducers, such as phenobarbitone
and DDT, induce similar responses in man and the rat and a dissimilar response in the mouse. Some have dangerously proposed that a critical assessment of the carcinogenic potential to a man of a chemical compound, where
variations in results between test species exist, can be obtained only from
epidemiological studies in man exposed to high levels of the chemical for long
periods. If this suggestion were to be taken seriously, then in view of the known
lengths of the latent periods of different industrial cancers in man, such a
wait-and-see attitude might well require a long period of many years before the
onset of an epidemic of cancer due to the chemical in question manifested itself.

Geliatly (1975) deplored the use of the term "hepatoma" and instead adocated the use of the term "hepatic parenchymal nodule" as though a change in name had the power to alter the nature of the lesion. He advanced the concept that the common liver tumor of the mouse represents a broad spectrum covering focal, nonneoplastic, cellular proliferation (nodular hyperplasia), benign parenchymal neoplasm (liver cell adenoma), and finally malignant parenchymal neoplasms (hepatocellular carcinoma). In analyzing the carcinogenic relevance of these different categories of hepatic lesions of the mouse to man, he classified 4-dimethylaminoazobenzene as a powerful carcinogen for man because it induced hepatocellular carcinomas in the mouse according to his classification. By contrast, when he fed the food additives Flavour G and Flavour F he classified the increased hepatic lesions caused by these agents almost exclusively as small nodules of hyperplasia.

The reasoning employed by some who classify the mouse hepatoma as a hyperplastic lesion is difficult to understand unless they mean to imply that such a lesion is a stage in the evolution of cancer. But not all authors imply this meaning. Geliatly (1975) is firm in his conviction that some hepatic lesions of the mouse are hyperplasias to begin with, and remain so and do not progress to cancer during the lifetime of the animal, but he adduced no convincing evidence to support this contention. As with many neoplasms of man and animals, the early stages of cancer may be innocuous-looking cellular proliferations. As the neoplastic condition progresses to its final stages, the lesion takes on patterns or appearances that pathologists commonly recognize as cancer. What some do not appreciate is that the process is cancer from its earliest inception.

All these various and varying opinions and the huge sums of money that are involved have changed the emphasis in the studies of the mouse liver tumor from a scientific pursuit to a contentious, legal matter. This has led to violent disputes among experimental pathologists, to arbitrary actions by regulatory federal agencies, and to litigation in the courts. In a recent court case, the judge was so confused by the conflicting testimony of the expert witnesses that he threatened to order them to fetch their histological preparations and microscopes into court so that he, the lawyers for the contending parties, and the jurors might look for themselves through the compound lenses of the microscope and make up their own minds about the neoplastic or nonneoplastic, malignant or nonmalignant nature of this common hepatic tumor of the mouse. As might be expected, this threat threw the scientific community into confusion. My conservative pathologist friends began to write memos calculated to dissuade the judge from implementing the threat. They pointed out that this had never happened before in a civil suit and if carried out would establish a precedent that could lead to all manner of mischief. I argued on the other side. I pointed out this could produce a hilarious scene. Picture the judge, in flowing robes, slipping down from the bench and adjusting his eyeglasses before peering through the microscope for a brief exposure to the practice of oncology. Standing by is the clerk of the court preparing a system for the proper indexing of the histological slides and for recording the diagnoses, first those made by the judge, followed by those made by the contending attorneys, and in turn those by the 12 jurors, some of whom may not have completed the sixth grade of elementary school. A clever librettist like W. S. Gilbert, viewing this hilarious scene, could produce a first rate comic opera comparable to his "Trial by Jury." But my argument went unheeded. Instead, my friends the pathologists, who were so upset that they failed to see the humor of the situation, proceeded with their memos which finally dissuaded the judge. Thus when the judge backed away from his threat the opportunity was lost to permit the court to decide once and for all the neoplastic or nonneoplastic, the benign or malignant nature of the lowly mouse liver tumor, a lesion as I have said that often is not as large as the tip of a man's finger.

7.1.2. Hepatoblastoma

The *hepatoblastoma*, although it occurs spontaneously and may be induced by treatment, must be considered apart from the common hepatic tumor of the mouse because of its specific histological appearances and its biological behavior. Turusov *et al.* (1973b) have emphasized its resemblance to the hepatoblastoma of man. When one considers that the common hepatic tumor of the mouse was first described almost 70 years ago, in 1908, it is surprising that the hepatoblastoma was not identified until 1959, 51 years later, especially since during the intervening years a vast literature had accumulated on mouse liver tumors. Dr. M. K. Deringer identified the first tumor in a (YBR × AKR)F$_1$ mouse with the lethal yellow gene (A^y), and Dr. T. B. Dunn, who examined the histological sections, described the tumor as an unusual liver tumor with rosette formations resembling tumors that occur in human infants (Deringer, 1970). Turosov *et al.* (1973b) described the pathological and biological features of hepatoblastoma which arose in 99 mice, and reviewed previous publications in which this neoplasm had been correctly diagnosed (Rice, 1973) and incorrectly diagnosed as cholangiocarcinoma (Reuber, 1967) and cholangioma (Vlahakis and Heston, 1971). Rice (1973) induced the tumor by prenatal feeding with ethylnitrosourea. The tumors, described by Reuber (1967) and Vlahakis and Heston (1971), arose spontaneously. Of the 99 hepatoblastomas described by Turusov *et al.* (1973b), 5 occurred in CF-1 mice, males only; 0.9% of these arose in untreated mice and 3.8% in mice fed DDT. Of the 75 tumors, 15 metastasized to the lungs and in one mouse also to a medistinal lymph node and wall of the bladder. The 24 hepatoblastomas found in both sexes of untreated (YBR × AKR)F$_1$ mice and (DBA/2 × YBR)F$_1$ mice represented a frequency of 6% of hepatic tumors in each group (Deringer, 1970). All of the hepatoblastomas were found in old animals, and in those adequately necropsied invariably associated with the common type of hepatoma.

The hepatoblastomas measure 1–1.5 cm in diameter and consist of red, grayish, or brownish nodules, with cysts and areas of necrosis or large hemorrhagic cysts with thick grayish walls.

Histologically, the hepatoblastomas found within or adjacent to the common type of mouse hepatoma are readily distinguished by the deep basophilic coloration of the neoplastic cells. The basic unit is an organoid complex composed of a central vascular channel lined with flat endothelium and containing blood elements. The channel is surrounded by several layers of elongated, hyperchromatic, deeply staining tumor cells arranged radially and/or concentrically. These cells resemble embryonal hepatic cells. At the periphery, a few layers of elongated cells separate one organoid complex from another. In most areas, the cells are arranged in rows, rosettes, sheets, or ribbons. Some tumor areas consist of thick trabecular or cordlike structures separated by sinusoidal spaces. The cells here are small, with round, less hyperchromatic nuclei and relatively more cytoplasm which stains acidophilically. These cells resemble fetal hepatocytes. Large solid masses of cells, in no particular arrangement, exhibiting a high mitotic index, are mingled with dark spindle-shaped cellular elements. Cavernous channels with a thin endothelial lining are frequent in most tumors. Sometimes the hepatoblastoma is encapsulated by fibrous tissue, while at other times neoplastic cells invade the surrounding tissues including both adjacent liver tissue and the tissue of other hepatomas. Thick septa transverse the tumor, and osteoid and bone have been identified. Regressive changes consist of hemorrhage, necrosis, calcareous deposits, acicular spaces, and pigment. The reticular fibers vary in amount and pattern. They are sometimes confined to the periphery of the organoid complex and at other times are seen among the tumor cells. With appropriate methods, bile canaliculi can be identified between rows or cords of tumor cells of various shapes and sizes.

The hepatoblastoma of the mouse resembles in many features the hepatoblastoma of man and rat, while other features are dissimilar. The hepatoblastoma occurs at different age periods in different species, in infancy in human beings and in old age in mice. In rats, it may occur at different age periods depending on the carcinogenic regimen. More of the mouse hepatoblastomas are of the embryonic cell type, while more of the human tumors are of the fetal cell type. Bone, cartilage, and skeletal muscle elements are regularly present in human hepatoblastomas, but bone is infrequent in the mouse tumor and cartilage and muscle have not been observed. The mouse hepatoblastoma is always associated with the ordinary hepatic tumor of the mouse, whereas in man there is no other tumor associated with the hepatoblastoma.

7.2. Rat

In 1929, following his graduation from medical school and 2 years' training in pathology, the late Dr. T. Yoshida, together with his mentor, Professor T. Sasaki, embarked on studies of the pathological effects of the ingestion of o-aminoazotoluene on the epithelial cells of different organs of a number of species of animals. In the course of these studies, young Yoshida noted that cancer had developed in the livers of some rats. He published this epoch-making discovery in 1932. Probably no animal model in cancer research has been so thoroughly investigated from so may points of view, by so many scientists, in so many lands as has this model discovered by Yoshida (1932).

Becker (1974) has this to say about "Hepatoma—Nature's Model Tumor":

> Primary hepatoma is a tumor of special interest in the field of human oncology. The study of primary hepatocellular carcinoma . . . has opened exploration of the role of naturally occurring carcinogens, the fetal manifestations of malignancy and the use of an organ physiology for diagnosis and therapy. It is no surprise, therefore, that this tumor has been the focus of a wide variety of experimental programs, nor that many of the findings which resulted from these investigations appear directly applicable to man.

The present discussion is concerned primarily with the morphology of rat hepatic cancers and with histopathogenesis, with what is known or assumed to be true concerning the pathological alterations that occur in the liver of rats subjected to different experimental procedures, and with some evaluation of the relationship of various types of lesions to each other and to the cancers that are induced. Although much has been revealed, much remains to be accomplished by histological study advantageously combined with other methods of approach to clarify the steps in the process of carcinogenesis.

Spontaneous tumors are rare in the liver of untreated rats. Snell (1965) found only two in a series of 488 untreated rats of different strains necropised at 3-month intervals. Both tumors were well-differentiated trabecular carcinomas and neither had metastasized. The rats were 27 months of age. Snell did not observe any of the so-called nodules or hyperplastic nodules or neoplastic nodules that nowadays are turning up with such frequency in control groups of rats in experiments dealing with tests of chemicals for carcinogenicity. The reason for this discrepancy is unclear at present but the need to resolve the matter is urgent because these so-called nodules now play an important role in court proceedings devoted to trials for banning or approving the introduction of certain chemicals into the human environment. The fine cytopathology and chemical composition of such lesions are presently under investigation.

The incidence of induced tumors of the liver and the latent period of their induction varies with the potency of carcinogen, the length of the period of feeding, the composition of the diet, the sex and strain of the animal, and its hormonal status. Tumors of the liver induced by potent carcinogens given in large dosage to rats subsisting on a low-protein, low-vitamin diet arise early, and are usually multiple, often numerous, and generally uniform in size as though having developed simultaneously in a cirrhotic liver. When small amounts of weak carcinogens are administered over a relatively long period of time to rats protected with a complete diet, not all animals develop tumors, and with those that do the liver may contain only a single prominent tumor and few or no small ones. On the other hand, a large solitary tumor may spread extensively through the liver via the veins and lymph vessels. The first tumors to develop are discrete lesions and may be undetectable to the naked eye. It is concerning the significance of these that there is so much disagreement and uncertainty. When visible, and while still small, the early tumor may be white, gray, reddish, tan, or yellow, or mixtures of these colors. Large discrete and confluent hemorrhagic, necrotic, and infarcted tumor masses may horribly deform the liver and displace and distort the

abdominal viscera and cause sudden death from massive intraperitoneal hemorrhage.

For my purposes I have found it useful to classify induced hepatic tumors under
four headings as follows: (1) trabecular carcinomatous pattern, (2) adenocarcinomatous pattern, (3) anaplastic carcinomatous pattern, and (4) hepatoblastoma
pattern. A sizable histological section of a tumor of the liver may exhibit one
prevailing pattern or combinations of different patterns and the greatest possible
diversity of combinations may be seen in multiple tumors occurring within the
same liver (Stewart and Snell, 1957).

7.2.1. Trabecular Carcinomatous Pattern

Trabecular carcinoma pattern (synonyms: hepatocellular carcinoma, hepatic-cell
carcinoma, liver cell carcinoma, hepatoma, hepatoma type I, hepatoma type II,
hepatoma malignant), the simplest type of induced tumor, is composed of cords
(plates, muralia) of cells that alternate with endothelial-lined blood vascular
channels that may be widely dilated. The well-differentiated trabecular carcinomas may closely resemble normal liver in structure. On the other hand,
trabecular carcinoma may be so poorly differentiated as to merge with anaplastic
carcinoma and its splindle-celled and scirrhous variants. Trabecular carcinoma
frequently blends into adenocarcinoma, the glands of which may be lined by
hepaticlike cells or by hyperchromatic cuboidal and columnar cells like those seen
in intestinal carcinomas. The cells of trabecular carcinomas may contain fat or
glycogen. There is evidence that the more slowly growing tumors may contain
large deposits of glycogen. The cells of a trabecular carcinoma may vary from
those hardly distinguishable from normal hepatic cells to large neoplastic cell
types that form wide, irregular cords, syncytial cell masses, or sheets of cells with
scarcely discernable sinusoidal vessels. Clara, phosphotungstic acid–hematoxylin,
and iron alum hematoxylin stains are useful for the demonstration of bile
canaliculi. In some tumors the canaliculi may contain bile thrombi. In the less
well-differentiated trabecular carcinomas, board, thick, cellular cords may alternate with dilated sinusoids, which lend an angiomatous appearance to such
tumors, although they are easily distinguishable from hemagiosarcomas.
Reticulum and collagen fibers are generally scanty.

7.2.2. Adenocarcinomatous Pattern

Adenocarcinomatous patterns differ from each other in morphology and staining
characteristics of the neoplastic cells that compose the glands, in the presence or
absence of mucus in the cells and lumens, and in the spatial and quantitative
relationships of glands, blood vessels, and stroma. A glandular pattern may
predominate within the tumor or be intermingled with the other patterns. A
carcinoma exhibiting a mixture of glands and trabeculae is generally composed of
hepaticlike cells that are essentially similar in all respects except in shape, the cells
of the trabecular formations being polygonal while those lining glands are
cuboidal and columnar. An entire such structure may be contained within a

continuous reticular and collagenic envelope, thus forming an organoid structure replicating the patterns of the normal liver, composed as it is of a cord of hepatic cells with an axial canaliculus in continuity with a miniature acinus, the collecting canaliculus. Such structures alternate with sinusoids. In adenocarcinomas that have an abundant connective tissue stroma and that may be quite scirrhous, the sinusoidal pattern is likely to be inconspicuous and the hyperchromatic cuboidal and columnar cells may be stratified or arranged in papillary formation. Such neoplastic cells may resemble more closely those of a scirrhous intestinal carcinoma than they do trabecular carcinoma cells, with which, however, they may be intermingled. The amount of mucus present is variable but may be so abundant as to justify a classification of mucinous adenocarcinoma. Some observers have designated this group of primary adenocarcinomas of the liver as cholangiocarcinoma, thereby implying an origin from intrahepatic bile ducts, not because the tumor cells look like bile duct cells but because they do not closely resemble hepatic cells. That such adenocarcinomas may look like intestinal carcinomas is not surprising, since cancer arising in an organ may duplicate embryological patterns, and in the case of the liver patterns of the foregut. So many mixtures of the intestinal-like and trabecular-like cells may be seen in the same tumor and within the same microscopic field that to unscramble them on the presumption of different histogenetic origins would be inconceivable. Comparing the patterns of mitochondria and golgi apparatus, adenocarcinomas of the liver resemble more closely those of hepatic parenchymal cells or of intestinal cells than they do those of bile duct cells. If the azo dyes and fluorenylamine compounds were carcinogenic for the perilobular bile ducts, they should induce neoplasms of the large intrahepatic and the extrahepatic bile ducts as well. No such neoplasms have been described. Moreover, the dyes combine chemically with the protein of the hepatic cells, and as observed by microscope it is with these cells that the action takes place, while the intrahepatic bile ducts remain inert.

It may be worthwhile to compare and contrast certain liver tumors of man and the rat. The type of carcinoma of the liver that is endemic in parts of the world such as Asia and sub-Saharan Africa is hepatic cell carcinoma. Hepatic cell carcinoma occurs predominantly in men, especially in Oriental and African men, and is usually associated with portal cirrhosis; while it is characterized by extensive venous invasion, extrahepatic metastases are surprisingly infrequent and inconspicuous. Contrast this neoplasm with biliary carcinoma. Biliary carcinoma ocurs more frequently in women than in men, does not show a racial predilection or a frequent association with portal cirrhosis, and although not so invasive within the liver frequently metastasizes widely. Carcinoma of the extrahepatic biliary tract in man is characterized by these same features, and histologically the neoplasms from these different segments of the biliary tree resemble each other. The pattern of neither tumor resembles or differentiates into hepatic cell carcinoma. In the rat, carcinoma of the extrahepatic and large intrahepatic bile ducts is virtually nonexistent. Those who derive chemically induced liver tumors from the small intrahepatic bile ducts need to support their contention not with hunches but with acceptable evidence. This they have not done.

7.2.3. Anaplastic Carcinomatous Pattern

Anaplastic carcinomatous pattern (synonyms: undifferentiated carcinoma, spindle-cell carcinoma, medullary carcinoma) may be dominant in some tumors or confined to parts of otherwise well-differentiated tumors. Some anaplastic carcinomas are composed of cells that are generally the same in size, shape, and staining reaction, whereas others are composed of cells of widely divergent appearance, many of them being large tumor giant cells, with single or multiple nuclei. Even though anaplastic tumors vary widely in the appearance of their cells and in their structural patterns, they often retain distinguishing characteristics that identify them as primary tumors of the liver. Mitotic figures may be numerous and often bizzare in form. The least-differentiated anaplastic tumors fail to reproduce either trabeculae or glands while sinusoidal vessels may be present infrequently and the stroma inconspicuous. Many anaplastic tumors are exceedingly vascular, and the blood vessels may be large and so immature that it is difficult to demonstrate an endothelial lining. Thrombi are frequent and large portions of the tumor become necrotic.

7.2.4. Hepatoblastoma Pattern

Hepatoblastoma pattern (synonyms: sarcomatous, mixed embryonic, fetal pattern) appears in rats treated with hepatic carcinogens. Besides the recognizable carcinomas described, sarcomas and neoplasms composed of fetal and embryoniclike liver tissues appear singly or in combination with the histologically more adult tumors. The cellular and tissue components that may appear in these primitive neoplasms include sarcomatous mesenchyme, fibrosarcoma, cartilage, osteoid and bone, foci of hematopoietic tissue, squamous cell epithelial pearls, young vascular tissue, and primitive hepatic cells. These last cells are of two types. One type is the small pale-staining, finely vacuolated cells of the fetal type that form irregular and curved cords that enclosed demonstrable axial canaliculi or tiny acinar structures. The other cell type is darkly staining, elongated, and spindle-shaped. Cells of this appearance occur in sheet formation within which it is often possible to demonstrate canalicular structures by special staining methods. This latter pattern of tumor is likely to be highly vascularized and some areas may appear as angiosarcoma. These neoplasms are comparable to the embryonic mixed tumor of infants and the hepatoblastoma which has been described in the livers of mice (p. 329) (Turusov *et al.*, 1973*b*). In a publication (Stewart and Snell, 1957) in which the similarities of the embryoniclike, heterotopic tissues of these primitive neoplasms of rats and infants were compared, opinions of others (Allison and Willis, 1956) about the origins of different cells and tissues were cited. The tumor of infants is considered to arise from common ancestral cells, those of a primitive hepatic blastoma comparable to the multipotent nephritic blastoma to which is traced the nephroblastomas of man. In the hepatoblastoma of infants, both the young epithelia and the bone appear to arise from undifferentiated cellular tissue. The composite structure of the hepatic mixed tumors can be explained on the double embryological origin of the mammalian liver, partly from endodermal epithelium and partly from mesenchyme. This would explain the divergent differentiation of the neoplasms into both epithelial and nonepithelial cells and tissue patterns. Both the hepatoblastomas and the nephroblastomas are populated with tissue patterns that indicate reversion to embryonic and fetal tissue structure respective to the organs in which they arise. Although striped muscle, bone, and cartilage may be found in both tumors, muscle is more common in nephroblastoma, while bone and cartilage are more common in hepatoblastoma.

7.2.5. Other Sarcomas

Sarcomas that arise from cysts of the liver of rats that have ingested the larva of the cat tapeworm are described on p. 339.

7.2.6. Spread, Transplantation, Histogenesis, Associated Lesions

Hepatic cancers spread throughout the liver and disseminate to other organs and tissues by infiltration, direct extension, tumor thrombosis, and tumor embolism. The lymphatic vessels and all the blood vascular systems of the liver play a role in these processes. Secondary tumor deposits within the liver may be confused with multiple primary foci. When tumor cells infiltrate the sinusoids and space of Disse, cords of neoplastic cells alternate with cords of residual cells to compose a picture of unusual appearance. The spleen is often directly invaded and tumor implants on the omenta, mesenteries, and diaphragm. Extrahepatic growths may be found in the nodes, pancreas, adrenal gland, kidney, stomach, testis, lung, and bone. The induction of tumors showing limited or widespread metastasis has been linked to specific hepatic carcinogens. As expected, the more anaplastic varieties of hepatic tumors metastasize earliest and more widely than those that are well differentiated, but at the same time I have seen metastases in the lung that were difficult to distinguish from the pattern of normal liver tissue.

Transplanted lines of hepatic cancers have been established in inbred strains of rats and have yielded studies of the utmost biological and chemical importance, especially with the Morris minimal-deviation tumors (Hruban *et al.*, 1971). The literature dealing with transplanted liver tumors is voluminous and a review of the subject goes beyond the restrictions set for this chapter. Early accounts were published in the cancer journals of this country in the 1940s and 1950s, while the extensive and important work of the Japanese investigators may be found in the issues of *Gann*.

In the rat, as in man, cirrhosis may be associated with liver cancer, but in no other species, certainly not in man, has the array of diverse lesions been described in livers in which tumors are arising. These lesions are much more numerous and variable in rats receiving potent carcinogens, whereas they may be minimal or absent when weak carcinogens are employed. The associated lesions are pigmentary deposits of different chemical nature, hyaline bodies, cellular inclusions, pseudotubules that result from the atrophy of hepatic cords, cysts and glandular formations of different histological types, foci of metaplastic pancreatic-type tissue, areas of adenofibrosis often miscalled cholangiofibrosis, and the so-called foci of altered hepatic cells and nodules.

Some years ago, I (Stewart, 1964) presented evidence from our own studies that indicated that pseudotubules arise from hepatic cords through a process of atrophy of hepatic cells. I also cited evidence from the studies of others to support the view that the cells of the pseudotubules convert to perfectly normal hepatic cells when the injurious agent that caused their formation is removed. Ogawa *et al.* (1974) in a study of the pseudotubules (the cells of the nonlumenized tubules, oval cells) that appear in the livers of rats during azo dye carcinogenesis, located many of the cells within the space of Disse, intermingled among clearly recognizable hepatocytes. Electron micrographs and histochemical methods revealed various intensities of glucose-6-phosphatase activity in the endoplastic reticulum and in the nuclear envelope of the oval cells. While Ogawa *et al.* (1974) speculated that the oval cells might differentiate into neoplastic cells, the deduction seems inescapable that the oval cells derive from hepatic cells.

Stewart and Snell (1957) described the development of adenofibrosis from hepatic cells, and Terao and Nakano (1974) identified the lesion of adenofibrosis in electron micrographs as typical intestinal cell metaplasia composed of goblet cells, enterochromaffin cells, and Paneth cells. Kimbrough (1973) documented metaplasia of hepatic cells to acinar pancreatic-type tissue in rats treated with aroclor. The foci of metaplastic pancreatic tissue were small and most often located near areas of adenofibrosis, but they also developed where the hepatic parenchyma was otherwise normal, sometimes immediately adjacent to blood vessels in the center of the liver lobule. The foci occurred in different areas of the liver and several might be seen in the same histological section. Stains for esterase and protein-bound tryptophan in the metaplastic cells yielded results identical to those of pancreatic exocrine tissue. Thus under the influence of carcinogens hepatic cells can undergo metaplasia in two directions, one to form intestinal-type cells and the other to form pancreatic acinar-type cells.

There is no disagreement that many cancers arise from nodules of recognizable hepatic cells which are now the subject of intensive study. Undoubtedly, liver tissue subjected to the influence of hepatic carcinogens undergoes repeated cyclical alternations during which a new generation of cells replaces degenerated and necrotic cells. The architecture is often distorted as a result of regeneration and fibrosis. During the course of these events, identifiable foci or nodules make their appearances and these are composed of cells that, with the light microscope, exhibit recognizable differences from those of the surrounding parenchyma. On December 11, 1974, a workshop convened by the Associate Chief, Experimental Pathology Branch, Carcinogenesis, DCCP, National Cancer Institute, NIH, considered the nomenclature of rat liver tumors and in particular three basic types of lesion. The "foci of cellular alteration" were given descriptive names only; although of controversial significance, they were considered to be part of the spectrum of tissue changes leading to the formation of nodules. The term "hyperplastic nodule" was changed to "neoplastic nodule" because the evidence presented and discussed at the workshop indicated that this lesion is a genuine neoplasm, induced by known carcinogens, and does not simply represent a hyperplastic state. "Hepatocellular carcinomas" were classified according to their morphological appearances and biological behavior.

In the livers of rats treated with hepatic carcinogens, Bannasch and colleagues (Bannasch, 1968; Bannasch and Amgerer, 1974; Bannasch et al., 1972) and Theodassion et al. (1971) distinguished foci of hypertrophied glycogen-rich cells that exhibited retarded proliferative abilities. This lesion they regarded as persistent and irreversible, apart from its frequent transformation into nodules of progressive neoplastic proliferation. They described the nodules as populated with glycogen-deficient hepatocytes showing disorganization of the ergastoplasm, acidophilic, basophilic, or hypertrophied cells, and fat-storing or glycogen-storing cells. Thus they believe that transformation of normal hepatic cells into cancer in the rat is not abrupt but a slow process which is characterized by histological and biochemical changes.

Bruni (1973), from his examination of electron micrographs, identified certain cells in the so-called early neoplastic nodule as similar to fetal hepatocytes. These cells differed from the surrounding hepatic cells by the absence or greatly reduced volume of the smooth endoplastic reticulum. Bruni (1973) interpreted this depletion as an expression of permanently arrested differentiation. He concluded that the altered cells represented the initial stage of tumor formation.

Becker and Klein (1971) and Becker et al. (1971) examined the mitotic activity and the chromosome patterns of the hepatocytes of the nodules that they considered to be lineally related to the eventual appearance of carcinoma (Teebor and Becker, 1971). They found the alternations in chromosome patterns to be few and rather difficult to correlate with the distinctive abnormal chromosome patterns of the fully developed hepatic cancers. They concluded that in the absence of morphological evidence perhaps the determining events of cancer take place at the molecular level.

Farber (1973) and Okita and Farber (1975) (also quoted by Farber, 1974) have described an antigen and biochemical markers that they believe will open up a new approach to the study of the early stages of liver cancer. The antigen is common to cells regarded as preneoplastic hepatocyte populations and to liver cancer induced by hepatic carcinogens.

α-Fetoprotein, which is of value in the diagnosis and clinical management of human liver cancer, is also elevated in the serum of rats with experimentally induced liver cancer. Attempts have been made to determine how long before the morphological appearance of the cancer the test becomes positive and which cells within the liver produce the fetal antigen (Kroes et al., 1973). Okita et al. (1975), using an immunofluorescence method, identified α-fetoprotein in some liver tumors and some hyperplastic nodules but not in all. Becker and Sell (1974), using a sensitive radioimmunoassay method, have shown that elevated levels of α-fetoprotein, formerly considered to correlate with the development of the cancer, actually appear within 2 wk following the start of a regimen of 2-AAF feeding, and are thus unrelated to cell injury or tissue alteration. If the suggestion of Becker and Sell (1974) is correct, that the elevation of the fetal protein in the serum results from derepression of protein synthesis, then this marker may be less valuable than anticipated for the identification of liver nodules that are suspected to be of a neoplastic nature.

Several have attempted to correlate the significance of the histological appearance of the early neoplastic lesion with the results of transplantation (Reuber and Odashima, 1967). Reuber and Firminger (1963) were among the first to do so and they employed the conventional methods of histopathology to classify by the light microscope the lesions as benign or as malignant. They transplanted fragments of each lesion to other rats. They reported a good correlation, although from time to time they were surprised. The lesions they classified histologically as "hyperplasia" and as a small "carcinoma *in situ*" usually did not grow when transplanted. Those lesions that did grow on transplantation, were relatively large, measuring 7–9 mm in diameter and were from rats that had ingested the carcinogen 2-FAA for 3–4 months. They hypothesized that the so-called hyperplastic lesion progressed to a transplantable cancer under the continued influence of the carcinogen.

While many elegant studies have been carried out on livers of rats treated with hepatic carcinogens, there is a paucity of studies on the livers of control rats. In some carcinogenicity tests, as many at 15% of the livers of control rats may show nodules which in the light microscope resemble those diagnosed as neoplastic lesions in the livers of the experimental rats. These lesions of the control rats raise the possibility that there are carcinogens in the environment to which the caged rats are exposed. It seems timely to determine whether the lesions in controls show the same cytomorphology and biochemical changes described for the similar-appearing lesions of experimental rats. Another control would be a truly hyperplastic lesion of the liver induced by an agent that does not induce carcinoma of the liver, if such an agent can be identified. In mice, Leduc and Wilson (1959b) have distinguished, described, and illustrated a lesion of the liver different from hepatic tumors that occurs in mice treated with carbon tetrachloride and which regresses when the carbon tetrachloride is withdrawn (p. 326). Another animal model in which to study comparative aspects of the early neoplastic liver nodule is the chicken, in which fully developed liver tumors may be induced in a short space of time, often less than 1 month following inoculation of the bird with the MC29 avian leukosis agent (p. 339). In this model, one could almost get a motion picture view of the processes that eventuate in cancer, with all events being telescoped into a short capsule of time.

7.3. Other Animals

Among the domestic animals, hepatic tumors are common in dogs, cats, cattle, and sheep but are less frequent in other species (Jackson, 1936; Jubb and Kennedy, 1970). In animals, hepatic carcinoma is usually not associated with cirrhosis, an association that is common in man. Malignant hepatic tumors have also been found in roe deer and some birds, and a few years ago this neoplasm reached epidemic proportions in rainbow trout caused by the aflatoxin contained in the food contaminated with *Aspergillus flavus* that the fish had ingested while

still at the hatchery (Ashley, 1973). These induced neoplasms in fish have all been
classified as hepatocellular carcinomas. This has raised the suspicion that similar
tumors so frequent in black Africans are due to ingested aflatoxins, and, while
there is evidence of contamination of food by *Aspergillus flavus*, the question is still
unresolved. The hepatic tumors that arise in pigs that have ingested aflatoxin are
usually not associated with cirrhosis. A number of carcinogenic chemicals are
effective hepatic carcinogens for the dog, including aflatoxin B1, 2-
acetylaminofluorene, diethylnitrosamine, and N-nitrosopiperedine. Hirao *et al.*
(1974) classified the canine tumors caused by diethylnitrosamine as of both
mesenchymal and epithelial types, the latter being similar to those observed in rats
treated with hepatic carcinogens. Lapis *et al.* (1973) have described primary
hepatic tumors that arose in chickens infected with MC29 avian leukosis agent. By
comparison with a latent period of several months required for chemical
carcinogens to induce liver tumors in rats, the liver tumors arose in the diseased
Duke chickens infected with the virus in from 1 to $1\frac{1}{2}$ months. There was no
associated cirrhosis. The tumors were of differing distinctive growth patterns,
similar in many respects to those of rats treated with chemical carcinogens. One of
the authors of this publication (Lapis *et al.*, 1973), Dr. J. W. Beard, allowed me to
examine a manuscript, since published (Beard, *et al.*, 1975), describing studies in
which by electron microscopy he convincingly demonstrated that the tumors of
the liver of the chickens arose from hepatic cells and not from bile duct cells. Lapis
et al. (1975) have established and maintained serial transplants of the viral-
induced hepatic carcinomas in the thigh muscles, subcutaneous tissue, and
abdominal cavity of other chickens.

There is an etiological relationship between infestation with *Opisthorchis
felineus* and the development of biliary duct carcinomas in cats. Fascioliasis, with
the attendant severe chronic inflammatory changes, may also—but rarely—
eventuate in biliary duct carcinoma in sheep and cattle. These associations are
reminiscent of the biliary duct carcinomas that are seen in people harboring an
infestation of *Clonorchis sinensis*, as in China. In rats *Cysticercus fasciolaris*, the larva
of the cat tapeworm, *Taenia crassicollis*, when administered orally, regularly
induces sarcomas that arise from the wall of cysts produced in the liver (Bullock
and Curtis, 1925). The large sarcomas implant on the peritoneum and metastasize
to the mediastinal lymph nodes and thoracic viscera. All such tumors are of
mesothelial origin and none arises from hepatic cells.

In domestic animals, epithelial tumors of the liver have been classified as benign
and malignant, hepatocellular and cholangiocellular histological types. The
cholangiomatous-type tumors are said to predominate in dogs and cats, whereas
those of the hepatocellular type predominate in sheep and cattle. The tumors
classified as cholangiocarcinomas are fibrous, firm and whitish, often pedunculated, and are composed of papillary glandular, sometimes cystic, structures that
are likely to contain mucus. The hepatocellular carcinomas of domestic animals
appear and behave much like those of man and the rat. The tumors of
domestic animals may be single and exceedingly large, or multiple and numerous,
spreading by way of the veins throughout the liver and metastasizing to the lungs

and portal lymph nodes; or they may extend directly through the capsule of the liver to invade diaphragm and stomach and implant on the peritoneum. With most tumors of the liver classifiable as trabecular carcinomas, it is not unusual to find canaliculi plugged with bile thrombi. Foci of hematopoiesis are also not uncommon, particularly in the liver tumors of young sheep and pigs.

Veterinary pathologists freely acknowledge difficulties in distinguishing large areas of so-called nodular hyperplasia from benign hepatoma and the latter from carcinoma. Nodular hyperplasia occurs commonly in old dogs in which the liver is otherwise normal. There are reports of the reclassification of the benign growths in instances after finding intravascular invasion or metastatic deposits. It is probable that many of those designated as hyperplastic or benign nodules are genuine neoplasms of a low grade of malignancy, which, without change in histological pattern, are perfectly capable of progressing to high grades of malignant neoplasms that metastasize.

Another error, one suspects, is that some hepatocellular carcinomas are incorrectly classified as cholangiocarcinomas simply on the basis of a predominant glandular pattern. Pathologists may fail to appreciate that hepatic cells constitute a glandular organ, the acini into which they pour their secretions being the intrabecular canaliculi and the collecting canaliculi. Under the influence of the neoplastic process, these conduits enlarge and become exaggerated so that instead of being the inconspicuous, tiny channels they are in the normal liver, they may form conspicuous glands or even cysts. In rats, where proper studies have been made of the cells lining such glandular and cystic spaces of liver neoplasms, the cells have frequently shown the subcellular constituents that are characteristics of normal hepatic cells. Hence many such glandular neoplasms derive from hepatic cells and not from the bile ducts. Although liver tumors may occur in young animals, particularly sheep and pigs, hepatoblastomas like those that occur in man, the mouse, and the rat have not been described in veterinary pathology. The tumors of young domestic animals appear to be composed of more mature cells than those that compose the hepatoblastoma, although they may show areas of hematopoiesis.

8. Tumors of the Mammary Gland

8.1. Rat

Investigators have noted the spontaneous occurrence of mammary gland tumors of rats since early in this century and their induction, first by estrogens, since the late 1930s. Noble and Cutts (1959) thoroughly reviewed the literature up to the date of their publication. Young and Hallowes (1973) published an elegantly illustrated, comprehensive description of the pathology of these neoplasms, their functional capabilities, transplantability, methods for their induction, comparability to neoplasms of other species including man, the dog, cat, and mouse, and the early changes as well as the structure, ultrastructure, and histochemistry of the normal mammary gland tissue of the rat. They classified the tumors and tumorlike lesions into four major categories: lobular hyperplasias, fibroepithelial tumors, carcinomas, and sarcomas. They expanded this simple classification to separate different groups of tumors depending on different mixtures and combinations of cellular elements, degree of cellular differentiation, pattern of cellular arrangement, and extent and relationship between the tumor cells and areas of necrosis. Thus they broke down the group of fibroepithelial tumors to include adenoma, fibroadenoma, and fibroma. Lobular hyperplasia, as the name implies, is characterized by increased size and number of mammary lobules, which although somewhat complex in structure are composed of acini that closely resemble those in the surrounding mammary tissue. In the lesions of lobular hyperplasia and the combinations of fibroadenoma, there is a tendency toward the replication of the normal relationships among secretion, epithelium, myoepithelium, and stroma. With the other neoplasms, however, this relationship is distorted by the overgrowth of the epithelium or the connective tissue or both. The fibrous tissue elements may predominate to the point that glandular structures are infrequent or have disappeared. Enzymatic activity in the epithelium is generally less than that of the normal gland, whereas enzymatic activity of the connective tissue is greater, particularly the activities of alkaline and adenosine mono-, di-, and triphosphatase.

8.1.1. "Fibroadenoma"

In the so-called *fibroadenoma* of the rat, the connective tissue as a rule surrounds ducts, giving the appearance of a pericanalicular structure. The intracanalicular pattern that predominates in women is infrequent in the rat. This mammary gland tumor of the rat, often referred to as benign because of its histological resemblance to benign tumors of women, fulfills some of the criteria for the evaluation of malignancy. Growth of the primary tumor is generally slow but progressive, the tumor may reach an enormous size, and it transplants successfully to syngeneic animals (Stewart *et al.*, 1959). According to Foulds' (1951) review of the studies made by various investigators, the structure of primary tumors of this type frequently differs from that considered typical of a fibroadenoma. The epithelial component may increase at the expense of the connective tissue so that the histological appearance is more like that of an adenoma or a secreting adenoma. During pregnancy and lactation, or after the administration of estrogens, secretory activity in the tumor cells may roughly parallel that of the surrounding mammary gland tissue. The tumor is thus responsive to a physiological stimulus in much the same way as is the normal tissue from which it derived. On the other hand, the connective tissue component may overgrow the epithelium to produce the pattern of a fibroma or, rarely, a sarcoma. Such changes are likely to occur in long-standing primary tumors of old rats. Possibly growth of the epithelial component of the tumor depends on estrogens which may be present in inadequate amounts in old rats.

When a mammary tumor of the fibroadenomatous type is transplanted to other rats, its histological pattern may be duplicated for many successive generations, or structural variations may occur. Like the primary tumor, and under similar hormonal conditions, the predominant pattern of the transplanted tumor may become that of an adenoma or a secreting adenoma. Infrequently and for reasons that are not understood, more extreme alterations may occur during transplantation. The epithelium may differentiate into squamous, sebaceous, or sweat gland type, and the connective tissue may show chondroid, osteoid, or adipose differentiation. Occasionally the lesion of chronic mastitis may be simulated. All these variations are temporary and reversible. However, if during transplantation the epithelial component is lost and a fibrous histological pattern develops, the change is permanent and the epithelial component never reappears. A transformation to sarcoma rarely occurs in primary mammary tumors but commonly occurs in transplanted ones. This change from fibroadenoma to fibroma and later to sarcoma may take place early or late in the course of serial transplantation. The alteration in structure may become completed within one transplant generation or it may require several generations. A comparable irreversible change in the epithelial component, leading through adenoma to carcinoma, occurs but rarely. Thus the same tumor, if seen at different stages in its evolution, might be diagnosed as an epithelial or a connective tissue growth, or as a mixed tumor, any of which might be considered to be benign or malignant. The plasticity and variability of structure and behavior of the fibroadenoma of the rat are thus accompanied, in serial transplantation, by a tendency to irreversible change toward a more stable and more aggressive tumor, and especially toward sarcoma. As assessed by Foulds (1951), fibroadenoma appears to be a tumor in a stage of uncompleted development; given time and opportunity, it changes into something different.

8.1.2. Carcinomas

Carcinomas include adenocarcinoma, papillary adenocarcinoma, anaplastic carcinoma, cribriform carcinoma, comedocarcinoma, and squamous cell carcinoma. From these titles, one can construct a mental image of the histological variations that have been classified. They are clearly described and splendidly illustrated in the publication of Young and Hallowes (1973). The basic histological pattern consists of glandlike structures lined by neoplastic epithelial cells surrounding a lumen. Variations include papillary projections into the lumen and formation of solid sheets of cells and secretion vacuoles within the cytoplasm of the cells and in the lumens of the gland spaces. Lipid droplets in the epithelial cells may become so numerous that the neoplasm resembles a liposarcoma. Rounded masses of cells that have undergone central necrosis account for the comedocarcinoma appearance, which type is usually associated with a cribiform carcinomatous pattern. A pattern of squamous cell carcinoma may occur independently or in association with undifferentiated carcinoma. With these different patterns, the neoplastic epithelial cells may show all the morphological variations that one associates with a malignant neoplasm. The tumors ulcerate, infiltrate, metastasize, and kill the host animal as may any malignant tumor. The stroma in the common form of

adenocarcinoma is usually minimal, although carcinomas are commonly inter-
sected by broad bands of fibrovascular stroma that is often infiltrated with
inflammatory cells. This feature, common in the rat, is rarely seen in the
mammary tumors of mouse or man. Within the same tumor, particularly if it is
large and generally in the different multiple tumors that develop in a single rat
treated with a carcinogen, various histological patterns of mammary neoplasm are
likely to be found. All variations from so-called fibroadenoma to carcinoma may
be found intermingled in the same tumor. During serial transplantation in
syngeneic animals, a well-differentiated carcinoma may convert to anaplastic
carcinoma or sarcoma. Enzymes like those present in normal mammary gland
tissue are also demonstrable in adenocarcinomas but their activity is variable in the
same and different tumors. Sarcoma may arise spontaneously as a rapidly growing
primary neoplasm of the mammary gland in old females, or as a "malignant"
transformation of the stroma of a so-called fibroadenoma. Occasionally, carcinosarcoma arises as a single tumor composed of both epithelial and mesenchymal elements, but this event is less frequent in rats than in mice.

Metastases are variable. Spontaneous tumors may metastasize, but apparently
infrequently. In my own experience, those induced with the fluorenylamine
compounds are highly malignant and metastasize. Pulmonary metastases have
been found in up to 8% of rats bearing estrogen-induced tumors. As expected,
metastases from induced tumors are more frequent in animals allowed to survive
their full life span.

In their review of published reports of spontaneous mammary tumors in rats,
Young and Hallowes (1973) concluded that rats of all strains may develop
mammary tumors, but the frequency is extremely variable in different strains and
even in the same strain maintained in different laboratories; usually only one
mammary gland is involved. The percentages of Sprague–Dawley females that
developed spontaneous mammary tumors have varied in different laboratories
from 25% to 55% to 100%; the corresponding figures from Wistar rats in different
laboratories varied between 6% and 30%. Most such mammary tumors arose in
females around 2 yr of age and were classified as benign; carcinomas were more
likely to arise in older rats. Both types are infrequent in males. Because of the
variability in tumor development, each colony should be carefully studied for
background data and this should be repeated at intervals because of the likelihood
of genetic drift with time.

The frequency of induced tumors, as with spontaneous tumors, varies with
strain of rat, the carcinogen and combinations of carcinogens employed, methods
of administration, age and sex of the animal, hormonal status, germfree status,
diet, and environment including sunlight and temperature. The effects of
juggling various factors may influence not only the development of mammary
tumors but also the histological type, dependency, progression, regression, and
metastases as well. It is possible to induce tumors in all mammary glands at nearly
the same time. Breeding females are more susceptible than virgins, while male rats
are relatively resistant. Pregnancy is associated with an increased growth rate
of the tumor; lactation arrests growth; resumption of growth coincides with

weaning. Pituitary hormones play an essential role in tumorigenesis, while gonadectomy reduces the incidence.

The inducing agents that have been commonly employed are hormones, chiefly estrogens and pituitary growth hormone, ionizing radiation, and chemicals, including the aminofluorenes and aromatic polycyclic hydrocarbons. Low doses of DMBA induce mostly fibroadenomas, while high doses induce carcinomas. Until recently, viruses have not been implicated in the induction of mammary tumors of the rat. Therefore, the report by Ankerst *et al.* (1974) that adenovirus 9 when injected into newborn Wistar/Furth female rats was followed by the appearance of mammary fibroadenomas is noteworthy. The authors speculated whether the involvement of adenovirus 9 in the induction of these tumors was direct or indirect, being mediated by a latent virus in the infected rats and becoming activated by the adenovirus type 9 genome. There are, as yet, no data that illuminate either speculation. In another report, a C-type virus isolated from a transplantable mammary gland adenocarcinoma of a rat and inoculated into neonatal rats led to an increase in the incidence of mammary tumors (Bogden *et al.*, 1974).

In comparative studies, much has been made of the similarities in structure, behavior, or function of mammary tumors of the rat, mouse, dog, cat, and man. In the case of the rat, some induced mammary tumors respond to hormone treatment by adrenalectomy, oophorectomy, hypophysectomy, and androgen therapy. Some spontaneous tumors of women also respond to these procedures and agents, but in both species some mammary tumors respond to none of these hormonal influences. There are many obscurities in comparative oncology, none more evident than in mammary neoplasia. Why, for instance, is cancer so much more frequent in the mammary glands of certain strains of rats and mice, why so rare in the udder of cows, and unheard of in the mammary gland of whales? A stated aim by the editors (1973) of the WHO/IARC publications that deal with the pathology of tumors in laboratory animals has been to adopt, whenever possible, the classification and terminology proposed by WHO's International Reference Centers for human tumors. One wonders if this is a worthy aim or whether it had been wise to introduce a terminology for animal tumors more fitting to the correlation of their structural appearance and known behavior. On several pages of the publication by Young and Hallowes (1973), excellent as it is otherwise, the resemblance between rat and human mammary neoplasms is emphasized, perhaps overemphasized. Such emphasis is likely to mislead investigators inexperienced in pathology to believe that rat mammary tumors are in all respects suitable laboratory models for human breast cancer. There are significant differences. The scirrhous carcinoma, the common breast tumor of women, has not been identified in any other species. Mammary cancers in women invariably metastasize if untreated, whereas in rats most spontaneous and many carcinogen-induced mammary carcinomas do not metastasize. Some rat mammary tumors having the histological appearance of "cancer" regress and disappear upon the removal of the initiating agent. Disappearance of mammary cancer in women happens so infrequently that when it does the host becomes a candidate for canonization for surely this is evidence of divine intervention. Should the same names be applied to neoplasms that behave so differently in these species?

Discussions of comparative pathology often underemphasize the dissimilarities of the neoplasms of rodents, canines, felines, and human beings. As stated previously, what is needed in experimental and comparative pathology is a series of workshops and studies by collaborative groups of pathologists, similar to those that the WHO International Reference Centers for human tumors have instituted. These centers bring together pathologists, with their slides and clinical, biological, and behavioral data, to work out acceptable definitions of cancer types in rodents and other laboratory animals.

8.2. Mouse

Historically, mammary gland tumors of the mouse are a further example of the nonuniversality of the criteria for benign and malignant lesions (p. 309). Apolant (1906), who published the first detailed histological study of mammary tumors in mice, distinguished benign from malignant forms using histological criteria that he relied on in his everyday work in clinical pathology. Later experience proved such criteria to be unreliable when applied to mouse mammary tumors. Nicod (1936) was the one who laid to rest the myth of the distinctions between benign and malignant mammary tumors of mice by showing that an apparently well-differentiated tumor may grow rapidly and metastasize early. Foulds (1949, 1956) followed up this conception by stating that where neither prognosis nor therapy is required, allocation to a benign or a malignant category may dull the perception of the innumerable morphological features of such tumors and their biological modifications such as progression and responsiveness. Refinements in classification of mammary tumors continued to be made and the most useful of these is that by Dunn (1959). In this, she pointed out that not all tumors always fit snugly into "the sorting scheme," as she aptly termed it.

Gross features are helpful in the distinction between mammary tumors and other neoplasms located in the subcutaneous area. Because of the large amount and wide extent of the mammary tissue that composes the five pairs of glands, the tumors may be found at almost any subcutaneous site on the body. The tumors of mice infected with the mammary tumor virus are usually multiple, arise at a relatively early age, and are likely to be evenly distributed among the different glands. In mice without the virus, the tumors appear at an older age and are located chiefly in the pectoral area. Mammary tumors are round, oval, smooth or coarsely nodular, well circumscribed, and easily shelled out of the bed they occupy. The incised surface is usually grayish-white and soft, with a central area of necrosis; keratinized areas appear white and flakey. A milky fluid may ooze from the cut surface or a reddish fluid from the numerous blood-filled spaces.

The histological classification of mammary tumors devised by Dunn (1959) makes possible correlations of age, strain, genetics, breeding, hormonal state, and etiology. While individual tumors may vary from one area to another and different tumors from the same individual may show different histological patterns, proportions of one or another histological type usually predominate under given conditions. The Dunn (1959) classification uses six categories.

8.2.1. Adenocarcinoma, Type A

One of the six categories—adenocarcinoma, type A—is composed of a tiny, uniform, orderly acinar structure lined by small cuboidal cells arranged in a single row surrounding lumens that may be round, elongated, or tubular. Although mitoses are rare, the tumor metastasizes and transplants readily. Small foci of squamous cells are not infrequent. Secretory activity or lactation is reflected in the vacuolization of the epithelial cells. The stroma is minimal. Type A tumors and the following type B are the tumors that most frequently arise in C3H mice infected with the mammary tumor virus.

8.2.2. Adenocarcinoma, Type B

Adenocarcinoma, type B, represents a multiform group of patterns, some of which may replicate the type A pattern while others are composed of papillary cyst formations, tubular structures, sheets, nests or cords of cells, large blood-filled spaces, and variable amounts of stroma which is sometimes abundant. A comedolike formation of large masses of cells encompassing a central area of necrosis may contribute to the variable patterns that this type of tumor may exhibit. Metastases of types A and B are commonly found in the lungs but are rare in lymph nodes, and are modified by such factors as multiplicity, duration, size, and rapidity of growth of the primary tumor. This is in contrast to human mammary cancer, which metastasizes earliest to regional lymph nodes and later widely throughout the body tissues, including particularly the bones. The regional lymph nodes of mice resist secondary deposits even when surrounded by a mammary cancer that has already metastasized to the lungs.

8.2.3. Adenocarcinoma, Type C

Adenocarcinoma, type C, is a distinctive tumor of uniform structure throughout. It is composed of multiple tiny cysts of various sizes lined by a single layer of cuboidal epithelial cells that are closely invested with myoepithelial cells which form a layer of varying thickness in different areas of the neoplasm. The spindle-shaped terminations of the myoepithelial cells fray out to blend with the sparse, edematous connective tissue stroma. The type C neoplasm occurs nearly always in old mice devoid of the mammary tumor virus, particularly mice of strains BALB/c and C3Hf, thus reflecting by its unique composition an etiology, which though not known, must be unusual (Heston and Deringer, 1952a; Heston *et al.,* 1956).

8.2.4. Adenoacanthoma

Adenoacanthoma is composed of glandular structures arranged in patterns like those of the type A or type B neoplasms intermingled with squamous cell carcinoma which may constitute 25% or more of the neoplasm. Whole-body irradiation and, as shown more recently, exposure to inhalation of vinyl chloride induce this neoplasm in great numbers.

8.2.5. Molluscoid Tumor

The molluscoid tumor, a variant of adenocanthoma, is an organoid tumor whose central area consists of radiating dilated tubules lined by stratified squamous epithelial cells, while the peripheral terminations of these tubules are composed of glandular formations. Some molluscoid tumors grow slowly or rapidly, disappear and reappear, and they invade and transplant easily.

8.2.6. Sarcoma and Carcinosarcoma

Sarcoma and the mesenchymal element of carcinosarcoma derive in whole or in part from the specialized connective tissue of the mammary gland. The sarcomatous element is classified as fibrosarcoma and may exhibit wide variations in the appearance of the neoplastic cells. The epithelial components are arranged in irregular, often elongated ductlike structures. These tumors may arise spontaneously in untreated mice and they may develop as the intermediate and terminal patterns following the serial transplantation of purely glandular tumors. Sarcomas and carcinosarcomas may constitute the chief patterns seen in mammary tumors that have been induced by the subcutaneous injection of carcinogenic polycyclic hydrocarbons or exposure to whole-body irradiation; they may appear as patterns of other tumors composed of glandular structures that have been induced by other etiological agents.

8.2.7. Miscellaneous Tumors

Miscellaneous tumors of different histological patterns develop, but Dunn (1959) found no distinctive forms that might warrant separate categories.

8.2.8. Components, Etiology, Histogenesis

Various components of different mammary tumors have been studied in detail, including lactation, secretion, mucus, iron deposition, infiltration of mast cells, and presence of stainable alkaline phosphatase along the borders of the gland lumens and endothelial-lined spaces as well as in myoepithelial cells.

Since the mammary tumor virus induces the fatal type A and type B tumors at an early age, few or none of the infected animals survive into old age. Mice freed of the mammary tumor virus that live to an old age may also develop type A and type B tumors, but in addition other tumors of different histological patterns arise. In other words, it is the proportionate numbers of types A and B mammary tumors that are reduced when the virus is absent. With the removal of the mammary tumor virus, the influence of genetic constitution becomes manifested by an increase in certain tumor types that are characteristic of particular inbred strains of mice. When potent doses of a carcinogenic polycyclic hydrocarbon are injected into the mammary fat pad of virus-free mice, carcinosarcoma and sarcomas arise, whereas when small doses are applied percutaneously a high percentage of the developing tumors exhibit a glandular pattern. Combinations of progestin and estrogen significantly increase the mammary tumors induced with the percutaneous application of methycholanthrene. Repeated pregnancies also increase mammary tumors in some strains of mice. Weekly implantation of hypophyses removed from other mice produce mammary cancer in virgin females free of the mammary tumor virus. It is possible to induce tumors in male mice by estrogens, chemical carcinogens, and X-irradiation.

The effect of environment, apart from genetic, viral, and immunological factors, on the spontaneous incidence of mammary tumors and hepatic tumors was recently demonstrated when C3H-A^{vy}fB mice were bred and reared in Australia. Mice of this strain maintained in the United States at the NCI laboratories in Bethesda exhibited a very high incidence of these neoplasms. When imported into Australia, the incidence declined to nearly zero in subsequent generations. However, when the mice in Australia were fed the diet provided in the United States, the incidence of mammary tumors increased, and was restored to the NCI level when the shavings of the Douglas fir were replaced by shavings of red cedar wood, the bedding used at NCI. The Australian authors (Sabine *et al.*, 1973) suggested that the bedding and diet used in the United States may contain carcinogens. In further speculations on this phenomenon, Schoental (1974) suggested two possible environmental carcinogenic agents. One, podophyllotoxin, known to induce liver tumors, is contained in the red cedar wood shavings; the other, estrogenic substances known to induce breast tumors, is present in the mouse food either as possible additive dietary contaminants or as natural estrogens from fungi that sometimes contaminate cereals. Heston (1975) tested these hypotheses and concluded that the poor health of the Australian mice, due to an inadequate diet and infestation with ectoparasites, accounted for the reduced incidences of mammary and hepatic tumors.

The precancerous process that precedes the development of cancer in high tumor strain mice is the so-called hyperplastic alveolar nodule. It arises within the mammary fat pads as an easily recognizable yellow nodule, due to its content of iron, and consists of a focus of lobuloalveolar development in a ductular area. The compact or loosely arranged proliferated alveoli consist each of a single row of cuboidal cells around a tiny lumen. The appearance of the nodule is modified by the nodule-inducing virus and by the factors that influence mammary tumor development, including the mammary tumor virus, genetics, hormones, chemicals, X-irradiation, and age and strain of mouse. The frequency of the nodules parallels the later development of mammary tumors, although only a fraction of the nodules progress to cancer during the lifetime of the animal. Several observers have described gradation between the hyperplastic alveolar nodule and mammary cancer (Medina, 1973).

8.3. Domestic Animals

The dog, among domestic animals, is the species most prone to develop mammary tumors. Dogs of both sexes develop tumors, but in the female mammary gland tumors are, next to cutaneous tumors, the most frequently occurring neoplasm. Mammary tumors also occur in the female cat, but their frequency is considerably less than in the dog. In other domestic animals, the cow, sow, ewe, and mare, mammary tumors are rare, and if they do arise they are likely to pursue a slow and indolent course (Jubb and Kennedy, 1970).

8.3.1. Dog

Mammary tumors of the dog, in comparison with those of all other species, present the most confusion in the various aspects and combinations of histological types of tissue that may comprise single or multiple tumors in one or more mammary glands of the same or different animals; in the lack of agreement concerning the histogenesis of the different cells and tissues that comprise the neoplasms; in their classification and nomenclature; in the assessment of malignancy; in the uncertainty about the relationship among hyperplastic, metaplastic, and neoplastic lesions; and in the dearth of follow-up data on animals once they have developed tumors.

The various types of well-differentiated and anaplastic cells and tissues that may comprise the mammary tumors of the dog are embryonic and adult hyaline cartilage, osteoid, bone, bone marrow with hematopoietic elements, connective tissue, fat, neural tissue, blood vessels and endothelial cells, nonsecretory and mucoid-secreting myoepithelial cells, reticular cells, mucus-secreting and nonsecretory glandular cells that may form acini, ducts, and cysts, squamous epithelial cells, and sebaceous cells. Different observers hold different views regarding the origin of these cellular and tissue elements. One theory holds that the interstitial tissue of the mammary gland produces the mesenchymal elements, that the epithelial cells produce the epithelial elements while myoepithelium gives origin to the reticular cells from which the mucoid and chondroid tissues may develop. Others have described transition forms between epithelial cells and cartilagenous elements and between the cartilagenous and osseous elements. Pulley (1973) has reported that the myoid, chondroid, and osteoid elements may arise from myoepithelial cells. As discussed elsewhere in this chapter, with neoplasms of other sites in different species including man there is support for the view that a single type of stem cell may give rise to neoplasms of different histological patterns. With the mammary gland tumors of dogs, more work is required to establish the validity of the views already expressed about the histogenesis of the various tissue types that compose them or new possibilities need to be revealed.

a. Mixed Tumor. Understandably, with the conglomeration of different types of cells and tissues that may be found in mammary tumors, the most frequent type is the mixed tumor, which comprises roughly 50–70% of all mammary tumors of the bitch (Misdorp et al., 1973; Moulton et al., 1970). With the so-called canine benign mixed tumors, those of mesenchymal pattern may be lipomas, fibromas, myofibromas, osteomas, and angiomas. The epithelial patterns, with variable amounts of stroma, include the adenomas composed of well-developed glandular areas that are classifiable papillary, cystic, pericanalicular, or intracanalicular. Most mixed tumors do not metastasize during the lifetime of the animal. In the absence of clinical follow-up and since the life of a dog is frequently foreshortened for humane or other reasons, the potential of mixed tumor to metastasize is unclear. In the absence of data, the error is calculated as being around 30%. It has been observed that a mixed mesenchymal neoplasm, at its primary site, may not have exhibited infiltrative growth or any commonly accepted histological criteria of malignancy such as increased mitotic activity or cellular anaplasia, yet may already have metastasized as a sarcoma. The statement is sometimes made that carcinoma or sarcoma has developed in a previously benign tumor. This has led to considerable uncertainty in the classification of mixed mammary tumors as benign, borderline, or malignant. Most of the efforts in this direction have been to develop criteria for classification on the basis of those established for man. However, with the mixed tumors of the dog, every criterion or group of criteria for the classification of benign neoplasms has been violated by the appearance of secondary deposits at a distant site. This exercise is full of surprises. The metastases of mixed tumors may be found widespread throughout the dog's body and may consist of one or more of the various types of tissue that compose the primary tumor. Generally, however, those mixed tumors of the dog that do metastasize do so as carcinomas.

b. Mammary Sarcoma. The classification of mammary sarcomas in the dog is based on histology and not histogenesis. In the bitch, mammary sarcomas or mixed mesenchymal neoplasms constitute roughly 13% of all mammary cancers and are therefore considerably more frequent than in women. They are also more frequent in the bitch than are carcinomas and may arise in relatively young dogs as compared with the age bracket in which the carcinomas arise, and they grow to a large size. Misdorp *et al.* (1971) did not concur in opinions expressed by other authors that most sarcomas arise from preexisting mixed tumors. Apart from a small group classified as sarcoma NOS, they subdivided the sarcomas with either osseous or cartilagenous differentiation into two separate entities of simple sarcoma and separated these types from combined sarcoma which exhibited multidifferentiation. The bone may be so dense in the osseous type of mammary sarcoma that the secondary deposits in bone may simulate by X-ray primary osteogenic sarcoma. They also recognized another group as fibrosarcomas, most of which they thought rather closely resembled the stromal type of mammary sarcoma that occasionally arises in women. The mammary sarcomas of bitches, compared with those of women, are more likely to metastasize to lymph nodes. However, the common type of cystosarcoma phylloides of women is very rarely encountered in dogs. In the study by Misdorp *et al.* (1971), 5 of 17 of the combined sarcomas which had metastasized exhibited an apparently benign appearance in the primary tumor, which is in line with a frequently repeated statement made in veterinary literature that mixed mesenchymal neoplasms that have a benign histological appearance may metastasize.

c. Carcinoma. Carcinomas are termed complex if they consist of cells resembling both secretory and myoepithelial cells. The complex tumors are considered to be less malignant than tumors of the simple type which consist of only one of these two types of cells (Hampe and Misdorp, 1974). The carcinomas in mixed tumors are classified as pure or mixed adenocarcinoma, solid carcinoma, squamous cell carcinoma, cystic carcinoma, ductal or acinar carcinoma, duplex adenocarcinoma (epithelial and myoepithelial cells), papillary, cribriform, cystic, and solid carcinoma, sebaceous cell carcinoma, mucinous carcinoma, spheroidal cell carcinoma, and spindle cell carcinoma (Misdorp *et al.*, 1972, 1973). The carcinomatous elements in the malignant mixed tumors may thus be extremely variable and may be intermingled with various patterns of sarcoma. While pure forms of mammary carcinoma have been described and are currently being diagnosed, characteristically within a single tumor classified as carcinoma there may be multidifferentiation. Sometimes, under these circumstances, the mixed elements are ignored and the classification is established on the basis of the predominant type of tissue. The pathologist faces two paradoxical problems. To his surprise, the benign-appearing mixed tumor containing epithelial elements may metastasize, while up to 50% of those he classifies as carcinoma may not. Some carcinomas at their primary site are located in contact with or in juxtaposition to benign-looking tumors. The lymph nodes and lungs are the most frequent sites of metastasis of carcinomas, remembering of course that sick animals are likely to be sacrificed, thus obviating full expression of the metastases.

d. Dysplastic, Proliferative, and Metaplastic Lesions. The large number of dysplastic, proliferative, and metaplastic lesions of diversified histological types that pathologists have encountered in the mammary glands of apparently normal bitches has for a long time created confusion and disagreement among different observers as to whether any or all or which ones are potentially or actually neoplastic (Jubb and Kennedy, 1970). Among the dysplasias, the lesions of the myxodysplasia group appear to be transitional between a proliferative lesion and mixed tumor. Dysplasias occur in dogs at a relatively young age, corresponding roughly with the ages of women when they develop cystic disease and fibroadenomas. The variety of histological patterns exhibited by apparently benign dysplasias may be imagined from the fact that one observer listed them under seven major divisions plus two subcategories of these, totaling nine separate categories.

e. Comparison With Human Tumors, Incidence, Etiology. The International Histological Typing of Breast Tumors in Man, prepared by Scarff and Torloni (1968) under the auspices of the World Health Organization, used 32 separate categories for their classification. Hampe and Misdorp (1974) used 52 categories to classify mammary tumors of the dog in the International Histological Classification of Tumours of Domestic Animals. These by no means reflect the complexity of the endeavor, because the mixed tumors were classified in two line items and definitely benign tumors were not always precisely separated into distinct, accurate categories apart from so-called apparently benign tumors. With human mammary tumors, the most-differentiated area is used for typing and the least-differentiated for grading. With the bitch, grading of tumors is not useful in prognosis. There is thus a contrast between the widely accepted, carefully worked out, and prognostically valuable classification of breast tumors of women and the failure to date to agree on any one of the several classifications that veterinary pathologists have worked out for the bitch. The mixed patterns of the epithelial tumors, the so-called complex carcinomas and the sarcomas and mixed tumors of the dog, are completely out of proportion to those of man. Mammary squamous cell carcinomas of different types also occur considerably more frequently in the dog, while the mucinous adenocarcinoma occurs less frequently; but, when the latter does occur, this neoplasm is biologically more malignant than in man. Paget's disease of the nipple, although not very common in women, is debatably not present in animals. The common histological type of breast cancer of women, scirrhous carcinoma, tumors that comprise the group of infiltrating duct carcinomas with productive fibrosis, comprise 70% of human mammary cancers. Carcinomas of dogs, according to Jabara (1970), present a much more variable picture than those in women. Virtually every tumor in Jabara's (1970) series showed different carcinomatous structures and each tumor had been classified by its quantitative dominating features. Those that were better differentiated reproduced the adenocarcinoma pattern. Strandberg and Goodman (1974) have stated their belief that some epithelial types of mammary tumors of the dog can be brought into relationship with the epithelial tumors of women. These are the lobular carcinoma and the lobular carcinoma *in situ*, which are reported to comprise 10% of all canine carcinomas. The authors have recommended these malignant epithelial mammary neoplasms of the dog as representing a close model for human cancer of the breast in morphology, behavior, and incidence.

Mammary gland tumors account for 25% of the neoplasms that develop in the dog. More than half of these arise in the posterior of the five pairs of glands. Thirty to fifty percent of dogs affected with mammary tumors also bear multiple growths, showing either the same or a different histological type in the same or different mammae. All mammary glands of any one dog may be involved with different histological types of tumors. Epidemiological studies have shown that mammary tumors of all types have a frequency rate around 200 per 100,000, making them the most common neoplasms of bitches. The frequency with which malignant mammary tumors occur in the bitch varies between 26% and 74% of mammary tumors depending on the criteria of the observer. However, when based on the observation of metastasis not more than 10% are judged to be malignant. Comparing tumors of the mammary gland in both sexes of canines and human beings, Schneider (1970) reported that canine age-adjusted incidence rates were 3 times higher in females and 16 times higher in males than in the corresponding sexes of human beings. Female age-specific rates increased at the same magnitude for both species until the start of the age of natural menopause in women; then the human rates continued to increase, but more slowly, while the canine rates increased as rapidly as they had before the dogs reached this comparable age. There are rather pronounced variations in the frequency of mammary cancer in women that are dependent on ethnic, cultural, or geographic variations, as illustrated by the high rate in Parsees and low rate in Hindus living on the subcontinent of India, the high rate in blacks in America contrasted with the low rate in sub-Saharan Africa, and the high rate in Chinese and Japanese women born and living in Hawaii as compared to the rates in the respective countries of their origin. These frequencies are usually associated with reciprocal frequencies of cancer of the cervix in these populations. Comparable differences for mammary tumors have not been recorded for the dog, although purebred dogs seem to be affected more often than mixed breeds; the purebred beagle bitches appear to be particularly susceptible, while boxers less often develop this neoplasm. Andersen (1965) followed 354 untreated laboratory beagles throughout their life span. Approximately 50% of the bitches developed mammary tumors, and mammary carcinomas caused 27% of the deaths.

To enrich our knowledge about mammary cancer in the dog is no longer a simple exercise in academia to be pursued with the left hand on alternate Thursdays. It is an urgent problem of the utmost practical importance since the bitch, with her mammary tumors, has now emerged as an animal model in a number of comparative studies of human breast cancer. As Strandberg and Goodman (1974) pointed out, the spontaneous tumors of the bitch have been used as models for devising new surgical procedures and for testing the effects of chemotherapeutic agents to be used in women. The beagle, in particular, has been employed in much of the research and development work leading to the formulation of the steroid contraceptive agents. How equate such studies in the dog, they ask, when so many of the canine mammary tumors are of the mixed type or sarcoma, whereas in women the prevalent neoplasm is the infiltrative scirrhous carcinoma? Endocrine hormones involved with the reproductive cycle play a role in mammary cancer in both species. The risk of cancer is reduced in women who have been subjected to artificial menopause and in those members of societies where marriage is early and children numerous. Likewise, the risk is prevented in bitches which are sprayed before puberty, and it is reduced by forced breeding compared to that for bitches that have few or no litters. It is evident that the mammary gland tissue of the bitch is extremely susceptible to the induction of tumors by progestins and the female beagle is the dog most frequently used to test drugs containing these hormones. In a report of a long-term study, Finkel and Berliner (1973) outlined the requirements of this system in drug testing based on their own studies. The palpable mammary nodules in the untreated control dogs were recorded. A number of dogs receiving different progesterone-related synthetic progestins at various dose levels up to 5 yr developed mammary tumors, some of which the authors diagnosed as benign and others as malignant; some of the latter metastasized. Nelson *et al.* (1973) also published a histological classification of the mammary nodules so induced in bitches.

If, as seems probable for the reasons stated, the bitch will be used more and more as a close model for women with breast cancer, a good deal of new knowledge needs to be developed. Follow-up studies of women with breast cancer using comparisons of clinical and pathological staging and histological patterns of the neoplasm with the postoperative course and length of survival of the patient have produced a body of extremely accurate and valuable prognostic information. This contrasts with the inaccuracy and paucity of information about mammary cancer in the dog. The surgical principle of excising the mammary cancer along with the affected lymph channels and nodes in continuity in woman has not been practiced to any extent in the bitch. In the woman the neoplasm is likely to involve one breast, whereas in the bitch multiple tumors are the rule, thus requiring more radical surgery. The superficial and deep lymphatic drainage is more complicated in the bitch, increasing the likelihood that affected lymph vessels will be incised, leaving behind secondary deposits in nodes. Clinical postoperative follow-up and the use of diagnostic X-rays to reveal neoplastic spread have been inadequately employed in the bitch; moreover, the bitch is likely to be destroyed for humane reasons, and because of the paucity of necropsies postmortem data are scanty. Thus there are wide gaps in the present knowledge of the malignant mammary tumors of dogs and even wider gaps in the comparisons of these with mammary tumors of women. However, a new endeavor that promises to provide much new and needed knowledge about mammary neoplasms of bitches is the establishment by the World Health Organization of an International Reference Center at Amsterdam for the collection of canine tumors and the data bearing on them.

8.3.2. Cat

In the cat, 80% or more of mammary tumors are carcinomas. The most commonly diagnosed is the papillary adenocarcinoma, while the less frequent histological types have been variously classified as solid, medullary, mucinous, undifferentiated, or anaplastic. Necrosis is often extensive. About 10% of mammary neoplasms are classified as adenomas or fibroadenomas, while sarcomas and mixed mesenchymal tumors, so common in dogs, are rare in cats. In general the mammary carcinoma of the cat grows rapidly from its onset; it commonly recurs postoperatively, and, even against the background of inadequate follow-up, early euthanasia, and paucity of reported necropsies, upwards of 30% of neoplasms have been reported to have metastasized. In a series of 61 carefully conducted necropsies of cats with metastatic mammary cancer, Misdorp (1972) reported that between 80% and 90% of the neoplasms had metastasized to the regional lymph nodes and the lungs, 25-30% to the pleura and the liver, and less than 2% to the skeleton. The arrangement of the lymphatic system draining the mammary glands, including the superficial and deep vessels and nodes, is similar in the cat and the dog. In the report by Weijer *et al.* (1972), the average age of the cat at first detection of a mammary tumor was 10.8 yr, the average delay until surgery 7 months, and the average postoperative survival 1 yr.

All agree that mammary neoplasms arise less frequently in the cat than the dog, but there have been rather wide variations in reported statistics on these neoplasms in the cat. They have been reported to constitute 10% or less of all tumors in the cat, but a figure as high as 50% has been reported in some series. They have been ranked third in frequency after lymphosarcoma and cutaneous neoplasms. Necropsies have shown that upwards of 25% of cats with mammary tumors have a second primary neoplasm at some site other than the mammary glands. Mammary tumors have been reported to arise more frequently in the anterior of the four pairs of mammary glands, but Weijer *et al.* (1972) found the site of the tumors, in their series, nearly equally distributed among the four pairs. In contrast to the dog, in which mammary tumors are usually multiple, feline mammary tumors tend to be single, and there is no predilection for any one breed.

Spaying of cats is not completely effective in the prevention of mammary cancer, although the neoplasm rarely develops in castrated males. Cats with ovaries intact have a sevenfold higher relative risk of mammary cancer than cats ovariectomized at or about puberty. Hayden and Nielsen (1971) have summarized the unresolved role of hormones in relation to the formation of mammary tumors in cats. The development of tumors in young cats and in mammary glands undergoing postlactation involution would suggest that prolonged stimulus with estrogen, or progesterone, or both, contributes to carcinogenesis. Ovarian hormones are, of course, not concerned in the induction of the cancers that arise in males and in ovariectomized females. In these, extraovarian sources of estrogen or progesterone or the interaction of other hormones possibly from the adrenal gland or pituitary gland may play a role. Thus the possible roles of the hormones including prolactin, progesterone, and estrogen in the initiation, progression, and regression of mammary tumors in the cat require further study. Allen (1973) has described 12 examples of fibroglandular proliferation of mammary gland tissue of intact female cats that regress with ovariectomy; the lesions histologically resemble fibroadenoma of women.

Although mammary tumors have been less extensively studied in the cat than in the dog judging from reports of such studies as have been made in the two species, certain comparisons emerge. The benign and malignant neoplasms are distinguished histologically with more assurance in the cat and the mammary carcinomas are more easily recognized as malignant neoplasms. Moreover, the histological appearances of the mammary adenocarcinomas of the cat are considerably more uniform from specimen to specimen. Some pathologists have attempted to grade the degree of malignancy of feline carcinomas into three, others into five categories and to correlate the different grades with manner of growth and tumor size to determine prognosis. Thus the grading of neoplasms in the cat for the purpose of prognosis is more useful than in the dog. It has been stated by some and denied by others that the cat may serve as a more suitable laboratory model than the dog for the comparative study of human mammary tumorigenesis since more of its tumors are carcinomas and resemble more closely some of the mammary tumors of women (Misdorp, 1964; Cotchin, 1957, 1959). Certainly, neither of these species reproduces the features of the scirrhous carcinoma, the common neoplasm of women, nor do the mouse or rat, both of which species have been proposed, at different times and by different observers, as laboratory models for human neoplasms. However, it will require some time for the accumulation of knowledge about mammary cancer in the two small species of domestic animals to reach the degree of sophistication already attained with the two rodent species. In comparable studies of the mammary gland tumors, histogenesis and histopathological classifications and multiplicity of tumors are important, as are the hormonal, physical, chemical, and viral agents that may initiate and promote them as well as their dependency on diet and different combinations of hormones. The cat has proved to be an extremely useful animal in many laboratory investigations, and perhaps after more comprehensive studies it will emerge as a proper model for some types or aspects of human mammary cancer.

8.4. Other Animals

Greene (1939) classified a series of familial mammary tumors in rabbits as of two distinct types. One type was distinguished by periods of engorgement in the mammary tissue that evolved into cystic mastitis and finally into neoplasm which exhibited a papillary glandular structure. The other type originated in clinically normal mammary gland tissue and was characterized by a purely adenomatous structure.

The few mammary gland tumors described in guina pigs untreated or subjected to whole-body radiation have been classified as benign or as adenocarcinomas which frequently metastasized.

From the few data available, the mortality rates for spontaneous mammary tumors of captive wild animals correspond somewhat to those of women. In a study in which postmortem records and other pertinent history were available, Lombard (1958) personally examined 13 mammary neoplasms found among 16,502 necropsies of mammals from four large zoological gardens and one that turned up among the necropsies of 688 primate animals at a medicobiological station. She collected reports of 25 additional mammary tumors of different species of mammals from seven zoological gardens and three research laboratories. The species comprised six orders of mammals: primates, carnivores, seals, marsupials, ungulates, and rodents. Approximately 90% of the neoplasms were of epithelial derivation, and of these the vast majority were carcinomas.

A few reports are available on the effects of the administration of hormones to monkeys. Kirschstein *et al.* (1972) reported a metastasizing duct cell carcinoma of the mammary gland of one of six rhesus monkeys treated with Enovid for 2 yr. Drill et al. (1974) administered oral contraceptives to 96 female rhesus monkeys for 5 yr, and although this treatment induced lactation and hypertrophy of the mammary gland tissue in some animals, none developed carcinoma. In an earlier study, Geschickter and Hartman (1959) described ductal hyperplasia, metaplasia, and acinar dilatation but no cancers in monkeys treated with estrogens.

9. Tumors of the Soft Tissues

There are some similarities but many differences between man and mouse in respect to the comparative aspects of soft tissue tumors. Much of what follows has been described elsewhere by the author (Stewart, 1975). In man, the hormonal status of the host may influence tumor growths to form and to regress. In mice, hormones are strong initiators of cancers of some sites, but their role as initiators of soft tissue neoplasms, apart from mammary sarcomas, is of little importance. Nevertheless, maturity, sex, and endocrine alteration (castration) may influence, to some extent, the development and histological pattern of soft tissue tumors in the mouse. With mice, genetics is frequently the determining factor that governs site, histological pattern, and incidence of spontaneous or induced soft tissue neoplasms. With man, heredity is rarely an overriding influence, although it plays a dominant role in von Recklinghausen's neurofibromatosis.

Nearly all of the chemically induced soft tissue neoplasms of mice are rapidly growing and do not exhibit the wide range of relatively benign or less malignant types that constitute the bulk of soft tissue neoplasms of man (Stewart, 1953a, 1975). Stout and Lattes (1967) estimated for man the ratio of benign to malignant soft tissue neoplasms as 6 : 1. With mice, soft tissue neoplasms of the benign type are exceedingly rare. The soft tissue neoplasms of man abound in identifiable tissue that clearly points to the source of origin, as reflected in the authoritative histological typing by Enzinger *et al.* (1969), which has 16 major groupings with an average of seven-plus subgroups per major group, amounting to well over 100 distinct classification categories. With mice, many tumors are so undifferentiated that the cell or cells of reference cannot be named with any degree of certainty, thus accounting for the large group of unclassified neoplasms. The common neoplasms of the mouse that are histologically identifiable fall into only a few simple major categories: fibrosarcoma, leiomyosarcoma, rhabdomyosarcoma, hemangioma, hemangioendothelioma, mixed carcinosarcoma (chiefly of mammary gland origin), malignant schwannoma, transformed tissue culture neoplasms and the debatable Moloney sarcoma virus (MSV) granulomatous tumors. Chondrosarcoma is infrequent in the mouse, and liposarcoma, granular cell myoblastoma, and tumors of lymph vessels are rare. Malignant schwannomas arise from peripheral nerves and ganglia, as for example those of the ear, mediastinum, abdominal region, and the cranial and spinal nerve roots. From the 1st two sites, the schwannomas may secondarily spread along the nerves that exit into the soft tissues and the tumors pursue a clinical course mimicking that of a primary neoplasm of soft tissues. Malignant schwannomas are more commonly encountered in mice and rats than in man. Synovial sarcoma, formerly considered to be exceedingly rare in rodents, has recently been shown to arise with high frequency at a number of different sites, chiefly the extremities of strain BALB/cf/Cd mice, in which it constitutes 12% of all neoplasms (Rabstein and Peters, 1973). In other strains of mice, this neoplasm is nearly unknown. Mesothelioma, a rapidly increasing neoplasm of man seen chiefly in persons exposed to asbestos, and a neoplasm that commonly arises in the tunica vaginalis testis of untreated old rats, particularly Buffalo strain rats, is rare in mice. Chabot *et al.* (1970) induced a high incidence of mesotheliomas of the peritoneum and pericardium by the injection of strain MC29 avian leukosis virus into these respective serosal-lined cavities of chicks. They described the animal model they developed as remarkably similar to the mesotheliomas of man and the bovine.

Lipoma, hibernoma, and liposarcoma, among the rarest of soft tissue neoplasms in the cat, rat, and the mouse, occur commonly in the dog and not uncommonly in man, while in the guinea pig liposarcoma constitutes upwards of 20% of the subcutaneous sarcomas induced with methylcholanthrene. The parakeet also commonly develops lipomas of the pectoral subcutaneous tissues.

The reasons why neoplasms of fat tissue occur in man, the parakeet, the dog, and the guinea pig and are so rare in the mouse, cat, and rat and why malignant hemangioendothelioma is common in the mouse, rat, and dog and rare in man are unsolved puzzles. Since it is believed that some soft tissue tumors of the same histological type may originate from different cells, possibly the neoplastic expression of adipose tissue in the mouse and rat is a fibrosarcoma. This concept has support from the studies in mice and rats, in which species chondrosarcomas and osteogenic sarcomas may arise in sites where bone or cartilage does not exist. The opposite of this is exemplified by the experiments of Franks *et al.* (1970), who reported that histologically similar neoplasms arose at the transplantation sites in host mice that had received inoculations of a variety of different tissue culture explants from syngeneic mice. For man, Stout and Lattes (1967) state that not all fibrosarcomas necessarily originate from fibroblasts but that other types of cells can function as facultative fibroblasts, including lipoblasts and histiocytes. If, as seems probable, the neoplastic expression of the lipoblast is fibrosarcoma in the mouse and liposarcoma in the guinea pig, then these two species are suitable models for studies of the comparative aspects of this problem.

Experimental pathologists are just now beginning to sort out from the heterogeneous group of fibrosarcomas of rodents a category of neoplasm that resembles those of man which Enzinger *et al.* (1969) classified as malignant fibrous histiocytoma, to which they assign a histiocytic origin. This neoplasm has a storiform pattern of malignant fibroblasts (formerly designated the "herringbone" pattern) interspersed with conspicuously malignant histiocytes and showing also xanthoma cells and inflammatory cells. We have identified a few such neoplasms in mice in the material at the Registry of Experimental Cancers. This was the prevalent histological pattern reproduced in the soft tissue neoplasms of rats that had received subcutaneous injections of carcinogenic plant extracts (Pradhan *et al.*, 1974). Pradhan *et al.* (1974) are, to my knowledge, the first to correctly diagnose malignant fibrous histiocytoma in rats, and they provided excellent descriptions and a convincing illustration of these tumors. Almost certainly, the viral transmissible ST feline sarcoma falls into this classification, although Snyder and Dungworth (1973) continue to classify it as fibrosarcoma. Snyder *et al.* (1970) identified the cell types of this neoplasm as fibroblasts and macrophages with infiltrated mast cells and lymphocytes. Some of the macrophages had foamy cytoplasm and contained phagocytosed material. By light and electron microscopy, they were able to trace intermediate cell forms between the macrophages and the interwoven bundles of neoplastic fibroblastic cells, leaving no doubt in their minds that the neoplasm originates from histiocytic-type cells. If my assessment of the histological classification of the ST feline sarcoma is correct, then abundant material is available for comparative pathology studies of the malignant fibrous histiocytoma, since the virus that transmits the neoplasm to cats also induces identical soft tissue neoplasms in rabbits, pigs, lambs, and both Old and New World nonhuman primates (Theilen *et al.*, 1970; Deinhardt *et al.*, 1970).

Thus, while a cell of one tissue type may give rise to a neoplasm classified as a different histological type, there are still other neoplasms which have not been traced with certainty to any specific type of cell or tissue. Some of these neoplasms are easily recognized under the microscope, although their origin has not been agreed upon and for all practical purposes remains unknown. A long-time example is the granular cell tumor (granular cell myoblastoma) that arises in man, the mouse, and the rat. Over the years, its origin has been traced to many different cell types with more confidence than objective proof. However, Sobel and Marquet (1974) have published convincing evidence from comparative studies that the granular cell tumor arises from an undifferentiated mesenchymal (fibroblastlike) cell and perhaps this will lay the dispute.

The group of fibrosarcomas, in their appearance, location, and behavior, also illustrates differences between man (Stout, 1948) and the mouse. In the mouse, the induced fibrosarcomas arise proportionally very frequently and are rapidly growing, highly malignant, and very cellular, many of the cells being atypical giant cells. In man, genuine fibrosarcomas are relatively uncommon, usually nonmetastasizing, and not highly malignant. Although in man they may be very cellular and show a disproportion in the relative size of individual cells, there are, as a rule, no mutinucleated giant cells. Indeed, so infrequent are multinucleated giant cells that their presence in a soft tissue neoplasm of man would, according to Stout and Lattes (1967), suggest a diagnosis of liposarcoma or rhabdomyosarcoma rather than fibrosarcoma. A disease characterized by a fibrous type of tumor, seen in man but not in the mouse, is the neurofibromatosis of von Recklinghausen. Among mammals, there is no known model for this disease, but Dawe (1973) has pointed out a resemblance to the neurogenic tumors of certain fish. Patients with von Recklinghausen's disease often have tumors arising in multiple regions of the soft parts and such tumors may grow slowly or cease to grow after a time and remain confined to the site of origin for decades or scores of years, or even for the lifetime of the patient. At any time in the course of the disease, one or more of the tumors may undergo sarcomatous transformation and kill the patient. In rats, many of the neoplasms ordinarily diagnosed as fibrosarcoma are so relatively benign in their behavior that Carter (1973) thinks they should be listed in some category other than sarcoma, which implies a malignant neoplasm.

Studies of neoplasms of fibrous and muscle origin in man have revealed a body of conflicting knowledge that might be tested in laboratory animals. With mice, it is known that the response of the soft tissues to the development of chemically induced neoplasms is considerably greater in neonates than in adults. Moreover, a difference depending on age has been shown in the proportions of the histological types of sarcomas induced. With subcutaneous injection of 3-methylcholanthrene into mice of two groups, one aged 2 wk and the other 6–12 months, leiomyosarcoma arose more frequently in the younger animals while fibrosarcoma was more frequent in the older animals. Few attempts have been made, however, to assess the behavioral differences of spontaneous soft tissue neoplasms of identical histological appearances in relation to the age of the animal or the anatomical site of origin. On the other hand, with the soft tissue neoplasms of man, given proper information and satisfactory biopsy material, it is possible for the pathologist to classify fairly accurately the majority of neoplasms and render a reasonable estimate of prognosis for any given patient. For example, the desmoid fibromatosis of the abdominal wall (desmoid tumor) is a well-recognized clinicopathological entity. Tumors with identical pathological features that arise from fascial structures elsewhere in the body, the so-called extra-abdominal desmoid tumors, are considerably more prone to infiltrate locally and to recur following resection than are the histologically similar tumors of the abdominal wall. Slye *et al.* (1917) described the histology of the spontaneous spindle cell sarcomas of the mice of the Slye stock as varying in appearance from well-differentiated, desmoidlike growths to large-cell sarcomas with uninuclear and multinuclear giant cells. However, they reported no correlations between the behaviors of the desmoidlike growths in relation to the site at which they arose.

Differences in behavior, depending on different factors, are also exhibited by neoplasms of muscle origin in patients. Given a benign-looking smooth muscle tumor of the subcutis, one can rest assured that local excision will cure the disease. But a tumor with the same histological appearance located in the retroperitoneum or deep in the tissues of the thigh may recur or even metastasize despite the perfectly benign-looking histology. With childhood neoplasms, many are less malignant than their counterparts in adults, although an exception to this general rule is the rhabdomyosarcoma, which is more malignant in children and has a different histological appearance. The alveolar type of rhabdomysarcoma may appear suddenly in a localized part of the body of a child, disseminate rapidly and widely, and pursue a relentlessly fatal course in the brief period of 2 months. The wide range of histological appearances of rhabdomyosarcomas of man is not recognized among rodent tumors, whether because these varieties of pattern do not exist or because they have not been searched for. Perhaps Sáxen (1953) touched on this problem when he stated that although he was unable to prove a direct connection between pleomorphic cells and myoblasts within a heterogeneous group of induced soft tissue neoplasms of mice, it seemed from appearances in the tumors that the muscle cells could be differentiating into malignant round cells and spindle cells. Thus there is the need for more careful study of the murine soft tissue sarcomas with a view to refinement of morphological classification and evaluation of behavioral characteristics.

The complexity of patterns of the mixed histological types of soft tissue neoplasms also differs somewhat in man from that of the mouse. There are additionally differences in mice depending on the site of origin and whether the neoplasm is spontaneous or induced. The various histological patterns that may be seen in neoplasms of the mouse that are induced by the subcutaneous injection of chemical carcinogens may depend on the initiation of the neoplastic process in different cell types that may come in contact with the carcinogen. This then may be followed by regression of one or another clone of cells or its overgrowth. Understandably, then, mixed histological types of tissue may occur in soft tissue neoplasms so induced in mice. However, the mixed soft tissue neoplasms of rodents do not exhibit the wide variety and the different combinations within a single neoplasm of the several distinctive mesenchymatous tissue elements commonly seen in soft tissue neoplasms of man. These may be fat, fibrous tissue, reticular tissue, smooth and striated muscle, bone, cartilage and blood vessels, variously maturely differentiated or anaplastic, benign, or malignant looking. Myxoid liposarcoma may contain, in different regions, mature adipose tissue, primitive mesenchyme, spindle cells that resemble fibrosarcoma, or even foci that resemble pleomorphic rhabdomyosarcoma. One wonders whether these mixtures of histologically different tissues are the result of metaplasia within the tumor that arose *ab initio* from a single cell type or whether each histological type of tumor tissue arose from its corresponding cell of reference. With such mixed soft tissue neoplasms of man one doesn't know.

Analogies may exist between some of the debatable tumorlike lesions of man and those of the mouse and the cat; if so, the experimental lesions of these latter species could be used for comparison with the spontaneous diseases in man. In children, in particular, considerable knowledge has accumulated on the morphology and behavior of pseudosarcoma, paradoxical fibrosarcoma, and the like, lesions considered not to represent genuine neoplastic processes. Yet some of the soft tissue tumors of fascia that are curable by simple excision may present a cytological and structural pattern as evil-looking histologically as the highly malignant soft tissue neoplasms. With mice, there also exists a category of lesions that biologically are somewhat comparable. These are the atypical granulomatous tumors with neoplastic-looking bizarre giant cells that arise in the soft tissues following injection of the Moloney sarcoma virus (MSV). The lesions induced by MSV tend to regress and disappear in immunologically competent mice, but may evolve into genuine neoplasms in mice that are immunologically incompetent. The ST feline sarcoma, which is also transmissible by a virus, behaves somewhat similarly. The tumors that arise in the soft tissues at the local site of injection of the ST virus in cats and that metastasize have the appearance of a malignant neoplasm. Yet with time and as the cats grow older, many of the induced lesions regress (Snyder and Dungworth, 1973). It would seem, therefore, that the respective diseases of these two laboratory animal species might serve as models for the debatable soft tissue tumorlike diseases of man.

A principal aim of modern comparative pathology is to develop or to reveal animal models that are suitable for studies of diseases of man. There are indications that possibilities exist with the soft tissue neoplasms of laboratory animals. The spontaneous neoplasms of mice range in frequency from nearly zero in some strains up to 5% or more in others. By use of appropriate experimetal conditions, profound influences can be brought to bear on the variations of induced neoplasms of the soft tissues. To date, at least two factors seem to have limited this aim. One is that soft tissue neoplasms of laboratory animals have been studied much less intensely than other neoplasms such as those of the breast, skin, lung, liver, hematopoietic tissues, and genital organs. The other factor is that some of those who have studied soft tissue neoplasms of laboratory animals seem to know little about soft tissue neoplasms of man. For the future, it is to be hoped that progress in the experimental field will narrow this gap so that the knowledge gained in the laboratory will soon reach the sophistication level long ago achieved by studies of soft tissue neoplasms of man. Thus the field of comparative pathology could immeasurably broaden our knowledge of soft tissue tumors of man.

10. Hemangiosarcoma (Malignant Hemangioendothelioma)

Apart from Kaposi's sarcoma, which has a geographic distribution that suggests a chemical or biological agent as its cause, hemangiosarcoma (malignant hemangioendothelioma) is among the least frequent of neoplasms encountered in man. However, the importance of this neoplasm has assumed large dimensions since its appearance, in December 1973, in workers in the plastics industry who had been exposed to the monomer vinyl chloride. Whether the polymers made from vinyl chloride or the resins, or combinations of these, or other agents released in the different processing procedures carried on in the industry are also carcinogenic for man is at present under investigation. The U.S. Occupational Safety and Health Administration is the regulatory agency responsible for the establishment of safe standards for workers who are exposed to the monomer vinyl chloride in their occupational environment. These workers turn out the polyvinyl chloride. In addition, there are workers who fabricate plastic products, the annual value of which amounts to over $60 billion a year. This gives some idea of the importance both to the individual and to the industry of a diagnosis of hemangiosarcoma. Pathologists can't afford to make mistakes. The discovery of no other industry-related neoplasm has precipitated as much national and worldwide activity in such a short period of time as the discovery that vinyl chloride causes hemangiosarcomas in the labor force of the plastics industry. In the 6 months following the discovery, three major conferences were held to consider the problems involved, two in this country and one at the World Health Organization's International Agency for Research on Cancer at Lyon, France. A defect revealed at these conferences was the frequent misdiagnosis of this neoplasm by the clinical pathologist who first examined the specimen. This mistake had been made in nearly all of the early cases occurring in this country and abroad, and the same mistake in diagnosis was reported to have been made in other cases described at the Lyon meeting. This is not too surprising since fewer than 25 cases of hemangiosarcoma are expected annually in the United States. Among the huge numbers of accessions of pathological specimens at the AFIP in Washington, there are only 66 cases of hemangiosarcoma in man. With many of these also, the lesion was misdiagnosed initially. It is important for the clinical pathologist to familiarize himself with this neoplasm since, considering the large labor force that has been exposed in the plastics industry over the past 30 odd years, we can reasonably expect new cases of hemangiosarcoma to appear in these workers. There is no other neoplasm, that I know of, where the ratio is so great between the paucity of cases of hemangiosarcoma in man and the great numbers in laboratory rodents and domestic animals, particularly the dog. The clinical pathologist would do well to familiarize himself with the large material and abundant literature dealing with the neoplasm in animals (Stewart, 1953a, 1975).

Experimental and veterinary pathologists prefer the term "hemangioen-dothelioma" to designate the malignant neoplasm of blood vessels and endothelial cells. Synonyms used interchangeably for this neoplasm are hemangiosarcoma, angiosarcoma, hemangioendothelial-sarcoma, and malignant hemangioen-dothelioma. Hemangioendothelioma is one of the most ubiquitous of histological types of neoplasm seen in animals. In the accessed material at the Registry of Experimental Cancers of the National Cancer Institute at Bethesda, hemangioen-dothelioma has been coded to 22 different organ and tissue sites in mice, rats, and hamsters. These are skin, subcutaneous connective tissues, skeletal muscle, retroperitoneal tissues, peritoneum, mesenteries and omenta, lung, pleura, stomach, intestine, pancreas, liver, adrenal gland, ovary, uterus, testis, penis, kidney, urinary bladder, lymph node, and spleen.

Spontaneous hemangiosarcoma is a common neoplasm of the dog. Waller and Rubarth (1967) published a careful description of the pathological features of this neoplasm as observed in 49 dogs from a total of 12,635 necropsies performed over a 25-yr period at the Royal Veterinary College, Stockholm. Based on these figures, the annual mortality rate in dogs was around 16 per 100,000; the male–female ratio was 3 : 1, and the Alsatian (German shepherd) followed by the boxer was the breed most commonly affected. The most frequent primary site to be involved by the neoplasm was the heart, 50%, followed by the liver, spleen, and peritoneum, each about 10%. The neoplasm was identified at 16 different primary or secondary organ and tissue sites in the Stockholm dogs. The histological descriptions of the canine neoplasm revealed the same similarities and variables described for this neoplasm in mice, rats, hamsters, and the human subjects that I have examined.

A number and variety of carcinogenic agents induce hemangioendotheliomas in laboratory animals. These include thorotrast, polycyclic hydrocarbons, ultraviolet light, azo dyes, urethan, and hydrazine, nitroso, and fluorenylamine compounds, and lately vinyl chloride also. Spontaneous hemangioendotheliomas have been described in many inbred strains of mice, and in one strain in particular, the HR/De (hairless) strain, a frequency of 24% has been reported (Deringer, 1956, 1962). When the animals of this strain were treated with o-aminoazotoluene, there was a two- to threefold increase. Among 788 neoplasms of various histological types found in the soft tissues of untreated strain C3H mice and its substrains, 23 or approximately 3% were identified as hemangioen-dothelioma (Dunn *et al.*, 1956). As compared with strain C3H mice, strain BALB/c mice proved to be considerably more susceptible to the induction of hemangioen-dothelioma of the peritoneum, mesentery, and mesenteric lymph nodes following the oral administration of 3-methylcholanthrene (Stewart, 1953a; White and Stewart, 1942). BALB/c mice are also more prone to develop hemangioen-dothelioma induced by other carcinogens, females being more susceptible than males, and the susceptibility of castrated males greater than that of intact males, indicating strain and sex influences. o-Aminoazotoluene, under different conditions of administration, is capable of evoking both hemangioen-dothelioma and sarcoma in several strains of mice (Andervont, 1950b).

The hemangioendotheliomas arise at a variety of different sites distant from site of application, whereas the sarcomas appear locally at the site of subcutaneous injection. Olive oil solutions of the dye induce both hemangioendothelioma and sarcoma, but the crystalline compound induces only hemangioendothelioma. When the crystalline material is injected subcutaneously into the axillary region, most of the induced hemangioendotheliomas arise in the interscapular fat; when injected subcutaneously at the base of the tail or mid-dorsally, or when administered orally, the majority of the neoplasms, which are hemangioendotheliomas, arise in the lungs. As with the azo dyes, the carcinogenic action of the nitroso compound dimethylnitrosame is somewhat dependent on the route of administration. When injected subcutaneously, dimethylnitrosamine induces more hemangioendotheliomas of soft tissues (not necessarily at the site of injection) than when administered orally. Hence juggling the agent, the solvent, and the routes of administration may influence the site and histological type of the neoplasm. These factors need to be taken into consideration in the development of plans for studies of the occurrence of hemangioendotheliomas in human populations working in the plastics industry.

Grossly, hemangioendotheliomas of rodents are distinguishable by their color, which is due to the presence of fresh, coagulated, or degenerated blood. The tumor masses may be cystic, sometimes firm, irregularly nodular, red, red-brown, or blackish. The peripheral limits may be sharply circumscribed by compressed collagenous tissue, but the neoplasms lack encapsulation and are invasive but ordinarily do not metastasize. In my own experiments, I have seen a few examples of metastasis, but one needs to be alert not to confuse primary tumors induced at multiple sites with metastases. The rupture of the fragile vessels of this neoplasm may result in fatal hemorrhage into a body cavity.

Microscopically, hemangioendotheliomas of rodents are composed of atypical blood vessel endothelium which forms both vascular channels and solid cellular masses. The degree of cellularity varies considerably, as do the size, shape, number, and appearance of the vascular channels. Some tumors or areas of tumors are composed almost exclusively of closely packed, thin-walled vascular channels of capillary, cavernous, or intermediate size. Other areas are chiefly cellular, with and without blood spaces, and the tumor cells may be flat, round, spindle-shaped, polygonal, greatly enlarged, or extremely irregular in form. The nuclei of the tumor cells may be single or multiple, irregular in shape and size, and often exceedingly large and excessively lobated, possessing large masses of dense chromatin. The mitotic figures, which are usually numerous, are frequently bizarre. A striking feature is the intravascular endothelial-cell proliferation, which may amount to a many-layered lining that partially or completely occludes the lumen. The vessels which do possess a lumen usually contain blood, sometimes thrombi, or collections of leukocytes. Throughout the tumor are areas of necrosis, inflammatory foci, hemorrhage, and blood pigment. Peripherally, there may be active invasion of the surrounding tissue or there may be a pseudocapsule of collagenous tissue, extensions from which compartmentalize the tumor. In the vascular areas, the reticulum fibers occupy a basement-membrane-like position in relation to the vessel wall, much like the relationship seen with normal vessels. In the cellular nonvascular areas, the reticulum fibers are few in number and surround relatively large cellular aggregations with little tendency to permeate among the tumor cells. This is a reliable criterion for distinguishing hemangiosarcoma from fibrosarcoma. Peripherally a wide, reactive, hemorrhagic zone surrounds the vascular tumor. This zone is usually devoid of neoplastic cells. Unless care is taken to include the center of the tumor mass in the material sectioned, the neoplastic nature of the lesion may be overlooked.

It is doubtful, as some observers have stated, that in mice hemangioma is the first stage of hemangioendothelioma. This debatable point needs further investigation. However, the microscopic appearances of the very early stages of hemangioendothelioma, the malignant neoplasm, "easily distinguish it" from hemangioma and have been described and illustrated in mice whose lesions were induced by oral administration of the polycyclic hydrocarbons (White and Stewart, 1942). A common necropsy finding in human subjects is hemangioma of the liver. If hemangioma were the initial stage of hemangiosarcoma, then this malignant neoplasm should evolve sufficiently frequently to appear quite often at necropsy instead of being the exceedingly rare neoplasm it is in man.

Following successive transplantations over long periods, the growth of the hemangioendothelioma in mice may appear as a blood-filled cyst. Within the walls of such a cyst are blood-filled, endothelial-lined channels similar to those of the neoplasm in the primary host. To retransplant requires excised tissue from immediately within the capsule. The transplants rarely yield metastases.

Of the cases of malignant hemangioendothelioma from human subjects that I have examined, all involved occupational exposure during life to vinyl chloride in the plastics industry. All subjects had hemangiosarcoma of the liver and one, in addition, had hemangiosarcoma of the serosa of the duodenum and another had hemangiosarcomas of four other sites, the mesentery, lung, heart, and kidney. In this last subject, the histological appearances of the neoplasms of the liver, heart, and kidney indicated them to be primary at these respective sites. It was, however, not possible to state whether those of the lung and mesentery were primary or secondary. The hemangiosarcomas of these human subjects closely resembled hemangiosarcomas that I have studied in laboratory animals. In the human cases, the hemangiosarcomas were multicentric within each of the primary sites. One could find foci in which only the blood vessels were dilated, and between the dilated vessels the cells of the particular organ were still recognizable as hepatic cell cords, cardiac muscle fibers, or renal tubules as the case might be. Here and there in the earliest neoplastic focus to be recognized, lining cells of the dilated vessels were darker than usual and more prominent due to increase in size, intensity of staining, and alteration in shape. The number of these dilated vessels and altered endothelial cells increased in different foci of tumor development just as one sees in the analogous tumors of laboratory animals. The altered endothelial cells proliferated to form several layers of lining cells on the inner surface of the dilated vessels. This led to the filling and subsequent occlusion of the vessel lumen or to the formation of a solid sheet of neoplasm in which vessels were less frequently identified or absent. The hepatic cells and liver cords between the dilated sinuses became compressed, atrophied, and disappeared, often to be replaced by fibrous tissue, ending in a dense hyaline stroma separating the neoplastic vessels. Perhaps this had sometimes led to the mistaken diagnosis of fibrosarcoma.

The human liver material that I reviewed showed large irregular patches of degeneration, necrosis, and fibrosis. The fibrosis may be perilobular and intralobular and there may be large superficial patches of fibrosis on the surface of the liver. I think the liver damage represents a separate toxic effect produced by the vinyl chloride apart from the carcinogenic effect of this agent. Long before the discovery of its carcinogenic effect, industrial physicians had recognized the toxic effects of vinyl chloride on the peripheral blood vessels and bones of workers in the plastics industry (Filatova and Antonyuzhenko, 1971). In our animal material, we may see hemangiosarcomas arising with little or no associated parenchymal damage, inflammation, or fibrosis in the organ or tissue site where the neoplasm has developed. An example is the hemangiosarcoma produced by urethan, which although carcinogenic is not particularly toxic. Other times, as for example with rats that ingest large doses of a powerfully toxic and carcinogenic fluorenylamine compound, the livers containing the areas of hemangiosarcoma frequently also show fibrosis, degeneration, and necrosis as well as other neoplasms of hepatic cell origin. Therefore, on the basis of my experience and taking into consideration different factors of etiology and latency periods, I consider the lesions of hemangiosarcoma of man and laboratory animals to be closely comparable.

Of the 66 cases of hemangiosarcoma accessed at the AFIP in Washington, and described at a meeting on vinyl chloride at the National Library of Medicine in May 1974, more than two-thirds of the livers had multiple nodules of neoplasm. In some specimens, these nodules were sometimes so large as to be palpable clinically. As in rats, there was the possibility for rupture of these superficial vascular tumors leading to hemoperitoneum. In the AFIP cases, cirrhosis was present in less than 15% of the specimens and when present was generally of the portal type. Here is a distinct difference from the vinyl chloride cases, in which the livers showed much surface fibrosis, as well as portal and intralobular fibrosis and focal proliferation of fibroblasts. Forty-five percent of the hemangiosarcomas from the AFIP material were said to have metastasized, while no more than one (and that only a possibility) of the vinyl chloride cases that I examined metastasized.

Several of the vinyl chloride cases also have had large spleens. These showed large lymph follicles, perifollicular hemorrhage, distension of splenic sinuses, and cellular thickening and fibrosis of the tissue between the dilated sinuses, all reminiscent of Banti's disease including portal hypertension. In laboratory animals with hemangiosarcoma of the liver, comparable splenic lesions are not observed. Rats treated with the fluorenylamine compounds may develop hyperplasia, hypertrophy, and fibrosis of the spleen (Morris et al., 1961), but to date these lesions have not been carefully compared with those of man.

Thus pathologists working in the area of experimental carcinogenesis and with veterinary material have had the opportunity over the years to examine hemangioendotheliomas at many sites in different species in contrast to the paucity of cases in man. This is a reversal of what generally obtains. Generally, the comparative pathologist carries out his studies of pathological conditions in animals by comparing the animal lesions with those of man. With many diseases, the corresponding lesions of man have been studied in larger numbers, in greater depth, and over a longer span of time. With hemangiosarcoma, the situation is reversed. Experimental and veterinary pathologists have had vastly more experience with this neoplasm than has the clinical pathologist. The logical conclusion is that, if the clinical pathologists are to progress rapidly in their understanding of hemangiosarcomas in people exposed to vinyl chloride, they would be well advised to enlarge their knowledge by studying the many neoplasms of this histological type that are now accessed in laboratories maintained by comparative pathologists.

11. References

ACKERKNECHT, E. H., 1953, *Rudolf Virchow, Doctor, Statesman, Anthropologist*, University of Wisconsin Press, Madison.

AKAMATSU, Y., WADA, F., AND IKEGAMI, R., 1969, Transplantation of spontaneous hepatomas in C3H mice; biological and biochemical studies, *Gann* **60**:145.

ALLEN, H. L., 1973, Feline mammary hypertrophy, *Vet. Pathol.* **10**:501.

ALLISON, R. M., AND WILLIS, R. A., 1956, An ossifying embryonic mixed tumor of an infant's liver, *J. Pathol. Bacteriol.* **72**:155.

ANDERSEN, A. C., 1965, Parameters of mammary gland tumors in aging beagles, *J. Am. Vet. Med. Assoc.* **147**:1653.

ANDERSEN, A., AND GUTTMAN, P., 1966, Lung neoplasms in whole-body X-irradiated beagles, in: *Lung Tumours in Animals* (L. Severi, ed.), pp. 359–368, Division of Cancer Research, Perugia.

ANDERVONT, H. B., 1950a, Studies on the occurrence of spontaneous hepatomas in mice of strains C3H and CBA, *J. Natl. Cancer Inst.* **11**:581.

ANDERVONT, H. B., 1950b, Induction of hemangioendotheliomas and sarcomas in mice with o-aminoazotoluene, *J. Natl. Cancer Inst.* **10**:927.

ANDERVONT, H. B., AND DUNN, T. B., 1952, Transplantation of spontaneous and induced hepatomas in inbred mice, *J. Natl. Cancer Inst.* **13**:455.

ANDERVONT, H. B., AND DUNN, T. B., 1955, Transplantation of hepatomas in mice, *J. Natl. Cancer Inst.* **15**:1513.

ANDERVONT, H. B., AND DUNN, T. B., 1962, Occurrence of tumors in wild house mice, *J. Natl. Cancer Inst.* **28**:1153.

ANKERST, J., JONSSON, N., KJELLEN, L., NORRBY, E., AND SJÖGREN, H. O., 1974, Induction of mammary fibroadenomas in rats by adenovirus type 9, *Int. J. Cancer* **13**:286.

APOLANT, H., 1906, Die epithelialen Geschwulste der Maus, *Arb. Koneglchu Inst. Exp. Ther.* **1**:7.

ASHLEY, L. M., 1973, Animal model: liver cell carcinoma in rainbow trout, *Am. J. Pathol.* **72**:345.

BAILLIE, SIMMS, WILLAN, SHARPE, HOME, PEARSON, ABERNETHY, AND DENMAN, 1806, Institution for investigating the nature of cancer, *Edinburgh Med. J.* **2**:382 (reprinted in *Int. J. Cancer* **2**:281, 1967).

BANNASCH, P., 1968, The cytoplasm of hepatocytes during carcinogenesis; electron and light microscopical investigations of the nitroso-morpholine-intoxicated rat liver, in: *Recent Results of Cancer Research*, Vol. 19, 105 pp., Springer, New York.

BANNASCH, P., AND ANGERER, H., 1974, Glykogen und Glukose 6-phosphatase wahrend der Kanzerisierung der Rattenleber durch N-Nitrosomorpholin, *Arch. Geschwulstforsch.* **43**:105.

BANNASCH, P., PAPENBURG, J., AND ROSSI, W., 1972, Cytomorphologische und morphometrische Studien der Hepatocarcinogenese, Z. Krebsforsch. 77:108.

BASHFORD, E. F., AND MURRAY, J. A., 1904, The significance of the zoological distribution, the nature of the mitoses, and the transmissibility of cancer, Br. Med. J. 1:269.

BEARD, J. W., HILLMAN, E. A., BEARD, D., LAPIS, K., AND HEINE, U., 1975, Neoplastic response of the avian liver to host infection with strain MC29 leukosis virus, Cancer Res. 35:1603.

BECKER, F. F., 1974, Hepatoma—Nature's model tumor, Am. J. Pathol. 74:179.

BECKER, F. F., AND KLEIN, K. M., 1971, The effect of L-asparaginase on mitotic activity during N-2-fluorenylacetamide hepatocarcinogenesis: Subpopulations of nodular cells, Cancer Res. 31:169.

BECKER, F. E., AND SELL, S., 1974, Early elevation of α_1-fetoprotein in N-2-fluorenylacetamide hepatocarcinogenesis, Cancer Res. 34:2489.

BECKER, F. F., FOX, R. A., KLEIN, K. M., AND WOLMAN, S. R., 1971, Chromosome patterns in rat hepatocytes during N-2-fluorenylacetamide carcinogenesis, J. Natl. Cancer Inst. 46:1261.

BITTNER, J. J., 1936, Some possible effects of nursing on the mammary gland tumor incidence in mice, Science 84:162.

BOGDEN, A. E., COBB, W. R., AHMED, M., ALEX, S., AND MASON, M. M., 1974, Oncogenicity of the R-35 rat mammary tumor virus, J. Natl. Cancer Inst. 53:1073.

BRUNI, C., 1973, Distinctive cells similar to fetal hepatocytes associated with liver carcinogenesis by diethylnitrosamine: Electron microscopic study, J. Natl. Cancer Inst. 50:1513.

BULLOCK, F. D., AND CURTIS, M. R., 1925, Types of cysticercus tumors, J. Cancer Res. 9:425.

BUTLER, W. H., 1971, Pathology of liver cancer in experimental animals, in: Liver Cancer, pp. 30–41, IARC Scientific Publication No. 1, Lyon.

CARTER, R. L., 1973, Tumours of the soft tissues, in: Pathology of Tumours in Laboratory Animals, Vol. I: Tumours of the Rat, Part I (V. S. Turusov, ed.), pp. 151–168, International Agency for Research on Cancer, Lyon.

CHABOT, J. F., BEARD, D., LANGLAIS, A. J., AND BEARD, J. W., 1970, Mesothelioma of peritoneum, epicardium and pericardium induced by strain MC29 avian leukosis virus, Cancer Res. 30:1287.

CLARKE, W. J., PARK, J. F., AND BAIR, W. J., 1966, Plutonium particle-induced neoplasia of the canine lung. II. Histopathology and conclusions, in: Lung Tumours in Animals (L. Severi, ed.), pp. 345–357, Division of Cancer Research, Perugia.

COTCHIN, E., 1957, Neoplasia in the cat, Vet. Rec. 69:425.

COTCHIN, E., 1959, Some tumours of dogs and cats of comparative veterinary and human interest, Vet. Rec. 71:1040.

CUBA-CAPARO, A., DE LA VEGA, E., AND COPAIRA, M., 1961, Pulmonary adenomatosis of sheep-metastasizing bronchiolar tumors, Am. J. Vet. Res. 22:673.

DAHME, E., 1966, Classification and nomenclature of the spontaneous lung tumours in animals, in: Lung Tumours in Animals (L. Severi, ed.), pp. 143–150, Division of Cancer Research, Perugia.

DAWE, C. J., 1973, Comparative neoplasia, in: Cancer Medicine (J. F. Holland and E. Frei, eds.), pp. 193–240, Lea and Febiger, Philadelphia.

DEINHARDT, F., WOLFE, L. G., THEILEN, G. H., AND STANLEY, P., 1970, ST-feline fibrosarcoma virus: Induction of tumors in marmoset monkeys, Science 167:881.

DERINGER, M. K., 1956, The effect of subcutaneous inoculation of 4-o-tolylazo-o-toluidine in strain HR mice, J. Natl. Cancer Inst. 17:533.

DERINGER, M. K., 1959, Occurrence of tumors, particularly mammary tumors in agent-free strain C3HeB mice, J. Natl. Cancer Inst. 22:995.

DERINGER, M. K., 1962, Response of strain HR/DE mice to painting with urethan, J. Natl. Cancer Inst. 29:1107.

DERINGER, M. K., 1970, Influence of the lethal yellow (A^y) gene on development of reticular neoplasms, J. Natl. Cancer Inst. 45:1205.

DRILL, V. A., MARTIN, D. P., HART, E. R., AND MCCONNELL, R. G., 1974, Effect of oral contraceptives on the mammary glands of rhesus monkeys: A preliminary report, J. Natl. Cancer Inst. 52:1655.

DUNN, T. B., 1959, Morphology of mammary tumors in mice, in: Physiopathology of Cancer 2nd ed. (F. Homburger, ed.), pp. 38–84, Hoeber, New York.

DUNN, T. B., HESTON, W. E., AND DERINGER, M. K., 1956, Subcutaneous fibrosarcomas in strains C3H and C57BL female mice and F1 and backcross hybrids of these strains, J. Natl. Cancer Inst. 17:639.

EDITORS, 1973, Introduction in: Pathology of Tumours in Laboratory Animals. Vol. 1: Tumours of the Rat (V. S. Turusov, ed.), p. ix, International Agency for Research on Cancer, Lyon.

EDWARDS, J. E., AND DALTON, A. J., 1942, Induction of cirrhosis of the liver and of hepatomas in mice with carbon tetrachloride, J. Natl. Cancer Inst. 3:19.

EDWARDS, J. E., DALTON, A. J., AND ANDERVONT, H. B., 1942, Pathology of a transplanted spontaneous hepatoma in a C3H mouse, *J. Natl. Cancer Inst.* **2**:555.

ELLERMANN, V., AND BANG, O., 1908, Experimentelle Leukämie bei Hühern, *Z. Hyg. Infektionskr.* **63**:231.

ENZINGER, E. M., LATTES, R., AND TORLONI, H., 1969, *Histological Typing of Soft Tissue Tumours* International Histological Classification of Tumours No. 3, World Health Organization, Geneva.

FARBER, E., 1973, Hyperplastic liver nodules, in: *Methods in Cancer Research* Vol. VII (H. Busch, ed.), pp. 345–370, Academic Press, New York.

FARBER, E., 1974, Pathogenesis of liver cancer, *Arch. Pathol.* **98**:145.

FIBIGER, J., 1919, On spiroptera carcinomata and their relation to true malignant tumors; with some remarks on cancer age, *J. Cancer Res.* **4**:367.

FILATOVA, V. S., AND ANTONYUZHENKO, V. A., 1971, Dynamics of hygienic working conditions and occupational disease incidence among workers in suspension polyvinyl chloride production over a number of years, *Gig. Tr. Prof. Zabol.* **15**:32 (NIH Libr. Transl. 74–352C).

FINKEL, M. J., AND BERLINER, V. R., 1973, The extrapolation of experimental findings (animal to man): The dilemma of the systemically administered contraceptives, *Bull. Soc. Pharmacol. Environ. Pathol.* **4**:13.

FOULDS, L., 1949, Mammary tumors in hybrid mice, growth and progression of spontaneous tumours, *Br. J. Cancer* **3**:345.

FOULDS, L., 1951, Experimental study of the course and regulations of tumour growth, *Ann. R. Coll. Surg. Eng.* **9**:93.

FOULDS, L., 1956, The histologic analysis of mammary tumors in mice, *J. Natl. Cancer Inst.* **17**:701.

FOULDS, L., 1969, *Neoplastic Development* Vol. 1, Academic Press, New York.

FOUTS, J. R., 1970, The stimulation and inhibition of hepatic microsomal drug-metabolizing enzymes with special reference to effects of environmental contaminants, *Toxicol. Appl. Pharmacol.* **17**:804.

FRANKS, L. M., CHESTERMAN, F. C., AND ROWLATT, C., 1970, The structure of tumours derived from mouse cells after "spontaneous" transformation *in vitro*, *Br. J. Cancer* **24**:843.

FUMIO, H., FUJISAWA, T., TSUBURA, E., AND YAMAMURA, Y., 1972, Experimental cancer of the lung in rabbits induced by chemical carcinogens, *Cancer Res.* **32**:1209.

GARDINER, M. R., ROYCE, R., AND BOKOR, A., 1965, Studies on *Crotalaria crispa* a newly recognized cause of Kimberley horse disease, *J. Pathol. Bacteriol.* **89**:43.

GELIATLY, J. B. M., 1975, The natural history of hepatic parenchymal nodule formation in a colony of C57BL mice with reference to effect of diet, Workshop on Murine Hepatomas, Lane End, Bucks, May 13–17, 1974 (publication pending).

GESCHICKTER, C. F., AND HARTMAN, C. G., 1959, Mammary response to prolonged estrogenic stimulation in the monkey, *Cancer* **12**:767.

GORER, P. A., 1940, The incidence of tumours of the liver and other organs in a pure line of mice (Strong's CBA strain), *J. Pathol. Bacteriol.* **50**:17.

GRASSO, P., AND CRAMPTON, R. F., 1972, The value of the mouse in carcinogenicity testing, *Food Cosmet. Toxicol.* **10**:418.

GREENE, H. S. N., 1939, Familial mammary tumors in the rabbit, clinical history, *J. Exp. Med.* **70**:147.

GROSS, L., 1951, "Spontaneous" leukemia developing in C3H mice following inoculation, in infancy, with AK-leukemic extracts or AK-embryos, *Proc. Soc. Exp. Biol. Med.* **76**:27.

GROSS, L., 1955, Induction of parotid carcinomas and/or subcutaneous sarcomas in C3H mice with normal C3H organ extracts, *Proc. Soc. Exp. Biol. Med.* **88**:362.

GUÈRIN, M., 1954, *Tumeurs Spontanées des Animaux de Laboratoire (Souris-Rat-Poule)*, 215 pp., Amedée Legrand et Cie, Paris.

HAMPE, J. F., AND MISDORP, W., 1974, Tumours and dysplasias of the mammary gland, *Bull. WHO* **50**:111.

HAYDEN, D. W., AND NIELSEN, S. W., 1971, Feline mammary tumours, *J. Small Anim. Pract.* **12**:687.

HESTON, W. E., 1975, Brief communication: Testing for possible effects of cedar wood shavings and diet on occurrence of mammary gland tumors and hepatomas in C3H-A^{vy} and C3H-A^{vy}fB mice, *J. Natl. Cancer Inst.* **54**:1011.

HESTON, W. E., AND DERINGER, M. K., 1952a, Test for a maternal influence in the development of mammary gland tumors in agent-free strain C3Hb mice, *J. Natl. Cancer Inst.* **13**:167.

HESTON, W. E., AND DERINGER, M. K., 1952b, Induction of pulmonary tumors in guinea pigs by intravenous injection of methylcholanthrene and dibenzanthracene, *J. Natl. Cancer Inst.* **13**:705.

HESTON, W. E., AND VLAHAKIS, 1961, Influence of the AY gene on mammary-gland tumors, hepatomas, and normal growth in mice, *J. Natl. Cancer Inst.* **26**:969.

HESTON, W. E., AND VLAHAKIS, G., 1968, C3H-A^{vy}—A high hepatoma and high mammary tumor strain of mice, *J. Natl. Cancer Inst.* **40:**1161.

HESTON, W. E., DERINGER, M. K., AND DUNN, T. B., 1956, Further studies on the relationship between the genotype and the mammary tumor agent in mice, *J. Natl. Cancer Inst.* **16:**1309.

HESTON, W. E., VLAHAKIS, G., AND DESMUKES, B., 1973, Effects of the antifertility drug Enovid in five strains of mice, with particular regard to carcinogenesis, *J. Natl. Cancer Inst.* **51:**209.

HIRANO, T., STANTON, M., AND LAYARD, M., 1974, Measurement of epidermoid carcinoma development induced in the lungs of rats by 3-methylcholanthrene-containing beeswax pellets, *J. Natl. Cancer Inst.* **53:**1209.

HIRAO, K., MATSUMURA, K., IMAGAWA, A., ENOMOTA, Y., HOSOGI, Y., KANI, T., FUJIKAWA, K., AND ITO, N., 1974, Primary neoplasms in dog liver induced by diethylnitrosamine, *Cancer Res.* **34:**1870.

HOCH-LIGETI, C., AND ARGUS, M. F., 1970, Effects of carcinogens on the lung of guinea pig, in: *Morphology of Experimental Respiratory Carcinogenesis* (P. Nettesheim, M. G. Hanna, Jr., and J. W. Deatherage, Jr., eds.), pp. 267–279, U.S. Atomic Energy Commission Division of Technical Information, Oak Ridge, Tenn.

HOWARD, E. B., 1970, The morphology of experimental lung tumors in beagle dogs, in: *Morphology of Experimental Respiratory Carcinogenesis* (P. Nettesheim, M. G., Hanna, Jr., and J. W. Deatherage, Jr., eds.), pp. 147–160, U.S. Atomic Energy Commission Division of Technical Information, Oak Ridge, Tenn.

HRUBAN, Z., MORRIS, H. P., MOCHIZUKI, Y., MERANZE, D. R., AND SLESERS, A., 1971, Light microscopic observations of Morris hepatomas, *Cancer Res.* **31:**752.

JABARA, A. G., 1970, Abnormalities of mammary growth—Hyperplasia and neoplasia, in: *Pathology of Domestic Animals* 2nd ed., Vol. 1 (K. V. F. Jubb, and P. C. Kennedy, eds.), pp. 569–573, Academic Press, New York.

JACKSON, C., 1936, The incidence and pathology of tumours of domesticated animals in South Africa, Onderstepoort *J. Vet. Res.* **6:**1.

JUBB, K. V. F., AND KENNEDY, P. C., 1970, *Pathology* of Domestic Animals, 2nd ed., Vol. 1, Academic Press, London.

KIMBROUGH, R. D., 1973, Pancreatic-type tissue in livers of rats fed polychlorinated biphenyls, *J. Natl. Cancer Inst.* **51:**679.

KIMBROUGH, R. D., AND LINDER, R. E., 1974, Induction of adenofibrosis and hepatomas of the liver in BALB/cJ mice by polychlorinated biphenyls (Aroclor 1254), *J. Natl. Cancer Inst.* **53:**547.

KIRSCHSTEIN, R. L., RABSON, A. S., AND RUSTEN, G. W., 1972, Infiltrating duct carcinoma of the mammary gland of a rhesus monkey after administration of an oral contraceptive: A preliminary report, *J. Natl. Cancer Inst.* **48:**551.

KORTEWEG, R., 1936, On the manner in which the disposition to carcinoma of the mammary gland is inherited in mice, *Genetica* **18:**350.

KREYBERG, L., 1967, *Histologic Typing of Lung Tumours*, International Histologic Classification of Tumours No. 1, World Health Organization, Geneva.

KROES, R., WILLIAMS, G. M., AND WEISBERGER, J. H., 1973, Early appearance of serum α-fetoprotein as a function of dosage of various hepatocarcinogens, *Cancer Res.* **33:**613.

KYRIAZIS, A. P., KOKA, M., AND VESSELINOVITCH, S. D., 1974, Metastatic rate of liver tumors induced by diethylnitrosamine in mice, *Cancer Res.* **34:**2881.

LAPIS, K., BEARD, D., AND BEARD, J. W., 1973, MC29 virus induced liver tumors in chickens. I. Light microscopic morphology and histogenesis of virus induced liver tumors, *Orvostudomany* **24:**229.

LAPIS, K., BEARD, D., AND BEARD, J. W., 1975, Transplantation of hepatomas induced in the avian liver by MC29 leukosis virus, *Cancer Res.* **35:**132.

LASKIN, S., KUSCHNER, M., AND DREW, R. T., 1970, Studies in pulmonary carcinogenesis, in: *Inhalation Carcinogenesis* (M. G. Hanna, Jr., P. Nettesheim, and J. R. Gilbert, eds.), pp. 321–351, U.S. Atomic Energy Commission Division of Technical Information, Oak Ridge, Tenn.

LEBLANC, M. U., 1858, Recherches sur le cancer des animaux, *Rec. Méd. Vét.* **35:**769, 902.

LEBLANC, M. U., 1859, Recherches sur le cancer des animaux, *Rec. Méd. Vét.* **36:**25.

LEDUC, E. H., AND WILSON, J. W., 1959a, A histochemical study of intranuclear inclusions in mouse liver and hepatoma, *J. Histochem. Cytochem.* **7:**8.

LEDUC, E. H., AND WILSON, J. W., 1959b, Transplantation of carbon tetrachloride-induced hepatomas in mice, *J. Natl. Cancer Inst.* **22:**581.

LEDUC, E. H., AND WILSON, J. W., 1959c, An electron microscope study of intranuclear inclusions in mouse liver and hepatoma, *J. Biophys. Biochem. Cytol.* **6:**427.

LIEBELT, A. G., LIEBELT, R. A., AND DMOCHOWSKI, L., 1971, Cytoplasmic inclusion bodies in primary and transplanted hepatomas of mice of different strains, *J. Natl. Cancer Inst.* **47:**413.

LIPPINCOTT, S. W., EDWARDS, J. E., GRADY, H. G., AND STEWART, H. L., 1942, A review of some spontaneous neoplasms in mice, *J. Natl. Cancer Inst.* **3:**199.

LITTLE, C. C., AND STRONG, L. C., 1924, Genetic studies on the transplantation of two adenocarcinomata, *J. Exp. Zool.* **41:**93.

LOMBARD, L. S., 1958, Mammary tumors in captive wild animals, in: *International symposium on Mammary Cancer* (L. Severi, ed.), pp. 605–616, Division of Cancer Research, Perugia.

LORENZ, E., JACOBSON, L. O., HESTON, W. E., SHIMKIN, M., ESCHENBRENNER, A. B., DERINGER, M. K., DONIGER, J., AND SCHWEISTHAL, R., 1954, Effects of long-continued total-body gamma irradiation on mice, guinea pigs, and rabbits. III. Effects on life span, weight, blood picture, and carcinogenesis and the role of the intensity of irradiation, in: *Biological Effects of External X and Gamma Radiation*, Part I (R. E. Zirkle, ed.), pp. 24–148, McGraw-Hill, New York.

McFADYEAN, J., 1891, The occurrence of tumours in the domesticated animals, *J. Comp. Pathol. Ther.* **4:**143.

McFARLAND, J., 1943, Mysterious mixed tumours of salivary glands, *Surg. Gynecol. Obstet.* **76:**23.

MEDINA, D., 1973, Preneoplastic lesions in mouse mammary tumorigenesis, in: *Methods in Cancer Research*, Vol. VII (H. Busch, ed.), pp. 3–53, Academic Press, New York.

MIGAKI, G., HEMBOLT, C. F., AND ROBINSON, F. R., 1974, Primary pulmonary tumors of epithelial origin in cattle, *Am. J. Vet. Res.* **35:**1397.

MISDORP, W., 1964, Malignant mammary tumors in the dog and the cat compared with the same in the woman, thesis, Rijksuniversiteit of Utrecht, Utrecht.

MISDORP, W., 1972, Quelques aspects comparatifs des cancer de la mamelle chez la chienne, la chatte et la femme, *Rec. Méd. Vét.* **148:**583.

MISDORP, W., COTCHIN, E., HAMPE, J. F., JABARA, A. G., AND VON SANDERSLEBEN, J., 1971, Canine malignant mammary tumors. I. Sarcomas, *Vet. Pathol.* **8:**99.

MISDORP, W., COTCHIN, E., HAMPE, J. F., JABARA, A. G., AND VON SANDERSLEBEN, J., 1972, Canine malignant mammary tumors. II. Adenocarcinomas, solid carcinomas and spindle cell carcinomas, *Vet. Pathol.* **9:**447.

MISDORP, W., COTCHIN, E., HAMPE, J. F., JABARA, A. G., AND VON SANDERSLEBEN, J., 1973, Canine malignant mammary tumors, III. Special types of carcinomas, malignant mixed tumors, *Vet. Pathol.* **10:**241.

MIYAJI, T., 1952, Some observations on the volume of the nucleus of spontaneous hepatomas in mice, *J. Natl. Cancer Inst.* **13:**627.

MOHR, W., ALTHOFF, J., AND PAGE, N., 1972, Tumors of the respiratory system induced in the common European hamster by *N*-diethylnitrosamine, *J. Natl. Cancer Inst.* **49:**595.

MONTESANO, R., SAFFIOTTI, U., FERRERO, A., AND KAUFMAN, D. G., 1974, Brief Communication: Synergistic effects of benzo[a]pyrene and diethylnitrosamine on respiratory carcinogenesis in hamsters, *J. Natl. Cancer Inst.* **53:**1395.

MORRIS, H. P., WAGNER, B., RAY, F. E., SNELL, K. C., AND STEWART, H. L., 1961, Comparative study of cancer and other lesions of rats fed *N,N*-2,7-fluorenylenebisacetamide or *N*-2-fluorenylacetamide, *Natl. Cancer Inst. Monogr.* **5:**1.

MOULTON, J. E., TAYLOR, D. O. N., DORN, C. R., AND ANDERSON, A. C., 1970, Canine mammary tumors, *Vet. Pathol.* **7:**289.

MÜLLER, J., 1838, Ueber den Feinern Bou und die Formen der krankhaften Geschwülste, 60 pp., Reimer, Berlin.

MURRAY, J. A., 1908, Spontaneous cancer in the mouse; histology, metastasis, transplantability and the relations of malignant new growth to spontaneously affected animals, Third Scientific Report, pp. 69–115, Imperial Cancer Research Fund, London.

National Cancer Institute Monograph, No. 31, 1969, Neoplasms and related disorders of invertebrate and lower vertebrate animals (C. J. Dawe and J. C. Harshbarger, eds.).

NELSON, L. W., WEIKEL, J. H., JR., AND RENO, F. E., 1973, Mammary nodules in dogs during four years' treatment with megestrol acetate or chlormadinone acetate, *J. Natl. Cancer Inst.* **51:**1303.

NETTESHEIM, P., AND HAMMONS, A. S., 1971, Induction of squamous cell carcinoma in the respiratory tract of mice, *J. Natl. Cancer Inst.* **47:**697.

NICOD, J. L., 1936, Essai de classification des cancers spontanés de la glande mammaire chez la souris blanche, *Bull. Assoc. Fr. Étude Cancer* **25:**743.

NIELSEN, S., 1966, Spontaneous canine pulmonary tumors, in: *Lung Tumours in Animals* (L. Severi, ed.), pp. 151–164, Division of Cancer Research, Perugia.

NIELSEN, S. W., 1970, Pulmonary neoplasia in domestic animals in: *Morphology of Experimental Respiratory Carcinogenesis* (P. Nettesheim, M. G. Hanna, Jr., and J. W. Deatherage, Jr., eds.), pp. 123–145, U.S. Atomic Energy Commission Division of Technical Information, Oak Ridge, Tenn.

NOBEL, T. A., NEUMAN, F., AND KLOPFER, W., 1969, Histologic patterns of the metastasis in pulmonary adenomatosis in sheep (Jaagsiekte), *J. Comp. Pathol.* **79**:537.

NOBLE, R. L., AND CUTTS, J. H., 1959, Mammary tumors of the rat: A review, *Cancer Res.* **19**:1125.

NOWINSKY, M., 1876, Zur Frage über die Impfung der krebsigen Geschwülste, *Centralbl. Med. Wiss.* **14**:790.

OGAWA, K., MINASE, T., AND ONOE, T., 1974, Demonstration of glucose 6-phosphatase activity in the oval cells of rat livers and the significance of the oval cells in azo dye carcinogenesis, *Cancer Res.* **34**:3379.

OKITA, K., AND FARBER, E., 1975, An antigen common to preneoplastic hepatocyte populations and to liver cancer induced by N-2-fluorenylacetamide, ethionine or other hepatocarcinogens, *Gann Monogr. Cancer Res.* (to be published).

OKITA, K., GRUENSTEIN, M., KLAIBER, M., AND FARBER, E., 1974, Localization of α-fetoprotein by immunofluorescence in hyperplastic nodules during hepatocarcinogenesis induced by 2–acetylaminofluorene, *Cancer Res.* **34**:2758.

PARK, J. F., CLARKE, W. J., AND BAIR, W., 1966, Plutonium particle-induced neoplasia of the canine lungs. I. Clinical and gross pathology, in: *Lung Tumours in Animals* (L. Severi, ed.), pp. 331–344, Division of Cancer Research, Perugia.

PERK, K., HOD, I., AND NOBEL, T. A., 1971, Pulmonary adenomatosis of sheep (Jaagsiekte). I. Ultra-structure of the tumor, *J. Natl. Cancer Inst.* **46**:525.

POUR, P., STANTON, M., KUSCHNER, M., LASKIN, S., AND SHABAD, L., 1975, Tumours of the respiratory tract, in *Pathology of Tumours in Laboratory Animals* Vol. I: Part II *Tumours of the Rat* (V. S. Turusov, ed.), International Agency for Research on Cancer, Lyon, (to be published).

PRADHAN, S. N., CHUNG, E. B., GHOSH, B., PAUL, B. D., AND KAPADIA, G. J., 1974, Potential carcinogens. I. Carcinogenicity of some plant extracts and their tannin-containing fractions in rats, *J. Natl. Cancer Inst.* **52**:1579.

PULLEY, L. T., 1973, Ultrastructural and histochemical demonstration of myoepithelium in mixed tumors of the canine mammary gland, *Am. J. Vet. Res.* **34**:1513.

RABSTEIN, L. S., AND PETERS, R. L., 1973, Tumors of the kidneys, synovia, exocrine pancreas and nasal cavity in BALB/cf/Cd mice, *J. Natl. Cancer Inst.* **51**:999.

Radionuclide carcinogenesis, *AEC Symp. Ser. Monogr.* No. 29, 1974 (C. L. Sanders, R. H. Busch, J. E. Ballou, and D. D. Mahlum, eds.), U.S. Atomic Energy Commission Division of Technical information, Oak Ridge, Tenn.

REUBER, M. D., 1967, Poorly differentiated cholangiocarcinomas occurring "spontaneously" in C3H and C3H × Y hybrid mice, *J. Natl. Cancer Inst.* **38**:901.

REUBER, M. D., 1971, Morphologic and biologic correlation of hyperplastic and neoplastic hepatic lesions occurring "spontaneously" in C3H × Y hybrid mice, *Br. J. Cancer* **25**:538.

REUBER, M. D., AND FIRMINGER, H. I., 1963, Morphologic and biologic correlation of lesions obtained in hepatic carcinogenesis in A × C rats given 0.025 percent N-2-fluorenyldiacetamide, *J. Natl. Cancer Inst.* **31**:1407.

REUBER, M. D., AND ODASHIMA, S., 1967, Further studies on transplantation of lesions in hepatic carcinogenesis in rats given 2-(diacetamido)fluorene, *Gann* **58**:513.

RICE, J., 1973, The biological behavior of transplacentally induced tumours in mice, in: *Transplacental Carcinogenesis* (L. Tomatis and W. Mohr, eds.), pp. 71–83, IARC Scientific Publication No. 4, Lyon.

RIGDON, R. H., 1966, Tumors produced by methylcholanthrene in the respiratory tract of the white Pekin duck, in: *Lung Tumours in Animals* (L. Severi, ed.), pp. 755–764, Division of Cancer Research, Perugia.

ROE, F. J. C., 1968, Carcinogenesis and sanity, *Food Cosmet. Toxicol.* **6**:485.

ROE, F. J. C., AND GRANT, G. A., 1970, Inhibition by germ-free status of development of liver and lung tumours in mice exposed neonatally to 7,12-dimethylbenz[a]anthracene tests: Implications in relation to tests for carcinogenicity, *Int. J. Cancer* **6**:133.

ROUS, P., 1910, A transmissible avian neoplasm (sarcoma of the common fowl), *J. Exp. Med.* **12**:696.

ROWLATT, C., FRANKS, L. M., AND SHERIFF, M. U., 1973, Mammary tumour and hepatoma suppression by dietary restriction on C3H-A^{vy} mice, *Br. J. Cancer* **28**:83.

SABINE, J. R., HORTON, B. J., AND WICKS, M. B., 1973, Spontaneous tumors in C3H-A^{vy} and C3H-A^{vy}fB mice: High incidence in the United States and low incidence in Australia, *J. Natl. Cancer Inst.* **50**:1237.

SÁXEN, E. A., 1953, On the factor of age in the production of subcutaneous sarcomas in mice with 20-methylcholanthrene, *J. Natl. Cancer Inst.* **14**:547.

SEATON, V. A., 1958, Pulmonary adenomatosis in Iowa cattle, *Am. J. Vet. Res.* **19**:600.

SCARFF, R. W., AND TORLONI, H., 1968, *Histologic Typing of Breast Tumours*, International Histological Classification of Tumours No. 2, World Health Organization, Geneva.

SCHILLER, A. L., 1970, Discussion, in *Morphology of Experimental Respiratory Carcinogenesis* (P. Nettesheim, M. G. Hanna, Jr., and J. W. Deatherage, Jr. eds.), p. 141, U.S. Atomic Energy Commission Division of Technical Information, Oak Ridge, Tenn.

SCHNEIDER, R., 1970, Comparison of age, sex, and incidence rates in human and canine breast cancer, *Cancer* **26**:419.

SCHOENTAL, R., 1974, Role of podophyllotoxin in the bedding and dietary zearalenone of spontaneous tumors in laboratory animals, *Cancer Res.* **34**:2419.

SCHREIBER, H., NETTESHEIM, P., LIJINSKY, W., RICHTER, C. B., AND WALBURG, H. E., 1972. Induction of lung cancer in germfree specific-pathogen-free, and infested rats by N-nitroso-hepatomethyleneimine: enhancement by respiratory infection, *J. Natl. Cancer Inst.* **49**:1107.

SHOPE, R. E., 1932, A transmissible tumor-like condition in rabbits, *J. Exp. Med.* **56**:793.

SLYE, M., HOLMES, H. F., AND WELLS, H. G., 1915, Spontaneous primary tumors of the liver in mice: Studies on the incidence and inheritability of spontaneous tumors in mice, *J. Med. Res.* **33**:171.

SLYE, M., HOLMES, H. F., AND WELLS, H. G., 1917, Primary spontaneous sarcoma in mice, *J. Cancer Res.* **2**:1.

SMITH, G. S., WALFORD, R. L., AND MICKEY, M. R., 1973, Lifespan and incidence of cancer and other diseases in selected long-lived inbred mice and their F1 hybrids, *J. Natl. Cancer Inst.* **50**:1195.

SNELL, K. C., 1965, Spontaneous lesions of the rat, in: *Pathology of Laboratory Animals* (W. E. Ribelin and J. R. McCoy, eds.), pp. 241–302, Thomas, Springfield, Ill.

SNYDER, S. P., AND DUNGWORTH, D. L., 1973, Pathogenesis of feline viral fibrosarcomas: Dose and age effects, *J. Natl. Cancer Inst.* **51**:793.

SNYDER, S. P., THEILEN, G. H., AND RICHARDS, W. P. C., 1970, Morphological studies on transmissible feline fibrosarcoma, *Cancer Res.* **30**:1658.

SOBEL, H. J., MARQUET, E., 1974, Granular cells and granular cell lesions, in: *Pathology Annual.* (S. C. Sommers, ed.), pp. 43–79, Appleton–Century–Crofts, New York.

STANTON, M. F., AND BLACKWELL, R., 1964, Induction of epidermoid carcinoma in lungs of rats: A "new" method based upon deposition of methylcholanthrene in areas of pulmonary infarction, *J. Natl. Cancer Inst.* **27**:375.

STANTON, M. F., BLACKWELL, R., AND MILLER, E., 1969, Experimental pulmonary carcinogenesis with asbestos, *Am. Ind. Hyg. Assoc. J.* **30**:236.

STANTON, M. F., MILLER, E., WRENCH, C., AND BLACKWELL, R., 1972, Experimental induction of epidermoid carcinoma in the lungs of rats by cigarette smoke condensate, *J. Natl. Cancer Inst.* **49**:867.

Stedman's Medical Dictionary, 1961, 20th ed., p. 737, Williams and Wilkins, Baltimore.

STEWART, H. L., 1953a, Tumors induced by subcutaneously injected carcinogens, in: *The Physiopathology of Cancer* (F. Homburger and W. Fishman, eds.), pp. 46–61, Hoeber–Harper, New York.

STEWART, H. L., 1953b, Endometrial carcinoma in the rabbit, in: *The Physiopathology of Cancer* (F. Homburger and W. Fishman, eds.), pp. 165–170, Hoeber-Harper, New York.

STEWART, H. L., 1964, Morphology, origin and fate of so-called pseudotubules of the liver, *Acta Unio. Int. Contra Cancrum* **20**:577.

STEWART, H. L., 1966a, Comparison of histologic lung cancer types in captive wild mammals and birds and laboratory and domestic animals, in: *Lung Tumours in Animals* (L. Severi, ed.), pp. 25–58, Division of Cancer Research, Perugia.

STEWART, H. L., 1966b, Pulmonary cancer and adenomatosis in captive wild mammals and birds from the Philadelphia Zoo, *J. Natl. Cancer Inst.* **36**:117.

STEWART, H. L., 1975, Tumours of the soft tissues, in: *Pathology of Tumours in Laboratory Animals*, Vol. II: *Tumours of the Mouse* (V. S. Turusov, ed.), International Agency for Research on Cancer, Lyon, (to be published).

STEWART, H. L., AND SNELL, K. C., 1957, The histopathology of experimental tumors of the liver of the rat: A critical review of the histopathogenesis, *Acta Unio Int. Contra Cancrum* **13**:770.

STEWART, H. L., SNELL, K. C., AND MORRIS, H. P., 1965, The combined effect of 3-methylcholanthrene and N,N'-2,7-fluorenylenebisacetamide on induction of cancer of the glandular stomach of the rat, *J. Natl. Cancer Inst.* **34**:157.

STEWART, H. L., SNELL, K. C., DUNHAM, L. J., AND SCHLYEN, S. M., 1959, Transplantable and transmissible tumors of animals, in: *Atlas of Tumor Pathology*, Section XII, Fasicle 40, 378 pp., Armed Forces Institute of Pathology, Washington, D.C.

STEWART, H. L., DUNN, T. B., SNELL, K. C., AND DERINGER, M. K., 1975. Tumors and proliferative lesions of the respiratory apparatus of mice, in: *Pathology of Tumours in Laboratory Animals* (V. S. Turusov, ed.), International Agency for Research on Cancer, Lyon, (to be published).

STEWART, S. E., 1955, Neoplasms in mice inoculated with cell-free extracts or filtrates of leukemic mouse tissues. I. Neoplasms of the parotid and adrenal glands, *J. Natl. Cancer Inst.* **15**:1391.

STICKER, A., 1902, Ueber den Krebs der Thier inbesondere uber die Emfanglichkeit der verschiedenen Hausthiearten und uber die Unterschiede des Thiere- und Menschenkrebses, *Arch. Klin. Chir.* **65**:616, 1023.

STOUT, A. P., 1948, Fibrosarcoma, the malignant tumor of fibroblasts, *Cancer* **1**:30.

STOUT, A. P., AND LATTES, R., 1967, Tumors of soft tissues in: *Atlas of Tumor Pathology* 2nd ser., Fasicle 1, Armed Forces Institute of Pathology, Washington, D.C.

STRANDBERG, J. D., AND GOODMAN, D. G., 1974, Animal model: Canine mammary neoplasia, *Am. J. Pathol.* **75**:225.

STRONG, L. C., AND SMITH, G. M., 1936, Successful transplantation of a hepatoma in mice, *Am. J. Cancer* **28**:112.

STÜNZI, H., 1973, Zur vergleichenden Pathologie des Lungenkarzinoms beim Haustier, *Pathol. Microbiol.* **39**:358.

TEEBOR, G. W., AND BECKER, F. F., 1971, Regression and persistence in hyperplastic hepatic nodules induced by N-2-fluorenylacetamide and their relationship to hepatocarcinogenesis, *Cancer Res.* **31**:1.

TERAO, K., AND NAKANO, M., 1974, Cholangiofibrosis induced by short-term feeding of 3'-methyl-4-(dimethylamino)-azobenzene: An electron microscopic observation, *Gann* **65**:249.

THEILEN, G. H., SNYDER, S. P., WOLFE, L. G., AND LANDON, J. C., 1970, Biological studies with viral induced fibrosarcomas in cats, dogs, rabbits and non-human primates, in: *Comparative Leukemia Research* (R. M. Dutcher, ed.), pp. 393–400, Karger, New York.

THEODASSION, A., BANNASCH, P., AND REUSS, W., 1971, Glykogen und endoplasmatische Reticulum der Leberzell mach hohen Dosen des Carcinogens N-nitrosomorpholine, *Virchows Arch. B* **7**:126.

THORPE, E., AND WALKER, A. I. T., 1973, The toxicity of dieldrin (HEOD). II. Comparative long-term oral toxicity studies in mice with dieldrin, DDT, phenobarbitone, β-BHC and γ-BHC, *Food Cosmet. Toxicol.* **11**:433.

TOMATIS, L., TURUSOV, V., DAY, N., AND CHARLES, R. T., 1972, The effect of long-term exposure to DDT on CF-1 *Int. J. Cancer* **10**:489.

TRAIN, R. E., 1974, Shell Chemical Co. *et al.*, consolidated aldrin/dieldrin hearing, *Fed. Reg.* **39**:37246.

TURUSOV, V. S., DAY, N. E.. TOMATIS, L., GATI, E., AND CHARLES, R. T., 1973a., Tumors in CF-1 mice exposed for six consecutive generations to DDT, *J. Natl. Cancer Inst.* **51**:983.

TURUSOV, V. S., DERINGER, M. K., DUNN, T. B., AND STEWART, H. L., 1973b, Malignant mouse-liver tumors resembling human hepatoblastomas, *J. Natl. Cancer Inst.* **51**:1689.

VLAHAKIS, G., AND HESTON, W. E., 1971, Spontaneous cholangiomas in strain C3H-A^{vy}fB mice and in their hybrids, *J. Natl. Cancer Inst.* **46**:677.

WALLER, T., AND RUBARTH, S., 1967, Hemangioendothelioma in domestic animals, *Acta Vet. Scand.* **8**:234.

WEIJER, K., HEAD, K. W., MISDORP, W., AND HAMPE, J. F., 1972, Feline malignant mammary tumors. I. Morphology and biology: Some comparisons with human and canine mammary carcinomas, *J. Natl. Cancer Inst.* **49**:1697.

WHITE, J., AND STEWART, H. L., 1942, Intestinal adenocarcinoma and intra-abdominal hemangioendothelioma in mice ingesting methylcholanthrene, *J. Natl. Cancer Inst.* **3**:331.

WHO, 1974, Veterinary Public Health: A review of the WHO programme—2, *WHO Chronicle* **28**:178.

YOSHIDA, T., 1932, Über die experimentelle Erzeugung von Hepatom durch die Fütterung *o*-Amidoazotoluol, *Proc. Jpn. Acad.* **8**:464.

YOUNG, S., AND HALLOWES, R. C., 1973, Tumours of the mammary gland, in: *Pathology of Tumours in Laboratory Animals*, Vol. I: *Tumors of the Rat* (V. S. Turusov, ed.), pp. 31–74, International Agency for Research on Cancer, Lyon.

11

Neoplasia in Poikilotherms

DANTE G. SCARPELLI

1. Introduction

A detailed knowledge of the incidence, distribution, and natural history of neoplasia throughout the animal kingdom is of central importance in gaining an understanding of cancer as a biological process. Examples of abnormal growth have been encountered in many taxonomic groups of animals and at every level of biological complexity. However, except for the mammals, the study of neoplasia, especially in the lower vertebrates, is to a large extent descriptive, haphazard, and incomplete. In this chapter, we will deal with some aspects of the biology of neoplasia in poikilotherms. As we shall see, this task becomes increasingly difficult as we approach the more primitive vertebrates and invertebrates because there are significant gaps in our knowledge of their biology and patterns of response to injury. Further, in more primitive forms of life, the precise classification of disturbances of tissue growth as neoplastic becomes increasingly difficult because of the vast structural and functional differences that separate these organisms from the more familiar and well-studied higher poikilotherms. This state of affairs has become particularly frustrating in recent years in view of the rapid advances in cell biology which emphasize the unity of basic organization and function throughout biological systems and the striking similarities of such. In this regard, it is worth recalling that many aspects of the inflammatory reaction observed in the water flea (*Daphnia*), as well as the sequential reactions of protein synthesis elucidated from biochemical studies of *Escherichia coli*, are directly applicable to these phenomena in higher animals, including the mammals, since they appear to have been copied with great fidelity throughout the evolutionary development of life. Thus it is quite probable that basic insights gained from the

DANTE G. SCARPELLI • Department of Pathology and Oncology, University of Kansas Medical Center, College of Health Sciences and Hospital, Kansas City, Kansas.

study of neoplasia and related disturbances of growth in poikilotherms will lead to a greater understanding of cancer in homeotherms.

2. The Distribution and Characteristics of Some Common Neoplasms in Poikilotherms

Since the initial description of adenocarcinoma in trout liver by Bashford (1904), there have been numerous reports of *bona fide* neoplasms in poikilotherms, especially the fishes, and to a lesser extent other lower vertebrates and invertebrates. Before briefly discussing the distribution of neoplasms in various classes of poikilotherms, it should be pointed out that gross differences in the incidence of neoplasia between one class and another may simply reflect the extent to which these have been carefully studied. The fishes, especially the teleosts, are a case in point, since they represent a major source of food for man. They have been examined very carefully and thus numerous neoplasms of all varieties have been encountered in them. Contrast this with the reptiles, most of which do not represent animals important to man; these have been studied in small numbers, in the main limited to captive animals in zoos. The amphibians, on the other hand, are used widely as laboratory animals and are intermediate between the fishes and reptiles in terms of the degree to which they have been studied and the apparent incidence and variety of neoplasms encountered in them.

2.1. Reptiles

Examples of neoplasia in the reptiles have been described in the three major orders. These include a variety of neoplasms both benign and malignant of epithelial and connective tissue origin such as adenocarcinoma of pancreas, bile duct, and kidney, malignant melanoma, osteogenic sarcoma, and lymphosarcoma. A curious exception is the apparent absence of neoplasms of hematopoietic origin in the turtles (chelonians); However, until more members of this order are studied, such a conclusion must be a tentative one. Benign cutaneous neoplasms deserve special mention because they are widely distributed among the reptiles, with the exception of the snakes (ophidians). Papillomas constitute the most common neoplasm encountered in the lizards (lacertilians) and turtles. The neoplastic nature of such lesions in the turtles is under some question since these are commonly associated with localized parasitic infestation, raising the possibility that fibroepithelial proliferation may represent a tissue reaction to the parasites. It bears mentioning that these lesions have a predominant fibrous component, while the epithelial component is characterized by moderate hyperplasia, and that, to date, all the lesions described have been benign. However, the presence of fibromatous lesions in the lungs of a green sea turtle (*Chelonia mydas*) without an associated localized parasitic infestation would suggest that some of these lesions may not be a reaction to injury, but may represent true neoplasms. Although a viral etiology has long been suspected, no virus has yet been isolated. In view of the

extensive pollution of the seas and oceans by a wide variety of chemcials from
industrial and other sources, one cannot rule out a chemical etiology. Papillomas
in lizards are more sessile, possess a less prominent fibrous component, and are
not commonly associated with cutaneous parasites. No transformation to malignant epithelial lesions has been documented, although, in contrast to the turtle,
squamous cell carcinomas have been described in the lizards.

2.2. Amphibians

A variety of benign and malignant neoplasms have been reported in various
members of the class Amphibia which include renal adenocarcinoma, hepatoma,
ovarian cystadenocarcinoma, nephroblastoma, melanoma, and lymphosarcoma.
Several of these are sufficiently unique or have served as models that have yielded
major contributions to our knowledge concerning the biology of cancer that they
deserve special mention. A renal adenocarcinoma of the leopard frog (*Rana*

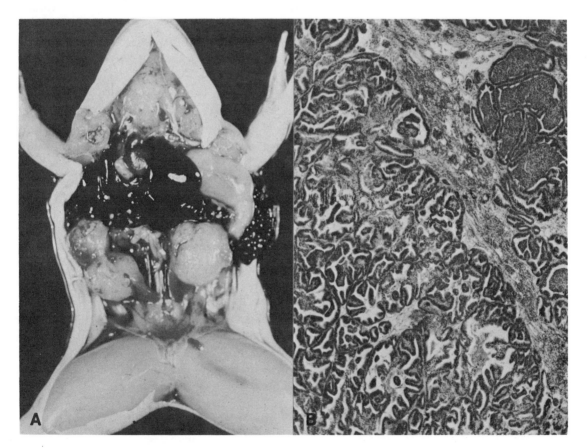

FIGURE 1. A: Bilateral renal adenocarcinoma in a leopard frog (*Rana pipiens*). (Accession No. 282 of the Registry of
Tumors in Lower Animals, Smithsonian Institution. Contributed by Katherine C. Snell.) B: The neoplasm consists of
moderately well-differentiated adenocarcinoma characterized by the nests of papillary epithelium on the left. A nodule of
less well-differentiated cells is present on the upper right. × 60. (Accession No. 172 of the Registry of Tumors in Lower
Animals, Smithsonian Institution. Contributed by Gladys S. King.)

pipiens) (Fig. 1), first studied extensively by Lucké (1934) and suggested by him to be caused by a virus, has captured the attention of many investigators over the years.

Histogenetic studies of the tumor, which arises in epithelium of the renal tubule, suggest that the earliest lesions are manifested as focal epithelial hyperplasia involving a few kidney tubules and ultimately progress to adenocarcinomas which tend to metastasize widely to adjacent organs, often filling the abdominal cavity. Histologically, the tumors show all gradations and patterns ranging from adenoma and cystadenoma to papillary adenocarcinoma. The viral etiology of this neoplasm was under serious question for many years due to the inconstant appearance of intranuclear inclusion bodies in the neoplastic epithelium.

A number of studies, especially those of Fawcett (1956) and Tweedel (1967), have clearly established that a herpes-type virus is involved. Further work has shown that the appearance of virus and concomitantly the intranuclear inclusions in tumor cells are favored by exposure of tumor-bearing frogs to low temperature (Rafferty, 1965). This explains the absence of intranuclear inclusions in tumor cells of summer frogs. Mizell and Zambernand (1965) have suggested that this may be an example of lysogeny where "cryptic" virus is activated by low temperature, a phenomenon well known in bacteriophage infection of bacteria but, except for the Lucké tumor, not yet encountered in other virally induced neoplasms. A careful epidemiological study by McKinnell (1969) of over 4000 feral frogs collected from North Dakota, South Dakota, Louisiana, and Minnesota revealed that the tumor is widespread in frogs originating in the north central United States, with a tumor prevalence rate of 4.4–5% among spring and fall adult leopard frogs, compared with a tumor prevalence of 0.14% for summer frogs. Analysis of tumor prevalence among frogs collected from 15 counties in Minnesota showed that a considerable variation existed in the geographic distribution of the tumor, with a prevalence as high as 14% in one county in contrast to absence of tumor in all frogs collected in nine of 15 counties. Furthermore, no tumors were seen in frogs collected from the Dakotas and Louisiana.

The mexican axolotl (*Ambystoma mexicanum*) is an amphibian that has yielded a number of spontaneous neoplasms of unusual variety such as a transplantable neuroepithelioma derived from olfactory epithelium (Brunst, 1967, 1969), benign testicular tumors resembling seminomas arising from spermatogonial epithelium (Humphrey, 1969), and melanomas which histologically resemble the blue nevus of higher vertebrates, including man. They are transplantable and exhibit local invasive properties; of additional interest is the fact that the tumors appear to have a genetic basis.

2.3. Fishes

The majority of neoplasms in the fishes have been encountered in teleosts, with relatively few examples occurring in the cartilaginous fishes (*Chondrichthyes*). Numerous cases of both benign and malignant neoplasms of epithelial and connective tissue origin have been reported in the fishes and have been amply described in several excellent reviews summarized in Table 1. The tumors include some that merit further discussion because they have been studied in greater detail and/or possess some interesting biological characteristics. One of the most studied neoplasms has been hepatocarcinoma of rainbow trout (*Salmo gairdneri*), first described by Wood and Larson (1961) in hatchery populations. The morphology of this tumor ranges from a well-differentiated trabecular variant to a more anaplastic tumor consisting of solid sheets of malignant hepatocytes (Fig. 2). The tumor invades intrahepatic portal veins, extends to involve adjacent organs, and may metastasize to the kidney, spleen, and gills by the hematogenous route. A potent dietary carcinogen, aflatoxin B_1 (AFB$_1$), a mycotoxin produced by certain strains of *Aspergillus flavus*, has been identified by Halver (1967). Careful attention to the conditions for preparation and storage of fish diets to preclude infection by *Aspergillus* has led to a virtual disappearance of spontaneous tumors in the fish hatchery industry. It is of interest to note that with very few exceptions hepatic carcinoma is limited to a single species of trout. Whether this is due to genetic resistance of other species of salmonids or to their inability to metabolize aflatoxin to its carcinogenic principle is unknown.

Close association of a tumor with a certain species, as in the case of hepatoma, has also been noted for several other varieties of tumors in fish (Schlumberger,

TABLE 1

Resource Bibliography on Neoplasms and Neoplastic-like Lesions in Poikilotherms

Phyla, subphyla, taxa	Reference
Invertebrates	Scharrer and Lochhead (1950)
	Johnson (1968)[a]
	Dawe (1968, 1969a)
	Sparks (1972)
	Harshbarger (1973)
	Dawe (1973)
Protozoa, coelenterates, platyhelminthes, annelids, sipunculids, and arthropods	Sparks (1969)
Protozoa	Van Wagtendonk (1969)
Insects	Harker (1963)
	Harshbarger and Taylor (1968)
Mollusks	Pauley (1969)
Invertebrates and lower vertebrates	Dawe and Harshbarger (1969)
	Scarpelli (1969)
Echinoderms, prevertebrates, and fishes	Wellings (1969)
Lower vertebrates	Lucké and Schlumberger (1949)
	Reichenbach-Klinke and Elkan (1965)
Fishes	Nigrelli (1954)
	Schlumberger (1958)
	Finkelstein (1960)
	Mawdsley-Thomas (1969, 1971)
Fishes, amphibians, and reptiles	Schlumberger and Lucké (1948)
	Balls (1962)
	Balls and Ruben (1964, 1968)
Amphibians	Mizell (1969)

[a] Annotated bibliography.

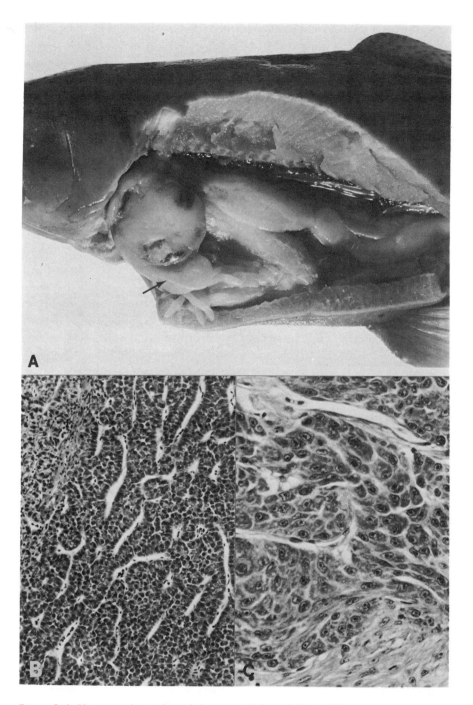

FIGURE 2. A: Hepatocarcinoma in a rainbow trout (*Salmo gairdneri*). This neoplasm was induced after 8 months of feeding a diet containing 6ppb aflatoxin B_1. Note that most of the liver has been replaced by neoplasm with only a small remnant of uninvolved liver remaining (arrow). B and C: Histological appearance of variants of hepatocarcinoma. B: Well-differentiated trabecular hepatoma with anastomotic cords of neoplastic hepatocytes. × 60. C: Poorly differentiated hepatoma. Note the mitotic figures and the bizarre-appearing tumor cells with large nuclei and nucleoli. × 350.

1957). Notable among these are the melanoma of swordtail–platyfish (*Xiphophorus*
helleri–Platypoecilus maculatus) hybrids (Häussler, 1928), peripheral nerve sheath
tumors of snappers (*Lutinidae*) and goldfish (*Auratus crassius*) (Lucké, 1942;
Schlumberger, 1952), lymphosarcoma in northern pike (*Esox lucius*) (Nigrelli,
1943), and adamantinomas, particularly in chinook salmon (*Oncorhynchus
tshawytscha*) (Schlumberger and Katz, 1956). The association of these tumors with
a particular species is probably the result of a complex of genetic as well as
environmental factors. Swordtail–platyfish hybrids have provided an excellent
model for the study of genetic factors in the induction of melanomas (Anders,
1967). These lesions, although appearing moderately undifferentiated histologically, seem to have a limited potential for extensive invasive growth. In addition to
genetic influences, the development of these tumors depends on certain environmental factors including sex hormones (Berg and Gordon, 1953; Siciliano *et al.*,
1971). The foregoing reports are unique since they represent rare instances
where fish have been employed in the study of genetics in cancer. This is because
inbred strains of fish have not been developed, although there are current efforts
under way to accomplish this. Peripheral nerve tumors appear as multiple sessile
nodules, most frequently on the dorsolateral aspect of the head, trunk, and caudal
fin (Fig. 3); these are soft and frequently show foci of hemorrhage and cystic
degeneration. Attempts to demonstrate physical continuity of such tumors with
nerves are rarely successful, but their dorsolateral localization correlates well with
the body areas of fish which are most richly innervated by nerves of the lateral line
sensory organs, neuromasts.

Approximately one-third of the tumors have a histological appearance characteristic of neurilemoma, consisting of multiple rows of palisading nuclei
interspersed with an edematous-appearing loose stroma containing stellate
mesenchymal cells. Occasionally the histological pattern shows dense bundles of
elongate fusiform cells without evidence of palisading, an appearance suggestive
of neurofibroma in which neurites can be demonstrated with special stains.

Classification of such neoplasms as nerve sheath tumors has been challenged by
Duncan and Harkin (1969) on the basis of ultrastructural findings which show
absence of basement membranes adjacent to tumor cells, a relationship characteristic of Schwann cells. However, this conclusion must be viewed with caution,
since goldfish (*A. crassius*) are also known to develop subcutaneous fibromas and
leiomyomas. Lymphosarcoma of northern pike (*E. lucius*), which has been
apparently successfully transmitted by inoculation of cell-free filtrates and is thus
presumed to be of viral origin (Mulcahy and O'Leary, 1970), appears to be rather
widespread, having been reported in Ireland and Canada. In Canada, the tumor
has also been found in another species of the Esocidae, the muskellunge.
Odontogenic tumors arise largely in salmonids (Schlumberger and Katz, 1956) as
multiple firm nodules along the dental arch of both upper and lower jaws. These
grow to a size that could seriously compromise normal nutrition. Histologically,
such neoplasms consist of glandlike spaces lined by columnar cells (ameloblasts)
derived from the enamel organ. Although the etiology remains unknown,
geographic and species localization suggest that it may be due to chemicals or

biological agents in the environment coupled with a special sensitivity of sal-monids.

Cutaneous neoplasms, ranging from focal epidermal hyperplasia and papillomas to infiltrating epidermoid carcinomas, are very numerous and, in contrast to hepatoma and the other tumors mentioned above, widely distributed among

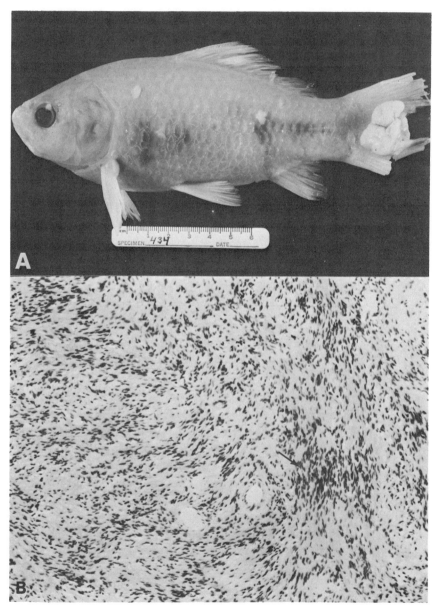

FIGURE 3. A: Peripheral nerve tumors in a goldfish (*Auratus crassius*) distributed as sessile masses involving the eye, lateral body surface, and tail fin. (Accession No. 434 of the Registry of Tumors in Lower Animals, Smithsonian Institution. Contributed by B. M. Levy.) B: Histological section of the tumor shows bundles of elongate fusiform cells, some of which are disposed into palisading arrays (arrow). × 175.

many species of fish. These lesions are of special interest because as a result of
rather extensive study several have been shown to probably be of viral origin. A focal epidermal hyperplasia of walleye (*Stizostedion vitreum*) from Lake Oneida in New York State (Walker, 1969), papillomas of the Atlantic eel (*Anguilla vulgaris*) (Wolf and Quimby, 1970), and papillomas of flathead sole (*Hippoglossoides elassodon*) (Wellings and Chuinard, 1964) appear to be associated with viral particles. Koch's postulates have not been fulfilled for any of these lesions by isolation of infectious agents from them and subsequent induction of identical lesions by experimental inoculation. Until this is accomplished, the relationship of these particles to cutaneous preneoplastic and neoplastic lesions in fish must remain tentative.

2.4. Primitive Vertebrates and Invertebrates

Lesions with gross and histological features of neoplasia have also been described in more primitive chordates, but to date these have been few—i.e., a tumor resembling a neurilemoma in an adult sea lamprey (*Petromyzon marinus*), an agnathous fish (Dawe, 1969a), and a chromaffinoma in an amphioxus (*Branchiostoma lanceolatum*), a cephalochordate (Stolk, 1961). In invertebrates, a subkingdom of animals long considered to be devoid of neoplasms, a variety of tumors have been described in recent years. The largest number have been encountered in bivalve mollusks; these include a wide range of neoplasms such as epitheliomas of the mantle (Wolf, 1969, 1971; Pauley and Sayce, 1972) and ovary (Barry and Yevich, 1972), sarcomas (Farley, 1969a; Couch, 1969; Farley and Sparks, 1970; Newman, 1972), leukemia-like hematopoietic tumors (Farley, 1969b; Farley and Sparks, 1970), and a lesion bearing close resemblance to a ganglioneuroma (Pauley *et al.*, 1968). The hematopoietic and sarcomatous neoplasms deserve special mention because their morphology and biological behavior suggest that they are quite probably true malignant neoplasms. The tumor cells appear to be quite primitive, exhibit numerous mitoses, invade normal tissues, and severely compromise the affected mollusks (Fig. 4). Insect neoplasms have been described exclusively in *Drosophila melanogaster* bearing either of the mutant genes *1(2)gl* and *1(2)gl⁴*. Neoplasms include a spontaneous noninvasive tumor arising in the imaginal disc tissue of larvae (Hadorn, 1969; Gateff and Schneiderman, 1969) and a neuroblastoma arising in brain which is invasive and transplantable (Gateff and Schneiderman, 1967, 1969).

It is clear from even just a cursory survey of the animal kingdom that lesions which qualify as neoplasms are widely distributed throughout the various taxonomic groups. The decreasing examples of unequivocal neoplasms in the invertebrates are no doubt due to (1) the paucity of systematic studies of large populations of invertebrates and (2) the failure to recognize certain lesions that are neoplastic equivalents which are missed because of the incompleteness of our knowledge of tissue structure and function in these primitive forms of life. As the various phyla of invertebrates are studied in greater detail, including the Insecta

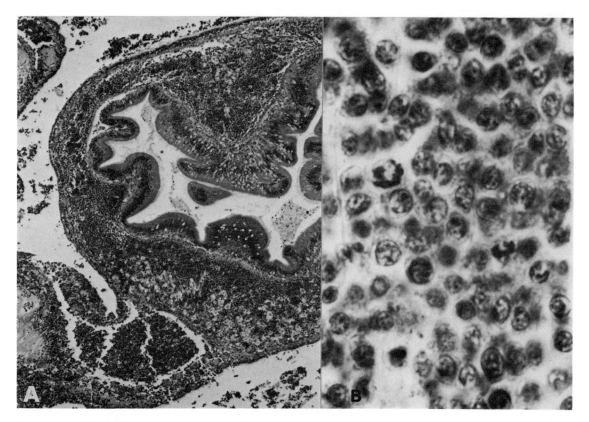

FIGURE 4. A: Histological section of the gut and surrounding connective tissue from an oyster (*Crassostrea virginica*), showing infiltration by numerous cells. × 85. B: A high magnification of an infiltrate shows it to consist of small mononuclear cells with coarse nuclear chromatin; several cells are in mitosis. × 1400. (Accession No. 224 of the Registry of Tumors in Lower Animals, Smithsonian Institution. Contributed by A. Farley.)

with its vast number of species, it is highly probable that many more examples of neoplasia will be found. A resource bibliography pertaining to neoplasms and related lesions in poikilotherms is summarised in Table 1 to assist those who wish to read more extensively.

3. Neoplasm or Reaction to Injury?

3.1. General Considerations

In the lower vertebrates and invertebrates, as in the higher vertebrates, the differential diagnosis of a localized area of swelling or a mass must include the defense reactions of inflammation and healing, as well as that of neoplasm. It is, in fact, all the more critical to rule out inflammation and healing in the diagnosis of a "tumor" in the lower vertebrates and invertebrates because in them reactions to injury commonly present as tissue masses and thus often mimic a neoplasm. Further, since many lower vertebrates and invertebrates are feral and often infected with virus and bacteria and/or infested with parasites, the possibility of tissue injury, inflammation, and reparative tissue reactions is quite high.

A brief consideration of the patterns of the inflammatory response and subsequent tissue healing in several selected but representative lower vertebrates and invertebrates emphasizes the importance of, and often difficulty in, differentiating between a tissue reaction to injury and a neoplasm.

Reptiles, amphibians, and fish possess cellular and humoral defense mechanisms which appear to be in general similar to those present in higher vertebrates. These include cell immigration, phagocytosis, antibody production, and activation of fibroblasts with attendant collagen formation. However, it must be pointed out that many important details still remain to be established. Bacteria, parasites, and certain foreign materials invoke an inflammatory response which, if sufficiently prolonged, can lead to the formation of giant cells and ultimately dense fibrous connective tissue which encapsulates and sequesters the inflammatory focus from the host. In instances where the lesions are large enough to cause local swelling or sufficiently diffuse to cause marked thickening, distortion, and induration of organs, a gross diagnosis of neoplasm is often made, only to be discarded when the lesions are studied histologically.

3.2. Selected Examples

3.2.1. Reptiles and Amphibians

In addition to the infestation of fibroepithelial papillomas in green sea turtles (*Chelonia mydas*) by leeches of genus *Ozobranchus* (Nigrelli, 1943) mentioned previously, another suborder of this class, the lizards, may show multiple small skin nodules that grossly resemble sessile papillomas which histologically prove to be focal areas of epidermal hyperplasia with hyperkeratosis secondary to heavy infestation by mites (Reichenbach-Klinke and Elkan, 1965).

In the amphibians, the lymphoreticular lesions of the South African toad (*Xenopus laevis*) and the Japanese (*Triturus pyrrhogaster*) and the crested (*T. cristatus*) newts, classified as lymphosarcomas, must be considered as suspect. Although the "tumors" of *X. laevis* and *T. pyrrhogaster* can be transplanted to other hosts, they are invariably associated with acid-fast bacilli (Dawe, 1969b, 1973), and in *T. pyrrhogaster* identical "tumors" of the lymphoreticular system can be induced by injections of mycobacteria cultured from spontaneous lesions. According to Dawe (1973), the disease in *T. cristatus* also falls in the category of an infectious granuloma. It is important to point out that the lymphoid tumor of *X. laevis* has received much attention and has been accepted as a true neoplasm for some time. Transmission of the disease by either cell-free material or whole cells devoid of acid-fast bacilli must be accomplished before this lesion can be accepted as a malignant neoplasm of lymphoreticular tissue. Multiple adenomas of the integument of the grass frog (*R. temporaria*) reported by Pflugfelder and Eilers (1959) proved ultimately to contain nematodes. Since the lesions were associated with a parasite and were benign, it is difficult to classify them as true neoplasms rather than as a tissue reaction to injury.

DANTE G.
SCARPELLI

3.2. Fishes

The best example of a lesion in fish which has been incorrectly classified as a neoplasm is lymphocystis, a chronic virus infection widely distributed among freshwater and marine species (Nigrelli, 1952). The lesions, usually located on the dorsal and tail areas and often involving the fins, vary from nodules several millimetres in size to large sessile masses which grossly resemble an aggressive neoplasm. The lesions consist of hypertrophied dermal fibroblasts measuring 300–2000 μm in diameter which have undergone a remarkable degree of nuclear enlargement (Fig. 5) secondary to elaboration of virus (Wolf *et al.*, 1966) in the cytoplasm (Walker, 1962). The masses regress spontaneously and mortality is low. Since cutaneous infection by myxosporidians in fish can also lead to marked epithelial hyperplasia (Nigrelli, 1948) which may simulate a neoplasm, all such lesions should be examined carefully to rule out their presence.

In the more primitive chordates, especially the invertebrates, the problem of distinguishing tissue reaction to injury from a true neoplasm becomes even more difficult due largely to the very significant gaps in our knowledge about the basic pathology of these life forms. A further complication is the fact that inflammation and healing in primitive chordates and invertebrates are predominantly cellular reactions and much more proliferative in nature than is often the case for the higher vertebrates. Thus tissue masses are a common finding in such animals and must be interpreted with considerable caution.

3.2.3. Invertebrates

In reading the literature of the invertebrate biologist and pathologist, one is struck by the large numbers of reports of so-called tumors which are clearly proliferative responses to infectious agents or foreign materials leading to the formation of a tumorlike mass. Cantacuzéne (1919) provided some of the earliest work concerning the nature of the inflammatory reaction and subsequent healing in the primitive chordates. He injected bacteria into the sea squirt (*Ascidia mentula*) and noted that the decreased numbers of bacteria in the blood were accompanied by increased numbers of ameboid leukocytes containing bacteria around the site of injection. He interpreted these correctly to represent phagocytes having ingested bacteria. Experiments of a similar nature by Thomas (1931) on the same species established that following the injection of bacteria an acute inflammatory reaction developed which led to abscess formation, localized and limited by the proliferation of mesenchymal cells, the entire complex giving rise to a small mass. In this and subsequent studies, the most intense phagocytosis was exhibited by large ameboid leukocytes.

In phyla such as Arthropoda, Mollusca, Annelida, and Platyhelminthes, there are certain interesting features of the reaction to injury which merit brief comment. In the Insecta subphylum of Arthropoda, the reaction to injury caused by bacteria and foreign bodies in the hemocoele is characterized by phagocytosis of the bacteria or foreign material by amebocytes and aggregation of amebocytes around the noxious material; finally, if the numbers of bacteria or foreign body

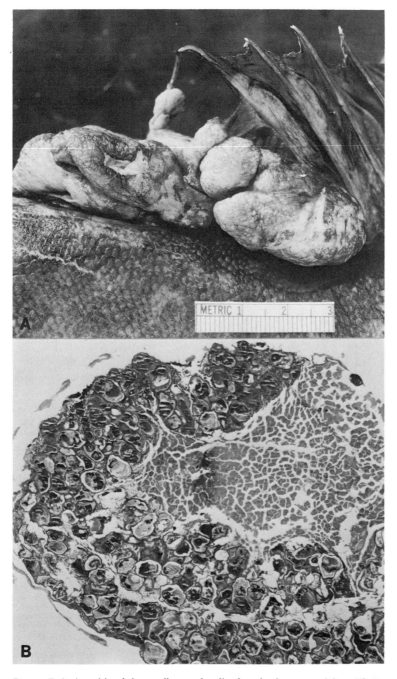

FIGURE 5. A: A multinodular sessile mass localized on the dorsum and dorsal fin in a ling cod (*Ophiodon elongatus*), due to infection with lymphocystis virus. B: Histological section of a nodule shows that the lesion consists of cystlike structures; these represent hypertrophied nuclei of individual dermal fibroblasts. The lack of invasion of the underlying muscle bundles attests to the nonmalignant behavior of this lesion. × 30. (Accession No. 106 of the Registry of Tumors in Lower Animals, Smithsonian Institution. Contributed by the Pacific Biological Station, Namaimo, British Columbia, Canada.)

are too large to be effectively removed by phagocytosis, amebocytes and other blood cells form a syncytial capsule around them (Salt, 1963, 1967) which may develop into a large mass. Not infrequently the cells comprising the capsule contain phagocytized melanin pigment. In fact, most forms of injury in insects are followed by proliferation and aggregation of blood cells. This, coupled with regeneration, gives rise to tissue masses which are frequently interpreted as tumors. Melanoma, a pigmented tumorlike condition of the fruit fly *Drosophila melanogaster*, which has been accepted as a true neoplasm for many years (Barigozzi, 1958), has many of the characteristics of a defensive tissue reaction consisting of nodule formation and encapsulation as described earlier. Further, these lesions, which appear during the larval stage, do not show progressive growth after pupation, are not invasive, and do not significantly shorten the life of affected flies. The foregoing indicates that these "melanomas" are not biologically analogous to the malignant melanomas in higher vertebrates.

In the Mollusca, especially the bivalves Pelecypoda, there are numerous reports of proliferative benign lesions of connective tissue (Sparks, 1972) which present as tissue masses and because of microscopic features cannot be classified as being neoplastic. These lesions are referred to as "tumorlike growths," and in a number of instances have been reclassified as focal hyperplastic reactions of unknown etiology. Since bivalves are filter-feeders and filter surprisingly large amounts of water during their lifetime, it is highly probable that they might ingest some noxious or foreign material which would incite connective tissue proliferation secondary to inflammation.

In a series of experiments on the earthworm (*Lumbricus terrestris*), Firminger *et al.* (1969) showed that the response of this organism to freezing injury leads to an intense proliferation of epithelial cells which "invade" the underlying circular muscle (Fig. 6) and extend into the coelomic cavity. As long as several months after injury, the healed segments have all the morphological characteristics of a neoplasm, but are clearly an extreme example of the potential of the reaction to injury in this species which could lead one to an erroneous diagnosis. In view of the foregoing, the so-called granular cell myoblastoma in *L. terrestris* described by Hancock (1961) may well represent the regenerative response of epithelium to injury and not a neoplastic transformation.

Finally, let us consider the flatworms (*Platyhelminthes*), since interesting tumorlike lesions have been described in the class Turbellaria. Turbellarians possess a remarkable ability to regenerate (Brøndsted, 1955) as evidenced by the fact that two halves of a transected planarian worm can regenerate into two complete worms. It may be that this regenerative property is, in some as yet unknown fashion, responsible for the high frequency of spontaneous localized tissue overgrowths as well as the apparent ease with which these can be induced experimentally. Two types of growth disturbances have been described. One, a spontaneous occurrence first described by Goldsmith (1939), consisted of the development of supernumerary body parts such as pharynx, head, and tail. According to Goldsmith, as many as eight heads were observed in one worm. The second type of "tumor" is less well organized, consisting of masses of disorganized

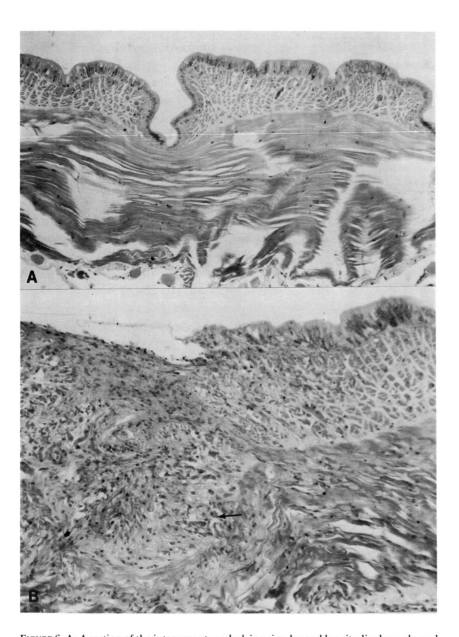

FIGURE 6. A: A section of the integument, underlying circular and longitudinal muscle, and connective tissue of an earthworm (*Lumbricus terrestris*). Note the clear demarcation between the integument and the muscle layers. × 110. B: A section of the integument and adjacent structures of the same animal as shown above from a site injured by focal exposure to cold 22 days prior to sacrifice. Note the mass of cells infiltrating the adjacent layers of muscle (arrow). This lesion, which mimics a neoplasm, is actually a florid proliferative response of host cells as part of the healing process. × 170. (Accession No. 158 of the Registry of Tumors in Lower Animals, Smithsonian Institution. Contributed by H. I. Firminger.)

cells which present as reddened swellings (Lange, 1966). Tumor-bearing worms were able to divide even when the "tumor" had become the largest part of the body. Furthermore, "tumorous" parts of the body were able to generate new heads at normal rates; eventually these parts and the tumor underwent lysis.

Similar lesions, especially multiple body parts, were induced by treating planarians with coal tar (Goldsmith, 1937) and, more recently, the polycyclic carcinogens 3,4-benzo[a]pyrene and 3-methylcholanthrene (Foster, 1963, 1969). It is of interest in this regard to recall that polycyclic carcinogens and steroids have also been shown to be potent inducers of differentiation in early embryos (Waddington, 1938), and that 3-methylcholanthrene induces supernumerary limbs in the regenerating limb of newts (Breedis, 1952). It may be that a somewhat analogous effect results from the interaction of polycyclic carcinogens with the apparently totipotent neoblasts of planarians. Although the supernumerary body parts and malformations encountered in planarians are somewhat reminiscent of teratomas in higher animals, the analogy may be more apparent than real. Despite the fact that these disturbances of tissue growth in planarians provide an interesting model to study regeneration and differentiation, it is difficult at present to classify them as neoplasms.

No discussion of abnormal tissue growth in invertebrates would be complete without mention of the fact that invertebrates such as some arthropods, echinoderms, annelids, and flatworms have the capacity to rid themselves of injured or diseased body parts by autotomy or self-amputation. Insects and crustaceans can shed only limbs, while annelids can rid themselves of whole body segments including the head. Flatworms, on the other hand, can autotomize a major part of their body and then regenerate the lost portion until a whole animal is formed. Mention is made of this phenomenon to point out that it might conceivably be a mechanism by which a neoplasm or its equivalent could be discarded by an animal; however, such an occurrence has yet to be documented.

The author hopes this brief consideration of the problems encountered in differentiating proliferative reactions to injury from neoplasm has not engendered a nihilistic attitude in the reader regarding the existence of neoplasia or its equivalent in primitive vertebrates and invertebrates, but rather that he will be extremely careful in his interpretation of proliferative lesions in them.

4. Etiological and Biological Perspectives

Efforts to elucidate the nature and extent of the various etiological agents responsible for neoplasms in lower vertebrates and invertebrates are an important aspect of comparative oncology from several points of view. The wide distribution of these animals in a myriad of terrestrial and aquatic ecosystems constitutes a sensitive biological sensor for the detection of carcinogenic agents in the environment. The phylogenetic and biological diversity represented in the lower vertebrates is an ideal substrate for a comparative study of cancer and related disorders. A detailed knowledge of the etiology and mechanisms of neoplasia in invertebrates, animals without a thymus, will provide excellent models for those studying the role of the thymus-dependent immune system in oncogenesis.

4.1. Chemical Carcinogens

While the induction of neoplasms by chemicals in higher vertebrates, including man, has been a prime focus of interest in cancer research for many years, similar studies in lower vertebrates and invertebrates have been largely neglected until recently. Such information is more than just of academic interest, since pollution of the land and especially water by an ever-growing number of chemical substances continues at an alarming rate. The foregoing, coupled with the fact that many organisms are capable of bioconcentrating substances in their environment, makes it possible that carcinogenic levels of a chemical could be reached and maintained. One is reminded in this instance of the bivalves mentioned earlier as filter-feeders that are well known for their remarkable ability to ingest and concentrate substances present in water to fairly high levels. Excellent examples of this are the accumulation of polycyclic hydrocarbons in barnacles (Zechmeister and Koe, 1952) and oysters (Cahnmann and Kuratsune, 1957), and more recently of polychlorinated biphenyls in lake trout (*Salvelinus namaycush*) (Bache *et al.*, 1972), and radionuclides of certain heavy metals in the blue mussels (*Mytilus edulis*) (Pentreath, 1973). To what extent exogenous chemical carcinogens are responsible for the induction of neoplasms in feral populations is not known.

Thus far, we have dealt largely with carcinogens from an exogenous source. Recent studies (Sander, 1967; Lijinsky, 1974) have established that nitrites can react with secondary and tertiary amines in the acid environment of the stomach to form nitrosamines, which are potent carcinogens. The presence of carcinogenic substances in lower vertebrate and invertebrate species used as a source of food by man would pose a considerable hazard.

4.1.1. Apparent Resistance of Amphibians

Numerous attempts to induce neoplasms in amphibians by means of chemicals have been reported (Lucké and Schlumberger, 1949), all of which were either unsuccessful or not sufficiently well documented to firmly establish that neoplasia did indeed occur. It is worth noting that in all instances polycyclic carcinogens were employed, which may not be potent for amphibians. Amputation of the forelimb and subsequent regeneration in the water newt (*Triturus viridescens*) apparently impose different conditions, since implantation of crystals of 3-methylcholanthrene into the blastema cap led to the development of sarcomas (Breedis, 1952), as well as supernumerary limbs mentioned previously. It is surprising that no systematic experiments utilizing the numerous other chemical carcinogens currently available such as alkylating agents, aromatic amines and amides, aliphatic nitrosamines and nitrosamides, halogenated aliphatic and alicyclic hydrocarbons, pyrrolizidine alkaloids, and the various aflatoxins have been carried out on amphibian animal models. In view of the promising results obtained with some of these agents in the fishes, such studies may prove interesting.

Before concluding this commentary on chemical carcinogenesis in amphibians, we should consider hairlessness, a special characteristic of the amphibian integument which has been implicated to explain its refractoriness to polycyclic carcinogens (Giovanella, 1969; Giovanella *et al.*, 1970). This suggestion is based on the fact that hairless Swiss mice are much more resistant to induction of cutaneous papillomas by the carcinogen 9,10-dimethyl-1,2-benzanthracene (DMBA) than their hair-bearing isogenic litter mates. Since binding of ^{3}H-labeled DMBA to DNA, RNA, and proteins of skin was identical in hairless and hair-bearing mice (Goshman and Heidelberger, 1967), it is postulated that cells of the pilosebaceous apparatus are the "only" cells in mouse skin capable of undergoing malignant transformation subsequent to repeated topical application of DMBA. The proponents of this view seemed to overlook the ease with which epidermoid carcinoma can be induced in the uterine cervix and vaginal epithelium of mice, which is totally devoid of hair follicles, by direct application of 3-methylcholanthrene (Scarpelli and von Haam, 1957). There must be other factors of equal or greater importance in amphibian skin which are responsible for its unresponsiveness to polycyclic carcinogens. Since this is an area in which there has been a dearth of systematic study, it would seem prudent in our present state of knowledge not to ascribe the resistance of amphibian integument to the absence of hair follicles and associated structures. The responsiveness of reptile and amphibian integument and other tissues to various organic and inorganic chemical carcinogens is an open question which certainly deserves further and more detailed study.

4.1.2. Susceptibility of Fishes

Successful experimental studies on the effects of chemical carcinogens on higher poikilotherms have thus far been limited largely to fish. Halver (1965, 1969) demonstrated that hepatic neoplasms could be induced in rainbow trout (*Salmo gairdneri*) by feeding a variety of substances that were known hepatocarcinogens in the rat and other higher vertebrates. Hepatomas were induced by 2-acetylaminofluorene (2-AAF), aminoazotoluene, *p*-dimethylaminoazobenzene, dimethylnitrosamine (DMN), urethan, thioacetamide, carbon tetrachloride, and tannic acid, among other compounds. The majority of these compounds gave rise to small intrahepatic tumors in a relatively small percentage of fish, with the exception of dimethylnitrosamine, which induced rapidly growing tumors with a propensity for metastasis. The neoplastic nature of the tumors was confirmed histologically and the majority were found to be hepatic carcinomas of adenomatous, trabecular, or mixed type. Since 2-AAF, which is a potent hepatocarcinogen in the rat, induced considerably fewer neoplasms in rainbow trout than expected, its metabolism was studied. It was found that while trout can hydroxylate 2-AAF to the 3-, 5-, and 7-hydroxy derivatives, it does not form the N-hydroxy derivative (Lotlikar *et al.*, 1967), which has been shown to be the proximate carcinogen in the

rat (Miller and Miller, 1969). These results demonstrate that in trout the
hydroxylated derivatives of 2-AAF other than the N-hydroxy metabolite may be
carcinogenic. Further, they emphasize the value of extending experimental
studies to include lower vertebrate animals including the fishes, which until a few
years ago (Buhler and Rasmusson, 1968) were considered incapable of drug
oxidation (Brodie and Maickel, 1962). In contrast to 2-AAF, DMN fed at a high
level induced hepatoma in 100% of fish. In experiments on a cyprinoid fish, the
zebra danio (*Brachydanio rerio*), Stanton (1965) induced hepatic carcinomas with
diethylnitrosamine added to aquarium water at levels of 10–20 ppm. Studies by
Magee (Halver, 1969) with tritiated DMN indicate that this carcinogen is
metabolized by trout in a fashion identical to that observed in the rat.

Careful dietary experiments by Wolf and Jackson (1967) established that
cottonseed flour free of aflatoxin B_1 also induced hepatoma in rainbow trout.
Subsequent studies (Lee *et al.*, 1968; Sinnhuber *et al.*, 1968) identified that
cyclopropenoid fatty acids (CPFAs) present in cotton seed (Phelps *et al.*, 1965) and
cottonseed meal, a major protein source in trout diets, markedly potentiated the
carcinogenicity of aflatoxin B_1. When aflatoxin B_1 was fed together with 200 ppm
of CPFA, a dose as low as 0.4 ppb of the carcinogenic mycotoxin was capable of
regularly inducing hepatoma. Scarpelli (1974) found that the methyl ester of
sterculic acid, a cyclopropenoid fatty acid, is a mitogen for hepatocytes both in
trout and in the rat. It is suggested that CPFAs potentiate the carcinogenic effects
of aflatoxin B_1 by stimulating DNA synthesis, subsequently increasing the mitotic
index of hepatocytes and thereby enhancing the opportunity for mutagenesis. At
present, it is not known whether sterculate is a promoter of tumor induction or a
cocarcinogen. The implication of foodstuffs derived from cotton seed in the
induction of cancer is of more than passing importance to man, since cotton seed
products such as meal are used as a major protein source for nutrition of poultry,
and oil and flour are ingested by large segments of the world population. The
preceding has been presented to point out that chemical carcinogenesis is a
complicated phenomenon in poikilotherms as it is in homeotherms.

The biology of trout hepatoma is intriguing from the following points of view.
The biological behavior of such liver neoplasms is strikingly reminiscent of
minimum-deviation hepatomas in rats by virtue of their slow growth, tendency to
metastasize late, and apparent ability to synthesize plasma protein (Scarpelli *et al.*,
1963). More recent immunoelectrophoretic studies of the reaction of hepatoma
serum with antibodies to normal trout serum indicate that although plasma
proteins are markedly elevated, such sera show absence of a slow-moving
component, probably an immunoglobulin (Scarpelli and Barth, unpublished
observations), indicating that even in such tumors deletions of normal function,
although relatively minor, do exist.

A phylogenetic study of the cholesterol feedback system in liver (Siperstein,
1965) in part corroborated and extended the earlier observations of Clayton
(1964) that the capacity for cholesterol synthesis is apparently lost in the
invertebrates. Further, he noted that in contrast to the normal liver of rat and
man, where feeding of cholesterol leads to an inhibition of cholesterol synthesis,

normal rainbow trout liver has apparently lost this feedback control mechanism. In this regard, normal trout liver resembles neoplastic liver tissue in higher animals, in that it continues to synthesize cholesterol although the trout is being fed a diet containing 5% cholesterol. It is noteworthy that apparently normal rainbow trout liver, which is very prone to neoplastic transformation, has a biological characteristic of neoplastic liver in higher animals. Further studies on the significance of this interesting biological fact may shed light on the relationship of metabolic feedback control mechanisms to the development of malignancy.

4.1.3. Invertebrates

Studies on the effects of chemical carcinogens on invertebrates have been singularly disappointing. The results have been largely negative except for a few instances where proliferative lesions have been induced. The most recent work in this area report focal hyperplasia of the gut in house fly (*Musca domestica*) larvae following feeding of derivatives of 2-fluorenamine (Cantwell *et al.*, 1966), and a similar reaction in the hepatopancreas of the crayfish (*Procambarus clarkii*) induced by exposure to dimethylnitrosamine (Harshbarger *et al.*, 1970). These lesions exhibited a very limited growth potential and could not be justly classified as neoplasms. The remarkable resistance of primitive vertebrates and invertebrates to chemical carcinogens is of interest since there is ample evidence that many of these animals, especially insects, are capable of drug metabolism by enzymatic pathways which include hydroxylation, a reaction known to convert certain compounds to potent carcinogens (Terriere, 1968). Moreover, it is well established that many carcinogens are mutagenic for lower animals such as *Drosophila* (Auerbach, 1949). How then can one explain the apparent ineffectiveness of chemical carcinogens? It may be related to the fact that more primitive animals have higher contents of nuclear DNA than do more specialized forms (Mirsky and Ris, 1951; Goin *et al.*, 1968) as well as extensive gene duplication, making them more resistant to mutations of DNA which subsequently lead to the development of neoplasia.

4.2. Viruses

The role of viruses as etiological agents for some neoplasms in a wide variety of animal hosts is well established and viral oncology has developed into one of the most active areas of cancer research. It bears mentioning that some of the key work in viral oncology has emanated from the study of poikilothermic vertebrates. The implication of viruses in poikilotherms is encountered in early literature describing epidermal papillomas in fish (Keysselitz, 1908; Fiebiger, 1909; Breslauer, 1916). In every instance, the neoplasms were limited to a species of fish often living either in the close confines of an aquarium or in a limited stretch of water and histologically resembled infectious warts of mammals (Fiebiger, 1909) or contained intranuclear or cytoplasmic inclusions suggestive of virus disease.

Unfortunately, no attempts were made to transmit the disease by inoculation of cell-free material. An interesting report by the Champys (1935) described a spontaneous cutaneous tumor with invasive properties in the Alpine newt (*Triturus alpestris*) which was transplantable. They suggested that an oncogenic virus might be responsible, but did not succeed in inducing the lesion with cell-free material, nor were intracellular inclusions described.

4.2.1. Sarcoma in a Viper

A case report (Zeigel and Clark, 1971) of a sarcoma in a Russell's viper (*Vipera russelli*) describes the first clearly documented association of a virus with neoplasia in a reptile. The authors succeeded in establishing a cell line derived from the spleen; after several passages, C-type particles were evident by electron microscopy. These were observed budding from the plasma membrane of tumor cells and were also found in a pellet of venom centrifuged at 80,000*g* for 30 min. The virus particles are morphologically similar to those associated with leukemias and other lymphoreticular neoplasms in a variety of murine and avian species. The results of further studies of this virus, especially its transmissibility and subsequent induction of sarcoma, are awaited with great interest.

4.2.2. Renal Adenocarcinoma in the Frog

Renal adenocarcinoma of the leopard frog, *R. pipiens* referred to earlier, has become a widely used model in tumor biology. The ultrastructural study by Fawcett (1956) described viruslike (90–100 nm) particles containing a 40-nm dense inner core. These were present both in the nucleus and in the cytoplasm, always associated with inclusion bodies, and were found only in frogs that had been captured during winter. Temperature sensitivity of the virus has been demonstrated by transplantation of summer tumor fragments in the anterior chamber of the eye of leopard frogs known not to carry the virus and maintaining them at a temperature of 7.5°C, whereupon virus particles developed in the tumor implants (Mizell *et al.*, 1968, 1969). The activation of previously latent virus in summer tumor tissue has also been accomplished *in vitro* with tumor fragments incubated at 7.5°C on agar slants (Breidenbach *et al.*, 1971). Converse experiments in which virus-laden winter tumor tissue was maintained at temperatures of 15–20°C showed that at 15°C virus replication soon ceased and that after 6 wk at this temperature virus was no longer detectable in winter tumor cells by electron microscopy (Skinner and Mizell, 1972). Clearly, the most elegant demonstration of the latent phase has been the identification of virus-specific messenger RNA in morphologically "virus-free" summer tumor cells by hybridization experiments (Collard *et al.*, 1973). This ideal model for detailed study of the latent phase of the virus–host cell relationship in which virus genome is present but not expressed until it is subjected to cold has been complicated by the demonstration of at least two additional viruses in the tumor cells (Rafferty, 1965; Granoff *et al.*, 1969). One of these, morphologically identical to the Lucké virus, can replicate in tissue culture of frog kidney and frog embryo cells, but apparently is not oncogenic

(Granoff *et al.*, 1969). Its precise role in tumor induction remains to be elucidated. A third virus often found in these cells is a small intranuclear virus (Lunger *et al.*, 1965) whose role is also unknown. It may be that one or both of these interact with the Lucké virus to effect the neoplasic transformation of renal epithelium in a manner similar to the "helper" virus in the Rous chicken sarcoma.

4.2.3. Lymphosarcoma in Northern Pike

An early report by Nigrelli (1947) on the occurrence of lymphosarcoma in 12 adult northern pike (*E. lucius*) in the New York Aquarium is of particular interest because the animals, all occupants of one tank, developed the disease during the period of 1 yr, suggesting that an infectious agent might be involved. Twenty-three years later, Mulcahy and O'Leary (1970) succeeded in transmitting the disease. The tumors most often arise in the head region, although other body areas are not exempt (Fig. 7). One is struck by the number of lesions that appear to arise in the branchial region, where a paired mass of lymphoid tissue, which is considered by some to be an analogue of the thymus, resides. The lesions, which are bulky, invasive, and tend to metastasize, consist of closely packed undifferentiated lymphoid cells supported by a fibrous stroma and delicate reticulum. Ultrastructural studies of spontaneous tumors and those induced by inoculation of cell-free filtrates derived from spontaneous tumors failed to show viral particles (Mulcahy *et al.*, 1970). These results must be regarded as preliminary. The rapid methodological developments in culture of fish cells and tissues, and the establishment of stable fish cell lines (Wolf and Quimby, 1969), will provide a powerful tool for future research on this interesting fish neoplasm. It would be of interest to know whether the incidence and development of the disease in fish could be modified by irradiation of the thymus, as is the case for the mouse.

4.2.4. Herpesvirus in a Bivalve Mollusk Susceptible to Neoplastic Diseases

Among the invertebrates, the recent discovery of a herpesvirus infection in *C. virginica* (Farley *et al.*, 1972), a species of bivalve mollusk which is also the host for a variety of malignant and benign neoplasms, is of considerable interest in light of the growing association of herpesvirus with neoplasia in higher animals. Although no relationship has yet been established between the virus and any neoplasm of oysters, one has only to recall the well-known latency of viruses to be circumspect in his approach to this question. The seasonal recrudescence in the winter months of two epizootic neoplasms in bivalve mollusks, a sarcoma in the oyster (*Ostrea lurida*) and the mussel (*Mytilus edulis*) and a gill carcinoma in the clam (*Macoma balthica*) (Farley, 1974), suggests that a temperature-sensitive agent such as a virus may be responsible in a manner analogous to the herpesvirus associated with the Lucké renal adenocarcinoma.

4.3. Immunity and Neoplasia

In recent years, it has become increasingly evident that in the higher vertebrates, including man, a close relationship probably exists between neoplasia and

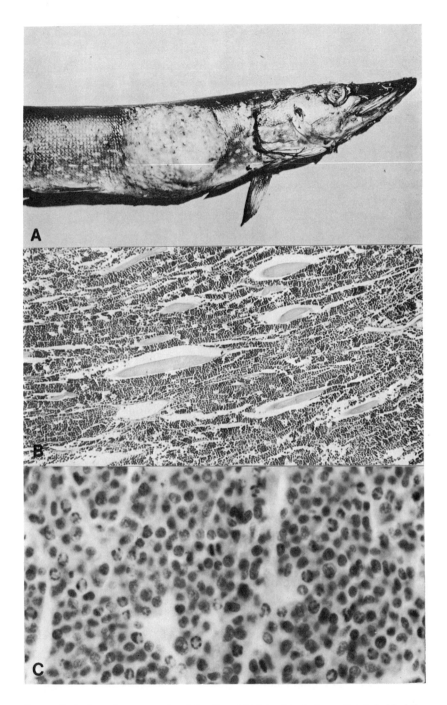

FIGURE 7. A: Lymphosarcoma involving the right lateral body immediately behind the gills in a northern pike (*Esox lucius*). (Courtesy of E. I. Sillman, University of Manitoba, Winnipeg, Canada.) B: A section of the neoplasm shows infiltration and separation of muscle fibers by dense sheets of small lymphocytes. × 60. C: At a higher magnification, the neoplastic cells appear as tightly packed uniform small lymphocytes; in the center of the field, a telophase mitotic figure is present. × 700.

immunity. An intimate relationship is suggested by the association of neoplasia with naturally occurring disease of immunological deficiency (Coleman *et al.*, 1961; Page *et al.*, 1963), protracted immunosuppressive therapy (Wilson *et al.*, 1968), and the waning immunity which accompanies involution of the thymus and thymic-dependent lymphoid system in aging (Gross, 1965; Stutzman *et al.*, 1968). These relationships between immunity and cancer have led to the view that the lymphoid system, especially that associated with cell-mediated immunity, functions as a monitor capable of identifying and eliminating cells including neoplastic cells with surface antigens that differ from those of the host's normal cells. According to Thomas (1959) and Burnet (1964), such a function of lymphoid tissue constitutes "immunological surveillance", which protects higher animals from the deleterious consequences attendant to malignant transformation of their somatic cells (see Chapt. 8, this volume).

4.3.1. Amphibian Models

In the lower vertebrates, two experimentally induced neoplasms have been reported in amphibians which could serve as excellent models to study the role of immunity in cancer. The first of these is the transplantable lymphosarcoma of the *A. mexicanum* induced after repeated skin allografting (DeLanney and Blacker, 1969). The tumors begin as localized lesions in grafts after third-set allografting reciprocally made between adult animals with $A^h C^h \times C^h \times C^h$ genotype for the histocompatibility factors A^h and C^h. The lymphosarcomas grow initially as solid tumors, reach a considerable size, and develop a leukemic phase terminally characterized by malignant lymphocytes in the peripheral blood. The neoplasm has been transplanted by either implants of solid tumor or liver, spleen, testis, whole blood, and buffy coat from tumor-bearing animals. Attempts to transmit the tumor by means of cell-free extracts have failed. The lymphosarcoma appears to be specific for the C^h strain; adult histoincompatible hosts do not support growth of the tumor or transmit it unless they are thymectomized early in the larval stage of development or made tolerant to the C^h strain prior to transplantation of the tumor. Animals of the C^h strain, which ordinarily would die from single implants of tumor, become immune following implantation of tumor into a limb with subsequent amputation 55 days later, suggesting the existence of a tumor-specific transplantation antigen.

A second promising model is that described by Schochet and Lampert (1969) of a plasma cell tumor arising in an adult female leopard frog following implantation of Lucké renal adenocarcinoma into the anterior chamber of the eye. The tumor arose in the thigh, infiltrated the thigh muscles, and consisted of plasma cells of varying degrees of differentiation. Most of these were immature and many were in mitosis. Electron microscopy showed a well-developed endoplasmic reticulum with dilated cisternae containing finely granular proteinaceous material. Some of the cells contained large osmiophilic cytoplasmic inclusions classified as Russell bodies. Tubular intracytoplasmic inclusions resembling those described by Fawcett (1956) and Zambernard *et al.* (1966) in Lucké renal adenocarcinoma cells were also encountered. Whether these particles represent a form of the herpesvirus or the other viruses which are present in the Lucké tumor and are primarily involved in the genesis of the plasma cell tumor remains to be determined. The possible immune aspects of this tumor model arise from the fact that similar neoplasms in BALB/c mice are induced by long-standing antigenic stimulation of the immune system (Potter and Boyce, 1962) and the possibility that tumor tissue in the anterior chamber may have served as a chronic antigenic stimulus. It may be that both an immunogenic mechanism and a viral one are involved.

4.3.2. Immunity and the Infrequency of Neoplasia in Invertebrates

In very primitive vertebrates such as the hagfish (*Eptratus stoutii*), an agnathan fish, and invertebrates which lack a thymus, a thymic-dependent lymphoid system, a capacity for acquired immunity (Papermaster *et al.*, 1964), and immunological surveillance, neoplasia seems to be rare. According to Good and Finstad (1969), this may be a reflection of the phylogenetic relationship among the lymphoid system, immunity, and malignancy. They expand on the theory of immunological surveillance and further postulate that the immune system evolved as an adaptation to protect higher animals from their high capacity to develop malignancy. The high capacity for malignant transformation is attributed to the fact that the evolutionary demands imposed on the genomes of higher animals by increased differentiation and specialization of cells have also increased the chance for errors of gene function and expression, some of which could lead to a loss of growth control. Thus, since the more primitive life forms represented in the lowest vertebrates and invertebrates are functionally more simple than the higher vertebrates, and often have a higher content of nuclear DNA and considerable gene repetition, redundancy, and stability, there is considerably less chance for spontaneous gene errors and little need for a system providing immunological surveillance. It follows then that such animals should be devoid of both immune systems and the capacity to develop malignancy.

While the hypothesis fits nicely with the current state of knowledge concerning immunity and neoplasia in primitive animals, our understanding of these areas of biology is still sufficiently incomplete that it would be best to withhold final judgment until more information becomes available. For example, although all the facets of immunity present in higher animals are not represented in invertebrates (Cushing, 1967), Cooper (1969) has shown that specific graft rejection, one of the components of acquired immunity, exists in annelid worms. Further, a naturally occurring hemagglutinin in the blood of the oyster (*C. virginica*) appears to play a role in the phagocytosis of red cells by oyster amebocytes (Tripp, 1966) in a fashion reminiscent of opsonins in higher animals; some species of invertebrates appear capable of producing bactericidal substances upon the injection of live or killed bacteria. Thus, although many aspects of acquired immunity are absent in invertebrates, at least one has remained, and several substances have been identified which, although not globulins, seem to be important humoral mediators of host defense against bacteria and foreign substances; these may represent primitive equivalents of an immune system. Finally, as mentioned earlier, the paucity of neoplasms in the many phyla that constitute the invertebrates may be more apparent than real, since these animals have not been as systematically and thoroughly studied as have the vertebrates.

4.4. Regeneration and Neoplastic Growth in Urodeles

The brilliant studies of Spemann (1918; Spemann and Mangold, 1924) established that the variety of differentiated growth in the embryo appears to be controlled by potent regional cellular and humoral factors that subsequently have been termed "individuation fields." In postembryonic life, individuation fields appear to be operative in controlling the events of regeneration of tail and limbs in urodeles and larval anurans; in fact, these have served as excellent models for its study. Some insight into the extent of control has been obtained by the following classical experiments; if the bone which is removed by amputation is replaced by bone from another kind of limb, the limb which is regenerated is identical to the original one. Replacement of the characteristic pigmented skin of urodeles by a sleeve of nonpigmented skin over the regenerating stump does not prevent the regenerate limb from being totally pigmented.

The concept of individuation fields stimulated Waddington (1935) and later Needham (1942) to suggest that neoplasia may represent an "escape" of tissue from the influence of such fields which have become weak or are absent in the adult. Needham (1942) elaborated further by suggesting that malignant neoplasms originating in anurans, which have a low capacity for regeneration and weak individuation fields, be implanted in regenerating limbs of urodeles which possess strong fields to ascertain whether growth of the neoplasm can be "mastered." Although one can find inconsistencies in such a theory as evidenced by the frequency of spontaneous malignancy in organs capable of regeneration and in young individuals, both of which presumably possess strong individuation fields, it has been tested experimentally. The results, although not conclusive, are worthy of consideration. The earliest work along these lines is that reported by Briggs (1942) in which the Lucké frog adenocarcinoma of kidney was transplanted at various sites into *R. pipiens* tadpoles. The implants grew to form tumors at all sites except the tail, where the implant regressed before the initiation of absorption at metamorphosis. Tumors in the subcutaneous tissue of the trunk survived metamorphosis. Metamorphic regression of tumor implanted in the tail was probably due to local changes which characterize this phenomenon such as activation of acid hydrolases and histolysis. It would be of interest to know whether regeneration of the tail secondary to amputation would affect growth of the tumor, since the effect of an individuation field would be maximal in this instance.

The experiments by Rose and Wallingford (1948) and Rose and Rose (1952) employing adult newts (*T. viridescens*) were more promising, since renal carcinoma implants appeared to regress during limb regeneration following amputation. However, these results are complicated by the fact that adult salamanders

tend to reject frog carcinoma tissue unless the antihistaminic pyribenzamine is
used, so that regression may have been on an immune basis rather than a field
effect. Similar experiments with the larval newts *Amblystoma maculatum* and *A.
opacum* by Ruben (1955) showed that frog renal carcinoma implants were not
affected by limb regeneration. However, details concerning the biological
behavior and ultimate fate of the tumor implants were not given; a comparison of
such data in normal newts with those undergoing limb regeneration would be of
interest. More recently, the question of the effects of individuation fields on tumor
differentiation and growth has been reopened by Seilern-Aspang and Kratochwil
(1963), who demonstrated that chemically induced cutaneous mucus gland
carcinomas of the newt *T. cristatus* localized beyond the first sacral vertebra
underwent differentiation and regressed following amputation of the tail, while
those on the trunk continued to grow. Further, Seilern-Aspang and Kratochwil
(1962) found that the behavior of such induced tumors varied depending on their
location; for example, 93% of tumors on the tail were not infiltrative, while 90% of
tumors on the trunk were so. Although these findings must be corroborated and
extended before they can be considered as established, they are of considerable
interest because they suggest that individuation fields may affect the differentiation and growth of neoplastic tissue, as well as offer a model for future study.
Studies of regeneration, field effects, and the subsequent behavior of neoplastic
cells with the tools of cell biology are long overdue.

4.5. Imaginal Disc Differentiation and Neoplasia in Insects

The complex biology of larval growth, metamorphosis, and adult growth in
holometabolous insects offers a unique opportunity to study the relation of
hormonal and other growth control mechanisms to cell differentiation and
neoplasia. Postembryonic larval development of insects consists of a series of
stages called instars, each separated from the next by a molt. This pattern pertains
until an adult or imago emerges at the final molt. Within the larva, the future adult
is concealed in a number of primordial cell groups called imaginal discs which are
without function in the larva and are programmed for forming the adult body.
The discs arise at definite sites during embryogenesis and consist of groups of
epithelial cells which appear strikingly similar morphologically. With the onset of
metamorphosis, cell division in the discs ceases and differentiation begins which
ultimately leads to formation of their corresponding imaginal structures in the
adult (Nothiger, 1972).

Hadorn (1966) found that the events of metamorphosis in imaginal discs of
Drosophila can be prevented by transplanting them directly into the abdomens of
adult flies. Under these conditions, mitotic division of imaginal disc blastema cells
continues indefinitely and they remain in an undifferentiated state, since they are
prevented from entering and passing through metamorphosis, which is a
requisite for imaginal differentiation. During his studies, he found that some of
the transplants developed into very rapidly growing blastemas which he called
"atelotypic lines" and filled the host's abdomen after only a few days' growth. Such

blastemas also lost their capacity for adult differentiation, test implants never reaching the final adult stage, indicating that they were not able to react normally to the hormones that induce metamorphosis. Imaginal eye-antennal discs transplanted *in vivo* for many generations (Gateff and Schneiderman, 1969) gave rise to an atelotypic blastema which was cultured for 80 transfer generations and behaved like a benign neoplasm. Imaginal discs from larvae with a mutant gene $1(2)gl^4$ on the second chromosome exhibit similar growth characteristics and behave as a benign neoplasm. An invasive neuroblastoma (Fig. 8) which is readily transplantable was also encountered in larvae with the mutant gene; this tumor eventually killed recipient host flies following transplantation. The responses of these aberrant cell lines to the hormonal changes which accompany metamorphosis are interesting and bear mention. Metamorphosis is thought to be characterized by the secretion of a group of steroid hormones called ecdysones

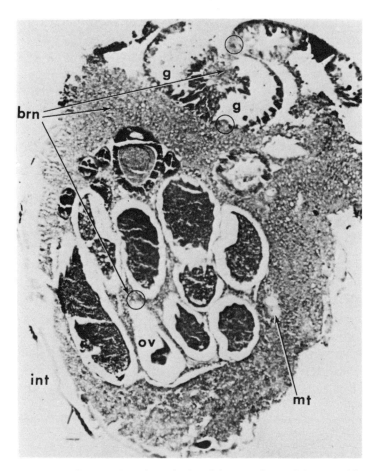

FIGURE 8. Cross-section through the abdomen of an adult *Drosophila melanogaster* fly bearing transplantable neuroblastoma from a $1(2)gl^4$ mutant. Note that the tumor (brn), which consists of uniform small cells, has grown beneath the integument (int), filled the coelomic cavity, surrounded the ovaries (ov) and malpighian tubules (mt), and invaded the gut (g). × 70. From Gateff and Schneiderman (1969).

accompanied by a decrease in the level of juvenile hormones, lipid substances, the most active being the terpene farnesol. Under these conditions, atelotypic and mutant disc cell lines stop dividing, although they do not differentiate into adult tissue. The neuroblastoma cells, on the other hand, continue to divide during and after metamorphosis, much like malignant neoplasms of higher animals, which also lose their capacity to respond to normal growth control mechanism.

Although the genesis of the benign neoplasms induced by repeated transplantation of imaginal discs is not known, studies on the hormonal control of normal imaginal disc development suggest that it may involve continuous hormonal stimulation, since ecdysone, which is present at high levels in larval stages, is capable of inducing DNA synthesis and mitosis and stimulating both RNA and protein synthesis (Fristrom, 1972).

The exciting results arising from imaginal disc transplantation are probably just a beginning, since application of this technique to *Drosophila*, a species whose genetics have been studied in great detail and which has served as a prime test object for mutation research, will eventuate in the development of many more types of aberrant transplantable blastemas and neoplasms.

4.6. Abnormal Growth in Hydra

Hydras, freshwater coelenterates, have long captured the attention of developmental biologists (Trembley, 1744) because of their extraordinary capacity to regenerate a new animal from parts of their gastric column. More recently, this has been accomplished with dispersed gastric column cells when these were allowed to reaggregate (Gierer *et al.*, 1972). Since cells of the gastric column give rise to a complete animal, such cells or their derivatives must be capable of expressing *all* the information contained in the genome. This totipotentiality is reflected in the apparent ease with which the organisms form bizarre monsters with multiple heads upon aggregation of dissociated normal cells. Eventually, such monsters separate to form normal animals. Permanent multiheaded animals occur spontaneously and can be induced by exposure to certain chemicals; such organisms exhibit surprisingly normal growth and behavior and are regarded as examples of a disturbance of normal programmed growth (Shostak and Tammariello, 1969). Numerous experiments have demonstrated that morphogenesis and differentiation of hydras during regeneration exhibit a polarity which appears to be under control of tissue nearest to the head region. Polarity of morphogenesis has been ascribed to a substance localized in the cytoplasm of hydra nerve cells (Schaller and Gierer, 1973) which presumably controls the direction of differentiation and leads to formation of a new head at the edge of tissue closest to the original head following transection.

An interesting giant mutant of *Chlorhydra viridissima* which arose in mass cultures undergoing sexual reproduction appears to have lost the property of polarity (Lenhoff *et al.*, 1969). Whereas bisected normal hydras regenerate a basal disc from the head-bearing apical region and the basal disc regenerates another head, the apical region of the mutant regenerates a second head, giving rise to a bipolar animal with a head at each end. When the apical segments of mutants are grafted to the basal half of normal hydras of the same species, the resultant hydra "heterocytes" are capable of budding and producing only mutant organisms which are both larger and heavier than normal *C. viridissima* hydras. Budding ceases about 23 days after initial grafting. If, after this time, the basal half of the heterocyte is replaced by engrafting a basal segment from another normal hydra, subsequent budding produces both mutant and normal-appearing hydras. Surprisingly, some of the normal-appearing hydras give rise to a progeny with phenotypic characteristics of the mutant. Furthermore, when normal-appearing hydras derived from heterocytes are maintained in culture for several weeks or more, they invariably assume the abnormal morphological characteristics of the mutant. Lenhoff *et al.* (1969) suggest that these experiments demonstrate that mutant somatic cells in the heterocyte spread through the animal and ultimately dominate the normal host tissues in a manner reminiscent of tumor growth. While this phenomenon is interesting and merits further study, such a suggestion is premature until more is known about cell population kinetics and cell-to-cell interaction of mutant and normal hydra cells in the heterocyte. For example, are normal hydra cells physically replaced by preferential growth of mutant ones, or are they "transformed" by a macromolecule such as DNA, a virus, or other factor(s) produced by and transferred from mutant cells? Answers to such questions will greatly clarify the nature and significance of the apparent dominance of mutant hydras. This primitive biological model system clearly illustrates the difficulties encountered when one tries to compare its abnormal growth characteristics with those of higher animal forms.

5. References

ANDERS, F., 1967, Tumour formation in platyfish–swordtail hybrids as a problem of gene regulation, *Experienta* **23**:1.

AUERBACH, C., 1949, Chemical mutagenesis, *Biol. Rev. Cambridge Philos. Soc.* **24**:355.

BACHE, C. A., SERUM, J. W., YOUNGS, W. D., AND LISK, D., 1972, Polychlorinated biphenyl residues: Accumulation in Cayuga Lake trout with age, *Science* **177**:1191.

BALLS, M., 1962, Spontaneous neoplasms in amphibia: A review and descriptions of six new cases, *Cancer Res.* **22**:1142.

BALLS, M., AND RUBEN, L. N., 1964, A review of the chemical induction of neoplasms in amphibia, *Experientia* **20**:241.

BALLS, M., AND RUBEN, L. N., 1968, Lymphoid tumors in amphibia: A review, *Prog. Exp. Tumor Res.* **10**:238.

BARIGOZZI, C., 1958, Melanotic tumors in *Drosophila, J. Cell. Comp. Physiol.* **52**:371.

BARRY, M. M., AND YEVICH, P. P., 1972, Incidence of gonadal cancer in the quahaug, *Oncology* **26**:87.

BASHFORD, E. F., 1904, The zoological distribution, the limitations in the transmissibility, and the comparative histological and cytological characters of malignant new growths, Imperial Cancer Research Fund, Scientific Report No. 1, pp. 3–36.

BERG, O., AND GORDON, M., 1953, Relationship of atypical pigment cell growth to gonadal development in hybrid fishes, in: *Pigment Cell Growth* (M. Gordon, ed.), pp. 43–72, Academic Press, New York.

BREEDIS, C., 1952, Production of accessory limbs and of sarcoma in the newt (*Triturus viridescens*) with carcinogenic substances, *Cancer Res.* **12**:861.

BREIDENBACH, G. P., SKINNER, M. S., WALLACE, J. H., AND MIZELL, M., 1971, *In vitro* induction of a herpes-type virus in "summer phase" Lucké tumor explants, *J. Virol.* **7**:679.

BRESLAUER, T., 1916, Zur Kenntnis der Epidermoidalgeschwülste von Kaltblütern, *Arch. Mikrosk. Anat.* **87**:200.

BRIGGS, R., 1942, Transplantation of kidney carcinoma from adult frogs to tadpoles, *Cancer Res.* **2**:309.

BRODIE, B. B., AND MAICKEL, R. P., 1962, Comparative biochemistry of drug metabolism, *Proc. First Int. Pharmacol. Meet.* **6**:299.

BRØNDSTED, H. V., 1955, Planarian regeneration, *Biol. Rev. Cambridge Philos. Soc.* **30**:65.

BRUNST, V. V., 1967, Tumors in amphibians. 1. Histology of a neuroepithelioma in *Siredon mexicanum*, *J. Natl. Cancer Inst.* **38**:193.

BRUNST, V. V., 1969, Structures of spontaneous and transplanted tumors in the axolotl (*Siredon mexicanum*), in: *Recent Results in Cancer Research (Special Supplement) Biology of Amphibian Tumors*, (M. Mizell, ed.), pp. 215–219, Springer, New York.

BUHLER, D. R., AND RASMUSSON, M. E., 1968, The oxidation of drugs by fishes, *Comp. Biochem. Physiol.* **25**:223.

BURNET, F. M., 1964, Immunological factors in the process of carcinogenesis, *Br. Med. Bull.* **20**:154.

CAHNMANN, H. J., AND KURATSUNE, M., 1957, Determination of polycyclic hydrocarbons in oysters collected in polluted water, *Anal. Chem.* **29**:1312.

CANTACUZÉNE, J., 1919, Etude dé une infection experimentale chez *Ascidia mentula*, *C. R. Soc. Biol.* **82**:1019.

CANTWELL, G. E., SHORTINO, T. J., AND ROBBINS, W. E., 1966, The histopathological effects of certain carcinogenic 2-fluorenamine derivatives on larvae of the house fly, *J. Invertebr. Pathol.* **8**:167.

CHAMPY, C., AND MLLE CHAMPY, 1935, Sur un épithélioma transmissible chez le triton, *Bull. Assoc. Fr. Etude Cancer* **24**:206.

CLAYTON, R. B., 1964, The utilization of sterols by insects, *J. Lipid Res.* **5**:3.

COLEMAN, A., LEIKIN, S., AND GUIN, G. H., 1961, Aldrich's syndrome, *Clin. Proc. Child. Hosp. Natl. Med. Cent.* **17**:22.

COLLARD, W., THORNTON, H., MIZELL, M., AND GREEN, M., 1973, Virus-free adenocarcinoma of the frog (summer phase tumor) transcribes Lucké tumor herpes virus specific RNA, *Science* **181**:448.

COOPER, E. L., 1969, Neoplasia and transplantation immunity in annelids, in: Neoplasms and Related Disorders of Invertebrate and Lower Vertebrate Animals (C. J. Dawe and J. C. Harshbarger, eds.), *Natl. Cancer Inst. Monogr.* **31**:655.

COUCH, J. A., 1969, An unusual lesion in the mantle of the American oyster, *Crassostrea virginica*, in: Neoplasms and Related Disorders of Invertebrate and Lower Vertebrate Animals (C. J. Dawe and J. C. Harshbarger, eds.), *Natl. Cancer Inst. Monogr.* **31**:557.

CUSHING, J. E., 1967, Invertebrates, immunology and evolution, *Fed. Proc.* **26**:1666.

DAWE, C. J., 1968, Invertebrate animals in cancer research, *Gann Monogr.* **5**:45.

DAWE, C. J., 1969*a*, Phylogeny and oncology, in: Neoplasms and Related Disorders of Invertebrate and Lower Vertebrate Animals (C. J. Dawe and J. C. Harshbarger, eds.), *Natl. Cancer Inst. Monogr.* **31**:1.

DAWE, C. J., 1969*b*, Some comparative morphological aspects of renal neoplasms in *Rana pipiens* and of lymphosarcoma in amphibia, in *Recent Results in Cancer Research (Special Supplement) Biology of Amphibian Tumors* (M. Mizell, ed.), pp. 429–440, Springer, New York.

DAWE, C. J., 1973, Comparative neoplasia, in: *Cancer Medicine* (J. F. Holland and E. Frei, eds.), pp. 193–240, Lea and Febiger, Philadelphia.

DAWE, C. J., AND HARSHBARGER, J. C., 1969, Neoplasms and Related Disorders of Invertebrate and Lower Vertebrate Animals, *Natl. Cancer Inst. Monogr.* **31**.

DELANNEY, L. E., AND BLACKER, K., 1969, Acceptance and regression of a strain-specific lymphosarcoma in Mexican axolotls, in: *Recent Results in Cancer Research (Special Supplement) Biology of Amphibian Tumors* (M. Mizell, ed.), pp. 399–408, Springer, New York.

DUNCAN, T. E., AND HARKIN, J. C., 1969, Electron microscopic studies of goldfish tumors previously termed neurofibromas and schwannomas, *Am. J. Pathol.* **55**:191.

FARLEY, C. A., 1969*a*, Sarcomatoid proliferative disease in a wild population of blue mussels (*Mytilus edulis*), *J. Natl. Cancer Inst.* **43**:509.

FARLEY, C. A., 1969*b*, Probable neoplastic disease of the hematopoietic system in oysters *Crassostrea virginica* and *Crassostrea gigas*, in: Neoplasms and Related Disorders of Invertebrate and Lower Vertebrate Animals (C. J. Dawe and J. C. Harshbarger, eds.), *Natl. Cancer Inst. Monogr.* **31**:541.

FARLEY, C. A., 1974, Epizootic neoplasia in bivalve mollusks, Twentyfirst International Cancer Congress **1**:219.

FARLEY, C. A., AND SPARKS, A. K., 1970, Proliferative diseases of hemocytes, endothelial cells, and connective tissue cells in mollusks, in: Comparative Leukemia Research 1969, *Bibl. Haematol. (Basel)* **36**:610.

FARLEY, C. A., BANFIELD, W. G., KASNIC, G., AND FOSTER, W. S., 1972, Oyster herpes-type virus, *Science* **178**:759.

FAWCETT, D. W., 1956, Electron microscope observations on intracellular virus-like particles associated with the cells of the Lucké renal adenocarcinoma, *J. Biophys. Biochem. Cytol.* **2**:725.

FIEBIGER, J., 1909, Über Hautgeschwülste bei Fischen nebst Bermerkungen uber die Pockenkranheit der Karpfen, *Z. Krebsforsch.* **7**:165.

FINKELSTEIN, E. A., 1960, Tumors of fish (in Russian), *Arkh. Patol.* **22**:56.

FIRMINGER, H. I., ANTOINE, S., AND ADAMS, E., 1969, Epithelioma-like lesion in *Lumbricus terrestris* after cold injury, in: Neoplasms and Related Disorders of Invertebrates and Lower Vertebrate Animals (C. J. Dawe and J. C. Harshbarger, eds.), *Natl. Cancer Inst. Monogr.* **31**:645.

FOSTER, J. A., 1963, Induction of neoplasms in planarians with carcinogens, *Cancer Res.* **23**:300.

FOSTER, J. A., 1969, Malformations and lethal growths in planaria treated with carcinogens, in: Neoplasms and Related Disorders of Invertebrate and Lower Vertebrate Animals (C. J. Dawe and J. C. Harshbarger, eds.), *Natl. Cancer Inst. Monogr.* **31**:683.

FRISTROM, J. W., 1972, The biochemistry of imaginal disk development, in: *The Biology of Imaginal Disks* (H. Ursprung and R. Nothiger, eds.), pp. 109–154, Springer, Berlin.

GATEFF, E., AND SCHNEIDERMAN, H. A., 1967, Developmental studies of a new mutant of *Drosophila melanogaster*: Lethal malignant brain tumor *(1(2)gl⁴)*, *Am. Zool.* **7**:760

GATEFF, E., AND SCHNEIDERMAN, H. A., 1969, Neoplasms in mutant and cultured wild-type tissues of *Drosophila*, in: Neoplasms and Related Disorders of Vertebrate and Lower Vertebrate Animals (C. J. Dawe and J. C. Harshbarger, eds.), *Natl. Cancer Inst. Monogr.* **31**:365.

GIERER, A., BERKING, S., BODE, H., DAVID, C. N., FLICK, K., HANSMANN, G., SCHALLER, H., AND TRENKNER, E., 1972, Regeneration of hydra from reaggregated cells, *Nature New Biol.* **239**:98.

GIOVANELLA, B., 1969, Skin carcinogenesis, mammals versus amphibia, in: *Recent Results in Cancer Research (Special Supplement) Biology of Amphibian Tumors* (M. Mizell, ed.), pp. 195–203, Springer, New York.

GIOVANELLA, B. L., LIEGEL, J., AND HEIDELBERGER, C., 1970, The refractoriness of the skin of hairless mice to chemical carcinogenesis, *Cancer Res.* **30**:2590.

GOIN, O. B., GOIN, C. J., AND BACHMANN, K., 1968, DNA and amphibian life history, *Copeia* **1968**:533.

GOLDSMITH, E. D., 1937, Production of supernumerary outgrowths in planarians by the application of ethyl alcohol, aniline oil and coal tar, *Anat. Rec.* **70**:134 (Suppl. 1).

GOLDSMITH, E. D., 1939, Spontaneous outgrowths in *Dugesia tigrina* (syn. *Planaria maculata*), *Anat. Rec. Suppl.* **75**:158.

GOOD, R. A., AND FINSTAD, J., 1969, Essential relationship between the lymphoid system, immunity, and malignancy, in: Neoplasms and Related Disorders of Invertebrate and Lower Vertebrate Animals (C. J. Dawe and J. C. Harshbarger, eds.), *Natl. Cancer Inst. Monogr.* **31**:41.

GOSHMAN, L. M., AND HEIDELBERGER, C., 1967, Binding of tritium-labeled polycyclic hydrocarbons to DNA of mouse skin, *Cancer Res.* **27**:1678.

GRANOFF, A., GRAVELL, M., AND DARLINGTON, R. W., 1969, Studies on the viral etiology of the renal adenocarcinoma of *Rana pipiens* (Lucké tumor), in: *Recent Results in Cancer Research (Special Supplement) Biology of Amphibian Tumors* (M. Mizell, ed.), pp. 279–295, Springer, New York.

GROSS, L., 1965, Immunological defect in aged population and its relationship to cancer, *Cancer* **18**:201.

HADORN, E., 1966, Konstanz, Wechsel und Typus der Determination und Differenzierung in Zellen aus männlichen Genitalscheiben von *Drosophila melanogaster* nach Dauerkultur *in vivo*, *Dev. Biol.* **13**:424.

HADORN, E., 1969, Proliferation and dynamics of cell heredity in blastema cultures of *Drosophila* in: Neoplasms and Related Disorders of Invertebrate and Lower Vertebrate Animals (C. J. Dawe and J. C. Harshbarger, eds.), *Natl. Cancer Inst. Monogr.* **31**:351.

HALVER, J. E., 1965, Hepatomas in fish, in: *Primary Hepatoma.* (W. J. Burdette, ed.), pp. 103–112, Utah Press, Utah.

HALVER, J. E., 1967, Crystalline aflatoxin and other vectors for trout hepatoma, in: *Trout Hepatoma Research Conference Papers* (J. E. Halver and I. A. Mitchell, eds.), pp. 78–102, Bureau of Sport Fisheries Wildlife Research Report No. 70.

HALVER, J. E., 1969, Aflatoxicosis and trout hepatoma, in: *Aflatoxin Scientific Background, Control, and Implications* (L. A. Goldblatt, ed.), pp. 265–306, Academic Press, New York.

HANCOCK, R. L., 1961, Neoplasms in *Lumbricus terrestris* L., *Experientia* **17**:547.

HARKER, J. E., 1963, Tumors, in: *Insect Pathology: An Advanced Treatise*, Vol. 1 (E. A. Steinhaus, ed.), pp. 191–213, Academic Press, New York.

HARSHBARGER, J. C., 1973, Invertebrate animals—What can they contribute to cancer research? *Fed. Proc.* **32**:2224.

HARSHBARGER, J. C., AND TAYLOR, R. L., 1968, Neoplasms of insects, *Ann. Rev. Entomol.* **13**:159.

HARSHBARGER, J. C., CANTWELL, G. E., AND STANTON, M. F., 1970, Effects of N-nitrosodimethylamine on the crayfish, *Procambarus clarkii*, in: *Proceedings: IV International Colloquium on Insect Pathology* (held in conjunction with The Society for Invertebrate Pathology, College Park, M., August 1970), pp. 425–430.

HÄUSSLER, G., 1928, Über Melanombildungen bei Bastarden von *Xiphophorus helleri* und *Platypoecilius maculatus* var. *rubra*, *Klin. Wochenschr.* **7**:1561.

HUMPHREY, R. R., 1969, Tumors of the testis in the Mexican axolotl (*Ambystoma*, or *Siredon mexicanum*), in: *Recent Results in Cancer Research (Special Supplement) Biology of Amphibian Tumors* (M. Mizell, ed.), pp. 220–228, Springer, New York.

JOHNSON, P. T., 1968, *An Annotated Bibliography of Pathology in Invertebrates Other Than Insects*, Burgess, Minneapolis.

KEYSSELITZ, G., 1908, Uber ein Epithelioma der Barben, *Arch. Protistenkd.* **11**:326.

LANGE, C. S., 1966, Observations on some tumors found in two species of planaria—*Dugesia etrusca* and *D. ilvana*, *J. Embryol. Exp. Morphol.* **15**:125.

LEE, D. J., WALES, J. H., AYERS, J. L., AND SINNHUBER, R. O., 1968, Synergism between cyclopropenoid fatty acids and chemical carcinogens in rainbow trout (*Salmo gairdneri*), *Cancer Res.* **28**:2312.

LENHOFF, H. M., RUTHERFORD, C., AND HEATH, H. D., 1969, Anomalies of growth and form in hydra: Polarity, gradients, and a neoplasia analog, in: Neoplasms and Related Disorders of Invertebrate and Lower Vertebrate Animals (C. J. Dawe and J. C. Harshbarger, eds.), *Natl. Cancer Inst. Monogr.* **31**:709.

LIJINSKY, W., 1974, Reaction of drugs with nitrous acid as a source of carcinogenic nitrosamines, *Cancer Res.* **34**:255.

LOTLIKAR, P. D., MILLER, E. C., MILLER, J. A., AND HALVER, J. E., 1967, Metabolism of the carcinogen 2-acetylaminofluorene by rainbow trout, *Proc. Soc. Exp. Biol. Med.* **124**:160.

LUCKÉ, B., 1934, A neoplastic disease of the kidney of the frog *Rana pipiens*, *Am. J. Cancer* **20**:352.

LUCKÉ, B., 1942, Tumors of the nerve sheaths in fish of the snapper family (*Lutianidae*), *Arch. Pathol.* **34**:133.

LUCKÉ, B., AND SCHLUMBERGER, H. G., 1949, Neoplasia in cold blooded vertebrates, *Physiol. Rev.* **29**:91.

LUNGER, P. D., DARLINGTON, R. W., AND GRANOFF, A., 1965, Cell–virus relationships in the Lucké renal adenocarcinoma: An ultrastructure study, *Ann. N.Y. Acad. Sci.* **126**:289.

MAWDSLEY-THOMAS, L. E., 1969, Neoplasia in fish—A bibliography, *J. Fish Biol.* **1**:187.

MAWDSLEY-THOMAS, L. E., 1971, Neoplasia in fish—A review, in: *Current Topics in Comparative Pathology*, Vol. 1 (T. C. Cheng, ed.), pp. 87–170, Academic Press, New York.

MCKINNELL, R. G., 1969, Lucké renal adenocarcinoma epidemiological aspects, in: *Recent Results in Cancer Research (Special Supplement) Biology of Amphibian Tumors* (M. Mizell, ed.), pp. 254–260, Springer, New York.

MILLER, J. A., AND MILLER, E. C., 1969, The metabolic activation of carcinogenic aromatic amines and amides, in: *Progress in Experimental Tumor Research*, Vol. 11 (F. Homburger, ed.), pp. 273–301, Karger, Basel.

MIRSKY, A. E., AND RIS, H., 1951, The desoxyribonucleic acid content of animal cells and its evolutionary significance, *J. Gen. Physiol.* **34**:451.

MIZELL, M., 1969, *Recent Results in Cancer Research (Special Supplement) Biology of Amphibian Tumors*, Springer, New York.

MIZELL, M., AND ZAMBERNAND, J., 1965, Viral particles of the frog renal adenocarcinoma: Causative agent or passenger virus? II. A promising model system for the demonstration of a "lysogenic" state in a metazoan tumor, *Ann. N.Y. Acad. Sci.* **126**:146.

MIZELL, M., STACKPOLE, C. W., AND HALPEREN, S., 1968, Herpes-type virus recovery from "virus-free" frog kidney tumours, *Proc. Soc. Exp. Biol. Med.* **127**:808.

MIZELL, M., STACKPOLE, C. W., AND ISAACS, J. J., 1969, Herpes-type virus latency in the Lucké tumor, in: *Recent Results in Cancer Research (Special Supplement) Biology of Amphibian Tumors* (M. Mizell, ed.), pp. 337–347, Springer, New York.

MULCAHY, M. F., AND O'LEARY, A., 1970, Cell-free transmission of lymphosarcoma in the northern pike *Esox lucius* L. (Pisces; Esocidae), *Experientia* **26:**891.

MULCAHY, M. F., WINQVIST, G., AND DAWE, C. J., 1970, The neoplastic cell type in lymphoreticular neoplasms of northern pike, *Esox lucius, Cancer Res.* **30:**2712.

NEEDHAM, J., 1942, *Biochemistry and Morphogenesis*, pp. 239–270, Cambridge University Press, Cambridge.

NEWMAN, M. W., 1972, An oyster neoplasm of apparent mesenchymal origin, *J. Natl. Cancer Inst.* **48:**237.

NIGRELLI, R. F., 1943, The occurrence of leeches, *Ozobranchus branchiatus* on fibro-epithelial tumors of marine turtles, *Chelonia mydas, Zoologica* **28:**107.

NIGRELLI, R. F., 1947, Spontaneous neoplasms in fishes. III. Lymphosarcoma in *Astyanax* and *Esox, Zoologica* **32:**101.

NIGRELLI, R. F., 1948, Prickle cell hyperplasia in the snout of the redhorse sucker, *Moxostoma aureolum*, associated with an infection by the myxosporidian *Myxobolus moxostomi, Zoologica* **33:**43.

NIGRELLI, R. F., 1952, Virus and tumors in fishes, *Ann. N.Y. Acad. Sci.* **54:**1076.

NIGRELLI, R., 1954, Tumors and other atypical cell growths in temperate fresh water fishes of North America, *Trans. Am. Fish. Soc.* **83:**262.

NOTHIGER, R., 1972, The larval development of imaginal discs, in: *The Biology of Imaginal Disks* (H. Ursprung and R. Nothiger, eds.), pp. 1–34, Springer, Berlin.

PAGE, A. R., HANSEN, A. E., AND GOOD, R. A., 1963, Occurrence of leukemia and lymphoma in patients with agammaglobulinemia, *Blood* **21:**197.

PAPERMASTER, B. W., CONDIE, R. M., FINSTAD, J., AND GOOD, R. A., 1964, Significance of the thymus in the evolution of the lymphoid tissue and acquired immunity, in: *The Thymus in Immunobiology* (R. A. Good and A. E. Gabrielsen, eds.), pp. 551–591, Hoeber-Harper, New York.

PAULEY, G. B., 1969, A critical review of neoplasia and tumor-like lesions in mollusks, in: Neoplasms and Related Disorders of Invertebrate and Lower Vertebrate Animals (C. J. Dawe and J. C. Harshbarger, eds.), *Natl. Cancer Inst. Monogr.* **31:**509.

PAULEY, G. B., AND SAYCE, C. S., 1972, An invasive epithelial neoplasm in a Pacific oyster, *Crassostrea gigas, J. Natl. Cancer Inst.* **49:**897.

PAULEY, G. B., SPARKS, A. K., AND SAYCE, C. S., 1968, An unusual internal growth associated with multiple watery cysts in a Pacific oyster (*Crassostrea gigas), J. Invertebr. Pathol.* **11:**398.

PENTREATH, R. J., 1973, The accumulation from water of ^{65}Zn, ^{54}Mn, ^{58}Co and ^{59}Fe by the mussel, *Mytilus edulis, J. Marine Biol. Assoc. U.K.* **53:**127.

PFLUGFELDER, O., AND EILERS, W., 1959, Auslösung von Adenomen in der Epidermis von *Rana temporaria* durch "*Filaria*" *rubella* Rudolphi, *Z. Parasitenkd.* **19:**101.

PHELPS, R. A., SHENSTONE, F. S., KEMMERER, A. R., AND EVANS, R. J., 1965, A review of cyclopropenoid compounds: Biological effects of some derivatives, *Poultry Sci.* **44:**358.

POTTER, M., AND BOYCE, C. R., 1962, Induction of plasma-cell myeloma in strain BALB/c mice with mineral oil and mineral oil adjuvents, *Nature (London)* **193:**1086.

RAFFERTY, K. A., 1965, The cultivation of inclusion-associated viruses from Lucké tumor frogs, *Ann. N.Y. Acad. Sci.* **126:**3.

REICHENBACH-KLINKE, H., AND ELKAN, E., 1965, *The Principal Diseases of Lower Vertebrates*, Academic Press, New York.

ROSE, S. M., AND ROSE, F. C., 1952, Tumor agent transformations in amphibia, *Cancer Res.* **12:**1.

ROSE, S. M., AND WALLINGFORD, H. M., 1948, Transformations of renal tumors of frogs to normal tissue in regenerating limbs of salamanders, *Science* **107:**457.

RUBEN, L. N., 1955, The effects of implanting anuran cancer into nonregenerating and regenerating larval urodele limbs, *J. Exp. Zool.* **128:**29.

SALT, G., 1963, The defense reactions of insects to metazoan parasites, *Parasitology* **53:**527.

SALT, G., 1967, Cellular defense mechanisms in insects, *Fed. Proc.* **26:**1671.

SANDER, J., 1967, Kann Nitrit in der menschlichen Nahrung Ursache einer Krebsentstehung durch Nitrosaminbildung sein? *Arch. Hyg. Bakteriol.* **151:**22.

SCARPELLI, D. G., 1969, A survey of some spontaneous and experimental disease processes of lower vertebrates and invertebrates, *Fed. Proc.* **28:**1825.

SCARPELLI, D. G., 1974, Mitogenic activity of sterculic acid, a cyclopropenoid fatty acid, *Science* **185:**958.

SCARPELLI, D. G., AND VON HAAM, E., 1957, Experimental carcinoma of the uterine cervix in the mouse: A gross and histopathologic study, *Am. J. Pathol.* **33:**1059.

SCARPELLI, D. G., GRIEDER, M. H., AND FRAJOLA, W. J., 1963, Observations on hepatic cell hyperplasia, adenoma and hepatoma of rainbow trout (*Salmo gairdneri*), *Cancer Res.* **23**:848.

SCHALLER, H., AND GIERER, A., 1973, Distribution of the head-activating substance in hydra and its localization in membranous particles in nerve cells, *J. Embryol. Exp. Morphol.* **29**:39.

SCHARRER, B., AND LOCHHEAD, M. S., 1950, Tumors in the invertebrates: A review, *Cancer Res.* **10**:403.

SCHLUMBERGER, H. G., 1952, Nerve sheath tumors in an isolated goldfish population, *Cancer Res.* **12**:890.

SCHLUMBERGER, H. G., 1957, Tumors characteristic for certain animal species: A review, *Cancer Res.* **17**:823.

SCHLUMBERGER, H. G., 1958, *Pathologie der Laboratoriumstiere* (P. Cohrs, R. Jaffe, and H. Meessen, eds.), Springer, Berlin.

SCHLUMBERGER, H. G., AND KATZ, M., 1956, Odontogenic tumors of salmon, *Cancer Res.* **16**:369.

SCHLUMBERGER, H. G., AND LUCKÉ, B., 1948, Tumors of fishes, amphibians, and reptiles, *Cancer Res.* **8**:657.

SCHOCHET, S. S., AND LAMPERT, P. W., 1969, Plasmacytoma in a *Rana pipiens*, in: *Recent Results in Cancer Research (Special Supplement) Biology of Amphibian Tumors* (M. Mizell, ed.), pp. 204–214, Springer, New York.

SEILERN-ASPANG, F., AND KRATOCHWIL, K., 1962, Induction and differentiation of an epithelial tumour in the newt (*Triturus cristatus*), *J. Embryol. Exp. Morphol.* **10**:337.

SEILERN-ASPANG, F., AND KRATOCHWIL, K., 1963, Die experimentelle Aktivierung der Differenzierungspotenzen entarter Zellen, *Wien Klin. Wochenschr.* **75**:337.

SHOSTAK, S., AND TAMMARIELLO, R. V., 1969, Supernumerary heads in *Hydra viridis*, in: Neoplasms and Related Disorders of Invertebrate and Lower Vertebrate Animals (C. J. Dawe and J. C. Harshbarger, eds.), *Natl. Cancer Inst. Monogr.* **31**:739.

SICILIANO, M. J., PERLMUTTER, A., AND CLARK, E., 1971, Effect of sex on development of melanoma in hybrid fish of the genus *Xiphophorus*, *Cancer Res.* **31**:725.

SINNHUBER, R. O., LEE, D. J., WALES, J. H., AND AYRES, J. L., 1968, Dietary factors and hepatoma in rainbow trout (*Salmo gairdneri*). II. Cocarcinogenesis by cyclopropenoid fatty acids and the effect of gossypol and altered lipids on aflatoxin-induced liver cancer, *J. Natl. Cancer Inst.* **41**:1293.

SIPERSTEIN, M. D., 1965, Comparison of the feedback control of cholesterol metabolism in liver and hepatoma, in: *Developmental and Metabolic Control Mechanisms and Neoplasia*, pp. 427–451, Williams and Wilkins, Baltimore.

SKINNER, M. S., AND MIZELL, M., 1972, The effect of different temperatures on herpesvirus induction and replication in Lucké Tumor explants, *Lab. Invest.* **26**:671.

SPARKS, A. K., 1969, Review of tumors and tumor-like conditions in protozoa, coelenterata, platyhelminthes, annelida, sipunculida, and arthropoda, excluding insects, in: Neoplasms and related disorders of invertebrate and lower vertebrate animals (C. J. Dawe and J. C. Harshbarger, eds.), *Natl. Cancer Inst. Monogr.* **31**:671.

SPARKS, A. K., 1972, Tumors and tumorlike conditions in invertebrates, in: *Invertebrate Pathology: Non Communicable Diseases*, pp. 271–371, Academic Press, New York.

SPEMANN, H., 1918, Ueber die Determination der ersten Organanlagen des amphibien Embryo. I–IV, *Arch. Entwicklungsmech.* **43**:448.

SPEMANN, H., AND MANGOLD, H., 1924, Über Induktion von Embryonalanlagen durch Implantation artfremder Organisatoren, *Arch. Entwicklungsmech.* **100**:599.

STANTON, M. F., 1965, Diethylnitrosamine-induced hepatic degeneration and neoplasia in the aquarium fish, *Brachydanio rerio*, *J. Natl. Cancer Inst.* **34**:117.

STOLK, A., 1961, Chromaffinoma in amphioxus, *Proc. K. Ned. Akad. Wer.* [Biol. Med.] **64C**:478.

STUTMAN, O., YUNIS, E. J., AND GOOD, R. A., 1968, Deficient immunologic functions of NZB mice, *Proc. Soc. Exp. Biol. Med.* **127**:1204.

TERRIERE, L. C., 1968, Insecticide–cytoplasmic interactions in insects and vertebrates, *Ann. Rev. Entomol.* **13**:75.

THOMAS, J.-A., 1931, Sur les réactions de la tunique d'*Ascide mentula* Müll. a l'inoculation de *Bacterium tumefaciens* Sm., *C. R. Soc. Biol.* **108**:694.

THOMAS, L., 1959, Discussion, in: *Cellular and Humoral Aspects of the Hypersensitive States* (H. S. Lawrence, ed.), pp. 529–532, Hoeber-Harper, New York.

TREMBLEY, A., 1744, *Mémoirès Pour Servir à l'Histoire d'un Genre de Polypes d'eau Douce, a' Bras en Forme de Cornes*, Leiden, Verbeek.

TRIPP, M. R., 1966, Hemagglutinin in the blood of the oyster *Crassostrea virginica, J. Invertebr. Pathol.* **8**:478.

TWEEDEL, K. S., 1967, Induced oncogenesis in developing frog kidney cells, *Cancer Res.* **27**:2042.

VAN WAGTENDONK, W. J., 1969, Neoplastic equivalents of protozoa, in: Neoplasms and Related Disorders of Invertebrate and Lower Vertebrate Animals (C. J. Dawe and J. C. Harshbarger, eds.), *Natl. Cancer Inst. Monogr.* **31**:751.

WADDINGTON, C. H., 1935, Cancer and the theory of organizers, *Nature (London)* **135**:606.

WADDINGTON, C. H., 1938, Studies on the nature of the amphibian organization centre. VII. Evocation by some further chemical compounds, *Proc. R. Soc. London Ser. B* **125**:365.

WALKER, R., 1962, Fine structure of lymphocystis virus of fish, *Virology* **18**:503.

WALKER, R., 1969, Virus associated with epidermal hyperplasia in fish, in: Neoplasms and Related Disorders of Invertebrate and Lower Vertebrate Animals (C. J. Dawe and J. C. Harshbarger, eds.), *Natl. Cancer Inst. Monogr.* **31**:195.

WELLINGS, S. R., 1969, Neoplasia and primitive vertebrate phylogeny: Echinoderms, prevertebrates, and fishes—A review, in: Neoplasms and Related Disorders of Invertebrate and Lower Vertebrate Animals (C. J. Dawe and J. C. Harshbarger, eds.), *Natl. Cancer Inst. Monogr.* **31**:59.

WELLINGS, S. R., AND CHUINARD, R. G., 1964, Epidermal papillomas with virus-like particles in flathead sole, *Hippoglossoides elassodon, Science* **146**:932.

WILSON, R. E., HAGER, E. B., HAMPERS, C. L., CARSON, J. M., MERRILL, J. P., AND MURRAY, J. E., 1968, Immunologic rejection of human cancer transplanted with a renal allograft, *New Engl. J. Med.* **278**:479.

WOLF, H., AND JACKSON, E. W., 1967, Hepatoma in salmonids: The role of cottonseed products and species differences, in: Trout Hepatoma Research Conference Papers (J. E. Halver and I. A. Mitchell, eds.), *Bur. Sport Fish. Wild. (U.S.) Res. Rep.* **70**:29.

WOLF, K., AND QUIMBY, M. C., 1969, Fish cell and tissue culture, in: *Fish Physiology*, Vol. III (W. S. Hoar and D. J. Randall, eds.), pp. 253–305, Academic Press, New York.

WOLF, K. E., AND QUIMBY, M. C., 1970, Virology of eel stomatopapilloma, *Progress in Sport Fishery Research, 1970,* pp. 94–95, U.S. Department of Interior Fish and Wildlife Service (Resource Publication 106), U.S. Government Printing Office, Washington, D.C.

WOLF, K., GRAVELL, M., AND MALSBERGER, R. G., 1966, Lymphocystis virus: Isolation and propagation in centrarchid fish cell lines, *Science* **151**:1004.

WOLF, P. H., 1969, Neoplastic growth in two Sydney rock oysters, *Crassostrea commercialis* (Iredale and Roughley), in: Neoplasms and Related Disorders of Invertebrate and Lower Vertebrate Animals (C. J. Dawe and J. C. Harshberger, eds.), *Natl. Cancer Inst. Monogr.* **31**:563.

WOLF, P. H., 1971, Unusually large tumor in a Sydney rock oyster, *J. Natl. Cancer Inst.* **46**:1079.

WOOD, E. M., AND LARSON, C. P., 1961, Hepatic carcinoma in rainbow trout, *Arch. Pathol.* **71**:471.

ZAMBERNARD, J., VATTER, A. E., AND MCKINNELL, R. G., 1966, The fine structure of nuclear and cytoplasmic inclusions in primary renal tumors of mutant leopard frogs, *Cancer Res.* **26**:1688.

ZECHMEISTER, L., AND KOE, B. K., 1952, The isolation of carcinogenic and other polycyclic aromatic hydrocarbons from barnacles, *Arch. Biochem. Biophys.* **35**:1.

ZEIGEL, R. F., AND CLARK, H. F., 1971, Histologic and electron microscopic observations on a tumor-bearing viper: Establishment of a "C"-type producing cell line, *J. Natl. Cancer Inst.* **46**:309.

ACKNOWLEDGMENT

The author is deeply indebted to Dr. John C. Harshbarger, Director, Registry of Tumors in Lower Animals, Museum of Natural History, Smithsonian Institution, for his generous assistance.

12

Plant Tumors

Armin C. Braun

1. Introduction

The neoplastic diseases of plants have not only had a long and interesting history but also have, over the years, served as model systems for studying the basic cellular mechanisms that underlie the tumorous state. The crown gall disease of plants was, for example, the first neoplastic disease in which the proximate cause was characterized experimentally (Smith and Townsend, 1907), a finding that preceded by 1 year the report of Ellermann and Bang (1908) on the transmissibility of fowl leukemia and by 3 years the report of Rous (1910) on the production of solid tumors in chickens with cell-free filtrates. Plant tumors were also among the earliest shown to be transplantable. Shortly after the turn of the century, C. O. Jensen—who because of his now classic investigations on the transplantability of first mouse and later rat cancers is generally considered to be the father of modern experimental cancer research—also demonstrated that the plant tumors with which he worked were transplantable (Jensen, 1910, 1918). He stated, moreover, that those plant tumors "remind one so much of malignant tumors in animals that a closer study of their biological relationships would undoubtedly be profitable" (Jensen, 1910). In comparing plant and animal tumors it must be recognized, however, that there are certain structural and functional differences commonly used to distinguish cancers in animals that are more or less restricted to animals. However, the most essential characteristic, namely, the ability of a cell to grow in an essentially unrestrained or autonomous manner in a host, on which all other diagnostic features ultimately depend, is equally capable of expression in all higher organisms since it is a characteristic feature of the cell itself. While differences in particulars clearly exist, plants can nevertheless be legitimately used as experimental test objects for attempts to uncover fundamental concepts that lead to an understanding of neoplastic growth generally.

Armin C. Braun • The Rockefeller University, New York, New York.

411

There are essentially two general aspects of the tumor problem in which studies on the relatively simple plant tumors can contribute in a meaningful way to an understanding of neoplastic growth. The first of these is concerned with a characterization of substances and mechanisms that underlie the capacity of a tumor cell for essentially unrestrained or autonomous growth within a host, while the second is concerned with the nature of the heritable cellular change that underlies the neoplastic state. The present discussion will deal essentially with these two areas and an attempt will be made to show how experimental findings obtained with plant tumor systems may have broader biological implications. For a more comprehensive account of these and other aspects of the plant tumor problem, the reader is referred to Braun (1972).

Plant tumors, like animal tumors, may be initiated by diverse physical, chemical, and biological agents. The present discussion will be limited to three well-studied plant tumor systems which have different and distinct proximate causes and which are therefore admirably suited to illustrate certain fundamental concepts that underlie the neoplastic state in plants. The first and most thoroughly studied of these diseases is the crown gall disease. This neoplastic disease is initiated by a tumor-inducing principle that is transmitted by a specific bacterium (Braun, 1943, 1947). The tumor-inducing principle, which appears to be a self-replicating entity of viral nature (Aaron–DaCunha, 1969; Meins, 1973; de Ropp, 1947), possesses the ability to regularly transform normal conditioned plant cells into tumor cells in short periods of time. Once the cellular transformation has been accomplished, the continued abnormal and autonomous proliferation of the tumor cells becomes an automatic process that is entirely independent of the inciting bacterium (Braun, 1943, 1947). An interesting relationship has been found to exist, moreover, between the ability of the tumor-inducing principle to transform normal plant cells into tumor cells and the stage in the normal cell cycle in which the cellular transformation occurs (Braun, 1952; Braun and Mandle, 1948). It is only those plant cells that have been rendered competent as a result of irritation accompanying a wound that can be transformed into tumor cells by the tumor-inducing principle (Braun, 1952). Tumors of the most rapidly growing type are initiated just before the first evidence of cell division is found in the normal wound-healing response (Braun, 1952; Lipetz, 1966). Whether the stage in the normal cell cycle that is vulnerable to transformation is the S phase, at which time chromosomal DNA is replicated, or whether it is the M or mitotic phase, during which period a reprogramming of the genetic information is believed to occur, is not as yet known.

The second neoplastic disease of plants that will be discussed is known as the Kostoff genetic tumors, which occur in interspecific crosses of certain plant species within the genus *Nicotiana* (Smith, 1972). When, for example, two plant species such as *Nicotiana glauca* and *N. langsdorffii* are crossed and the seed of the hybrid is sown, the resulting plants commonly grow normally during the period of their active growth and in the absence of irritation. However, when the hybrid plants reach maturity and terminal growth ceases, a profusion of tumors invariably arise spontaneously from all parts (roots, stem, leaves, and flowers). The tumors arise at points of irritation and result from a chromosomal imbalance in all cells of the

hybrid. Unlike in the crown gall disease, no exogenous agent is involved in the
inception or maintenance of the tumorous state in this instance. These hybrid
tumors have their counterparts in animal pathology. The most thoroughly
studied examples of this type are the melanomas that develop regularly in the
platyfish × swordtail crosses in fish (Gordon, 1958) and the tumors that develop in
crosses between the wild mouse and an inbred strain of the domestic mouse (Little,
1947).

A third neoplasm that will be discussed is one that arises spontaneously in
culture, a phenomenon commonly referred to as habituation. Normal plant cells,
like normal animal cells, may acquire neoplastic properties when isolated from a
host and grown in culture. Habituated cells, like crown gall tumor cells and cells of
the Kostoff genetic tumors, are transplantable and are thus true tumors (Limasset
and Gautheret, 1950).

A feature common to all true plant tumor cells is that they are far less fastidious
in their growth requirements in culture than are comparable normal cell types.
The tumor cells, regardless of the initiating cause, grow profusely and indefinitely
on a simple, chemically defined culture medium composed only of mineral salts,
sucrose, and vitamins that does not support the continued growth of normal cells
of the type from which the tumor cells were derived. The question that arises,
therefore, is why true plant tumor cells should be less fastidious in their growth
requirements than are comparable normal cell types. An answer to that question
will require a precise characterization of the substances and mechanisms that
regulate normal cell growth and division as well as an understanding of the
manner in which those mechanisms become persistently altered during the
transition from a normal cell to a tumor cell.

2. The Development of Autonomy

2.1. The Regulation of Cell Growth and Division

If an understanding of the tumor problem is to be achieved, the experimental
oncologist will have to explain why neoplastic cells divide persistently and in an
essentially unrestrained manner in their hosts and why such cells may invade
underlying normal tissues and metastasize to distant sites while the growth of all
normal cells is precisely regulated. These are dynamic problems that, as indicated
above, will ultimately find their explanations in terms of substances and mechanisms that are involved in the regulation of growth. Growth in all higher organisms
results either from an enlargement of cells or from the combined processes of cell
enlargement and cell division. How, then, are these fundamental growth processes regulated? An abundance of evidence obtained from both plant and animal
material indicates that in any proliferating population of cells the individual
members proceed through a cell cycle which consists of an integrated series of
closely related biochemical events that begin in early interphase and culminate in

the division of one cell into two. The capacity of cells to regulate this sequence of events is apparent. It has, in fact, been suggested that any cell that does not divide is a cell that is blocked at some point on the pathway to division (Mazia, 1961). This means, of course, that in any persistently dividing population of cells, such as those found in tumors, all of the naturally occurring blocks in the cell cycle have been persistently removed, thus enabling such cells to grow and divide continuously in an otherwise suitable environment. What then are these arrest points in the normal cell cycle and how may they be removed? They include the G_1 phase block, at which point the cycle is most commonly arrested, the S phase block, which is determined, in many instances at least, by the absence of a cytoplasmic initiator of chromosomal DNA synthesis, the G_2 phase block, from which cells enter mitosis directly without again replicating their chromosomal DNA, and finally the block that occurs between mitosis and cytokinesis. This last arrest point is evidenced most clearly by the rather common occurrence in both animals and plants of binucleate and/or multinucleate cells in which mitosis has occurred without corresponding cell division. The question that arises, then, is how the several arrest points that regulate the normal cell cycle are persistently removed during the transition from a normal cell to a tumor cell.

2.2. Specific Substances Involved in the Regulation of Growth

Insight into this problem in the plant tumor field followed an understanding of the factors and mechanisms that regulate normal cell growth and division. Growth in all animals and plants results either from an enlargement of cells or from the combined processes of cell enlargement and cell division. These fundamental growth processes are controlled in higher plant species by the quantitative interaction of two growth-regulating substances (Braun and Naf, 1954; Jablonski and Skoog, 1954). The first of these is the plant growth hormone auxin (β-indole-3-acetic acid). This substance is concerned with cell enlargement and with chromosomal DNA replication (Das *et al.*, 1958; Simard, 1971). Auxin, in turn, acts synergistically with the cell division factor(s) to promote growth accompanied by cell division. The chemistry and mode of action of the cell-division-promoting factor(s) will be considered later in this chapter. That a fundamentally similar regulatory mechanism may be concerned in animal cells as well is suggested by a report showing that two substances, one of which is involved in chromosomal DNA synthesis while the second acts synergistically with the first, promote cell division in BHK-21 cells grown in a serum-free medium (Shodell, 1972). The second substance, like the cell-division-promoting factor in plants, is ineffective in encouraging either chromosomal DNA replication or cytokinesis in the absence of the first substance. Thus although the specific regulatory substances in animals and plants may differ in particulars, the basic mechanisms that underlie the regulation of cell proliferation may, in fact, be similar in cells of members of the two kingdoms. This might be expected since dividing cells of animals and plants go through precisely the same stages in the normal cell cycle and show the same arrest points in that cycle.

That auxin and the cell-division-promoting factor(s) play a central role in the development of a capacity for autonomous growth of all true plant tumor cells is evidenced from the results of a number of different experimental approaches. First, plant tumor cells grow profusely and indefinitely on a simple, chemically defined basic culture medium that does not support the growth of normal cells of the type from which the tumor cells were derived. The normal cells commonly require an exogenous source of either one or both of the two growth-regulating substances if cell growth and division are to occur in culture. It has been reported, moreover, that when mature differentiated parenchyma cells, in which the biosynthetic systems responsible for the production of auxin and the cell division factor(s) are strongly repressed, are transformed into crown gall tumor cells, both biosynthetic systems are activated and the tumor cells synthesize the two growth-regulating substances (Braun, 1956). Finally, the auxin and cell-division-promoting factor(s) have been isolated from crown gall tumor tissues and have been characterized chemically. The chemical nature and mode of action of these growth-regulating substances will be considered later.

2.4. *Evidence That the Persistent Activation of Normally Repressed Biosynthetic Systems Results in Autonomy*

The transformation of a normal cell to a rapidly growing, fully autonomous tumor cell in the crown gall disease is not a one-step process but takes place gradually and progressively over a 3- to 4-day period (Braun, 1947, 1951, 1958). When, for example, the transformation process is permitted to proceed for 34 h, after which time it is stopped by thermal treatment, very slowly growing tumors develop in a host. A 60-h exposure of plant cells to the tumor-inducing principle results in the formation of tumors that grow at a moderate rate, while tumors initiated in 72–96 h grow very rapidly in their hosts. Sterile tissues isolated from the three types of tumors described above and planted on a basic culture medium retain indefinitely their characteristic growth patterns (Braun, 1958). This, then, is an interesting example of tumor progression in which different grades of neoplastic change can be obtained at will. Since the three types of tumor cells retained indefinitely in culture their characteristic growth patterns, they appeared admirably suited and were used for a study of the factors required for rapid autonomous growth (Braun, 1958). In those studies, the fully autonomous, rapidly growing tumor cell transformed during a 72- to 96-h period was used as the standard. This cell type can synthesize in optimal or near optimal amounts all of the essential growth substances required for continued rapid growth from mineral salts, sucrose, and vitamins present in the basic culture medium. The moderately fast growing tumor cell transformed in a 60-h period required that the basic medium be supplemented with glutamine, inositol, and the cell enlargement hormone auxin to achieve a growth rate comparable to that of the fully autonomous tumor cell grown on the basic culture medium. The very slowly growing tumor cell required, in addition to glutamine, inositol, and auxin, a purine and pyrimidine as well as asparagine for rapid growth in culture. Normal cells did not grow at all on the basic culture medium. Thus, although the difference between the three types of tumor cells is a quantitative difference since all three grow indefinitely but at different rates on the basic medium, the difference between the tumor cells and the normal cells is qualitative. An analysis of the substances required for the rapid growth of normal cells in culture showed that they were the same as those required for the rapid growth of the most slowly growing tumor cell, with one exception. The normal cells possessed an absolute exogenous requirement for a cell-division-promoting factor. All three types of tumor cells had acquired, as a result of the transformation process, a capacity to synthesize that factor. This, then, would appear to represent a fundamental difference between a normal plant cell and a plant tumor cell since the continued production of the cell division factor by the tumor cells keeps those cells dividing persistently provided that the other essential biosynthetic systems are also functional. This study demonstrates then that as a result of the transition from a normal cell to a fully autonomous tumor cell a series of quite distinct but well-defined biosynthetic systems, which represent the entire area of metabolism concerned with cell growth and division, become progressively and persistently activated and the degree of activation of those systems within a cell determines the rate at which a tumor cell grows.

The biosynthetic systems shown to be persistently activated in a plant tumor cell can be divided operationally into two groups. In the first are auxin and the cell-division-promoting factor(s). These two substances establish the pattern of metabolism within a cell that is concerned with cell growth and division. It is these two substances that remove all of the naturally occurring blocks in the normal cell cycle. The fact that they are synthesized persistently by the tumor cells not only establishes but also maintains indefinitely in those cells the patterns of metabolism concerned with cell growth and division. The products of the other biosynthetic systems shown to be persistently activated in a plant tumor cell are required for the production by those cells of the mitotic and enzymatic proteins, the nucleic acids, and, in the case of inositol, the membrane systems of the cell. These metabolites are required to permit the expression of the pattern of metabolism concerned with cell growth and division that is established in a cell by auxin and the cell-division-promoting factor(s).

2.5. Evidence for an Extensive Activation of Biosynthetic Systems as a Result of the Neoplastic Transformation

It is clear from what has been stated above that there is an extensive and persistent activation of biosynthetic systems whose products are concerned rather specifically with cell growth and division as the result of the transformation of a normal plant cell to a tumor cell. That such activation of normally repressed biosynthetic systems is not limited to those concerned with cell growth and division is evidenced by the finding that crown gall tumor cells synthesize other substances that their normal counterparts either do not produce or synthesize in limited amounts. Interesting examples of this are found in three amino acid analogues, lysopine [N^2-(d-1-carboxyethyl)-l-lysine] (Lioret, 1956), octopine [N^2-(d-1-carboxyethyl)-l-arginine] (Ménagé and Morel, 1965), and nopaline [N^2-(1,3-dicarboxypropyl)-l-arginine] (Goldmann et al., 1969).

2.6. Changes in the Properties of the Membrane Systems That Influence Autonomy

The question to be considered next is what are the cellular mechanisms that are concerned in the persistent activation of the biosynthetic systems shown to be responsible for the development of a capacity for autonomous growth of plant tumor cells. Although the entire answer to that is by no means as yet available, studies have shown that during the transition from a normal cell to a rapidly growing, fully autonomous tumor cell progressive changes in the properties of the membrane systems of the cell occur (Braun and Wood, 1962; Wood and Braun, 1961, 1965). Fully transformed tumor cells take up ions and certain organic solutes very efficiently from dilute solutions as compared to their normal counterparts. Certain specific ions (K, NO_3, PO_4, and NH_3) have been found, moreover, to fully activate five and, in part, six of the seven essential biosynthetic systems shown to be rendered functional as a result of the transformation of a normal plant cell to a crown gall tumor cell. Only the system for synthesizing cell division factor and, in part, the inositol-producing system were not affected specifically by the ions studied. It was possible to cause normal cells to grow rapidly and mimic for the time being the fully autonomous tumor cells by simply raising the concentration of specific ions in the culture medium and supplementing that medium with a cell-division-promoting factor and inositol. The exogenous requirements for glutamine, asparagine, purines, and pyrimidines needed for the rapid growth of normal cells in a basic culture medium could therefore be completely replaced by increased levels in that medium of certain specific ions provided that inositol and a cell division factor were present in the medium. The changes observed in the properties of the tumor cell membranes appeared to be concerned with permeability changes rather than with energy-requiring active transport systems. The changes in the properties of the membrane systems that occur during the transition from a normal cell to a fully autonomous, rapidly growing crown gall tumor cell would appear significant since they permit the activation by ions of a large segment of metabolism concerned with cell growth and division.

2.7. The Nature and Mode of Action of the Cell-Division-Promoting Factors

It is clear from what has been written thus far that the cell-division-promoting factor(s) plays a central role in the development of a capacity for autonomous growth of plant tumor cells since it is the continued production of that factor(s) by the tumor cells that keeps those cells dividing persistently.

Two distinct classes of cell-division-promoting factors have now been isolated from tissues of higher plant species. The first of these are the 6-substituted adenylyl cytokinins, of which kinetin (6-furfurylaminopurine) may be considered the prototype (Miller *et al.*, 1956). Although this substance has not been found to occur naturally, other 6-substituted adenylyl cytokinins possessing similar biological activity have been isolated not only from higher plant species but from animals and microorganisms as well (Hall, 1970). These compounds, which are found to be present immediately adjacent to the anticodon in certain tRNAs, commonly contain an isopentenyl group at the 6-position of the adenine moiety. When these compounds are removed either enzymatically or chemically from the tRNA, they possess cell-division-promoting activity in plants. One 6-substituted purine, which has been given the trivial name of zeatin, [N^6-(*trans*-4-hydroxy-3-methyl-2-butenyl]adenine, and the riboside of that compound have been found to occur as free substances in certain plant tissues (Letham, 1963). Whether a specific pathway for the synthesis of a substance such as zeatin or its riboside exists in cells of higher plant species or whether those compounds are always derived as a result of tRNA turnover is not yet known. These 6-substituted adenylyl derivatives have been given the trivial name cytokinins.

A second chemically quite distinct class of naturally occurring cell-division-promoting factors has been isolated from both normal and tumor cells of taxonomically very different plant species. Physical and chemical studies suggest that they are substituted hypoxanthines that contain glucose as the sugar moiety (Wood *et al.*, 1974). These are therefore very different compounds from the 6-substituted adenylyl cytokinins and they have been given the trivial name cytokinesins. The question that arises, therefore, is how members of two different classes of compounds can both be effective in promoting cell division when used in association with an auxin. This question appears to have been resolved by the finding that when normal parenchyma cells, which require an exogenous source of a cell division factor for growth, are forced into rapid growth with a 6-substituted adenylyl cytokinin such as kinetin in an otherwise suitable culture medium they synthesize cytokinesin I (Wood and Braun, 1967). This finding led to the suggestion that the 6-substituted adenylyl cytokinins exert their biological effects by inducing the synthesis of the cytokinesins and that it is the cytokinesins that are directly involved in promoting cell growth and division. Thus the biosynthetic systems responsible for the production of the cytokinesins may be temporarily activated by a 6-substituted adenylyl cytokinin such as kinetin or they may be persistently activated as a result of the cellular transformation. Since the cytokinesins are substituted hypoxanthines and hence purinones and since the methylxanthines such as theophylline, theobromine, and caffeine are also purinones and are known to be cAMP(3′ : 5′) phosphodiesterase inhibitors, an attempt was made to determine whether the cytokinesins, like certain of the methylxanthines, are also inhibitors of the cAMP(3′ : 5′) phosphodiesterases and thus possibly exert their biological effects as regulators of cAMP(3′ : 5′) metabolism. It was found in those studies that cytokinesin I is perhaps the most potent naturally occurring inhibitor of not only plant but also animal (bovine brain) cAMP(3′ : 5′) phosphodiesterases yet described (Wood *et al.*, 1972). The 6-substituted adenylyl cytokinin zeatin riboside is by comparison a poor inhibitor of those enzymes, suggesting again that these two classes of compounds are functioning in different ways to exert their biological effects. If, therefore, cAMP(3′ : 5′)* is somehow concerned with regulation of cell division in higher plant species, it should be possible to replace the cell-division-promoting effects of the 6-substituted adenyl cytokinins and the cytokinesins with either cAMP(3′ : 5′) or a more stable derivative of that compound (Wood and Braun, 1973). The results of those studies showed that although cAMP(3′ : 5′) itself was ineffective in promoting cell growth and division the 8-bromo derivative of that compound could completely replace the cell-division-promoting activity of both the adenylyl cytokinins and the cytokinesins (Wood and Braun, 1973). The 8-bromo derivative of cAMP(3′ : 5′) was shown to be far more resistant to degradation by the cAMP(3′ : 5′) phosphodiesterases than was cAMP(3′ : 5′), and it was found to be at least as effective as cAMP(3′ : 5′) in the cAMP(3′ : 5′)-dependent histone phosphorylation reaction (Muneyama *et al.*, 1971). It thus appears to be a stable, biologically active form of cAMP (3′ : 5′). The 8-bromo derivative either could function to replace cAMP(3′ : 5′) in cellular metabolism or, because it is a stable structural analogue of cAMP(3′ : 5′), could act as a stable competitive inhibitor to the natural compound for binding sites on the phosphodiesterases and thus serve to protect the cAMP(3′ : 5′) synthesized by the plant cells (Wood and Braun, 1973).

A study of the intracellular levels of cAMP(3′ : 5′) in normal plant cells during the cell enlargement and cell division phases of the cell cycle demonstrated that the intracellular levels of cAMP(3′ : 5′) are determined by the plant hormone auxin, which it should be recalled is concerned with cell enlargement and chromosomal DNA replication. A correlation was found to exist, moreover, between the intracellular levels of cAMP(3′ : 5′) (Lundeen *et al.*, 1973) and chromosomal DNA replication (Simard, 1971). Whether this finding represents a causal relationship or merely a correlation is not yet known. The results of these studies nevertheless suggest that the plant hormone auxin determines the intracellular levels of cAMP(3′ : 5′) in this system and that the cytokinesins protect cAMP(3′ : 5′) synthesized by the cell during certain critical stages of the cell cycle by virtue of their acting as potent inhibitors of the cAMP(3′ : 5′) phosphodiesterases. A pertinent question that remains unanswered is the precise role that cAMP(3′ : 5′) plays not only in the regulation of cell division but, as we shall see later, also in cytodifferentiation.

All these studies indicate, then, that plant tumor cells acquire a capacity for autonomous growth as a result of the persistent activation of normally repressed biosynthetic systems whose products are concerned with cell growth and division. There is little to be found in the animal literature that argues strongly against similar mechanisms being involved in those systems.

* Recent studies suggest that the compound isolated from plant tissues and referred to here as cAMP(3′ : 5′) is probably a biologically active derivative of cAMP(3′ : 5′) rather than cAMP(3′ : 5′) itself.

3. The Heritable Cellular Change That Underlies the Tumorous State in Plants

3.1. The Usefulness of Plant Tumor Systems for Studying the Heritable Cellular Change

The next question to consider then is the nature of the heritable cellular change that results in the activation of the essential biosynthetic systems shown to be persistently unblocked in plant tumor cells. This could, in principle at least, involve a change in the integrity of the genetic determinants present in the nucleus of a cell in which a loss or permanent rearrangement of some of the nuclear DNA occurs. Thus the loss through mutation of, for example, a regulatory gene(s) could account for the observations. It is also possible that chromosomal imbalances may occur during the transition from a normal cell to a tumor cell, leading to an upset in the balance between those genes that determine growth and those concerned with the regulation of growth. The neoplastic state might also result from the addition of new genetic information following infection by an oncogenic virus. Finally, the transformation process, like normal development, might simply involve stable changes in the expression of the genetic information that is normally present in the nucleus of a cell. Because of certain unique characteristics inherent in plants and plant tumor systems, the use of those systems as experimental models permits a clear decision to be made from among the several possibilities listed above. The two properties that are characteristic of dicotyledonous plant species and that are useful in studying the nature of the heritable cellular change that underlies tumorigenesis are the following: (1) The manner in which such plant species grow. Primary growth of these species results from the rapid division, subsequent elongation, and finally differentiation of the meristematic cells at the extreme apex of a root or a shoot. (2) Totipotentiality of the somatic cells of certain higher plant species. The progeny of single differentiated somatic cells are capable of developing into normal, fully fertile plants (Steward *et al.*, 1964; Vasil and Hildebrandt, 1965). By combination of these two properties it has now become possible to achieve a normalization of the tumorous state in a number of different plant tumor systems and thus gain insight into the basic cellular mechanisms that underlie the heritable cellular change in those instances.

In any attempt to characterize the nature of the heritable cellular change that underlies tumorigenesis it must be recognized that the genetic information present in the nucleus of a cell must be implicated in directing cellular metabolism. The important question is not, therefore, whether that information is implicated, for it clearly is, but rather whether the heritable cellular change involves a permanent alteration of a mutational type involving a change in the integrity of that information, or whether it is epigenetic in nature and is concerned merely with a persistent change in the expression of that information. This distinction could perhaps be resolved most convincingly by demonstrating that the tumorous state is a reversible process leading to a normalization of a tumor cell. This, in turn,

would require a demonstration that all of the necessary genetic information is 421
inherently present in all normal cells and requires only to be persistently activated PLANT
to account for the establishment and maintenance of the tumorous state. That this TUMORS
may, in fact, be true appears well illustrated in the case of a neoplastic situation
known as habituation that was described briefly above.

3.2. Habituation

When normal cells are excised from a plant and grown in culture, they may
acquire, as do animal cells, neoplastic properties. In plant cells this results from a
newly acquired capacity to synthesize persistently the two growth-regulating
substances, an auxin and a cell-division-promoting factor(s)—which, it will be
recalled, establish the pattern of metabolism concerned with cell growth and
division—as well as those metabolites and vitamins that permit that pattern to be
expressed. The biosynthetic systems shown to be newly activated in the case of
habituation may become persistently unblocked individually, or more than one or
all may become activated more or less simultaneously. When all of the biosynthetic
systems are activated, the cells behave in every respect like typical plant tumor
cells. These newly acquired properties of habituated cells may be retained
indefinitely. This, then, represents a heritable cellular change that is highly stable
and occurs in the absence of any recognizable oncogen. Of interest in this
connection is a preliminary report suggesting that habituation for a single factor,
in this instance the cell-division-promoting factor, occurs with a frequency
between 2 and 3 orders of magnitude greater than that found for spontaneous
randomly occurring somatic mutations at any given gene locus (Binns and Meins,
1973). Although, as indicated, this heritable cellular change is highly stable and
was believed by some to be irreversible, it has now been found to be a completely
reversible process with the use of a significant number of cloned cell lines (Binns
and Meins, 1973; Lutz, 1971). These cloned habituated cell lines commonly grow,
as do typical plant tumor tissues, in a completely unorganized manner. When
however, those lines were placed on a special inductive medium, they formed
shoots and those shoots were isolated and placed on a medium that favored root
formation. The small plantlets that developed were then grown to maturity and
many flowered and set fertile seed. Since this phenomenon is completely
reversible, the results of these studies provide the ultimate proof that the
tumorous state, in plants at least, may arise and be perpetuated indefinitely as a
result of persistent changes in gene expressions. In this instance, nothing has been
added, deleted, or permanently rearranged. Thus we see that all of the genetic
information necessary for the establishment and maintenance of the tumorous
state is present in the normal cell genome, and since the tumorous state is
regularly reversible under special experimental conditions one does not have to
postulate drastic changes of a mutational type to account for the continued
abnormal and autonomous proliferation of a tumor cell. Any new genetic
information that is added to a cell as a result of infection by an oncogenic virus may

perhaps be looked upon as somehow persistently activating the segment of the host cell genome that is concerned with continued cell growth and division rather than coding specifically for one or more substances that are required for the autonomous proliferation of a tumor cell. Here, then, we have an example of a highly stable heritable cellular change that may be perpetuated indefinitely in a persistently dividing population of cells and that, unlike somatic mutation, is completely reversible under special experimental conditions. This system would appear to be ideally suited for an in-depth study of the substances and mechanisms that underlie this type of heritable cellular change.

3.3. The Kostoff Genetic Tumors

A second neoplastic disease of plants in which a reversal of the tumorous state has been demonstrated experimentally involves tumors of genetic origin, the so-called Kostoff tumors, that arise regularly and spontaneously in large numbers on certain interspecific hybrids within the genus Nicotiana (Smith, 1972). When, for example, two plant species such as Nicotiana glauca ($2n = 24$) and N. langsdorffii ($2n = 18$) are crossed and the seed of the hybrid ($2n = 21$) is sown, the resulting plants commonly develop normally during the period of their active growth. Once the F_1 hybrid plants reach maturity, however, a profusion of tumors arise spontaneously from all parts of them.

It was recently found that when differentiated leaf cells of the two parent species were isolated and grown separately in culture and the progeny of those cells then mixed together to permit fusion to occur, the amphiploid hybrid ($2n = 42$) grew profusely on a minimal culture medium that did not support the continued growth of leaf cells or of fused cells of either parent (Carlson et al., 1972). The amphiploid hybrid was thus behaving like a typical plant tumor cell in its growth characteristics on a minimal medium. When these hybrid cells were cultured further they organized tumor shoots, and when those shoots were tip-grafted to the N. glauca parent they not only grew in a completely organized manner and ultimately flowered and set fertile seed but also developed spontaneous tumors at the site of the graft union. This experimental test system demonstrates then that, despite serious chromosomal imbalance in all cells of the hybrid plant, the same abnormal karyotype can give rise on the one hand to morphologically perfectly normal-appearing plants that flower and set fertile seed while that same abnormal karyotype can on the other hand give rise to neoplastic growths. These two metastable states are completely and readily reversible in both directions. The experiments described above would appear to provide a model for the so-called chromosomal imbalance theory of cancer which postulates that tumors arise as the result of an upset in the balance between the genes that determine growth and those that are concerned with the regulation of growth (Bloch-Shtacher et al., 1972). The experiments carried out with the plant hybrids show then that despite serious chromosomal imbalance the neoplastic state is reversible. These studies would appear significant and provide strong support for the concept that the tumorous state, like normal developmental processes, may stem from persistent changes in the expression of a genetically equivalent but, in this instance, abnormal genome.

3.4. The Crown Gall Disease

A third plant tumor system, which differs from the other two in that a self-replicating entity of viral nature is almost certainly involved etiologically, is the crown gall disease. The typical crown gall tumor cell is characterized by rapid powers of proliferation and rather limited powers of differentiation, while these tissues never organize such structures as roots or shoots when maintained on conventional media in culture. It was discovered, however, that if totipotential cells found in certain plant species were transformed to a moderate degree but not fully there was produced, in place of the characteristic unorganized tumor, a complex overgrowth or teratoma (Braun, 1953). The teratoma was composed of a chaotic assembly of tissues and organs that showed varying grades of morphological development. Sterile tissue excised from the morphologically abnormal but organized structures and planted in culture grew profusely and indefinitely on a minimal culture medium, as did typical crown gall tumor cells. These teratoma-derived tumor cells differed from the typical crown gall cells in that they retained indefinitely in culture a capacity to organize tumor buds and shoots. When shoots from cloned teratoma cell lines were isolated and forced into rapid but organized growth as a result of a series of tip-graftings to healthy stock plants that were morphologically distinguishable from the grafted shoots, some of those shoots gradually recovered from the tumorous state and some of those flowered and set fertile seed (Braun, 1959, 1974). A second related phenomenon and one that involves a suppression of the tumorous state rather than a recovery from that state has now been observed in the crown gall disease. When tumor shoots that develop from cloned lines of teratoma tissues are grafted to the tops of appropriate plants of the same species, the stems and leaves that develop from those shoots may appear normal. Such stems and leaves may be perfectly organized and contain all of the diverse differentiated cell types that characterize their normal counterparts. The cells of such teratoma stems and leaves are clearly not exhibiting neoplastic properties and they appear by all generally accepted criteria to be both histologically and functionally normal. Yet when such specialized cell types are isolated from the teratoma and planted in culture they again assume their neoplastic properties. The results of these studies indicate, then, that the substances and mechanisms that govern the growth and differentiation of cells during the normal course of development can completely suppress the tumorous state, leading to the differentiation of specialized cells, tissues, and organs that appear structurally and functionally to be normal in every respect.

The results of all of these studies suggest then that the neoplastic state, like normal developmental processes, may stem from epigenetic modifications involving the persistent and selective activation or suppression of specific genes. The implication of all of this is that the genetic information in the nucleus of a neoplastic cell need not, as was believed for so many years, be irreversibly fixed but may instead be manipulated experimentally to give rise to a normal phenotype.

3.5. Specific Substances and Mechanisms Involved in the Reprogramming of Genetic Information with a Resulting Loss of Neoplastic Properties

The pertinent question here concerns the nature of the specific substances and mechanisms that regulate nuclear gene expression in normal and tumor cells. Again, plants may provide a model to gain insight into that question. It is a common observation that plant tumors of many different kinds growing not only in a host but also as cloned lines in culture contain terminally differentiated cells that are known as tracheary elements. These tracheary elements result from an attempt by the tumor tissue to vascularize and they are components of the normal vascular (xylem) system. Since the potentialities for this form of cytodifferentiation are clearly present in cells of many if not all plant tumors and since this represents a form of terminal differentiation with a resulting loss of neoplastic properties, an attempt was made to understand the substances and mechanisms underlying this type of cytodifferentiation (Basile *et al.*, 1973). The question to consider here is whether, if this type of differentiation were completely understood, it would be possible to program all the cells of plant tumors in such a way that they would become terminally differentiated with a loss of their neoplastic properties. Since the basic cellular mechanisms that underlie tracheary element formation are probably similar in normal and tumor cells, an attempt was made to study their induction in normal systems first. It had been found that when excised parenchyma cells of Romaine lettuce were treated with auxin and the 6-substituted adenylyl cytokinin kinetin the parenchyma cells differentiated into tracheary elements in large numbers (Dalessandro and Roberts, 1971). Since kinetin is not a naturally occurring substance but a man-made artifact, an attempt was made to replace the inductive effects of kinetin with other chemically distinct substances which, if shown to be effective, might provide insight into the basic cellular mechanisms that underlie this type of cytodifferentiation. It was found in that study that both cytokinesin I, which, it will be recalled, is a potent inhibitor of cAMP($3' : 5'$) phosphodiesterases, and the 8-bromo derivative of cAMP($3' : 5'$), which is a stable derivative of cAMP($3' : 5'$), were highly effective in inducing the formation of tracheary elements in the presence of auxin (Basile *et al.*, 1973). Since cAMP($3' : 5'$) itself when used in association with theophylline was also effective, the results obtained in this study suggest that cAMP($3' : 5'$) is somehow importantly involved in the induction and/or expression of this form of terminal differentiation that results in the loss of neoplastic properties when it occurs in plant tumor cells. The problem remaining is to define the precise role that cAMP($3' : 5'$) plays in this type of cytodifferentiation. A number of examples of animal cancer cells that differentiate regularly and spontaneously into nonmalignant cell types with a partial or occasional complete self-healing of the tumors are discussed in the previous volume. If the cellular mechanisms underlying all of

these phenomena were thoroughly understood, it seems not unlikely that the
expression and suppression of the malignant state could be obtained at will in a
significant number of tumors not only in plants but in animals as well. Such an
approach, if properly exploited, might ultimately lead to entirely new and more
rational methods of therapy.

ACKNOWLEDGMENT

Certain of these studies were supported in part by a research grant (NIH Grant
CA-13808) from the National Cancer Institute, U.S. Public Health Service.

4. *References*

AARON-DACUNHA, M. I., 1969, Sur la libération, par les rayons X, d'un principe tumorigène contenu
dans les tissus de crown gall de tabac, *C. R. Acad. Sci. Paris Ser. D* **268**:318.

BASILE, D. V., WOOD, H. N., AND BRAUN, A. C., 1973, Programming of cells for death under defined
experimental conditions: Relevance to the tumor problem, *Proc. Natl. Acad. Sci. U.S.A.* **70**:3055.

BINNS, A., AND MEINS, F., JR., 1973, Habituation of tobacco pith cells for factors promoting cell division
is heritable and potentially reversible, *Proc. Natl. Acad. Sci. U.S.A.* **70**:2660.

BLOCH-SHTACHER, N., RABINOWITZ, Z., AND SACHS, L., 1972, Chromosomal mechanism for the
induction of reversion in transformed cells, *Int. J. Cancer* **9**:632.

BRAUN, A. C., 1943, Studies on tumor inception in the crown-gall disease, *Am. J. Bot.* **30**:674.

BRAUN, A. C., 1947, Thermal studies on the factors responsible for tumor initiation in crown gall, *Am.
J. Bot.* **34**:234.

BRAUN, A. C., 1951, Cellular autonomy in crown gall, *Phytopathology* **41**:963.

BRAUN, A. C., 1952, Conditioning of the host cell as a factor in the transformation process in crown
gall, *Growth* **16**:65.

BRAUN, A. C., 1953, Bacterial and host factors concerned in determining tumor morphology in crown
gall, *Bot. Gaz.* **114**:363.

BRAUN, A. C., 1956, The activation of two growth-substance systems accompanying the conversion of
normal to tumor cells in crown gall, *Cancer Res.* **16**:53.

BRAUN, A. C., 1958, A physiological basis for autonomous growth of the crown-gall tumor cell, *Proc.
Natl. Acad. Sci. U.S.A.* **44**:344.

BRAUN, A. C., 1959, A demonstration of the recovery of the crown-gall tumor cell with the use of
complex tumors of single-cell origin, *Proc. Natl. Acad. Sci. U.S.A.* **45**:932.

BRAUN, A. C., guest editor, 1972, *Plant Tumor Research*, Vol. 15 of *Progress in Experimental Tumor
Research*, 235 pp., Karger, Basel.

BRAUN, A. C., 1975, The cell cycle and tumorigenesis in plants, *Results and Problems in Cell
Differentiation*, Vol. 7, *The Cell Cycle and Cell Differentiation*, (J. Reinert and H. Holtzer, eds.), pp.
177-196, Springer, Berlin.

BRAUN, A. C., AND MANDLE, R. J., 1948, Studies on the inactivation of the tumor-inducing principle in
crown gall, *Growth* **12**:255.

BRAUN, A. C., AND NAF, U., 1954, A non-auxinic growth-promoting factor present in crown gall tumor
tissue, *Proc. Soc. Exp. Biol. Med.* **86**:212.

BRAUN, A. C., AND WOOD, H. N., 1962, On the activation of certain essential biosynthetic systems in
cells of *Vinca rosea* L., *Proc. Natl. Acad. Sci. U.S.A.* **48**:1776.

CARLSON, P. S., SMITH, H. H., AND DEARING, R. D., 1972, Parasexual interspecific plant hybridization,
Proc. Natl. Acad. Sci. U.S.A. **69**:2292.

DALESSANDRO, G., AND ROBERTS, L. W., 1971, Induction of xylogenesis in pith parenchyma explants of
Lactuca, *Am. J. Bot.* **58**:378.

DAS, N. K., PATAU, K., AND SKOOG, F., 1958, Autoradiographic and microspectrophotometric studies of DNA synthesis in excised tobacco pith tissue, *Chromosoma* **9**:606.

DE ROPP, R. S., 1947, The growth-promoting and tumefacient factors of bacteria-free crown-gall tumor tissue, *Am. J. Bot.* **34**:248.

ELLERMANN, V., AND BANG, O., 1908, Experimentelle Leukämie bei Hühnern, *Zentralbl. Bakteriol. Parasitenkd. Abt. 1: Orig.* **46**:595.

GOLDMANN, A., THOMAS, D. W., AND MOREL, G., 1969, Sur la structure de la nopaline métabolite anormal de certaines tumeurs de crown-gall, *C. R. Acad. Sci. Paris Ser. D* **268**:852.

GORDON, M., 1958, A genetic concept for the origin of melanomas, *Ann. N.Y. Acad. Sci.* **71**:1213.

HALL, R. H., 1970, N^6-(Δ^2-Isopentenyl)adenosine: Chemical reactions, biosynthesis, metabolism, and significance to the structure and function of tRNA, *Prog. Nucleic Acid Res. Mol. Biol.* **10**:57.

JABLONSKI, J. R., AND SKOOG, F., 1954, Cell enlargement and cell division in excised tobacco pith tissue, *Physiol. Plant.* **7**:16.

JENSEN, C. O., 1910, Von echten Geschwülsten bei Pflanzen, in: *Deuxième Conférence Internationale pour l'Etude du Cancer, Tenue a Paris du Ler au 5 Octobre 1910*, pp. 243–254, Félix Alcan, Éditeur, Paris.

JENSEN, C. O., 1918, Undersøgelser vedrørende nogle svulstlignende dannelser hos planter, *K. Vet. Landbohoejsk. Aarsskr.* **1918**:91.

LETHAM, D. S., 1963, Zeatin, a factor inducing cell division isolated from *Zea mays*, *Life Sci.* **2**:569.

LIMASSET, P., AND GAUTHERET, R., 1950, Sur le caractère tumoral des tissus de tabac ayant subi le phénomène d'accoutumance aux hétèro-auxines, *C. R. Acad. Sci. Paris* **230**:2043.

LIORET, C., 1956, Sur la mise en évidence d'un acide aminé non identifié particulier aux tissus de "crown-gall," *Bull. Soc. Fr. Physiol. Vég.* **2**:76.

LIPETZ, J., 1966, Crown gall tumorigenesis. II. Relations between wound healing and the tumorigenic response, *Cancer Res.* **26**:1597.

LITTLE, C. C., 1947, The genetics of cancer in mice, *Biol. Rev. Cambridge Philos. Soc.* **22**:315.

LUNDEEN, C. V., WOOD, H. N., AND BRAUN, A. C., 1973, Intracellular levels of cyclic nucleotides during cell enlargement and cell division in excised tobacco pith tissues, *Differentiation* **1**:255.

LUTZ, A., 1971, Morphogenetic aptitudes of tissue cultures of unicellular origin, in: *Colloq. Internat. Centre Nat. Recherche Sci (Paris), No. 193, Les Cultures de Tissus de Plantes* (Proceedings of the Second International Conference Plant Tissue Culture, Strasbourg, France, July 6–10, 1970), pp. 163–168, Centre National de la Recherche Scientifique, Paris.

MAZIA, D., 1961, Mitosis and the physiology of cell division, in: *The Cell*, Vol. 3, (J. Brachet and A. E. Mirsky, eds.), pp. 77–412, Academic Press, New York.

MEINS, F., JR., 1973, Evidence for the presence of a readily transmissible oncogenic principle in crown gall teratoma cells of tobacco, *Differentiation* **1**:21.

MÉNAGÉ, A., AND MOREL, G., 1965, Sur la présence d'un acide aminé nouveau dans les tissus de crown-gall, *C. R. Acad. Sci. Paris* **261**:2001.

MILLER, C. O., SKOOG, F., OKUMURA, F. S., VON SALTZA, M. H., AND STRONG, F. M., 1956, Isolation, structure and synthesis of kinetin, a substance promoting cell division, *J. Am. Chem. Soc.* **78**:1375.

MUNEYAMA, K., BAUER, R. J., SHUMAN, D. A., ROBINS, R. K., AND SIMON, L. N., 1971, Chemical synthesis and biological activity of 8-substituted adenosine 3′,5′-cyclic monophosphate derivatives, *Biochemistry* **10**:2390.

ROUS, P., 1910, A transmissible avian neoplasm (sarcoma of the common fowl), *J. Exp. Med.* **12**:696.

SHODELL, M., 1972, Environmental stimuli in the progression of BHK/21 cells through the cell cycle, *Proc. Natl. Acad. Sci. U.S.A.* **69**:1455.

SIMARD, A., 1971, Initiation of DNA synthesis by kinetin and experimental factors in tobacco pith tissues *in vitro*, *Can. J. Bot.* **49**:1541.

SMITH, E. F., AND TOWNSEND, C. O., 1907, A plant-tumor of bacterial origin, *Science* **25**:671.

SMITH, H. H., 1972, Plant genetic tumors, *Prog. Exp. Tumor. Res.* **15**:138.

STEWARD, F. C., MAPES, M. O., KENT, A. E., AND HOLSTEN, R. D., 1964, Growth and development of cultured plant cells, *Science* **143**:20.

VASIL, V., AND HILDEBRANDT, A. C., 1965, Differentiation of tobacco plants from single, isolated cells in microcultures, *Science* **150**:889.

WOOD, H. N., AND BRAUN, A. C., 1961, Studies on the regulation of certain essential biosynthetic systems in normal and crown-gall tumor cells, *Proc. Natl. Acad. Sci. U.S.A.* **47**:1907.

WOOD, H. N., AND BRAUN, A. C., 1965, Studies on the net uptake of solutes by normal and crown-gall tumor cells, *Proc. Natl. Acad. Sci. U.S.A.* **54**:1532.

WOOD, H. N., AND BRAUN, A. C., 1967, The role of kinetin (6-furfurylaminopurine) in promoting division in cells of *Vinca rosea* L., *Ann. N.Y. Acad. Sci.* **144**:244.

WOOD, H. N., AND BRAUN, A. C., 1973, 8-Bromoadenosine 3′ : 5′-cyclic monophosphate as a promoter of cell division in excised tobacco pith parenchyma tissue, *Proc. Natl. Acad. Sci. U.S.A.* **70:**447.

WOOD, H. N., LIN, M. C., AND BRAUN, A. C., 1972, The inhibition of plant and animal adenosine 3′ : 5′-cyclic monophosphate phosphodiesterases by a cell-division-promoting substance from tissues of higher plant species, *Proc. Natl. Acad. Sci. U.S.A.* **69:**403.

WOOD, H. N., RENNEKAMP, M. E., BOWEN, D. V., FIELD, F. H., AND BRAUN, A. C., 1974, A comparative study of cytokinesins I and II and zeatin riboside: a reply to Carlos Miller, *Proc. Natl. Acad. Sci. U.S.A.* **71:**4140.

Index